A Clinical Guide to Orthopedics

A Clinical Guide to Orthopedics

Editor: Solomon Willis

AMERICAN
MEDICAL PUBLISHERS
www.americanmedicalpublishers.com

AMERICAN
MEDICAL PUBLISHERS
www.americanmedicalpublishers.com

Cataloging-in-Publication Data

A clinical guide to orthopedics / edited by Solomon Willis.
p. cm.
Includes bibliographical references and index.
ISBN 978-1-63927-839-8
1. Orthopedics. 2. Orthopedics--Diagnosis. 3. Orthopedics--Treatment. I. Willis, Solomon.
RD731 .C55 2023
617.3--dc23

American Medical Publishers,
41 Flatbush Avenue,
1st Floor, New York,
NY 11217, USA

ISBN 978-1-63927-839-8 (Hardback)

Contents

Preface

The main aim of this book is to educate learners and enhance their research focus by presenting diverse topics covering this vast field. This is an advanced book which compiles significant studies by distinguished experts in the area of analysis. This book addresses successive solutions to the challenges arising in the area of application, along with it; the book provides scope for future developments.

Orthopedics is the branch of surgery concerned with the treatment of conditions involving the skeletal system and its interconnecting parts. The musculoskeletal system comprises parts including bones, muscles, joints, tendons, and ligaments. Orthopedics is focused on treating several complications and conditions, such as bone fractures, back pain, neck pain, carpal tunnel syndrome, congenital conditions, and joint pain from arthritis. Arthroscopic surgery is a common type of minimally invasive orthopedic surgery. It is used to diagnose and treat problems in the knee joint. The surgery for knee replacement is broadly categorized into two types, namely, total knee replacement and partial knee replacement. Total knee replacement is used to remove and replace the entire damaged knee joint with metal components. This book provides comprehensive insights into the field of orthopedics. It will also provide interesting topics for research which interested readers can take up. Researchers and students actively engaged in this field will find this book full of crucial and unexplored concepts.

It was a great honour to edit this book, though there were challenges, as it involved a lot of communication and networking between me and the editorial team. However, the end result was this all-inclusive book covering diverse themes in the field.

Finally, it is important to acknowledge the efforts of the contributors for their excellent chapters, through which a wide variety of issues have been addressed. I would also like to thank my colleagues for their valuable feedback during the making of this book.

Editor

1

The Comparison of Inflammatory Cytokines between Spinal and General Anesthesia following Changes in Ischemic Reperfusion due to Tourniquet during Lower Limb Surgery

Mahmoud Ganjifard,[1] **Samaneh Kouzegaran**,[2] **Reza Abdi**,[3] **Mohsen Naseri**,[4] **Elahe Allahyari**,[5] **Amir Sabertanha**,[1] **and Batool Zeinali**[1]

[1]*Department of Anesthesia, Faculty of Medicine, Birjand University of Medical Sciences, Birjand, Iran*
[2]*Clinical Immunology and Allergy, Faculty of Medicine, Birjand University of Medical Sciences, Birjand, Iran*
[3]*Department of Orthopedics, School of Medicine, Ghaem Hospital, Mashhad University of Medical Sciences, Mashhad, Iran*
[4]*Cellular and Molecular Research Center, Birjand University of Medical Sciences, Birjand, Iran*
[5]*Social Determinants of Health Research Center, Department of Epidemiology and Biostatistics, Faculty of Health, Birjand University of Medical Sciences, Birjand, Iran*

Correspondence should be addressed to Amir Sabertanha; amirsaber63@gmail.com and Batool Zeinali; dr.ba_zeinaly@yahoo.com

Academic Editor: Francesco Liuzza

Background and Objective. The injuries caused by reperfusion of blood can lead to significant adverse effects after surgery. This study aimed to compare the effects of spinal and general anesthesia on inflammatory cytokines following changes in ischemic reperfusion due to tourniquet in lower limb surgeries. *Methods.* In this randomized controlled clinical trial, 34 patients with lower limb surgery admitted at the orthopedic ward of Imam Reza Hospital, Birjand, Iran, were selected by the available sampling method. They were randomly divided into two groups as follows: general anesthesia ($n = 17$) and spinal anesthesia ($n = 17$). Venous blood samples were taken from the patients of both groups at baseline (before the use of tourniquet) and 12 and 24 hours after reperfusion. Interleukin-6 (IL-6), tumor necrotizing factor-α (TNF-α), high-sensitivity C-reactive protein (hs-CRP), and ferritin were measured and recorded. The data were analyzed using independent t-test, chi-square, and repeated measure at the significant level of 0.05. *Results.* The results showed that hs-CRP and IL-6 significantly increased during the study ($p < 0.001$); however, the mean changes of TNF-α and ferritin were not significant during the study. Moreover, none of the inflammatory cytokines indicated significant differences between these two study groups ($p < 0.05$). *Conclusion.* According to the results, the use of tourniquet can lead to inflammation, and the inflammation is similar in both groups.

1. Introduction

The use of tourniquet is an integral part in various methods of organ surgery, which is more commonly used in orthopedic surgery to reduce blood loss and improve vision in the surgical field [1]. Although new tourniquets have been designed in terms of the principles to reduce the incidence of possible complications, their usage is still associated with specific local complications such as neurological paralysis, vascular injury, and compartment syndrome [2, 3]. In addition, ischemia-reperfusion due to the tourniquet, which can lead to ischemia-reperfusion injury (IRI), is an important complication following surgery [4, 5]. IRI phenomenon leads to specific hemodynamic and metabolic responses, and the hallmarks are systemic and local inflammatory reactions. Although ischemic reperfusion is necessary to prevent irreversible cellular injury, reperfusion itself can more increase tissue injury compared to ischemia alone [6].

General and spinal anesthesia are widely used in orthopedic surgery resulting in varying amounts of oxygen to the patient as well as systemic inflammatory responses [7]. The results of a randomized controlled experiment showed that spinal anesthesia (SA) significantly reduced postoperative vascular complications (deep vein thrombosis, pulmonary embolism, and heart attack), bleeding, and infection and caused ventilation/perfusion mismatch and failure [8]. It is assumed that the improvement in postoperative death is due to a change in the "stress response" induced during the surgery using spinal anesthesia [9]. Interleukin-6 (IL-6) levels, as a valid index for systemic inflammatory response, are related to the extent of reperfusion injury [10, 11]. It has been reported that elevated IL-6 levels are delayed by neutrophil apoptosis and are associated with modulating the epithelial permeability in the air paths [12, 13]. In patients undergoing lower limb reperfusion/ischemia in aortic surgery, IL-6 and IL-8 levels have been shown to be associated with increased protein permeability in the lungs and also significant impairment of gas exchange [14, 15]. However, recent studies have shown that plasma malondialdehyde (MDA), IL-6, and IL-8 levels can rise, compared to baseline, between two and 24 hours after the tourniquet opens, and in patients undergoing very minor surgery the tourniquet opens after 6 hours; plasma MDA, IL-6, and IL-8 levels reached baseline; however in few studies, the effect of spinal and general anesthesia on systemic inflammatory responses was compared among patients with IRI. Therefore, methods reducing the severity of this response are useful in certain high-risk individuals. Along with interleukins, several markers such as high sensitivity C-reactive protein (hs-CRP) and ferritin have also been identified as enhancing markers in response to inflammation, though the changes following ischemia-reperfusion injury have been studied in very few studies [16, 17]. According to the studies done before, time-dependent closure of the tourniquet leads to ischemic changes in distal tissues to the tourniquet closure site [18–20]. After opening the tourniquet and reperfusion, ischemic products cause systemic inflammatory changes and inflammatory cytokines release. The release of these cytokines as well as the increase of body temperature can delay the patient wound healing, cause morbidity, and increase hospitalization [21]. Since spinal anesthesia reduces the discharge of catecholamines from the nerve terminal in the lower limbs, and regarding the role of catecholamines in cellular metabolism processes [22], it seems that preclosure tourniquet in spinal anesthesia can play an important role in reducing cellular metabolism processes and result in a preconditioning against tourniquet-induced ischemia [23]. According to the performed studies, the use of anesthetic medicines also slightly reduces cell metabolism and can reduce the ischemic changes induced by tourniquet [24, 25]. Therefore, this study aimed to compare the effects of general and spinal anesthesia on inflammatory cytokines (interleukin-6 and tumor necrotizing factor-α (TNF-α)) and acute phase proteins including hs-CRP and ferritin induced by changes in ischemic reperfusion, due to pneumatic tourniquet during lower limb surgery.

2. Patients and Method

In this randomized controlled clinical trial, 34 patients undergoing lower limb surgery hospitalized in orthopedic ward of Imam Reza Hospital in Birjand, Iran, from December 2018 to July 2019 were selected by available sampling method. The inclusion criteria were as follows: (1) Patients with American Society of Anesthesiologists score of 1–2; (2) age ranging from 25 to 65 years; (3) lower limb surgery by the use of tourniquet; (4) use of tourniquet on one of the lower limbs; (5) absence of any vascular, respiratory, or kidney failure, liver function disturbance, and diabetic disease; (6) using no antioxidant or anti-inflammatory drug. The exclusion criteria of the study were as follows: (1) duration of surgery lower than 60 min and more than 90 min; (2) need of second surgery; (3) patients unwillingness to participate in the study at any stage of the study; (4) the death of patients. The current study was ethically approved by Medical Ethics Committee of Birjand University of Medical Sciences (ir.bums.rec.1396.178). The study was performed in terms of the principles of the Declaration of Helinski. Eligible patients were selected and after explaining the purpose of the study and assuring patients that the information will remain confidential and also after obtaining informed consent, the patients were included in the study. Since some patients were discharged from the hospital prior to taking supplementary samples, measurement of the studied factors was performed in 34 samples. Qualified patients (34 patients) were randomly divided into two groups as follows: general anesthesia ($n = 17$) and spinal anesthesia ($n = 17$). This sample size had acceptable power according to α: 0.05 and β: 0.8.

In both groups, intravenous cannulation with catheter 18 was performed on the peripheral veins of the upper limbs, and then 500 mL of normal saline was injected. In the general anesthesia group, anesthesia was induced with 1 mg of midazolam (30 to 50 mg/kg), 2 μg/kg of fentanyl, 0.5 mg/kg of atracurium, and 2 mg/kg of propofol. For maintenance of anesthesia, propofol at a dose of 100 μg/kg was used per minute, which can be increased to 200 μg/kg as needed. Atracurium was repeated every 30 minutes at one-quarter of the initial dose. In the case of hypotension, 500 mL of normal saline was first injected, 10 mg of ephedrine was intravenously injected if hypotension was more than 20% baseline, and blood pressure was precisely controlled with fluid therapy and inotropes. In the spinal anesthesia group, the patients were in the sitting position and we performed prep and drap of the third and fourth lumbar midline with Quincke needle number 25 treated with 2.5 mL bupivacaine 0.5% spinal anesthesia. The sensory level was checked using a needle every two minutes. When the sensory level reached the 12th lumbar vertebra, the bed position was returned to neutral, and then the surgical team was allowed to begin surgery.

The intravenous blood samples of the patients in both groups were taken at three times (8 to 10 mL each time), including before tourniquet application (baseline) and 12 and 24 hours after reperfusion. The samples were frozen after centrifugal plasma separation in order to be analyzed at the same time. IL-6 and TNF-α were determined by ELISA using Diaclone kits (French) in terms of the manufacturer's instructions. hs-CRP was also quantitated and recorded by immune turbidimetry using ZellBio GmbH kit and Fertin [26] by chemiluminescence using validated standard kits in the laboratory (monobind, USA).

After anesthesia and spinal anesthesia, tourniquet up to 150 mmHg of systolic blood pressure was inflated to prevent blood flow to the limb undergoing surgery (approximately 90 minutes). In order to control the mean arterial blood pressure and normal temperature, we used warm fluid. If arterial pressure is 20% lower than baseline during surgery, it indicates a reduction in blood pressure. A single dose of 5 mg intravenous ephedrine was administered as a bolus dose to regulate the blood pressure and continued to increase by one milligram to return blood pressure to the baseline. When postoperative bleeding occurred, the volume was replaced with salt solution rather than blood products. The duration of closure of tourniquet, the volume of topical anesthetic medicines, and the dose of ephedrine were recorded.

It should be noted that this study was a double-blind one in which the data were collected and recorded by an anesthesia resident who was blinded to the type of intervention. The surgeon and the anesthesiologist were the same in all procedures. The data were analyzed by the researcher who was unaware of the patient groups' classification and results of blood samples related to the type of intervention.

The data were analyzed using SPSS version 22. At first, Kolmogorov-Smirnov test was used to test the normal distribution of the study variables. Then, Chi-square and independent t-test were used to compare demographic information and cytokine's level in the two groups, respectively. In order to compare the patterns of inflammatory cytokines during the study period in study groups, repeated measure was used. The significance level was considered $p < 0.05$.

3. Results

The mean age and standard deviation of patients in general and spinal anesthesia were 28.65 ± 7.12 and 36.24 ± 14.33 years, respectively ($p = 0.06$). The mean of weight in two groups had no significant difference; 88.2% (15 cases) and 82.4% (14 cases) of general and spinal anesthesia were male, respectively. Also, 6% and 17.6% of the patients of general and spinal anesthesia had the history of medicine consumption. Duration of tourniquet closure in 58.8% of the patients of general anesthesia group and 82.4% of patients of spinal anesthesia group was more than 60 minutes; however, this difference was not statistically significant ($p = 0.13$). The two groups had similar history of previous disease ($p = 0.61$).

According to Table 1, the pattern of changes of inflammatory cytokines has no significant difference between the two studied groups ($p > 0.05$). Furthermore, TNF-α and ferritin showed no significant changes in both groups (p TNF-$\alpha = 0.23$ and p Fer $= 0.14$). However, hs-CRP and IL-6 had a significant ascending pattern ($p < 0.001$). Figure 1 shows that the ascending pattern during the study period for hs-CRP and IL-6 has a quadratic function.

The mean changes of IL-6 at different times in the two groups of general and spinal anesthesia showed no statistically significant difference. Mean changes in serum TNF-α level before and after 12 hours and before and after 24 hours indicated that no significant difference was found between the two methods of spinal and general anesthesia. No significant difference was observed in the means of serum ferritin level between two groups of spinal and general anesthesia.

4. Discussion

Induction of anesthesia by drugs influenced the immune system by affecting immune cells in perioperative period. These effects on immune cells, including T-lymphocytes, B-lymphocytes, macrophages, natural killer cells, and leukocytes, were investigated [27, 28]. The results of the present study showed that the mean serum level of hs-CRP in patients of both studied groups had no significant difference; however, the mean serum hs-CRP level changes during the study period showed significant difference.

Hughes et al. in a study investigated leukocyte activity and changes in inflammatory and coagulation markers caused by ischemia-reperfusion injury following tourniquet closure of the forearm [29]. They studied 10 healthy volunteers who had no history of heart disease at a 24-hour interval. The blood samples of the subjects were taken at baseline, 10 min after ischemia, and 5, 15, 30, and 60 min and 24 h after reperfusion. The results showed that the level of CRP concentration increased during the ischemia compared to baseline, and the maximum peak was at 15 min after reperfusion and reduced by passing 24 h from reperfusion; and at the same time, it was higher than the baseline [29].

Eroğlu et al. compared the effects of general and spinal anesthesia on systemic inflammatory response in patients undergoing total knee joint replacement surgery. The study results showed that, in both groups, CRP levels significantly increased 24 hours after surgery compared to the time of operation; however, no significant difference was found between the two groups [30], which is consistent with the results of the present study.

The results of the present study showed that the mean serum levels of IL-6 significantly increased over time in patients in both general and spinal anesthesia; however, the mean serum levels of IL-6 were not significantly different between the two groups of general and spinal anesthesia. The study results of Eroğlu et al. showed that IL-6 levels were significantly increased in two groups by passing 24 hours from surgery compared to baseline, but no significant difference was found between these two groups [30], which is consistent with the results of the present study. IL-6 and hs-CRP are cytokines and are more sensitive to inflammatory changes in the body and can rapidly respond.

The mean serum TNF-α level had no significant changes in both groups and during the study period. Halladin et al. conducted a study entitled "lower limb ischemia and reperfusion injuries in healthy volunteers by inflammatory and oxidative markers" and exposed 10 male volunteers to lower limb ischemia for 20 minutes [31]. They performed muscle biopsies, and blood samples were taken at 5, 15, 30, 60, and 90 minutes after tourniquet closure. The results showed that no significant increase was observed in MDA muscle biopsy after reperfusion. Oxidative plasma levels and pro- and anti-inflammatory parameters (ascorbic acid,

Table 1: The pattern of changes of inflammatory cytokines during the study period and between groups.

	General anesthesia			Spinal anesthesia			p value*	p value+
	Before	12 hours later	24 hours later	Before	12 hours later	24 hours later		
hs-CRP	3132.29 ± 2318.46	4404.53 ± 2102.69	4225.82 ± 2187.66	4822.94 ± 1393.18	5345.41 ± 603.76	5673.65 ± 431.05	<0.001	0.28
IL-6	14.03 ± 24.42	64.01 ± 79.47	37.04 ± 55.09	18.57 ± 29.09	56.28 ± 42.99	31.80 ± 24.18	<0.001	0.58
TNF-α	7.42 ± 2.88	33.15 ± 89	8.10 ± 3.53	9.02 ± 1.10	8.61 ± 2.38	6.54 ± 1.80	0.23	0.25
FER	74.29 ± 49.29	82.72 ± 44.74	78.66 ± 33.12	158.94 ± 177.77	138.51 ± 106.81	116.02 ± 85.19	0.14	0.07

*p value for the main effect. +p value for the interaction effect. Mauchly's W for hs-CRP (p value) = 0.92 (0.30). Mauchly's W for IL-6 (p value) = 0.43 (<0.001). Mauchly's W for TNF-α (p value) = 0.004 (<0.001). Mauchly's W for FER (p value) = 0.17 (<0.001). Significance of the bold value is < 0.05.

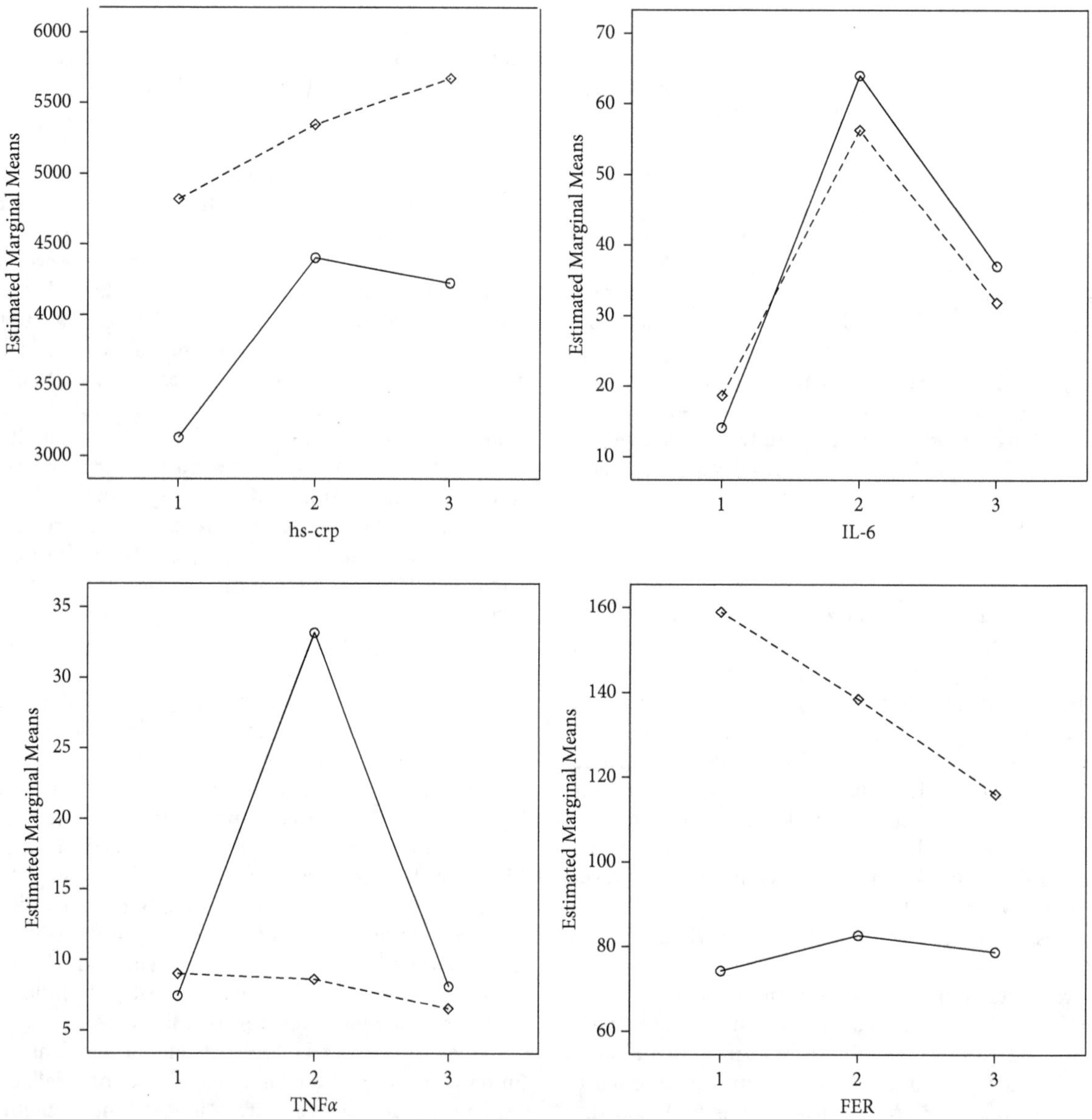

Figure 1: The pattern of changes of hs-CRP, IL-6, TNF-α, and ferritin [26] during the study period in two groups. Solid line and dash line show the general and spinal anesthesia, respectively.

dihydroascorbic acid, TNF, IL-1β, IL-6, and TNF-R) were not significantly different after reperfusion compared to baseline. They concluded that lower limb ischemia for 20 minutes has not caused ischemia-reperfusion injury in healthy volunteers [31], which is in some parts inconsistent with the results of the present study. In the present study, the closing time of tourniquet was longer than 60 minutes for most of the patients, whereas in a study by Halladin et al. [31]

tourniquet closing time was 20 minutes and they concluded that this time was short for producing and/or increasing the inflammatory markers. Probably the difference in the results of the present study and this study may be due to the duration of the tourniquet closure.

The results of various studies have shown that IL-6 levels significantly increased by passing 4 and 24 hours from reperfusion; however, TNF-α and IL-1 levels showed no significant increase during this period. In these studies, the closing time of tourniquet was 60 to 120 minutes [8, 31, 32].

Kamat et al. conducted a study on patients undergoing hand surgery. In these patients, the tourniquet was closed in the arm and inflated with 250 mmHg of Mercury, and also the duration of surgery was 116 ± 16 minutes. Accordingly, during surgery, tissue and blood samples were taken from the site of surgery at baseline and 2 and 10 minutes after reperfusion, and inflammatory factors were evaluated. The results showed that cytokines, IL-6, IL-7, IL-17, and TNF-α significantly increased at baseline after 10 min [33]. Secretion of proinflammatory (IL-6, Il-8, IL-1, and TNF-α) and anti-inflammatory (IL-10) cytokines was influenced by anesthesia. General anesthesia affects the levels of interferon Gamma (IFN-γ) and TNF-α [28].

The results of an experimental study showed that the highest TNF-α response to severe ischemia-induced injury occurred one minute after reperfusion and reached the control level after 10 minutes [34]; and in patients undergoing IL-6, it increased 30 to 60 minutes after surgery and changes in concentration significantly increased after 2 to 4 hours [35].

According to the results of the present study, it can be said that the maximal level of IL-6 in both groups was in 12 hours after surgery. Surgery or trauma induces a stress response, which protects the body. A regional anesthesia blocks neuroendocrine response but could not eliminate the cytokine response [36]. Secretion of IL-1 and TNF-α is the initiation of cytokine response, which induces the production of other cytokines, especially IL-6 as the reason of the systemic change [36]. The results of the present study showed that the mean serum fer level in patients of both groups and over time was not significantly different. By performing extensive searches in available databases such as SID, Magiran, Iranmedx, and Pubmed no study was found to have evaluated the level of fer in patients after opening tourniquet and reperfusion; therefore, it was not possible to compare this part of the results of the present study with other studies.

In the current study, the effect of drain use was not investigated due to lower rate of its application that might be useful for investigation in other studies as it increases the chance of inflammation [37]. Using tourniquet reduces intraoperative hemorrhage, allows better visualization of the surgeon, a is bloodless site, and finally reduces the surgery duration [5]. Also, it can be said that, in a healthy person under 50 years of age, tourniquet should not be closed for more than 2 hours [38]. The rate of two hours is reasonable, because after this period of ischemia, progressive venous acidosis will be developed in the site affected by the tourniquet [39]. An ischemic organ reperfusion is essential to prevent irreversible tissue injuries [40]. The injuries caused by reperfusion of skeletal muscles produce a variety of reactive oxygen species (ROS) and proinflammatory cytokines, which not only affect the muscles, but also cause injuries due to reduced blood flow to the organs [32, 41]. The lower limb ischemia-reperfusion injury can cause local injuries and severe abnormalities of the excreting organs including the lungs and kidneys [41]. Moreover, no hip replacement surgeries were performed in the current study.

4.1. Limitation. Because spinal anesthesia required patient consent, the emphasis was not on young people due to headaches. So the mean age of spinal anesthesia went up.

5. Conclusion

The pattern of hs-CRP, IL-6, TNF-α, and fer of the patients in both groups showed similar trend. The significant change of hs-CRP and IL-6 was observed over time. According to the results of the present study, the use of tourniquet leads to inflammation, and the inflammation is similar in both groups. In order to prevent the possible complications, it is suggested that, in the future studies, the amount of bleeding should be measured and compared between two methods. Moreover, the effect of drain use in the knee surgery is worth investigating. Considering the effect of duration of tourniquet closure on changes in inflammatory factors, it is recommended to conduct studies on patients with ischemia for 30 to 35 minutes and also on samples with reperfusion between 4 and 5 hours after reperfusion. Moreover, the use of disposable instrument was suggested in future studies to investigate the inflammatory responses.

Disclosure

This study was registered in the clinical trial system with code IRCT20150308021383N10. Mahmood Ganjifard and Samaneh Kouzegaran are the co-first authors.

Authors' Contributions

Mahmood Ganjifard and Samaneh Kouzegaran have contributed equally to the design of the study.

Acknowledgments

This study is related to thesis no. 455178 with the support of the research deputy of Birjand University of Medical Sciences.

References

[1] M. E. Baki, H. Uygun, B. Arı, and H. Aydın, "Bilateral femoral neck insufficiency fractures in pregnancy," *Joint Diseases and Related Surgery*, vol. 25, no. 1, pp. 60–62, 2014.

[2] E. Hirvensalo, H. Tuominen, M. Lapinsuo, and H. Heliö,

"Compartment syndrome of the lower limb caused by a tourniquet," *Journal of Orthopaedic Trauma*, vol. 6, no. 4, pp. 469–472, 1992.

[3] M. M. Yassin, D. W. Harkin, A. A. Barros D'Sa, M. I. Halliday, and B. J. Rowlands, "Lower limb ischemia-reperfusion injury triggers a systemic inflammatory response and multiple organ dysfunction," *World Journal of Surgery*, vol. 26, no. 1, pp. 115–121, 2002.

[4] S. Kahraman, K. Kilinç, D. Dal, and K. Erdem, "Propofol attenuates formation of lipid peroxides in tourniquet-induced ischaemia-reperfusion injury," *British Journal of Anaesthesia*, vol. 78, no. 3, pp. 279–281, 1997.

[5] M. Mathru, D. J. Dries, L. Barnes, P. Tonino, R. Sukhani, and M. W. Rooney, "Tourniquet-induced exsanguination in patients requiring lower limb surgery," *Anesthesiology*, vol. 84, no. 1, pp. 14–22, 1996.

[6] C. D. Collard and S. Gelman, "Pathophysiology, clinical manifestations, and prevention of ischemia-reperfusion injury," *Anesthesiology*, vol. 94, no. 6, pp. 1133–1138, 2001.

[7] C. Gonano, U. Leitgeb, C. Sitzwohl, G. Ihra, C. Weinstabl, and S. C. Kettner, "Spinal versus general anesthesia for orthopedic surgery: anesthesia drug and supply costs," *Anesthesia and Analgesia*, vol. 102, no. 2, pp. 524–529, 2006.

[8] A. Rodgers, N. Walker, S Schug et al., "Reduction of postoperative mortality and morbidity with epidural or spinal anaesthesia: results from overview of randomised," *BMJ*, vol. 321, no. 7275, p. 1493, 2000.

[9] H. Kehlet, "Modification of responses to surgery by neural blockade," *Neural Blockade in Clinical Anesthesia and Management of Pain*, Lippincott Williams and Wilkins, Philadelphia, PA, USA, 1998.

[10] R. M. H. Roumen, T. Hendriks, J. van der Ven-Jongekrijg et al., "Cytokine patterns in patients after major vascular surgery, hemorrhagic shock, and severe blunt trauma relation with subsequent adult respiratory distress syndrome and multiple organ failure," *Annals of Surgery*, vol. 218, no. 6, pp. 769–776, 1993.

[11] S. Spielmann, T. Kerner, O. Ahlers, D. Keh, M. Gerlach, and H. Gerlach, "Early detection of increased tumour necrosis factor alpha (TNFα) and soluble TNF receptor protein plasma levels after trauma reveals associations with the clinical course," *Acta Anaesthesiologica Scandinavica*, vol. 45, no. 3, pp. 364–370, 2001.

[12] W. L. Biffl, E. E. Moore, F. A. Moore, and C. C. Barnett, "Interleukin-6 delays neutrophil apoptosis via a mechanism involving platelet-activating factor," *The Journal of Trauma, Injury, Infection, and Critical Care*, vol. 40, no. 4, pp. 575–579, 1996.

[13] C. G. Persson, "Plasma exudation in the airways: mechanisms and function," *European Respiratory Journal*, vol. 4, no. 10, pp. 1268–1274, 1991.

[14] C. Adembri, E. Kastamoniti, I. Bertolozzi et al., "Pulmonary injury follows systemic inflammatory reaction in infrarenal aortic surgery," *Critical Care Medicine*, vol. 32, no. 5, pp. 1170–1177, 2004.

[15] P. G. Raijmakers, A. B. Groeneveld, J. A. Rauwerda, G. J. Teule, and C. E. Hack, "Acute lung injury after aortic surgery: the relation between lung and leg microvascular permeability to 111indium-labelled transferrin and circulating mediators," *Thorax*, vol. 52, no. 10, pp. 866–871, 1997.

[16] C. A. Camargo, J. F. Madden, W. Gao, R. S. Selvan, and P. Clavien, "Interleukin-6 protects liver against warm ischemia/reperfusion injury and promotes hepatocyte proliferation in the rodent," *Hepatology*, vol. 26, no. 6, pp. 1513–1520, 1997.

[17] R. G. Branco and P. C. R. Garcia, "Ferritin and C-reactive protein as markers of systemic inflammation in sepsis," *Pediatric Critical Care Medicine*, vol. 18, no. 2, pp. 194–196, 2017.

[18] E. Bostankolu, H. Ayoglu, S. Yurtlu et al., "Dexmedetomidine did not reduce the effects of tourniquet-induced ischemia-reperfusion injury during general anesthesia," *The Kaohsiung Journal of Medical Sciences*, vol. 29, no. 2, pp. 75–81, 2013.

[19] M. Terry, "Campbell's operative orthopedics," *Journal of the American Medical Association*, vol. 301, no. 3, pp. 329-330, 2009.

[20] R. Turan, H. Yagmurdur, M. Kavutcu, and B. Dikmen, "Propofol and tourniquet induced ischaemia reperfusion injury in lower extremity operations," *European Journal of Anaesthesiology*, vol. 24, no. 2, pp. 185–189, 2007.

[21] D. Özkan, T. Akkaya, A. Yalcindag et al., "Propofol sedation in total knee replacement," *Der Anaesthesist*, vol. 62, no. 7, pp. 537–542, 2013.

[22] L. Lin, L. Wang, Y Bai et al., "Pulmonary gas exchange impairment following tourniquet deflation: a prospective, single-blind clinical trial," *Orthopedics*, vol. 33, no. 6, p. 395, 2010.

[23] M. A. Gropper, R. D. Miller, L. I Eriksson et al., *Miller's Anesthesia, 2-Volume Set E-Book*, Elsevier Health Sciences, Amsterdam, Netherlands, 2019.

[24] E. Mas, A. E. Barden, T. B. Corcoran, M. Phillips, L. J. Roberts II, and T. A. Mori, "Effects of spinal or general anesthesia on F2-isoprostanes and isofurans during ischemia/reperfusion of the leg in patients undergoing knee replacement surgery," *Free Radical Biology and Medicine*, vol. 50, no. 9, pp. 1171–1176, 2011.

[25] T. Clementsen and O. Reikerås, "Cytokine patterns after tourniquet-induced skeletal muscle ischaemia reperfusion in total knee replacement," *Scandinavian Journal of Clinical and Laboratory Investigation*, vol. 68, no. 2, pp. 154–159, 2008.

[26] S. S. Signorelli, G. Oliveri Conti, A. Zanobetti, A. Baccarelli, M. Fiore, and M. Ferrante, "Effect of particulate matter-bound metals exposure on prothrombotic biomarkers: a systematic review," *Environmental Research*, vol. 177, Article ID 108573, 2019.

[27] C. A. Akdis, "Therapies for allergic inflammation: refining strategies to induce tolerance," *Nature Medicine*, vol. 18, no. 5, pp. 736–749, 2012.

[28] A. Jafarzadeh, M. Hadavi, G. Hassanshahi, M. Rezaeian, and R. Vazirinejad, "General anesthetics on immune system cytokines: a narrative review article," *Anesthesiology and Pain Medicine*, vol. 10, no. 4, Article ID e103033, 2018.

[29] S. F. Hughes, B. D. Hendricks, D. R. Edwards, S. S. Bastawrous, G. E. Roberts, and J. F. Middleton, "Mild episodes of tourniquet-induced forearm ischaemia-reperfusion injury results in leukocyte activation and changes in inflammatory and coagulation markers," *Journal of Inflammation*, vol. 4, no. 1, pp. 12–18, 2007.

[30] M. Eroğlu, S. Kokulu, H. B. Koca, M. E. Demirboğan, E. D. Baki, and Ö Özcan, "The effects of general and spinal anesthesia on systemic inflammatory response in patients undergoing total knee arthroplasty," *Joint Diseases and Related Surgery*, vol. 27, no. 3, pp. 153–159, 2016.

[31] N. Halladin, S. Ekeløf, M. Alamili et al., "Lower limb ischaemia and reperfusion injury in healthy volunteers measured by oxidative and inflammatory biomarkers," *Perfusion*, vol. 30, no. 1, pp. 64–70, 2015.

[32] H. Ruksana, D. R. Solanki, and M. I. Mathru, "Inflammatory

and redox responses to ischaemia/reperfusion in human skeletal muscle," *Clinical Science*, vol. 107, no. 5, pp. 497–503, 2004.

[33] P. Kamat, B. Juon, B. Jossen, T. Gajanayake, R. Rieben, and E. Vögelin, "Assessment of endothelium and inflammatory response at the onset of reperfusion injury in hand surgery," *Journal of Inflammation*, vol. 9, no. 1, p. 18, 2012.

[34] A. Steensberg, C. P. Fischer, C. Keller, K. Møller, and B. K. Pedersen, "IL-6 enhances plasma IL-1ra, IL-10, and cortisol in humans," *American Journal of Physiology—Endocrinology And Metabolism*, vol. 285, no. 2, pp. E433–E437, 2003.

[35] D. J. Whitehead and S. J. MacDonald, "TKA sans tourniquet: let it bleed: opposes," *Orthopedics*, vol. 32, no. 9, p. 680, 2011.

[36] T. G. Senapathi, I. M. Widnyana, M Wiryana et al., "Effectiveness of low-dose intravenous ketamine to attenuate stress response in patients undergoing emergency cesarean section with spinal anesthesia," *Journal of Pain Research*, vol. 9, pp. 689–692, 2016.

[37] M. Basilico, R. Vitiello, F. Liuzza et al., "Efficacy of postoperative drainage in total knee arthroplasty: review of the literature," *Orthopedic Reviews*, vol. 12, no. 1, p. 8663, 2020.

[38] E. F. S. Wilgis, "Observations on the effects of tourniquet ischemia," *The Journal of Bone and Joint Surgery*, vol. 53, no. 7, pp. 1343–1346, 1971.

[39] H. K. Eltzschig and C. D. Collard, "Vascular ischaemia and reperfusion injury," *British Medical Bulletin*, vol. 70, no. 1, pp. 71–86, 2004.

[40] H. Esme, H. Fidan, T. Koken, and O. Solak, "Effect of lung ischemia-reperfusion on oxidative stress parameters of remote tissues," *European Journal of Cardio-Thoracic Surgery*, vol. 29, no. 3, pp. 294–298, 2006.

[41] H. Yoshida, H. Yanai, Y. Namiki, K. Fukatsu-Sasaki, N. Furutani, and N. Tada, "Neuroprotective effects of edaravone: a novel free radical scavenger in cerebrovascular injury," *CNS Drug Reviews*, vol. 12, no. 1, pp. 9–20, 2006.

Predicting the Effect of Bilateral Pelvic Osteotomy on Sagittal Alignment Correction and Surrounding Muscles: A Mathematical Model

Vahhab Zarei,[1] Sharon C. Yson,[2] Joan E. Bechtold,[3] and Jonathan N. Sembrano[4]

[1] *PhD Student, University of Minnesota, 2450 Riverside Ave. S R200, Minneapolis, MN 55454, USA*
[2] *Spine Research Associate, University of Minnesota, 2450 Riverside Ave. S R200, Minneapolis, MN 55454, USA*
[3] *Vice Chair, Research, Gustilo Professor of Orthopaedic Research, Department of Orthopedic Surgery, University of Minnesota, 2450 Riverside Ave. S R200, Minneapolis, MN 55454, USA*
[4] *Associate Professor, Department of Orthopaedics, University of Minnesota, 2450 Riverside Ave. S R200, Minneapolis, MN 55454, USA*

Correspondence should be addressed to Sharon C. Yson; scyson@umn.edu

Academic Editor: Allen L. Carl

Study Design. Mathematical Model. *Objectives.* To investigate the relationship between pelvic osteotomy opening angle (OA) and its effect on spinopelvic sagittal parameters as well as the resting length of surrounding muscles. *Methods.* Predictive equations correlating OA with spinopelvic parameters were derived using geometric relationships. A geometric model calculated spinopelvic parameters (SVA, pelvic incidence [PI], PT, and T1 pelvic angle [TPA]) produced by progressively increasing the OA. These values were compared to optimal balance criteria in the literature. Four muscles crossing the osteotomy site were evaluated: Gluteus Medius (GMED), Gluteus Maximus (GMAX), Piriformis (P), and Tensor Fascia Lata (TFL). Insertion points were obtained from an OpenSim software model. GMAX and GMED were subdivided into 3 (anterior, middle, and posterior). *Results.* OA correlated negatively with PI, TPA, and SVA and positively with PT. From baseline SVA of 22 cm, OA 21° reduced SVA to 5cm. OA 23° reduced TPA to 14°. OA 30° increased PT to 20°. OA 26° decreased PI-LL to 10°. OA range of 26°-30° resulted in optimal sagittal deformity correction. OA correlated with SR positively for TFL and anterior GMED and negatively for the rest of muscles. For this OA, the SR approximately decreased 6%, 5%, 6%, 8%, and 5% for posterior GMED, anterior GMAX, middle GMAX, posterior GMAX, and P, respectively. It increased 8% and 4% for anterior GMED and TFL, respectively. *Conclusion.* Predictive relationships between osteotomy OA and spinopelvic parameters were shown, providing proof of concept that sagittal balance may be achieved via pelvic osteotomy.

1. Introduction

Surgeons have known for many years that a flattened lumbar lordosis (flatback syndrome) has adverse effects on surgical outcome. Lazennec et al. (2000) recognized that fusion should not only be the main goal of lumbar spine surgery; they have shown that failure to restore normal sagittal alignment correlated with postfusion pain [1]. However, it was not until the mid-2000s when Glassman et al. demonstrated clear statistical correlation between sagittal alignment and outcomes as measured by validated tools that primacy was placed on restoring and/or preserving sagittal alignment when performing spinal fusion surgery [2]. Even in patients who present with coronal deformity (i.e., scoliosis), sagittal alignment was still shown to be significantly more predictive of clinical outcome compared to coronal deformity correction [3].

Since then, Schwab et al. have formulated objective radiographic goals for surgeons to aim for when performing these surgeries. Among these are the approximation of pelvic incidence (PI) and lumbar lordosis (LL) (PI – LL < 9°), with reduction of compensatory posterior pelvic tilt (PT < 20°) and neutralization of sagittal vertical axis (SVA < 5 cm) [4]. More recently, Protopsaltis et al. introduced the T1 pelvic angle (TPA) and proposed an additional radiographic measurement goal (TPA < 14°) [5]. In the past few years,

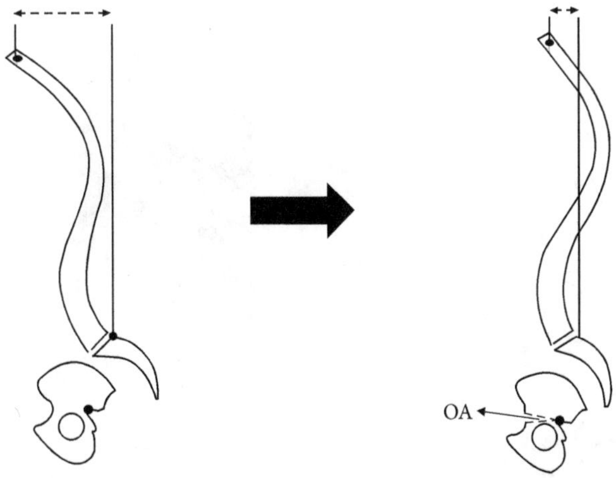

FIGURE 1: Schematic representation of the sagittal view of the spinopelvis system showing proposed bilateral pelvic osteotomy (BPO) procedure. Osteotomy will be performed caudal to SIJ but above the hip joints. A small change in pelvis opening angle (OA) will result in considerable sagittal vertical axis (SVA) correction.

spine surgeons have been more commonly requesting for full-spine standing (lateral) radiographs, both for preoperative planning and for postoperative evaluation, with inclusion of the femoral heads, to facilitate measurement of the aforementioned sagittal parameters.

An adverse consequence of increased emphasis on sagittal alignment correction has been the concomitant increase in multilevel fusion surgery and complex osteotomies (e.g., pedicle subtraction osteotomy), with resultant increased cost and morbidity. Over a span of a decade (2000-2010), the average charge per inpatient admission increased by approximately 230% and 190% for Medicare and private insurance, respectively [6]. Surgery for adult spinal deformities is technically demanding and has high complication rates [7, 8].

We propose a potential alternative to spinal osteotomies for spinal realignment surgery by creating the fulcrum of rotational correction more caudally at the pelvis, thus providing a longer lever arm to bring the head back in a balanced position. In other words, a greater change to the sagittal vertical axis could be produced by a relatively smaller angular change at the pelvic osteotomy site. To avoid injuries to the thecal sac and nerve roots within the spinal canal as well as to the sacroiliac joints (SIJ), we propose that the osteotomy be performed caudal to the SIJ but above the hip joints. These would be bilateral opening wedge osteotomies (BPO) from the anterior inferior iliac spine (AIIS) to the sciatic notch on each side of the pelvis. The posterior cortex along the sciatic notch will serve as the fulcrum of rotation in the sagittal plane. Figure 1 schematically shows how this osteotomy will be performed.

The objective of this study was to evaluate the capability of our proposed pelvic osteotomy to correct spinal sagittal malalignment using a mathematical predictive model. Osteotomy opening angle effects on sagittal spinopelvic parameters as well as resting length of muscles crossing the osteotomy site were examined. This study lays the groundwork for stepwise implementation of BPO for sagittal plane realignment in human patients.

2. Methods

2.1. Part A: Assessment of Sagittal Alignment after Virtual Bilateral Pelvic Opening Wedge Osteotomies. To evaluate the effect of BPO on sagittal alignment, predictive equations correlating pelvis opening angle (OA) with spinopelvic parameters were derived. These equations are based on anatomic landmarks (femoral head, BPO fulcrum, S1 endplate, and C7-T1 vertebral bodies) as shown in Figure 2(a). To demonstrate feasibility, a lateral full-spine X-ray of one patient with sagittal deformity (Figure 2(b)) was used identify the location of these points. Spinal curvature was assumed to remain fixed (i.e., to represent rigid spinal deformity). Predictive equations correlating OA with spinopelvic parameters were derived using trigonometric-geometric relationships:

$$SVA = L\sin(T1SPA) + L'\cos(\alpha_4 - OA)$$

$$TPA = T1SPA - \alpha_5 - \beta + \frac{\pi}{2}$$

$$PI = \sin^{-1}\left(\frac{\sin(\alpha_2 + OA)}{\sqrt{1 + k^2 - 2k\cos(\alpha_2 + OA)}}\right) + \alpha_1 \quad (1)$$

$$PT = PI + \frac{\pi}{2} - \alpha_1 - \alpha_3 + OA$$

where

$$\beta = \sin^{-1}\left(\frac{\sin(\alpha_2 + OA)}{\sqrt{1 + k'^2 - 2k'\cos(\alpha_2 + OA)}}\right)$$

$$T1SPA = \sin^{-1}\left(\frac{\sin(\alpha_6 + OA)}{\sqrt{1 + k''^2 - 2k''\cos(\alpha_6 + OA)}}\right) + \alpha_5 - \frac{\pi}{2} \quad (2)$$

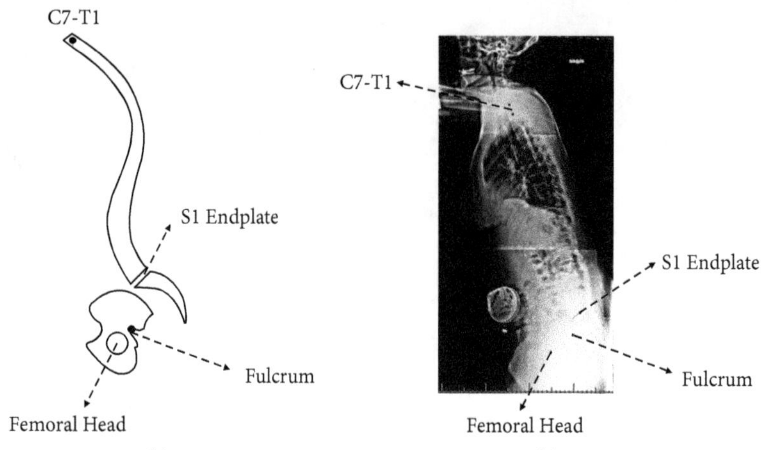

FIGURE 2: Diagram of the sagittal view of the spinopelvic system showing landmark points used to measure angles and distances used in the predictive equations (a). The location of these points was identified and measured in an actual full sagittal spine X-ray (b).

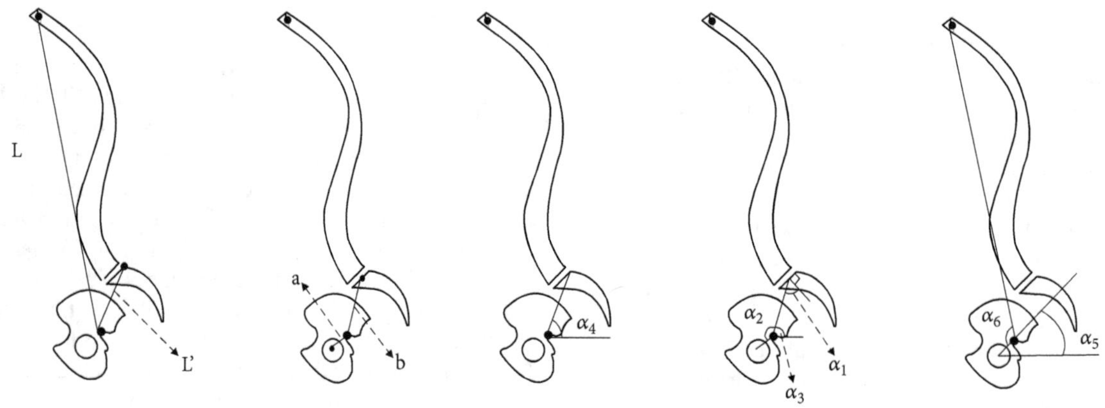

FIGURE 3: Lateral spine diagram showing angles used in the predictive equation.

And

$$k = \frac{b}{a}$$
$$k' = \frac{a}{b} \quad (3)$$
$$k'' = \frac{a}{L}$$

These equations are expressed in terms of OA, as well as patient-specific distances and angles (Figure 3). These lengths and angles can be easily calculated based on landmark points shown in Figure 2.

Changes of SVA, TPA, PT, and PI-LL with OA were plotted in figures based of which the acceptable range of OA can be specified. The allowable OA was confined to satisfy these conditions:

$$\begin{gathered} -50mm < SVA < 50mm \\ TPA < 14^\circ \\ PT < 20^\circ \\ PI - LL < 9^\circ \end{gathered} \quad (4)$$

2.2. Part B: Effect of Osteotomy on Involved Muscles. Aside from spinopelvic parameters, muscles passing across the osteotomy site are also under influence of BPO, as their resting length change because of the relative changes in their insertion points. Four muscles which cross the osteotomy site were studied: gluteus maximus (GMax), gluteus medius (GMed), tensor fasciae latae (TFL), and piriformis (P).

™GMax and GMed are relatively wide muscles and they may undergo shortening or lengthening depending on location over their span. Thus, each of them was subdivided into

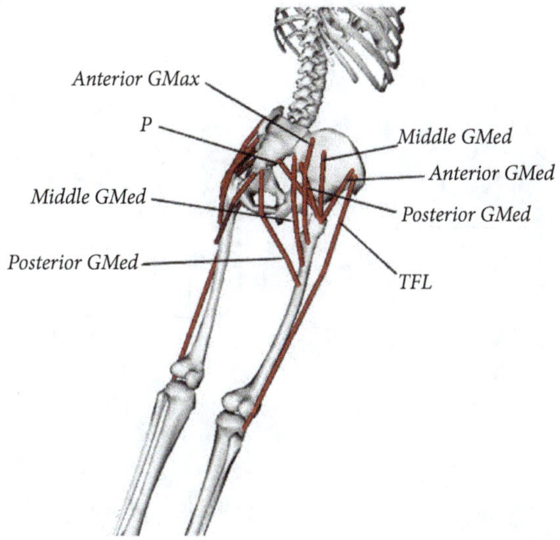

FIGURE 4: Schematic diagram of surrounding pelvic and hip muscles evaluated in the proposed procedure [9].

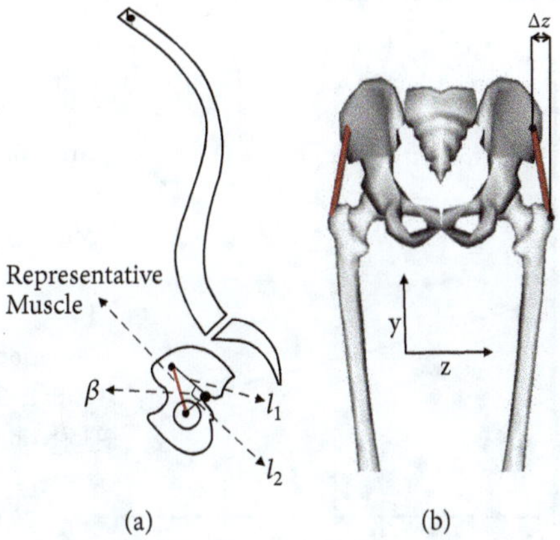

FIGURE 5: Sagittal Representation of the spine (a) and posterior representation of the pelvis and hip (b) showing lengths l_1, l_2, Δz, and angle β used in the predictive equation for muscle length. These parameters are different for each muscle segment. The red line represents a muscle segment [9].

three sections (named anterior, posterior, and middle), each assigned a uniform initial length (Figure 4). All of the muscle segments are considered as one dimensional longitudinal part.

A predictive equation was derived based on basic trigonometric laws to postoperatively estimate the length of each muscle:

$$d = \sqrt{l^2 + \Delta z^2} \tag{5}$$

where d is the muscle length and:

$$l = \sqrt{l_1^2 + l_2^2 - 2l_1 l_2 \cos(\beta + OA)} \tag{6}$$

l_1, l_2, Δz, and angle β in the equations are shown in Figure 5, with the z axis defined perpendicular to the sagittal plane. Since these parameters vary for different subjects and it is not possible to quantify them with spine X-ray images, OpenSim [9] software was utilized. OpenSim is an open source muscle modeling software from which muscle segment lengths were estimated.

Muscle-stretch ratio (SR) is defined as the ratio of new muscle length over initial length where L_0 is initial length and λ is the stretch ratio:

$$\lambda = \frac{d}{L_0} \tag{7}$$

Finally, this stretch ratio for each muscle was plotted with OA, to check if it exceeds the critical stretch ratio in the literature (25%). Shortening muscles, that is muscle whose insertion points become closer after surgery, are assumed to be safe, as they do not generate any stress.

3. Results

The linear relationships between osteotomy opening angle (OA) and selected sagittal spinopelvic radiographic parameters are shown on Figure 6. OA correlated negatively with PI,

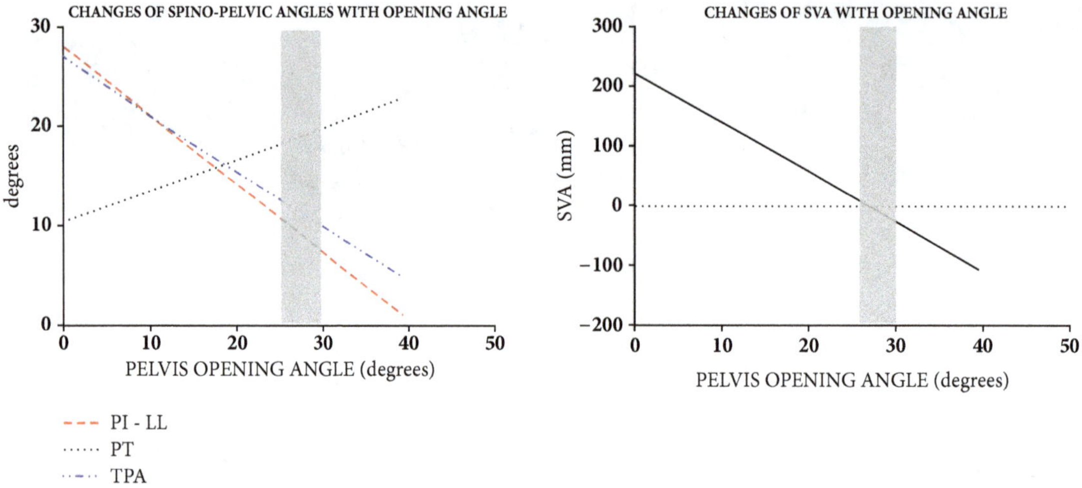

FIGURE 6: Graphs showing the relationship of osteotomy opening angle (OA) with spinopelvic parameters and SVA. The grey area represents the range of opening angles where optimal sagittal deformity correction is achieved.

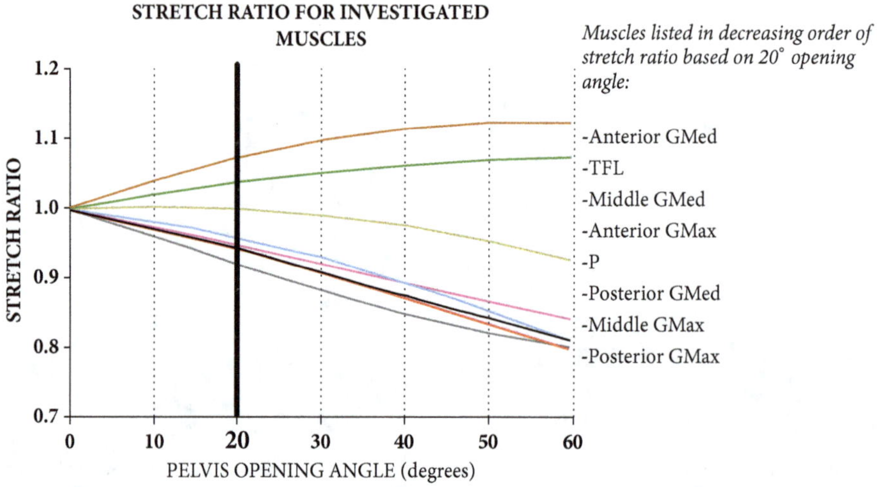

FIGURE 7: Graph showing the correlation of pelvis opening angle (OA) and the stretch ratio (SR) of selected muscle segments.

TPA, and SVA and positively with PT. From baseline SVA of 22 cm, a 21° OA reduced SVA to 5 cm. A 23° OA reduced TPA to 14°. A 30° OA increased PT to 20°. A 26° OA decreased PI-LL to 10°. Thus, an OA range of 26° to 30° resulted in optimal sagittal deformity correction. Within this range, PI decreased by 19°-21° from baseline.

As can be seen in Figure 6, the nonlinear relations for spinopelvic parameters, as shown as predictive equations, yield to linear correlations for the practical range of opening angles. For the specific patient examined in this paper, the alignment parameters have the following linear correlations:

$$\begin{aligned} SVA &= -8.3OA + 223.8 \\ PI &= -0.7OA + 54.4 \\ PT &= 0.3OA + 10.4 \\ TPA &= -0.6OA + 27.0 \end{aligned} \quad (8)$$

where SVA is in mm and OA, PI, PT, and TPA are in degrees. OA correlation with muscle SR is shown in Figure 7. OA correlated positively with muscle SR for the tensor fascia latae (TFL) and the anterior portion of the gluteus medius (anterior GMed); it correlated negatively with SR for the other muscles, including the anterior, middle, and posterior portions of the gluteus maximus (anterior, middle, and posterior GMax), the middle and posterior portions of the gluteus medius (middle and posterior GMED), and the piriformis (P). At a preselected 20° OA, muscle SR decreased by 6%, 5%, 6%, 8%, and 5% for posterior GMed, anterior GMax, middle GMax, posterior GMax, and P, respectively, and increased by 8% and 4% for anterior GMed and TFL, respectively. There was no SR change for middle GMed.

4. Discussion

In this study we primarily sought to examine the feasibility of a proposed pelvic osteotomy procedure in producing effective spinal sagittal alignment change via geometric mathematical modeling. Specifically, we looked at the relationships between pelvic osteotomy opening angle and commonly used spinopelvic radiographic parameters and calculated the amount of opening angle necessary to bring these parameters within the range of what is considered acceptable in the literature. Secondarily, the relationships between osteotomy opening angle and resting length of muscles spanning the osteotomy site, as characterized by the muscle-stretch ratio, was examined.

Predictive relationships between pelvic osteotomy OA and spinopelvic parameters were shown in our mathematical model, thus providing proof of concept that sagittal alignment may be achieved via pelvic osteotomy. Because of the negative correlation between osteotomy opening angle and PI, TPA and SVA, a minimum OA can be defined based on the lowest OA that would still correct these 3 parameters to acceptable levels. On the other hand, because of the positive correlation between osteotomy opening angle and PT, a maximum OA can be defined based on the highest OA beyond which PT would likely become unacceptable. Thus an acceptable or target range of OA can be deduced from the model. In the example used for the study, the minimum and maximum OA were 26° and 30°, respectively, thus providing a 4° range of acceptable OA. It should be pointed out, however, that these values were arrived at by modeling based on a single patient's radiograph. Thus, the ideal 26-30 degree range of opening angle is specific only to this patient. Given the wide spectrum of deformity, each patient would have his/her own range of ideal opening wedge angle.

There are other limitations to our study that should be discussed. (1) While we looked at the potential effects of bilateral pelvic osteotomies on spinal sagittal parameters, we have not performed such a procedure on actual patients for sagittal deformity correction. Thus, we are unable to make specific recommendations on aspects such as fixation method, type of bone graft, need for postoperative immobilization, and weight-bearing status. We speculate that the posterior iliac cortex should be preserved in order to maintain stability, that fixation has adequate rigidity to allow bed to chair transfers and ideally even weight-bearing, and that the bone graft should also have strong structural properties for supplemental stability. These will be the focus of future studies. (2) The assumption of a rigid spine may not be true for most cases of sagittal deformity. This may, however, hold true in cases where previous multilevel fusion was performed, whether the fusion was (a) the cause of the deformity ('iatrogenic flatback') or (b) performed for the deformity but inadequate correction was achieved.

There are important differences between our pelvic osteotomy procedure and conventional spinal osteotomies in terms of their effects on individual spinopelvic parameters and how spinal alignment is achieved. In conventional spine deformity surgery, correction is mainly effected on lumbar lordosis (LL), whereas pelvic incidence (PI) is regarded as a fixed parameter [10–12]. By performing the osteotomy in the pelvis, however, the fixed relationship between the hip joint and the sacrum is disrupted, and correction is effected instead on pelvic incidence. In this scenario, the lumbar lordosis is presumed to be a fixed parameter, such as in cases with prior multilevel fusion. With either method, matching between PI and LL is ultimately accomplished, either by increasing LL (traditional spinal osteotomy) or by decreasing PI (pelvic osteotomy).

Recently, Bodin and Roussouly from France published their case series on the use of Salter type osteotomy and sacral pedicle subtraction osteotomy to correct sagittal spine deformities [13]. The majority of their cases were diagnosed with spondyloptosis. Prior to surgery on actual patients, they performed mathematical modeling by doing virtual osteotomies on pelvic x-rays to predict the effect of the procedure on PI. They reported that, with Salter osteotomy, there is an inverse correlation between opening angle and PI. The same trend can be seen with our model. However, in addition to PI change, we also evaluated the effect of the osteotomy opening angle on SVA, TPA, and PT. Perhaps the foremost difference between the two models is that Bodin and Roussouly's was derived by performing virtual osteotomies on X-ray images and our predictive equations were based on fundamental geometric principles.

Another recent case study discussed the use of posterior sacral osteotomies to correct a fixed iatrogenic spinopelvic deformity. The technique involved longitudinal osteotomies through the sacral ala and derotation of the sacrum to achieve the desired pelvic incidence. At one year after surgery, the patient reportedly maintained a balanced sagittal alignment [14].

While the osteotomy we propose is in many respects similar to the Salter innominate osteotomy, it is fundamentally different in both its goal and the mechanism by which it is achieved. As with Salter, a linear osteotomy is created from the anterior surface of the ilium above the acetabulum towards the sciatic notch. An anterior opening wedge is then created with the fulcrum along the sciatic notch. The Salter osteotomy is meant to provide better coverage for the femoral head by redirecting the acetabulum; this is achieved by creating a pivot point at the pubic symphysis in addition to the posterior fulcrum. Thus, in order for this osteotomy to achieve the desired effect, it is by definition a unilateral osteotomy (even though subsequent authors have reported on bilateral Salter osteotomies). On the other hand, our pelvic osteotomy has the goal of correcting sagittal deformity by retroverting the superior portion of the pelvis. Thus, by definition this has to be performed bilaterally, and the correction achieved simultaneously.

We acknowledge that spinal osteotomies are effective and well-established procedures in the spine surgeon's armamentarium. Our conceptualized bilateral pelvic osteotomy is not meant to supplant these more traditional procedures, but rather to present it as a possible alternative in certain situations. These may include (1) previous multilevel fusion as mentioned above; (2) ankylosed spine in absence of previous surgery (e.g., ankylosing spondylitis); and (3) cases of abnormally high pelvic incidence (~> 75 degrees) where creating lumbar hyperlordosis to achieve PI-LL matching may not be deemed desirable because of potential concerns with symptomatic stenosis and facet degeneration. Lastly, if future studies are able to show that a pelvic osteotomy procedure is a smaller physiological hit to the body compared to spinal 3-column osteotomy surgery, patients with poor medical status who cannot tolerate the latter may be considered as candidates for pelvic osteotomy instead.

Whether planning for sagittal correction via spinal osteotomy or pelvic osteotomy, it is important to note that a posteriorly tilted pelvis (high PT) causes partial correction of the SVA. Therefore, the whole image has to be rotated anteriorly to 'correct' PT prior to planning the osteotomy; this step unmasks the true extent of the deformity without the mitigating effects of posterior pelvic tilt. Failure to rotate the image results in under-correction of the deformity.

An important limitation of our mathematical model is in terms of predicting final pelvic tilt (PT) and sagittal vertical axis (SVA). Unlike PI, LL, and TPA, PT and SVA are significantly affected by the position of the hip joint in the sagittal axis. Posterior rotation or extension of the hip joint produces posterior pelvic tilt or retroversion, a primary compensatory mechanism in the presence of sagittal deformity. By correcting the deformity, it is presumed that there will be concomitant normalization of PT. However, unlike LL (in spinal osteotomy) or PI (in pelvic osteotomy) this is not directly locked in position during surgery. Potential factors that may prevent PT normalization despite deformity correction may include hip extension contracture, hip flexion weakness and hip joint stiffness.

Because all the muscles that cross the pelvic osteotomy site also cross and help position the hip joints, we also examined the relationship between osteotomy opening angle and resting length of selected muscles, expressed as the individual muscle-stretch ratio (SR). Our model showed relationships between OA and individual muscle SR. In general, muscles that cross the osteotomy site anterior to the fulcrum of rotation at the osteotomy site tend to lengthen with opening of the osteotomy (tensor fascia latae and anterior gluteus medius), and posterior muscles tend to shorten (anterior, middle and posterior gluteus maximus, posterior gluteus medius and piriformis). Because the gluteus medius and maximus muscles have very broad muscle bellies, they were likely to experience differential lengthening or shortening of their fibers at different points in the muscles; thus, these muscles were divided each into anterior, middle and posterior portions. It is worth noting that because the gluteus medius spans the length of the osteotomy, the anterior portion of the muscle lengthens, the middle portion stay relatively isometric, and the posterior portion shortens with increasing opening of the osteotomy. Despite our ability to show effects of osteotomy angle on muscle SR, we cannot say whether there would be a measurable or clinically relevant effect on muscle function and body posture. It is, however, unlikely that pelvic osteotomy within the calculated recommended range to correct spinal alignment will adversely affect muscle function since our maximum SR (8% for anterior GMed) is substantially less than the reported critical SR value (25.4%) beyond which muscle function is significantly affected in animal models [15]. Lastly, this model does not take into account muscle effects of iatrogenic injury during surgery and of postoperative physical therapy.

A pelvic osteotomy procedure may also have unintended consequences on the hip joint(s); this may either be in terms of (a) position of the hip (cup ante/retroversion) or (b) potential acetabular surface deformation given osteotomy's proximity to the acetabulum. The former may lead to increased predisposition to hip instability/dislocation, particularly in the presence of total hip arthroplasty. This was touched upon by a recent publication showing decreased cup anteversion (which may lead to increased risk of prosthetic hip dislocation) after spinal deformity correction [16]. Whether the latter (b) issue will become clinically manifest is unknown. While there are pelvic osteotomies developed and currently utilized to mold or reconfigure the acetabulum for hip dysplasia, these are only performed in the very young patient population; it is unlikely that such reconfiguration also occurs in adult hips, although violation and subsequent weakening of the periacetabular subchondral bone is a possibility and cause of concern.

For mathematical modeling purposes, it was assumed that the spine is completely rigid. While this may hold true for clinical conditions such as ankylosing spondylitis, advanced multilevel spondylosis with autofusion and, perhaps more commonly, patients who have had extensive fusion surgery, it is much more difficult to predict how a mobile/flexible spine would respond to bilateral anterior opening wedge pelvic osteotomies. We hypothesize that there may still potentially be a role for such an osteotomy in patients who have an abnormally high pelvic incidence (~> 75°) and preferably prior to onset of degenerative changes at the lower lumbar levels secondary to chronic compensatory hyperlordosis. While we intuitively suspect that an osteotomy aimed at decreasing the pelvic incidence would lead to concomitant decrease (relaxation) of lumbar hyperlordosis without leading to a negative change in sagittal vertical axis, this is not supported by our mathematical model, as it does not take into account spinal flexibility

In summary, we have evaluated the feasibility of our proposed bilateral anterior opening wedge pelvic osteotomy as an alternative to traditional spinal osteotomy procedure for sagittal plane deformity correction. Using a geometric mathematical model, we demonstrated direct relationships between pelvic osteotomy opening angle and commonly used spinopelvic radiographic parameters (negative correlation with PI, SVA, and TPA; positive correlation with PT). In our model, we were able to accomplish correction of spinopelvic parameters to within accepted goals, thus demonstrating proof of concept that spinal alignment may be achieved by pelvic osteotomy in the setting of sagittal deformity. Lastly, we demonstrated effects of osteotomy opening angle on resting muscle lengths (expressed by individual muscle-stretch ratio) of selected muscles crossing the osteotomy site and hip joint.

Disclosure

This study was present at the Orthopaedic Research Society Meeting in 2016.

References

[1] J. Lazennec, S. Ramaré, N. Arafati et al., "Sagittal alignment in lumbosacral fusion: relations between radiological parameters and pain," *European Spine Journal*, vol. 9, no. 1, pp. 47–55, 2000.

[2] S. D. Glassman, K. Bridwell, J. R. Dimar, W. Horton, S. Berven, and F. Schwab, "The impact of positive sagittal balance in adult spinal deformity," *The Spine Journal*, vol. 30, no. 18, pp. 2024–2029, 2005.

[3] M. D. Daubs, L. G. Lenke, K. H. Bridwell et al., "Does correction of preoperative coronal imbalance make a difference in outcomes of adult patients with deformity?" *The Spine Journal*, vol. 38, no. 6, pp. 476–483, 2013.

[4] F. Schwab, A. Patel, B. Ungar, J.-P. Farcy, and V. Lafage, "Adult spinal deformity-postoperative standing imbalance: how much can you tolerate? An overview of key parameters in assessing alignment and planning corrective surgery," *The Spine Journal* vol. 35, no. 25, pp. 2224–2231, 2010.

[5] T. Protopsaltis, F. Schwab, N. Bronsard et al., "The T1 pelvic angle, a novel radiographic measure of global sagittal deformity, accounts for both spinal inclination and pelvic tilt and correlates with health-related quality of life," *Journal of Bone and Joint Surgery - American Volume*, vol. 96, no. 19, pp. 1631–1640, 2014.

[6] I. McCarthy, R. Hostin, M. O'Brien, R. Saigal, and C. P. Ames, "Health Economic Analysis of Adult Deformity Surgery," *Neurosurgery Clinics of North America*, vol. 24, no. 2, pp. 293–304, 2013.

[7] W. W. Schairer, A. Carrer, V. Deviren et al., "Hospital readmission after spine fusion for adult spinal deformity," *The Spine Journal*, vol. 38, no. 19, pp. 1681–1689, 2013.

[8] J. K. Scheer, J. A. Tang, J. S. Smith et al., "Cervical spine alignment, sagittal deformity, and clinical implications: A review," *Journal of Neurosurgery: Spine*, vol. 19, no. 2, pp. 141–159, 2013.

[9] S. L. Delp, F. C. Anderson, A. S. Arnold et al., "OpenSim: open-source software to create and analyze dynamic simulations of movement," *IEEE Transactions on Biomedical Engineering*, vol. 54, no. 11, pp. 1940–1950, 2007.

[10] J. C. Le Huec, S. Aunoble, L. Philippe, and P. Nicolas, "Pelvic parameters: origin and significance.," *European spine journal : official publication of the European Spine Society, the European Spinal Deformity Society, and the European Section of the Cervical Spine Research Society*, vol. 20, pp. 564–571, 2011.

[11] P. Roussouly and C. Nnadi, "Sagittal plane deformity: an overview of interpretation and management," *European Spine Journal*, vol. 19, no. 11, pp. 1824–1836, 2010.

[12] J. Legaye, G. Duval-Beaupère, J. Hecquet, and C. Marty, "Pelvic incidence: a fundamental pelvic parameter for three-dimensional regulation of spinal sagittal curves," *European Spine Journal*, vol. 7, no. 2, pp. 99–103, 1998.

[13] A. Bodin and P. Roussouly, "Sacral and pelvic osteotomies for correction of spinal deformities," *European Spine Journal*, vol. 24, no. 1, pp. 72–82, 2014.

[14] M. Czyz, S. Forster, J. Holton, B. Shariati, D. J. Clarkson, and B. M. Boszczyk, "New method for correction of lumbosacral kyphosis deformity in patient with high pelvic incidence," *European Spine Journal*, vol. 26, no. 8, pp. 2204–2210, 2017.

[15] W. E. Garrett Jr., M. R. Safran, A. V. Seaber, R. R. Glisson, and B. M. Ribbeck, "Biomechanical comparison of stimulated and nonstimulated skeletal muscle pulled to failure," *The American Journal of Sports Medicine*, vol. 15, no. 5, pp. 448–454, 1989.

[16] A. J. Buckland, J. Vigdorchik, F. J. Schwab et al., "Acetabular Anteversion Changes Due to Spinal Deformity Correction: Bridging the Gap between Hip and Spine Surgeons," *Journal of Bone and Joint Surgery - American Volume*, vol. 97, no. 23, pp. 1913–1920, 2014.

3

Autologous Bone Marrow-Derived Chondrocytes for Patients with Knee Osteoarthritis

Mir Sadat-Ali, [1,2] Abdallah S. AlOmran, [1,2] Sulaiman A. AlMousa, [1,2] Hasan N. AlSayed, [1,2] Khalid W. AlTabash, [1,2] Mohammed Q. Azam, [3] Tarek M. Hegazi, [2,4] and Sadananda Acharya [2,5]

[1]*Department of Orthopaedic Surgery, Imam AbdulRahman Bin Faisal University, Dammam, Saudi Arabia*
[2]*King Fahd Hospital of the University, AlKhobar, Saudi Arabia*
[3]*Orthopaedic Surgery, All India Institute of Medical Sciences, Rishikesh, India*
[4]*Radiology, Imam AbdulRahman Bin Faisal University, Dammam, Saudi Arabia*
[5]*College of Public Health, Imam AbdulRahman Bin Faisal University, Dammam, Saudi Arabia*

Correspondence should be addressed to Mir Sadat-Ali; drsadat@hotmail.com

Academic Editor: Paulo Adriano Schwingel

Background and Objective. The aim of this study was to compare the effect of autologous bone marrow-derived chondrocytes (ABMDCs) with pharmacological management of osteoarthritis of knee (OAK) and assess the benefit of the two in the improvement of pain relief, functional betterment, and quality of life (QOL). *Patients and Methods.* A prospective, randomized study was undertaken in patients with OAK grades II and III of Kellgren–Lawrence grading (KLG) in two groups. Group I had 5 million of intra-articular ABMDC in the affected joint, and Group II continued the nonsteroidal anti-inflammatory drugs (NSAIDs) and physical therapy as needed. Before the treatment, patients were meticulously examined and data were entered for age, sex, Body Mass Index (BMI), Visual Analogue Scale (VAS), Modified Knee Society Score-Short Form (MKSSSF), and QOL. Patients were followed up for 3, 12, and 24 months to assess efficacy, safety, and tolerability. To assess the cartilage regeneration of the damaged cartilage, magnetic resonance imaging (MRI) was used. *Results.* There were a total of 60 patients who were followed up. Three patients in Group II were removed from the analysis as they underwent total knee arthroplasty (TKA). A notably significant improvement was noticed in the ABMDC group on all scores of VAS and MKSSSF with $P < 0.0001$. The control group continued to be dissatisfied with the treatment they were taking. *Conclusions.* This study reveals that a single injection of 5 million of ABMDC was efficient in reducing the symptoms, improving the functional score and betterment of QOL.

1. Introduction

Osteoarthritis of the knee (OAK) is usually due to aging process, and many factors influence the severity of the disease. The prevalence of OAK of the knee is unknown, but recently, it was reported that over 12.5% of the population over 45 years of age suffer from OAK. [1] The incidence of OAK in Saudi Arabian population was found to be up to 3.5% [2, 3], but recent reports indicate that the prevalence of clinical OAK increased many folds to 13% [4] and radiological OA of knee to 53% in males and 60.9% in females [5].

The OAK is traditionally managed using nonsteroidal anti-inflammatory drugs (NSAIDs), physical therapy, and nutritional supplements [6–12]. The response to such treatment is not always absolute and requires steroid and hyaluronic acid injections and arthroscopic joint washout with diverse degrees of pain relief [13, 14].

In the recent past, incidence of OAK has increased, but no new modes of management have been added apart from the symptomatic treatment with NSAIDs and physical therapy. OAK progresses slowly, leading to joint destruction and reduction in quality of life and eventually ending with total knee arthroplasty (TKA). The management of OAK by the way of arthroplasty is expensive and complicated. Complications of TKA include vascular and neural injury, instability, malalignment, stiffness, joint infection, tibiofemoral dislocation, wear and tear of the polyethylene insert, osteolysis, implant loosening, and revisions [15].

Cell-based therapies particularly mesenchymal stromal cells (MSCs) for repair of the damaged cartilage and relief of pain have been tried in experimental animals with excellent results. MSCs for repair of damaged cartilage and for relief was used in sheep model with good outcome [16]. Jo et al. [17] reported that after injecting MSCs into the osteoarthritic knee, follow-up at 3, 6, and 12 months showed improvement in function and total relief of pain of the knee joint without causing adverse events and reduced cartilage defects by regeneration of the cartilage, which was similar to hyaline cartilage histologically. Soler et al. [18] reported the outcome of autologous MSCs in patients with grades II and III of Kellgren–Lawrence grading and found that a single intra-articular injection of the MSCs was safe and gave complete pain relief with improved quality of life with signs of cartilage repair based on the MRI.

There is increasing prevalence of OAK among Saudi Arabian population with the number of total knee arthroplasty procedures on the rise even in young patients, and many patients are left to suffer and the disease progression occurs, when other alternatives are available. Keeping this in mind to find an alternate and safe treatment, we decided to perform this pilot study using ABMDC as a single intra-articular knee injection of 5 million cells and to compare it with the standard treatment in the same cohort population.

2. Methods and Patients

This is a prospective, open-label, single-dose, clinical trial of injection of chondrocytes of 10^5 culture expanded cells. The study was approved by the Institutional Review Board of Imam AbdulRahman Bin Faisal University, Dammam, vide IRB-2018-01-314, dated 19/12/2018, and informed written consent was taken from all the patients before staring the treatment plan. All procedures in this study were conducted in accordance with the guidelines as laid down by the Institutional Review Board of Imam AbdulRahman Bin Faisal University, Dammam. The sample size was based on the ClinicalTrials.gov Identifier NCT03818737 (Multicenter Trial of Stem Cell Therapy for Osteoarthritis (MILES)) [19].

The objective of the study is to assess the benefits of autologous bone marrow-derived chondrocyte injection in patients with OAK and to assess safety, efficacy, and tolerability of this treatment. Efficacy was measured using the Visual Analogue Scale for pain, Short Knee Society score, pain at rest, pain on movement, satisfaction with daily life, and quality of life. The inclusion criteria were patients being between 45 and 70 years of age, diagnosed with OAK for at least 12 months based on American College of Rheumatology (ACR) criteria, and unsatisfied with conservative therapy of NSAIDs and physiotherapy. Patients should be able to communicate with the researchers and answer to the questionnaires, agreeing to participate and signing informed consent voluntarily.

The first 30 patients who agreed to be part of the chondrocyte treatment were part of Group I, and all second patients (30) who were being treated conservatively were Group II patients. The exclusion criteria were past knee intra-articular steroid/hyaluronic acid injection within the last 3 months, any knee surgery within the last 6 months, pregnancy and breast-feeding (women of childbearing age need the pregnancy test), mental disorders, and drug dependency. Patients were divided into two groups.

2.1. Bone Marrow Aspiration. Under general anesthesia, 20 cc of bone marrow was aspirated from the patients' iliac crest following standard procedures. The aspirate was added to a sterile bone marrow transplantation medium (Hanks' Balanced Salt Solution with 10,000 units/mL of penicillin, 10,000 μg/mL of streptomycin, and 25 μg/mL of amphotericin B). The samples were properly labeled and were immediately transported to the stem cell laboratory under ice-cold conditions.

2.2. MSC Separation and Expansion. Bone marrow in the transportation medium was overlaid on approximately 20 ml of sterile Ficoll-Paque Plus (Merck KGaA, Darmstadt, Germany) taken in a conical centrifuge tube (Sarstedt AG & Co, Nümbrecht, Germany) and centrifuged in a swing bucket centrifuge (Sorvall ST8, Thermo Fisher Scientific, Massachusetts, USA) at 2000 rpm for 5 minutes at 4°C. The resultant layer containing mononuclear cells were siphoned out and seeded onto a T75 tissue culture flask (Greiner Bio-One GmbH, Frickenhausen, Germany) at the rate of 5000 cells/cm [2]. Approximately 20 ml of the MSC culture medium (CTS™ StemPro™ MSC SFM, Thermo Fisher, Massachusetts, USA) was added, and the flask was incubated at 37 C, with 5% CO_2 and 95% RH in a CO_2 incubator. Adherent cells were cultured, and the process was continued with change of the medium every second day till cells became confluent. The cells were trypsinised, harvested, and used for chondrocyte differentiation. A portion of the cells was used for cell characterization using MSC specific antibodies in a flow cytometer (Human MSC Phenotyping Kit from Miltenyi Biotec (Auburn, CA, USA)). Positive expression of CD73, CD90, and CD105 and negative for CD45 were confirmed.

2.3. Chondrocyte Differentiation. The MSC cell aggregate was added to micro-mass culture using the MSC culture medium on a 90 mm cell culture dish (Nunc, Denmark). After two hours of adding the MSCs, the medium was washed off and fresh chondrocyte differentiation medium (CTS StemPro MSC medium supplemented with 10^{-7} M dexamethasone, 1 μM ascorbate-2-phosphate, 1% sodium pyruvate, and 10 ng/ml transforming growth factor-beta 1 (TGF-β1), Thermo Fisher, Massachusetts, USA)) was added [20]. The micro-mass culture was allowed to differentiate for 21 days with medium changes for every third day. The cells were harvested at the end of the culture and were characterized for the expression of MMP13 using a flow cytometer.

2.3.1. Intervention. Group I received ABMDC cell suspension which was prepared in 0.5 cc of sterile NSS at the rate of 1 × 10 [6] cells/body weight of the patient. The cell suspension was injected intra-articularly in the affected joint as a single-dose injection. Group I participants did not receive any further treatment including physical therapy.

In Group II, we continued the NSAIDs and physical therapy as needed. Before the treatment, patients were meticulously examined and data were entered for age, sex, Body Mass Index (BMI), Visual Analogue Scale (VAS), Modified Knee Society Score-Short Form (KSSSF), and QOL. Patients were followed up for 3, 12, and 24 months. Figure 1 gives the CONSORT flow chart.

2.3.2. Statistical Analysis. The data was entered in the database and analyzed using SPSS (Statistical Package for the Social Sciences), version 25.0, Chicago, Illinois. A P value of <0.05 was considered statistically significant with a confidence interval (CI) of 95%.

3. Results

A total of 60 patients were included and followed up (Figure 1). Three patients in Group II were removed from the analysis as they underwent total knee arthroplasty. All patients were followed for 3, 12, and 24 months. In 30 patients (treatment group), a single ABMDC of 5 million cells was injected. A control group of 27 patients were treated with NSAIDs, physical therapy, and Durolane, a hyaluronic acid injection. The demographic data of patients in groups I and II were similar before the treatment was instituted. Table 1 shows all the parameters assessed including age, KL grading, VAS, MKSSSF, QOL, daily living, and pain at movement with no statistically significant difference except for pain at rest which was significantly higher in group I at P value < 0.0009. There were no adverse effects in group I, but in group II, 1 patient (3.7%) had local cellulitis which was treated by oral antibiotics.

4. Clinical Efficacy

A robust improvement was observed in the ABMDC group on all scores of pain relief, VAS, QOL, MKSSSF, pain at rest, pain on movement, and assessment of daily life with a P value of <0.0001 for all parameters. The improvement was significant from 3 months onwards and continued for the period of follow-up of 24 months. The MKSSSF score at baseline was the control group that continued to suffer and be dissatisfied with the treatment (Table 2). The MKSSSF score at baseline in Group I was 37.40 ± 6.46 and consistently improved till the last follow-up at 24 months to 82.18 ± 3.79. The change from the baseline to the 1st follow-up at 12 months was statistically significant at $P < 0.0001$, and between 12 months and 24 months, the P value was <0.0003. In Group II, at the start of the study, the Modified Knee Scoring Score Short Form was 39.34 ± 6.83; at 12 months, it was 42.31 ± 5.72, and at 24 months, it was 40.15 ± 5.88. At baseline and 12 months, $P < 0.0892$ and at 24 months, $P < 0.6424$.

5. Radiological Outcomes

Kellgren–Lawrence grading and the assessment of the joint space width were not performed. The initial MRI examinations were studied and showed varying levels of cartilage defect, and a follow-up MRI showed healed cartilage defect. The regenerated cartilage appeared leveled and smoother (Figure 2).

6. Discussion

Our preliminary study showed that ABMDC intra-articular injection in KL II and III grade knees showed an excellent improvement compared to the patients in the standard treatment protocol. All of the three parameters tested in the ABMDC group, VAS, QOL, and MKSSSF, showed significant improvements compared to the control group over 24 months. We did not observe any apparent early or late adverse events due to the ABMDC intra-articular injection. Radiological improvement was noticed on evaluation by a follow-up MRI with evidence of the regenerated articular cartilage and disappearance of the depression of the cartilage as seen in the pretreatment MRI.

The initial report of Orozco and his colleagues [21] on clinical efficacy and safety of autologous human bone marrow-derived stem cells in OAK showed that there were a significant decrease in the knee pain and improved changes on the MRI scans. Vega et al. [22] and Gupta et al. [23] used allogenic bone marrow-derived stem cells and compared those with hyaluronic acid injections and reported functional improvement and no adverse events in the patients receiving stem cell injections. A recent systematic review and meta-analysis confirmed positive conclusions about clinical efficacy of MSCs to treat pain and decreased function in knee OA [24]. Park et al. [25] used a combination of composite of allogeneic umbilical cord blood-derived mesenchymal stem cells and hyaluronate hydrogel for cartilage regeneration in OA patients and reported a 7-year follow-up. They reported that the VAS and International Knee Documentation Committee scores improved at 6 months and that this improvement remained at 7 years of follow-up. The reported mechanism by which bone marrow stromal cells reduce the pain and regenerate the cartilage is by differentiating into chondrocytes or by conversion of the remaining prochondrocytes into mature chondrocytes [23]. The main function of the chondrocytes is to produce extracellular matrix and collagen I and II in the process of repairing the damaged cartilage. There is enough evidence that aging has a detrimental effect on stem cells in quality and quantity and hence self-healing is low [26].

In our study, we bypassed the route of mesenchymal stem cells and directly used 10^6 million autologous chondrocytes and found that the clinical effect was observed within weeks and secondly there was improvement in all the tested parameters, which were found to be better than the conservative methods of treatment. We did not encounter any risks involved in using the autologous chondrocytes, and we felt patients were more serene in using their own cells rather than allogeneic material. Moreover, in an earlier

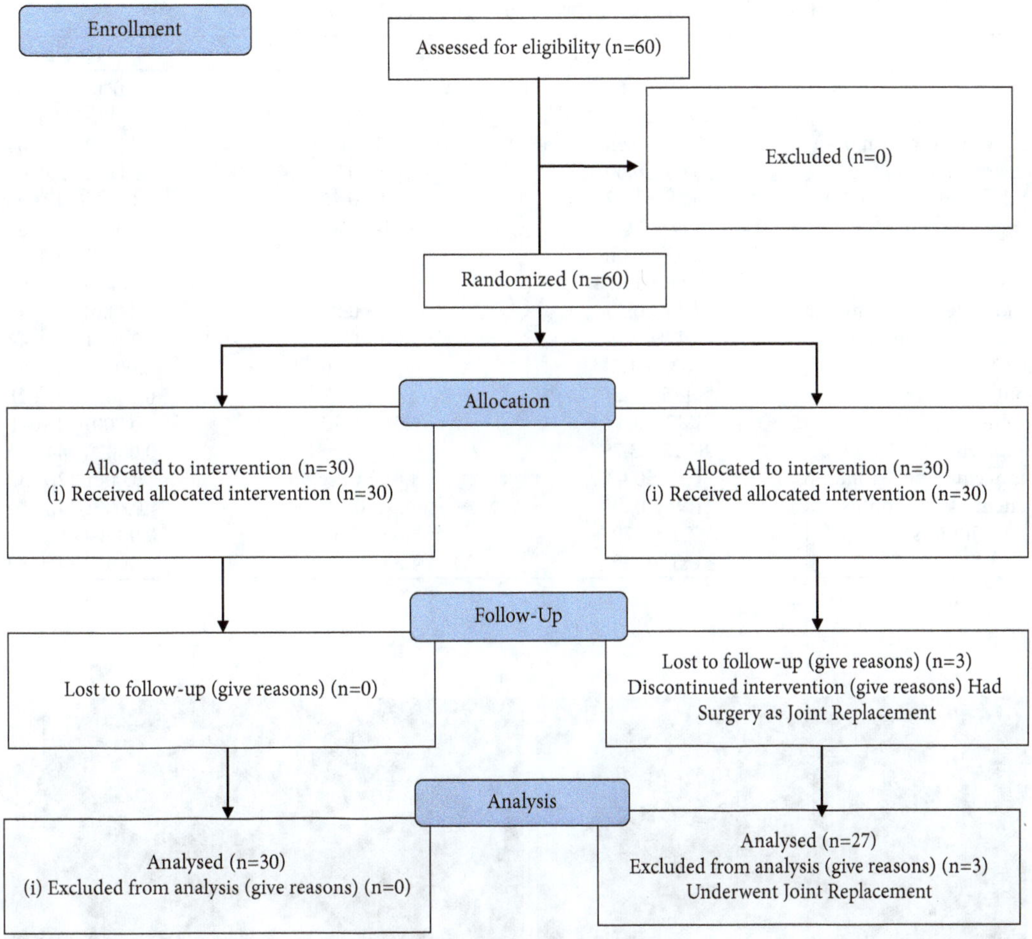

FIGURE 1: CONSORT flow diagram.

TABLE 1: Demographic data of baseline characteristics.

	ABMDC-group I	Conservative therapy-group II	*P* value
Age (years)	56.18 ± 6.56	56.75 ± 5.77	0.7302
Males	9	14	0.5
Females	24	16	0.2
KL grades II and III	18	16	0.2
Visual Analogue Scale*	6.65 ± 0.09	6.96 ± 1.1	0.1294
Modified Knee Scoring Score-Short Form**	37.40 ± 6.46	39.34 ± 6.83	0.2753
Pain at rest*	3.46 ± 0.50	3.85 ± 0.6	0.009
Pain on movement*	7.0 ± 0.87	7.15 ± 0.88	0.6682
Daily living*	4.49 ± 0.75	4.34 ± 0.97	0.5141
Quality of life (QOL)*	4.87 ± 1.09	5.25 ± 1.13	0.0716

*Score out of 10 and **score out of 100.

study, we used ABMDC for healing of the torn meniscus with convincing results [27].

A year ago, osteoarthritis was reported to be the fourth leading cause of chronic disability in the world [28] and is still being treated by conservative methods using nonsteroidal anti-inflammatory drugs (NSAIDs) and intra-articular injections. All the treatments have their limitations and long-term complications [29–31]. Even though our results and other meticulous analysis show that the overall results of the MSCs/chondrocyte treatment of OAK in both efficacy and safety are steps ahead and far superior to the conservative management, still this type of treatment is seen with skepticism and cynicism even among the treating physicians.

The limitations of our study are small size and absence of pretreatment and posttreatment arthroscopy to assess the cartilage repair, with the strength of the study being a matched group with three different parameters compared. In conclusion, our randomized control study persuades us to

Table 2: Comparison between groups at 3, 12, and 24 months.

Parameters	ABMDC-group I	Conservative therapy-group II	P value (95% CI)
VAS at 3 months	3.09 ± 0.64	6.75 ± 0.84	0.0001 (3.2659 to 4.0541)
MKSSSF at 3 months	57.48 ± 8.18	38.87 ± 6.33	0.0001 (−22.5247 to −14.6953)
Pain without movement at 3 months	3.37 ± 0.49	4.34 ± 0.6	0.0001 (0.6804 to 1.2596)
Pain on movement at 3 months	3.65 ± 0.60	7.09 ± 0.73	0.0001 (3.0867 to 3.7933)
Daily living at 3 months	5.28 ± 1.02	4.59 ± 0.75	0.0056 (−1.1698 to −0.2102)
QOL at 3 months	7.9 ± 0.64	4.81 ± 0.89	0.0001 (−3.4985 to −2.6815)
VAS at 12 months	2.59 ± 0.06	6.71 ± 0.72	0.0001 (3.8558 to 4.3842)
MKSSSF at 12 months	72.68 ± 13.15	42.31 ± 5.72	0.0001 (−35.860 to −24.880)
Pain without movement at 12 months	2.43 ± 0.50	4.5 ± 0.8	0.0001 (1.7196 to 2.4204)
Pain on movement at 12 months	2.47 ± 0.55	7.06 ± 0.71	0.0001 (4.2547 to 4.9253)
Daily living at 12 months	5.625 ± 1.21	4.75 ± 0.76	0.0021 (−1.4185 to −0.3315)
QOL at 12 months	8.175 ± 0.59	4.81 ± 0.89	0.0001 (−3.7621 to −2.9679)
VAS at 24 months	1.87 ± 0.42	6.34 ± 0.70	0.0001 (4.1671 to 4.7729)
MKSSSF at 24 months	82.18 ± 3.79	40.15 ± 5.88	0.0001 (−44.630 to −39.430)
Pain without movement at 24 months	1.75 ± 0.43	4.81 ± 0.64	0.0001 (2.7732 to 3.3468)
Pain on movement at 24 months	1.91 ± 0.39	6.9 ± 0.58	0.0001 (4.7300 to 5.2500)
Daily living at 24 months	7.4 ± 0.79	5.03 ± 0.82	0.0001 (−2.7976 to −1.9424)
QOL at 24 months	8.5 ± 0.50	4.34 ± 0.86	0.0001 (−4.5289 to −3.7911)

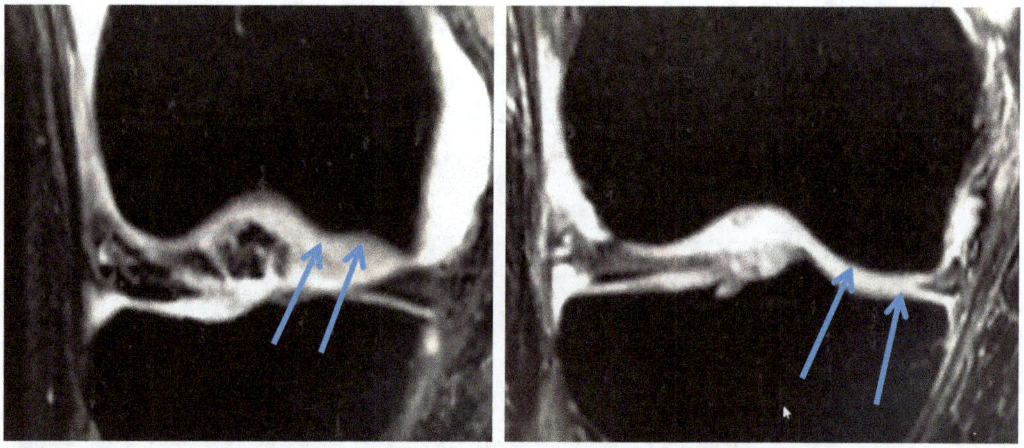

(a)

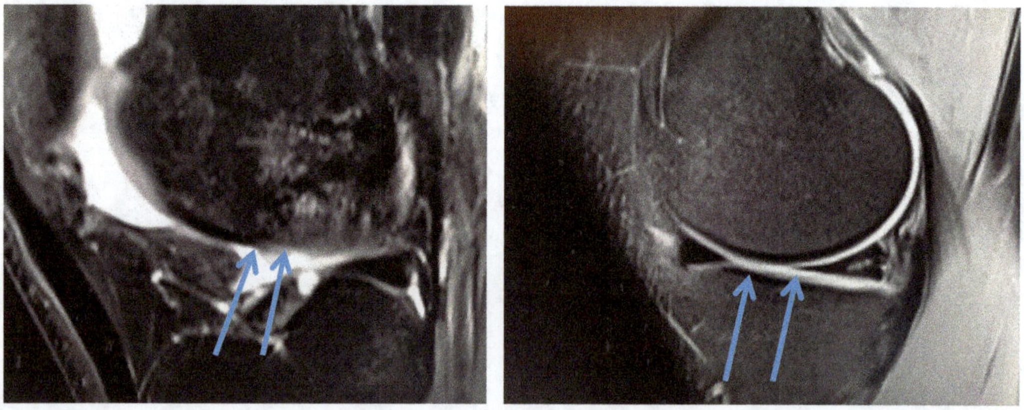

(b)

Figure 2: (a) AP view of the MRI of the knee joint showing depression in the femoral condyle (blue arrows) due to the damaged cartilage which completely recovered post injection of ABMDC. (b) Lateral view of the MRI of knee joint with erosion of the cartilage of the femoral condyle and post-injection regeneration of the damaged cartilage (blue arrows).

state that ABMDC is a better mode and option of treatment of OAK of KL grades II and III and it should be offered to the patients if the facilities exist to give such treatment.

7. Conclusions

Our study confirmed that a single injection of 5 million ABMDCs was efficient in reducing the symptoms and improving the functional score and betterment of QOL. We believe that such studies should be carried out nationwide to limit the progression of the OAK and improve the QOL of patients as they age.

Consent

Informed written consent was obtained from all patients before aspiration of the bone marrow and injection of the ABMDC in the affected knee joint. Patients gave consent for their anonymized information to be published and presented.

References

[1] K. Jordan and P. Croft, "The prevalence and history of knee osteoarthritis in general practice: a case–control study," *Family Practice*, vol. 22, no. 1, pp. 103–108, 2005.

[2] M. Sadat-Ali, Y. Al-Gindan, M. Al-Mousa, A. Al-Rubaish, and E. Al-Omari, "Osteoarthritis of the knee among Saudi Arabian security forces personnel," *Military Medicine*, vol. 161, no. 2, pp. 105–107, 1996.

[3] A. Ahlberg, B. Linder, and T. A. Binhemd, "Osteoarthritis of the hip and knee in Saudi Arabia," *International Orthopaedics*, vol. 14, no. 1, pp. 29-30, 1990.

[4] A. S. Al-Arfaj, S. R. Alballa, S. S. Al-Saleh et al., "Knee osteoarthritis in Al-Qaseem, Saudi Arabia," *Saudi Medical Journal*, vol. 24, no. 3, pp. 291–3, 2003.

[5] A. Al-Arfaj and A. A. Al-Boukai, "Prevalence of radiographic knee osteoarthritis in Saudi Arabia," *Clinical Rheumatology*, vol. 21, no. 2, pp. 142–145, 2002.

[6] M. S. M. Persson, J. Stocks, G. Varadi et al., "Predicting response to topical non-steroidal anti-inflammatory drugs in osteoarthritis: an individual patient data meta-analysis of randomized controlled trials," *Rheumatology*, vol. 59, no. 9, pp. 2207–2216, 2020.

[7] D. G. Wolff, C. Christophersen, S. M. Brown, and M. K. Mulcahey, "Topical nonsteroidal anti-inflammatory drugs in the treatment of knee osteoarthritis: a systematic review and meta-analysis," *The Physician and Sportsmedicine*, vol. 4, pp. 1–11, 2021.

[8] C. Zeng, M. Doherty, M. S. M. Persson et al., "Comparative efficacy and safety of acetaminophen, topical and oral non-steroidal anti-inflammatory drugs for knee osteoarthritis: evidence from a network meta-analysis of randomized controlled trials and real-world data," *Osteoarthritis and Cartilage*, vol. 29, no. 9, pp. 1242–1251, 2021.

[9] N. Kakatum, P. Pinsornsak, P. Kanokkangsadal, B. Ooraikul, and A. Itharat, "Efficacy and safety of sahastara remedy extract capsule in primary knee osteoarthritis: a randomized double-blinded active-controlled trial," *Evidence-based Complementary and Alternative Medicine*, vol. 2021, Article ID 6635148, 2021.

[10] A. Askari, S. A. Ravansalar, M. M. Naghizadeh et al., "The efficacy of topical sesame oil in patients with knee osteoarthritis: a randomized double-blinded active-controlled non-inferiority clinical trial," *Complementary Therapies in Medicine*, vol. 47, Article ID 102183, 2019.

[11] M. Anvari, H. Dortaj, B. Hashemibeni, and M. Pourentezari, "Application of some herbal medicine used for the treatment of osteoarthritis and chondrogenesis," *Iranian Traditional Medicine*, vol. 5, no. 3, pp. 126–149, 2020.

[12] M. Sadat-Ali, I. Al-Habdan, and A. Y. El-Hassan, "? is there an alternative to NSAIDs and cox-2 inhibitors in the management of osteoarthritis of knee," *Ostetoporosis International*, vol. 17, no. 1, p. 192, 2006.

[13] X. Chevalier, "Intra-articular treatments for osteoarthritis: new perspectives," *Current Drug Targets*, vol. 11, no. 5, pp. 546–560, 2010.

[14] A. Kirkley, T. Birmingham, R. Litchfield et al., "Arthroscopic surgery did not provide additional benefit to physical and benefit to physical and medical therapy for osteoarthritis of the knee," *Journal of Bone and Joint Surgery American Volume*, vol. 91, no. 5, p. 1281, 2009.

[15] W. L. Healy, C. J. Della Valle, R. Iorio et al., "Complications of total knee arthroplasty standardized list and definitions of the knee society," *Clinical Orthopaedics and Related Research*, vol. 471, no. 1, pp. 215–220, 2013.

[16] M. Caminal, C. Fonseca, D. Peris et al., "Use of a chronic model of articular cartilage and meniscal injury for the assessment of long-term effects after autologous mesenchymal stromal cell treatment in sheep," *New Biotech*, vol. 31, no. 5, pp. 492–498, 2014.

[17] C. H. Jo, Y. G. Lee, W. H. Shin et al., "Intra-articular injection of mesenchymal stem cells for the treatment of osteoarthritis of the knee: a proof-of-concept clinical trial," *Stem Cells*, vol. 32, no. 5, pp. 1254–1266, 2014.

[18] R. Soler, L. Orozco, A. Munar et al., "Final results of a phase I-II trial using ex vivo expanded autologous mesenchymal stromal cells for the treatment of osteoarthritis of the knee confirming safety and suggesting cartilage regeneration," *The Knee*, vol. 23, no. 4, pp. 647–654, 2016.

[19] "Multicenter trial of stem cell therapy for osteoarthritis (MILES)," 2021, https://www.clinicaltrials.gov.

[20] L. A. Solchaga, K. J. Penick, and J. F. Welter, "Chondrogenic differentiation of bone marrow-derived mesenchymal stem cells: tips and tricks," *Mesenchymal Stem Cell Assays and Applications*, vol. 698, pp. 253–278, 2011.

[21] L. Orozco, A. Munar, R. Soler et al., "Treatment of knee osteoarthritis with autologous mesenchymal stem cells: a pilot study," *Transplantation*, vol. 95, no. 12, pp. 1535–1541, 2013.

[22] A. Vega, M. A. Martín-Ferrero, F. Del Canto et al., "Treatment of knee osteoarthritis with allogeneic bone marrow mesenchymal stem cells: a random-ized controlled trial," *Transplantation*, vol. 99, no. 8, pp. 1681–1690, 2015.

[23] P. K. Gupta, A. Chullikana, M. Rengasamy et al., "Efficacy and safety of adult human bone marrow-derived, cultured, pooled, allogeneic mesenchymal stromal cells (Stempeucel®): preclinical and clinical trial in osteoarthritis of the knee joint," *Arthritis Research & Therapy*, vol. 18, no. 1, p. 301, 2016.

[24] P. Xia, X. Wang, Q. Lin, and X. Li, "Efficacy of mesenchymal stem cells injection for the management of knee osteoarthritis:

a systematic review and meta-analysis," *International Orthopaedics*, vol. 39, no. 12, pp. 2363–2372, 2015.

[25] Y.-B. Park, C.-W. Ha, C.-H. Lee, Y. C. Yoon, and Y.-G. Park, "Cartilage regeneration in osteoarthritic patients by a composite of allogeneic umbilical cord blood-derived mesenchymal stem cells and hyaluronate hydrogel: results from a clinical trial for safety and proof-of-concept with 7 Years of extended follow-up," *Stem Cells Translational Medicine*, vol. 6, no. 2, pp. 613–621, 2017.

[26] A. S. I. Ahmed, M. H. Sheng, S. Wasnik, D. J. Baylink, and K.-H. W. Lau, "Effect of aging on stem cells," *World Journal of Experimental Medicine*, vol. 7, no. 1, pp. 1–10, 2017.

[27] H. N AlSayed, M. Sadat-Ali, F. Z Uddin, F. M Alani, and S. Acharya, "Outcome of bone marrow derived chondrocyte injection for meniscal injuries: a preliminary study," *Trends in Medicine*, vol. 18, no. 5, pp. 1–4, 2018.

[28] D. J. Hunter and S. Bierma-Zeinstra, "Osteoarthritis," *The Lancet*, vol. 393, no. 10182, pp. 1745–1759, 2019.

[29] B. Caldwell, S. Aldington, M. Weatherall, P. Shirtcliffe, and R. Beasley, "Risk of cardiovascular events and celecoxib: a systematic review and meta-analysis," *Journal of the Royal Society of Medicine*, vol. 99, no. 3, pp. 132–140, 2006.

[30] C. H. Evans, V. B. Kraus, and L. A. Setton, "Progress in intra-articular therapy," *Nature Reviews Rheumatology*, vol. 10, no. 1, pp. 11–22, 2014.

[31] K. A. Campbell, B. J. Erickson, B. M. Saltzman et al., "Is local viscosupplementation injection clinically superior to other therapies in the treatment of osteoarthritis of the knee: a systematic re- view of overlapping meta-analyses," *Arthroscopy: The Journal of Arthroscopic & Related Surgery*, vol. 31, no. 10, pp. 2036–2045, 2015.

4

Comparison of Accuracy in Expert Clinical Examination versus Magnetic Resonance Imaging and Arthroscopic Exam in Diagnosis of Meniscal Tear

Seyed Ali Hashemi,[1] Mohammad Reza Ranjbar,[1] Mohammad Tahami,[1] Reza Shahriarirad,[2,3] and Amirhossein Erfani[2,3]

[1]*Research Center for Bone and Joint Diseases, Department of Orthopedic Surgery, Chamran Hospital, Shiraz University of Medical Sciences, Shiraz, Iran*
[2]*Student Research Committee, Shiraz University of Medical Sciences, Shiraz, Iran*
[3]*Thoracic and Vascular Surgery Research Center, Shiraz University of Medical Sciences, Shiraz, Iran*

Correspondence should be addressed to Reza Shahriarirad; r.shahriari1995@gmail.com

Academic Editor: Benjamin Blondel

Background. Many clinical tests and diagnostic studies have been developed to increase the clinician's ability to accurately diagnose disorders of the knee. Torn menisci or ligamentous structures within the knee cause significant pain and disability and thus require expeditious management. This study was conducted to evaluate the accuracy of clinical examination in comparison with MRI examination and with the help of arthroscopic examination as the gold standard in the diagnosis of meniscal tears. *Method.* All of the arthroscopic surgery candidates, presenting symptoms of meniscal or cruciate ligament lesions, referring to Namazi and Chamran hospitals, Shiraz, Iran, were included in this study. Clinical examination (including McMurray test, Apley test, and 20 Thessaly test) was performed before the arthroscopy, and the results were recorded in special forms. Magnetic resonance imaging (MRI) results were also added. Then, arthroscopy was performed, declaring the definite diagnosis, and the results were compared to the results obtained from both tests and MRI. Statistical analysis was performed using SPSS software. *Results.* 86 patients with a mean age of 27 years old, including 63 (73%) male and 23 (27%) female, were studied. 57 (66%), 19 (22%), and 10 (12%) injuries were caused by sports, twisting, or trauma, respectively. Arthroscopic results showed 32 meniscal tears, of which 28 (87%) and 4 (13%) were in medial and lateral menisci, respectively, including 10 bucket handle, 17 longitudinal, and 5 of other types (transverse, oblique, radial) of injuries. Comparing MRI results to arthroscopic results, we had 2 false-positive and 2 false-negative cases. 62 cases of McMurray test results were accurate; 15 and 9 cases were reported false positive and false negative, respectively. 60 cases of Apley test results were accurate; 16 and 10 cases were reported false positive and false negative, respectively. 78 cases of Thessaly test results were accurate; 5 and 3 cases were reported false positive and false negative, respectively. Comparing Thessaly test results to McMurray and Apley showed statistical significance ($P < 0.05$). Comparing Thessaly test results to MRI showed no statistical significance ($P = 0.151$), while comparing McMurray and Apley test results to MRI showed statistical significance ($P < 0.01$). *Conclusion.* Clinical examination, performed by an experienced examiner, can have equal or even more diagnostic accuracy compared to MRI to evaluate meniscal lesions. In this study, the Thessaly test has been approved as a reliable clinical test in the diagnosis of meniscal tears.

1. Introduction

Diagnosis of acute knee injuries has long been one of the issues discussed in orthopaedic sources. Many clinical trials and diagnostic studies have been conducted to increase the ability of physicians to correctly diagnose knee problems [1–3]. Since ruptured meniscus or ligamentous structures in the knee cause significant pain and disability, these lesions require prompt and accurate treatment and management. Due to the devastating consequences of meniscus injuries in patients, especially for those injured during exercise, timely and accurate diagnosis of these injuries is essential [4].

The necessity of surgery after meniscus injury is significantly determined by initial physical examination along with other diagnostic tests. A comprehensive examination should include a full description of the injury, palpation of the injury site, and a selection of specific tests. Athletes with meniscus tears usually describe a pop-like sound when redirecting in a sprint, such as twisting the heel of the foot with or without colliding with another player [5].

Joint line tenderness and effusion are also manifestations of meniscal injury. Palpation of the knee along the axis may have indefinite results in predicting meniscus ruptures with an acute ACL injury, with a specificity of 34.5% and sensitivity of 44.9% based on internal axis palpation and a specificity of 49.1% and sensitivity of 57.6% for external axis palpation. In cases where the ACL is unaffected, tenderness along the joint line more accurately (77%) identifies meniscal ruptures [5].

The main tests required to treat patients with symptoms so far include palpation of the joint border, McMurray test, Apley grind test, and Thessaly test [6, 7].

Arthroscopy is the gold standard of diagnosis in traumatic injuries to the knee joint. Arthroscopy, although highly accurate, is an invasive and expensive intervention that requires hospitalization and general or regional anesthesia, but it can also impose complications on an open surgery, such as infections, neurological and vascular injuries, and injury to the intra-articular elements of the knee [8, 9]. With 1,200 knee arthroscopies a year and rising, a noninvasive diagnostic tool that requires no intra-articular approach could minimize the potential risks of arthroscopy and reduce the numbers of needed arthroscopies [10]. Although the diagnostic significance of a physical examination by an experienced clinician has been evaluated in various studies [10, 11], further studies are justified for whether or not it could be favored over other diagnostic methods. Therefore, this study was conducted to evaluate the accuracy of clinical examination in comparison with MRI examination and with the arthroscopic examination as the gold standard in the diagnosis of meniscal tears.

2. Materials and Methods

This cross-sectional descriptive study was performed on all patients who referred to Shahid Chamran and Namazi hospitals of Shiraz with any signs of trauma to the meniscus or cruciate ligament, whether due to accidents or athletic trauma, and who were candidates for arthroscopic surgery. The study protocol was approved by the Ethics Committee of the Shiraz University of Medical Sciences.

Participants were selected by available sampling from patients who referred to Shahid Chamran and Namazi hospitals. Patients with trauma due to accidents or athletic trauma who were candidates for meniscus or cruciate ligament arthroscopic surgery were enrolled in our study. Patients who had positive examination in favor of meniscus injury and who had a clinical complaint were treated with arthroscopy, regardless of the MRI result. Also, patients who had imaging results in favor of meniscus injury with normal physical examination who underwent arthroscopy were included in the study. Eventually, 86 patients were enrolled in our study. All cases that had a history of knee surgery, knee arthroscopy, repair of ligaments or meniscus, or history of meniscectomy, either in total or partial, were excluded from the study.

Examinations were performed with competence by an experienced orthopaedic surgeon, with no knowledge of the patients' MRI results, before performing arthroscopy. All performed clinical examinations and the patient characteristics were entered in prepared specific forms for this purpose. Eventually, MRI results were added. The tests used in this study included the McMurray test, the Apley test, and the 20-degree Thessaly test. Then, the MRI images of each patient were examined by a qualified diagnostic radiologist expert and their results were reported. Finally, arthroscopy was performed by an experienced and qualified orthopaedic surgeon and with the help of his assistants; results were recorded as a definitive diagnosis; comparing the results with the results obtained from the tests and MRI, true positives and negatives and false positives and false negatives were obtained.

Statistical analysis was performed using SPSS (version 18; SPSS Inc., Chicago, IL, USA) and McNemar and chi-square (X^2) tests. The findings of this study were evaluated using descriptive statistics and sensitivity, specificity, accuracy, positive predictive value (PPV), and negative predictive value (NPV). The chi-square and McNemar tests, each based on their use, were used to compare the findings of the tests and MRI. Finally, the results of the comparison with P value less than 0.05 were considered statistically significant.

3. Results

In this study, 86 patients were enrolled with a mean age of 27 years (range: 15 to 45 years). Table 1 demonstrates the frequency and location, along with the types of injury findings by arthroscopy in our study.

Arthroscopic results revealed 32 cases of meniscus rupture, of which 28 (87%) were medial meniscus injuries and 4 (13%) were lateral meniscus injuries. Of these, 23 (72%) were male and 9 (28%) were female, with 13 (41%) cases of left knee injuries and 19 (59%) cases of right knee injury. Arthroscopy also showed a wide range of injuries including 10 bucket handle injuries, 17 longitudinal injuries, and 5 other types including transverse, oblique, and radiated or radial injuries.

Concerning the MRI imaging protocols and comparing them with the results of arthroscopy, the accurate results included 82 cases of which 30 (34.88%) were positive and 52 (60.48%) were negative. Among the 4 reported error cases, we had 2 false positives (2.32%) and 2 false negatives (2.32%). Of the two false positives, one had a longitudinal rupture and the other radial rupture; among the two false positives, one was a longitudinal rupture and the other was bucket handle.

TABLE 1: Frequency and location, along with the types of injury findings by arthroscopy in patients with meniscus injury.

	Frequency	Percent
Age		
15 to 25 years	22	25.58
25 to 35 years	45	52.32
35 to 45 years	19	22.10
Gender		
Male	63	73
Female	23	27
Cause of injury		
Exercise	57	66
Trauma/torsion	19	22
Accidental injuries	10	12
Location		
Right knee	53	61.6
Left knee	33	38.4
Arthroscopy injury		
Medial meniscus injury	28	87
Lateral meniscus injury	4	13
Bucket handle tear	10	31.25
Longitudinal tear	17	53.12
Transverse/oblique/radial tear	5	15.63

Using descriptive statistics, the sensitivity, specificity, and diagnostic accuracy of MRI were calculated to be 93.7 (79.2–99.1), 96.3 (2–99.4), and 95.35%, respectively.

Among the 86 cases examined, the results were as follows.

62 of all McMurray test cases were accurate. Of the 24 errors, 15 were false positive, of which 3 were in the lateral meniscus and 12 in the medial meniscus, and 9 cases, including 1 in the lateral meniscus and 8 in the medial meniscus, were reported false negative.

Sixty out of all Apley test cases were accurate. Of the 26 errors, 16 were false positive, 2 of which were in the lateral meniscus and 14 in the medial meniscus, and 10, including 1 in the lateral meniscus and 9 in the medial meniscus, were reported false negative.

78 of all Thessaly test cases were correct. Of the 8 errors, 5 were false positive, 1 in the lateral meniscus and 4 in the medial meniscus. However, among the false positives, one was discoid meniscus and another involving articular cartilage injury. Also, 3 cases, including 0 in the lateral meniscus and 3 in the medial meniscus, were reported false negative. Table 2 demonstrates the frequency of rupture types in false-negative and false-positive examinations.

Using descriptive statistics methods for McMurray, Apley, and Thessaly tests, sensitivity, specificity, accuracy, positive predictive value (PPV), and negative predictive value (NPV) were reported, as shown in Table 3.

4. Discussion

This study showed that the diagnostic power of experts' physical examination and MRI was high in meniscus injuries, although there were some differences. For example, the diagnostic power of MRI was higher than that of the tests performed on physical examination (McMurray, Apley, and Thessaly tests), as the results also showed greater sensitivity, specificity, and diagnostic accuracy of MRI than these tests, and among these tests, the diagnostic power of the Thessaly test was higher than that of the other two tests, as presented by higher sensitivity, specificity, accuracy, and positive and negative predictive values which were reasons to support this claim.

The results of our study in this area are in contrast to the results of a study by Navali et al. [12], which also emphasizes the high diagnostic power of experts' physical examination and MRI in meniscus injuries, but point to the importance of physical examination over MRI in their study, which is emphasized in the results of their study and also supported by other studies [7, 13–16].

Contrary to these studies, a study by Nikolaou et al. [17] acknowledges less diagnostic power of physical examination than MRI, which is consistent with the results of the present study. However, studies have shown that if a physical examination is performed by well-skilled and qualified personnel, it can produce results with accuracy similar to MRI, which can then be used as an appropriate diagnostic tool [12].

In general, the results of physical examinations for the diagnosis of lateral meniscus lesions were superior to those of medial meniscus. However, Navali's study points to the superiority of physical examination in the diagnosis of medial meniscus injuries [12].

In a meta-analysis by Wang et al., the international specificity and sensitivity of MRI of meniscal tears were 95.0% (95% confidence interval (CI): 91.0–97.0%) and 80.0% (95% CI: 66.0–89.0%) in lateral meniscal tears and 90.0% (95% CI: 85.0–95.0%) and 92.0% (95% CI: 88.0–95.0%), respectively [18].

In a study by Yan et al. [19], as in our study, MRI was introduced as a sensitive method for diagnosis of meniscus rupture. Although in a study by Ben-Galim et al. [20], false positives reported in MRI diagnosis were reported 65% for medial meniscal rupture and 43% for lateral meniscal rupture but has been recommended alongside physical examination due to high diagnostic accuracy and high negative predictive value. However, in our study, false-positive MRI cases accounted for only 2.32% of the cases, which confirms this method due to its high diagnostic accuracy (95.35%).

The surgeon can decide, solely relying on the clinical examination, whether further examination via MRI is necessary or whether the patient can be admitted for surgery. Lack of practice and experience in the examiners leads to variable accuracy in this decision. Bohnsack et al. [21] established that an experienced examiner can diagnose effectively by only clinical examination, in which in their study a clinical examination executed by an experienced surgeon was 80% precise for diagnosing lateral meniscal tears and 93% accurate for detecting medial meniscal tears while for the least experienced examiner in their study, which was a fourth-year resident, the clinical examination was 80% accurate for diagnosing lateral meniscal tears and 73% accurate for identifying medial meniscal tears. This linked to an MRI accuracy of 83% for both lateral and

Table 2: Frequency of rupture types in false-negative and false-positive examinations.

	False negative			False positive	
	Type of injury				
	Bucket handle	Longitudinal	Transverse/oblique/radial	Medial meniscus	Lateral meniscus
Thessaly	1	1	1	4	1
McMurray	2	5	2	12	3
Apley	2	6	2	14	2

Table 3: Sensitivity, specificity, accuracy, positive predictive value, and negative predictive value in Thessaly, McMurray, and Apley tests.

Type of test	Accuracy (%)	Negative predictive value (%)	Positive predictive value (%)	Specificity (%)	Sensitivity (%)
Thessaly	90.69	94.2	85.3	90.7 (79.7–96.9)	90.6 (75.0–97.9)
McMurray	72.09	81.3	60.5	72.2 (58.5–83.5)	71.9 (53.3–86.2)
Apley	69.77	79.2	57.9	70.4 (59.4–82)	68.7 (50–83.9)

The results of the comparison of the Thessaly test with each of the McMurray and Apley tests were statistically significant ($P < 0.001$); also, the McMurray and Apley tests were compared with each other with no significant difference ($P = 0.267$). Findings from each of the Thessaly, McMurray, and Apley tests were also compared with the MRI results, which unlike the McMurray and Apley tests, were not statistically significant for the Thessaly test ($P = 0.151$).

medial meniscal tears. Therefore, their results showed that a clinical examination performed by an experienced surgeon is more valuable than an MRI scan in the diagnosis of meniscal injuries [7].

In a study by Karachalios et al. [22], they reported a 20-degree Thessaly test with diagnostic accuracy of 94% in the diagnosis of medial meniscal rupture and 96% accuracy in the diagnosis of lateral meniscal rupture as well as small false positive and negative values, introducing the test as the first-line in clinical screening for meniscal rupture and has been recommended as a suitable alternative to costly MRI.

The results of comparing the Thessaly test with each of the McMurray and Apley tests were also statistically significant ($P < 0.001$), indicating the superiority of the Thessaly test over others. As also shown in our study, the rest of the indices (sensitivity of 90.6%, specificity of 90.7%, accuracy of 90.69%, and positive and negative predictive values 85.3 and 94.2) were also higher in this test compared to the two other tests. In a study by Harrison et al. [23] on 116 patients (with 66 Thessaly positive test cases), they reported a 90.3% sensitivity, 97.7% specificity, and 88.8% diagnostic accuracy for the Thessaly test and has been introduced as a valid test in the detection of meniscal rupture, which can replace older tests. As can be seen, the results of this study are consistent with our study. Also, the McMurray and Apley tests were compared in our study, with no statistically significant difference ($P = 0.267$). It should be noted that the error rates of these two tests were almost similar, nevertheless, considerably higher than the Thessaly test. The Karachalios study also highlights false positives in tests such as McMurray [22].

5. Conclusion

Many clinical trials and diagnostic studies have been conducted to increase the ability of physicians to correctly diagnose meniscus injuries. One noninvasive alternative to arthroscopy to diagnose meniscus injuries is MRI, which is used today to diagnose meniscus injuries before performing arthroscopic and surgical examinations. The present study showed that MRI with high sensitivity and specificity and significant diagnostic power could be useful in the diagnosis of meniscal ruptures and knee ligaments.

Performing a rigorous physical examination by an experienced examiner has the diagnostic power equal to or better than MRI in the determination of meniscal lesions. In this review, it was found that the Thessaly test can also be used as an appropriate physical examination to detect meniscal rupture in comparison with other tests.

Consent

The patients' records were anonymized and deidentified prior to analysis. Confidentiality of the details of the subjects was assured.

Disclosure

The study was the subject of the MD dissertation of Mohammad Reza Ranjbar.

Authors' Contributions

SH designed the study. MR collected the data and carried out the statistical analysis. RS and AE drafted the manuscript. SH revised and proofread the manuscript. All authors read and approved the final version of the manuscript.

Acknowledgments

This work was financially supported by the Office of the Vice Chancellor for Research of the Shiraz University of Medical Sciences. The technical assistant of staff in Chamran and Namazi hospitals is acknowledged.

References

[1] R. Crawford, G. Walley, S. Bridgman, and N. Maffulli, "Magnetic resonance imaging versus arthroscopy in the diagnosis of knee pathology, concentrating on meniscal lesions and ACL tears: a systematic review," *British Medical Bulletin*, vol. 84, no. 1, pp. 5–23, 2007.

[2] D. Shakoor, R. Kijowski, A. Guermazi et al., "Diagnosis of knee meniscal injuries by using three-dimensional MRI: a systematic review and meta-analysis of diagnostic performance," *Radiology*, vol. 290, no. 2, pp. 435–445, 2019.

[3] R. Sah, L. Bin, V. K. Sah, and K. S. Dhami, "Approach to meniscal tear by clinical examination and its management: a review," *Yangtze Medicine*, vol. 03, no. 3, pp. 195–211, 2019.

[4] M. D. Chivers and S. D. Howitt, "Anatomy and physical examination of the knee menisci: a narrative review of the orthopedic literature," *The Journal of the Canadian Chiropractic Association*, vol. 53, no. 53, pp. 319–33, 2009.

[5] T. Brindle, J. Nyland, and D. L. Johnson, "The meniscus: review of basic principles with application to surgery and rehabilitation," *Journal of Athletic Training*, vol. 36, no. 36, pp. 160–9, 2001.

[6] E. A. Makris, P. Hadidi, and K. A. Athanasiou, "The knee meniscus: structure-function, pathophysiology, current repair techniques, and prospects for regeneration," *Biomaterials*, vol. 32, no. 30, pp. 7411–7431, 2011.

[7] E. Ercin, I. Kaya, I. Sungur, E. Demirbas, A. A. Ugras, and E. M. Cetinus, "History, clinical findings, magnetic resonance imaging, and arthroscopic correlation in meniscal lesions," *Knee Surgery, Sports Traumatology, Arthroscopy*, vol. 20, no. 5, pp. 851–856, 2012.

[8] B. Friemert, Y. Oberländer, W. Schwarz et al., "Diagnosis of chondral lesions of the knee joint: can MRI replace arthroscopy?" *Knee Surgery, Sports Traumatology, Arthroscopy*, vol. 12, no. 1, pp. 58–64, 2004.

[9] K. Irie, T. Yamada, and K. Inoue, "A comparison of magnetic resonance imaging and arthroscopic evaluation of chondral lesions of the knee," *Orthopedics*, vol. 23, no. 6, pp. 561–564, 2000.

[10] B. Munk, F. Madsen, E. Lundorf et al., "Clinical magnetic resonance imaging and arthroscopic findings in knees: a comparative prospective study of meniscus anterior cruciate ligament and cartilage lesions," *Arthroscopy: The Journal of Arthroscopic & Related Surgery*, vol. 14, no. 2, pp. 171–175, 1998.

[11] L. Wee, "A comparison of accuracy between clinical history, physical examination and magnetic resonance imaging and arthroscopy in the diagnosis of meniscal and anterior cruciate ligament tears," *Journal of Orthopaedic Science*, vol. 5, no. 3, p. e8, 2008.

[12] A. M. Navali, M. Bazavar, M. A. Mohseni, B. Safari, and A. Tabrizi, "Arthroscopic evaluation of the accuracy of clinical examination versus MRI in diagnosing meniscus tears and cruciate ligament ruptures," *Archives of Iranian Medicine*, vol. 16, no. 16, pp. 229–32, 2013.

[13] A. E. Jah, S. Keyhani, R. Zarei, and A. K. Moghaddam, "Accuracy of MRI in comparison with clinical and arthroscopic findings in ligamentous and meniscal injuries of the knee," *Acta Orthopaedica Belgica*, vol. 71, no. 2, pp. 189–196, 2005.

[14] T. Madhusudhan, T. Kumar, S. Bastawrous, and A. Sinha, "Clinical examination, MRI and arthroscopy in meniscal and ligamentous knee Injuries–a prospective study," *Journal of Orthopaedic Surgery and Research*, vol. 3, no. 1, p. 19, 2008.

[15] G. K. Miller, "A prospective study comparing the accuracy of the clinical diagnosis of meniscus tear with magnetic resonance imaging and its effect on clinical outcome," *Arthroscopy: The Journal of Arthroscopic & Related Surgery*, vol. 12, no. 4, pp. 406–413, 1996.

[16] G. Arıcan, A. Özmeriç, Ö Şahin, S. İltar, and K. B. Alemdaroğlu, "Should we prefer magnetic resonance imaging to physical examination in meniscal tears," *The Journal of Knee Surgery*, 2019.

[17] V. S. Nikolaou, E. Chronopoulos, C. Savvidou et al., "MRI efficacy in diagnosing internal lesions of the knee: a retrospective analysis," *Journal of Trauma Management & Outcomes*, vol. 2, no. 1, p. 4, 2008.

[18] W. Wang, Z. Li, H. M. Peng et al., "Accuracy of MRI diagnosis of meniscal tears of the knee: a meta-analysis and systematic review," *The Journal of Knee Surgery*, 2019.

[19] R. Yan, H. Wang, Z. Ji, and Y. Guo, "Predicted probability of meniscus tears: comparing history and physical examination with MRI," *Swiss Medical Weekly*, vol. 141, no. 4950, 2011.

[20] P. Ben-Galim, E. L. Steinberg, H. Amir, N. Ash, S. Dekel, and R. Arbel, "Accuracy of magnetic resonance imaging of the knee and unjustified surgery," *Clinical Orthopaedics and Related Research*, vol. 447, pp. 100–104, 2006.

[21] M. Bohnsack, O. Rühmann, A. Sander-Beuermann, and C. Wirth, "Comparison of clinical examination with NMR spectroscopy in the diagnosis of meniscal lesions in daily practice," *Zeitschrift Fur Orthopadie und ihre Grenzgebiete*, vol. 137, no. 1, pp. 38–42, 1999.

[22] T. Karachalios, M. Hantes, A. H. Zibis, V. Zachos, A. H. Karantanas, and K. N. Malizos, "Diagnostic accuracy of a new clinical test (the thessaly test) for early detection of meniscal tears," *The Journal of Bone & Joint Surgery*, vol. 87, no. 5, pp. 955–962, 2005.

[23] B. K. Harrison, B. E. Abell, and T. W. Gibson, "The thessaly test for detection of meniscal tears: validation of a new physical examination technique for primary care medicine," *Clinical Journal of Sport Medicine*, vol. 19, no. 1, pp. 9–12, 2009.

5

Initial Rotational Instability of the Tapered Wedge-Shaped Type Cementless Stem

Yosuke Iwamoto,[1,2] Hiroaki Kijima,[1,2] Hiroshi Tazawa,[2] Natsuo Konishi,[2] Hitoshi Kubota,[2] Shin Yamada,[1,2] Takayuki Tani,[2] Keiji Kamo,[2] Norio Suzuki,[2] Yoshihiko Okudera,[2] Masashi Fujii,[1,2] Ken Sasaki,[2] Tetsuya Kawano,[2] Itsuki Nagahata,[1,2] Naohisa Miyakoshi,[1] and Yoichi Shimada[1,2]

[1]*Department of Orthopedic Surgery, Akita University Graduate School of Medicine, 1-1-1 Hondo, Akita 010-8543, Japan*
[2]*Akita Hip Research Group, 1-1-1 Hondo, Akita 010-8543, Japan*

Correspondence should be addressed to Yosuke Iwamoto; iwa_motio55@yahoo.co.jp

Academic Editor: Panagiotis Korovessis

Background. Because the tapered wedge-shaped type cementless stem has a small anteroposterior width and a low occupation rate in the medullary space, postoperative rotational instability and stem subsidence due to inadequate proximal fixation are concerns. The purpose of this study was to clarify the relationship between the rotational instability of the tapered wedge-shaped type cementless stem and femoral canal shape. *Methods.* A total of 61 primary total hip arthroplasties with the tapered wedge-shaped type cementless stem Accolade® TMZF (11 males, 50 females; mean age 60 years) from January 2012 to June 2015 who underwent computed tomography before surgery and within 4 weeks and 1 year after surgery were evaluated. The preoperative femoral neck anteversion angle, preoperative femoral canal flair index, the degree of postoperative stem subsidence within 1 year after operation, and the degree of rotational change in the stem setting angle within 1 year after operation were investigated. *Results.* The mean preoperative femoral neck anteversion angle was $32.2^\circ \pm 17.8^\circ$ (0°–69°), and the mean preoperative canal flair index was 3.68 ± 0.58 (2.44–5.55). There were no stem subsidence cases within 1 year after operation. The mean degree of rotational change in the stem from immediately to 1 year after surgery was $-0.4^\circ \pm 1.7^\circ$ (-3°–3°). There was no significant correlation between the canal flair index and the rotational change in the stem. In addition, the mean difference between the preoperative femoral neck anteversion angle and the stem rotational angle immediately after surgery was only $1.3^\circ \pm 5.3^\circ$ (-29°–15°). *Conclusions.* In all cases, including stove-pipe cases, the degree of rotational change in the Accolade® TMZF stem from immediately to 1 year after surgery was within 3°. In other words, regardless of femoral canal shape, the tapered wedge-shaped type cementless stem has little initial rotational instability.

1. Introduction

The tapered wedge-shaped type cementless stem is based on the concept of mediolateral fixation of the metaphysis. There has been a report that its initial fixation is good because it is resistant to settling and rotation by being pressed while compressing the surrounding cancellous bone [1]. Other reports indicated that it is possible to preserve cancellous bone because the shoulder part of such a stem is reduced, the anteroposterior width is narrow, and there are few perioperative complications such as intraoperative fracture [2, 3]. In addition, progression of proximal femoral atrophy due to stress shielding is considered mild because load is applied proximally to the femur due to the shorter length of the stem and the distal taper to block excessive distal fixation [4]. On the contrary, when the tapered wedge-shaped type cementless stem is inserted, for example, to stove-pipe type femoral canal cases, there is a fear of postoperative rotational instability and stem subsidence due to inadequate proximal fixation because its anteroposterior width is small, and the medullary space occupancy rate of such stems is low [5].

However, there has been no report of a detailed investigation of the initial rotational instability of the tapered wedge-shaped type cementless stem. In order to evaluate the rotational angle of the stem setting in detail, it is impossible to evaluate it only by radiography; it is necessary to evaluate it using axial images of computed tomography (CT). By evaluating stem rotational instability in detail using CT, the initial rotational instability of such stems, for example, for stove-pipe-type femurs due to osteoporosis, can be compared with cases in which such stems are used for canal-type femurs. In other words, by evaluating the degree of rotational change in the stem setting angle after surgery, it is possible to clarify the condition in which rotational instability of the tapered wedge-shaped type cementless stem is likely to occur, and it becomes possible to clarify the criteria for using such stems. Therefore, the purpose of this study was to clarify the relationship between rotational instability of the tapered wedge-shaped type cementless stem and the femoral canal shape type.

2. Materials and Methods

A total of 61 primary total hip arthroplasty (THA) cases with the tapered wedge-shaped type cementless stem Accolade® TMZF (Stryker Orthopaedics, Mahwah, New Jersey, USA) from January 2012 to June 2015 in a single hospital and who underwent CT (Revolution CT, Cytiva, Tokyo, Japan) before, within 4 weeks, and 1 year after surgery were evaluated. Thus, this is the retrospective study.

And all surgeries were operated by a single surgeon, and all surgical approaches used the direct lateral approach. The patients' average age was 60 years (range, 32–80 years); 11 were male, and 50 were female. The mean follow-up period was 2.7 years (13–44 months).

The preoperative femoral neck anteversion angle, preoperative femoral canal flair index (CFI), the degree of postoperative stem subsidence within 1 year after surgery, and the degree of rotational change in the stem setting angle within 1 year after surgery were investigated.

The preoperative femoral neck anteversion angle was the angle on the axial CT images from the line connecting the posterior projecting point of the distal medial and lateral condyles of the femur (posterior condylar axis) to the line of the femoral head-neck axis just beneath the femoral head (Figure 1) [6]. Preoperative medullary canal shape was evaluated using the canal-flare index (CFI). [7] Stem subsidence was judged on X-ray by whether the stem 1 year after operation moved distally more than 2 mm compared with the position of the stem on X-ray immediately after surgery.

The stem rotational setting angle was measured as the axis of the anterior/posterior stem on axial CT images with reference to the posterior condylar axis, and the degree of rotational change in the stem setting angle immediately to 1 year after surgery was evaluated (Figure 2) [8].

In addition, clinical outcomes were evaluated by the Japanese Orthopaedic Association Hip Score (JOA score) [9] to quantify hip function and by the Japanese Orthopaedic Association Hip Disease Evaluation Questionnaire (JHEQ) [10] to evaluate patient-reported outcomes.

The patients and their families were informed that data from the case would be submitted for publication and gave their consent. Patients and their families were also informed and agreed to have a CT scan before and immediately after surgery and one year after surgery and the associated increase in radiation dose. Approval was given by the institutional review board.

3. Results

The mean preoperative femoral neck anteversion angle was $32.2^\circ \pm 17.8^\circ$ (0°–69°), and the mean preoperative CFI was 3.68 ± 0.58 (2.44–5.55). There were 2 champagne-flute cases (CFI > 4.7), 7 stove-pipe cases (CFI < 3), and 52 normal canal-type cases.

There were no cases of stem subsidence within 1 year after surgery. The mean stem rotational angle was $30.7^\circ \pm 16.1^\circ$ (-6°–60°) immediately after surgery and $30.1^\circ \pm 16.2^\circ$ (-8°–61°) 1 year after surgery. The mean degree of rotational change in the stem from immediately to 1 year after surgery was $-0.4^\circ \pm 1.7^\circ$ (-3°–3°).

There was no significant correlation between the CFI and rotational change in the stem setting angle ($r = -0.21$, $p = 0.2338$, Spearman's rank correlation coefficient) (Figure 3). In addition, the mean difference between the preoperative femoral neck anteversion angle and the stem rotational angle immediately after surgery was only $1.3^\circ \pm 5.3^\circ$. In almost all cases, the stem was set at the same angle as the preoperative femoral neck anteversion angle. The JOA and JHEQ scores were significantly improved from preoperative (49.3 and 23.8, respectively) to postoperative (84.7 and 58.6) (all $p < 0.0001$, Wilcoxon rank sum test) (Figures 4 and 5).

There was no correlation between the improvement rate of the JOA score and rotational change in the stem setting angle ($r = 0.01$ $p = 0.7336$, Spearman's rank correlation coefficient) and no significant correlation between the JHEQ score improvement rate and rotational change in the stem setting angle ($r = -0.01$ $p = 0.6890$, Spearman's rank correlation coefficient).

4. Discussion

Few reports have evaluated the rotational angle of the stem with the passage of time from immediately to 1 year after surgery. Evaluation of the change in the stem rotational angle in detail using the axial CT images in the present study showed that the tapered wedge-shaped type cementless stem maintained rotational stability irrespective of the canal shape.

There have been many reports of good middle-to-long clinical outcomes of tapered wedge-shaped type cementless stems [1, 11]. Thus, this stem type is one of the most commonly used types of cementless stems at present.

However, there are reports of stem sinking and rotated dislocation cases [2] or of intraoperative femoral fracture cases that were thought to be the result of attempting to achieve more stable stem setting [3]. It has also been suggested that one cause of this instability is the

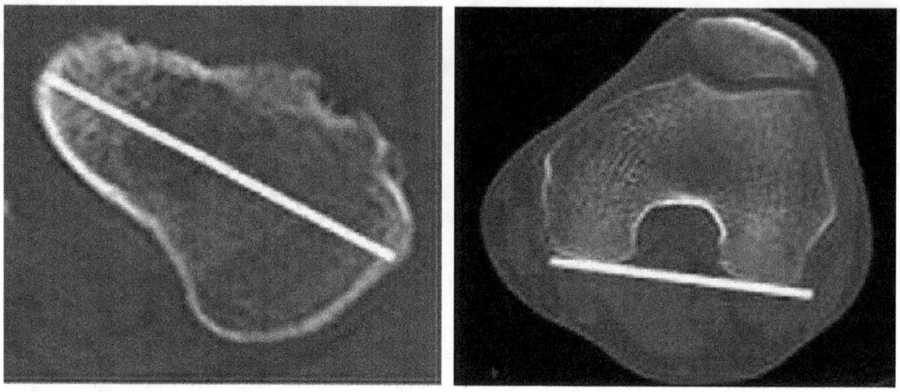

FIGURE 1: Femoral neck anteversion angle. The femoral neck anteversion angle is measured by identifying the femoral head-neck axis from the CT horizontal section slice just beneath the femoral head, with reference to the posterior condylar axis.

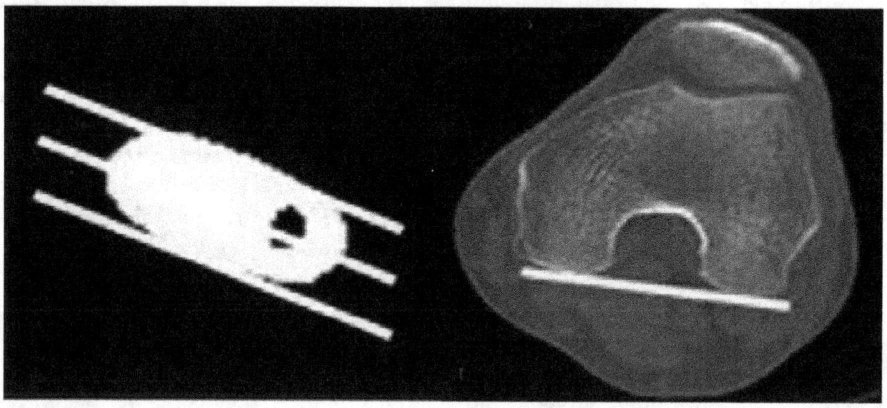

FIGURE 2: Stem rotation setting angle. The stem rotation setting angle is measured using the rotation axis of the stem from the anterior/posterior stem in the CT horizontal section with reference to the posterior condylar axis.

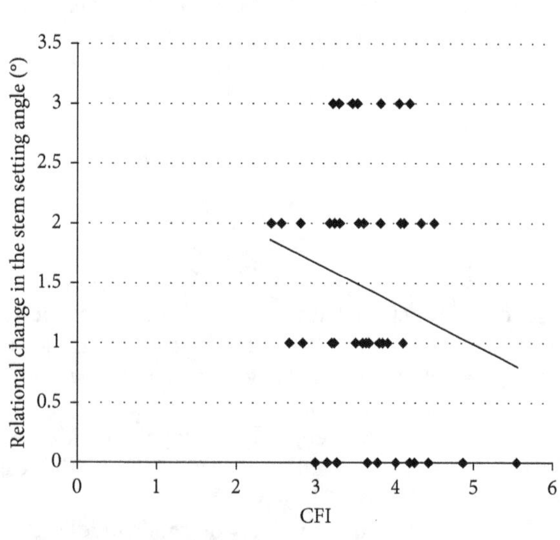

FIGURE 3: Correlation between the CFI and rotational change in the stem setting angle. There is no significant correlation between the CFI and rotational change in the stem setting angle ($r = -0.21$, $p = 0.2338$, Spearman's rank correlation coefficient).

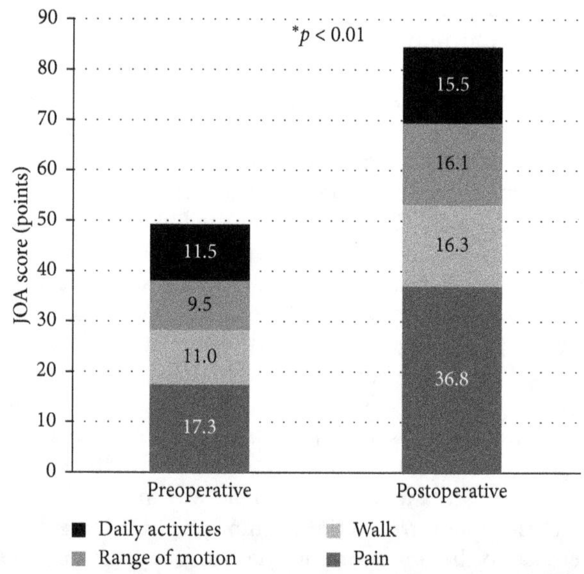

FIGURE 4: Preoperative and postoperative JOA scores. The JOA score is significantly improved from the preoperative mean of 49.3 to the postoperative mean of 84.7 ($p = 0.7336$, Wilcoxon rank sum test).

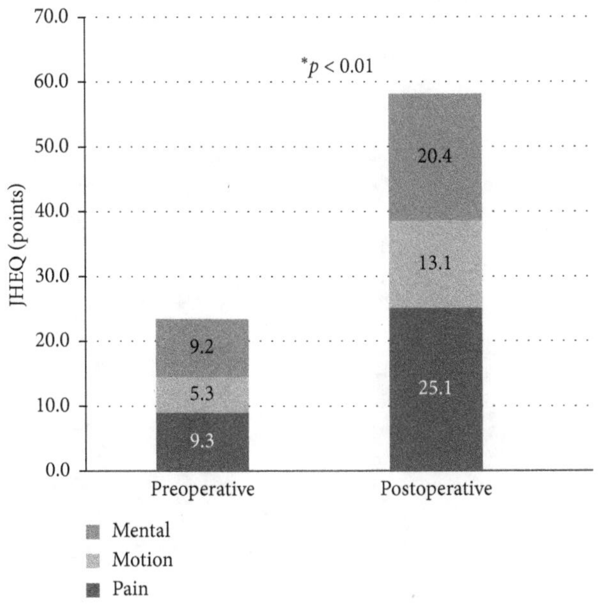

FIGURE 5: Preoperative and postoperative JHEQ scores. The JHEQ is significantly improved from the preoperative mean of 23.8 to the postoperative mean of 58.6 ($p = 0.6890$, Wilcoxon rank sum test).

rotational instability due to the small anteroposterior width and the low occupation rate in the medullary space. However, the rotational change in the stem setting angle at 1 year after surgery of Accolade® TMZF was very small in all cases, including stove-pipe cases, in the present study.

In the case studied in present research, the stems were inserted at the same anteversion angle of the femoral neck, and no effort has been made to change the rotation angle of the stem to a different anteversion angle than the patient's femoral neck. As a result, the stem fits in the area with the widest mediolateral widths; thus, the rotational instability did not occur, no matter how small the anteroposterior width of the stems was.

One of the limitations of this study is the accuracy of measurement on CT images. In this study, measurements of the femoral neck anteversion anterior angle and the stem rotation setting angle were performed using axial CT images. Measurement error is considered to occur due to differences in limb positioning during CT imaging [10]. It has also been reported that the femoral neck anteversion angle varies depending on the slice by a few millimetres [8]. However, Sugano et al. [8] reported no significant difference in the difference of the femoral neck axis taken by 3-dimensional CT although the mean measurement difference is only 1.4°, and the femoral neck axis measured with the slice just below the femoral head does not differ significantly [8]. Since the stem rotational angle was measured in the present study, it could be measured more accurately than femoral neck anteversion.

Current study did not take into account the patient's physique and the effects of postoperative rehabilitation. These were also the limitation of this study. Although there were no significant obesity cases included in this study, it is undeniable that allowing full weight-bearing early in the postoperative period may cause rotational instability in such cases.

Other limitations are that all cases were only from a single hospital, and the number of cases was small. Because the surgical technique was almost constant without performing intraoperative version control in the present study, the stem was set at the same angle in the femoral neck anteversion angle in almost all cases. If a similar investigation were to be conducted at other facilities in which the surgeons perform a "stem intraoperative version control procedure" under another concept or if similar investigations were to be performed with larger numbers of cases with the same procedure, more cases with rotational instability might be found. Identifying such cases will lead to the establishment of better indication criteria and stem setting technique of tapered wedge-shaped type cementless stems. This study provides the first step to that end.

5. Conclusion

In all cases, including stove-pipe canal cases, the rotational change in the Accolade® TMZF stem from immediately to 1 year after surgery was within 3°. Thus, the tapered wedge-shaped type cementless stem has little initial rotational instability, regardless of femoral canal shape type.

Acknowledgments

The authors gratefully acknowledge Yoichi Shimada (Department of Orthopedic Surgery, Akita University Graduate School of Medicine) for his advice. The authors also thank the Akita Hip Research Group (AHRG) for providing advice.

References

[1] P. F. Sharkey, T. J. Albert, E. L. Hume, and R. H Rothman, "Initial stability of a collarless wedge-shaped prosthesis in the femoral canal," *Seminars in Arthroplasty*, vol. 1, no. 1, pp. 87–90, 1990.

[2] V. Pellegrini Jr., S. Hughes, and C. Evarts, "A collarless cobalt-chrome femoral component in uncemented total hip arthroplasty. Five- to eight-year follow-up," *The Journal of Bone and Joint Surgery. British Volume*, vol. 74-B, no. 6, pp. 814–821, 1992.

[3] J. Parvizi, K. S. Keisu, W. J. Hozack, P. F. Sharkey, and R. H. Rothman, "Primary total hip arthroplasty with an uncemented femoral component," *The Journal of Arthroplasty*, vol. 19, no. 2, pp. 151–156, 2004.

[4] K. Yamaguchi, K. Masuhara, K. Ohzono, N. Sugano, T. Nishii, and T. Ochi, "Evaluation of periprosthetic bone-remodeling after cementless total hip arthroplasty," *The Journal of Bone and Joint Surgery-American Volume*, vol. 82, no. 10, pp. 1426–1431, 2000.

[5] H. J. Cooper, A. P. Jacob, and J. A. Rodriguez, "Distal fixation of proximally coated tapered stems may predispose to a failure of osteointegration," *The Journal of Arthroplasty*, vol. 26, no. 6, pp. 78–83, 2011.

[6] N. Sugano, P. C. Noble, and E. Kamaric, "A comparison of alternative methods of measuring femoral anteversion," *Journal of Computer Assisted Tomography*, vol. 22, no. 4, pp. 610–614, 1998.
[7] P. C. Noble, J. W. Alexander, L. J. Lindahl et al., "The anatomic basis of femoral comportment design," *Clinical Orthopaedics and Related Research*, vol. 235, pp. 148–165, 1988.
[8] L. D. Dorr, Z. Wan, A. Malik, J. Zhu, M. Dastane, and P. Deshmane, "A comparison of surgeon estimation and computed tomographic measurement of femoral component anteversion in cementless total hip arthroplasty," *The Journal of Bone & Joint Surgery*, vol. 91, no. 11, pp. 2598–2604, 2009.
[9] M. Kuribayashi, K. A. Takahashi, M. Fujioka, K. Ueshima, S. Inoue, and T. Kubo, "Reliability and validity of the Japanese Orthopaedic Association hip score," *Journal of Orthopaedic Science*, vol. 15, no. 4, pp. 452–458, 2010.
[10] T. Matsumoto, A. Kaneuji, T. Ichiseki et al., "Japanese orthopaedic association hip disease evaluation Questionnaire (JHEQ): a patient-based evaluation tool for hip-joint disease. The subcommittee on hip disease evaluation of the clinical outcome committee of the Japanese orthopaedic association," *Journal of Orthopaedic Science*, vol. 17, no. 1, pp. 25–38, 2012.
[11] J. R. McLaughlin and K. R. Lee, "Total hip arthroplasty with an uncemented tapered femoral component," *The Journal of Bone & Joint Surgery*, vol. 90, no. 6, pp. 1290–1296, 2008.

6

Advancing Simulation-Based Orthopaedic Surgical Skills Training: An Analysis of the Challenges to Implementation

Kivanc Atesok,[1] Shepard Hurwitz,[2] Donald D. Anderson,[3] Richard Satava,[4] Geb W. Thomas,[3] Ted Tufescu,[5] Michael J. Heffernan,[6] Efstathios Papavassiliou,[1] Steven Theiss,[7] and J. Lawrence Marsh[3]

[1]*Harvard University, Beth Israel Deaconess Medical Center, Department of Neurosurgery, Boston, MA, USA*
[2]*University of North Carolina, Department of Orthopaedic Surgery, Chapel Hill, NC, USA*
[3]*University of Iowa, Department of Orthopaedics and Rehabilitation, Iowa City, IA, USA*
[4]*University of Washington, Department of Surgery, Seattle, WA, USA*
[5]*University of Manitoba, Section of Orthopaedic Surgery, Winnipeg, MB, Canada*
[6]*Children's Hospital of New Orleans, LSU Health Science Center, Department of Orthopaedic Surgery, New Orleans, LA, USA*
[7]*University of Alabama at Birmingham, Department of Orthopaedic Surgery, Birmingham, AL, USA*

Correspondence should be addressed to Kivanc Atesok; kivanc.atesok@utoronto.ca

Academic Editor: Allen L. Carl

Simulation-based surgical skills training is recognized as a valuable method to improve trainees' performance and broadly perceived as essential for the establishment of a comprehensive curriculum in surgical education. However, there needs to be improvement in several areas for meaningful integration of simulation into surgical education. The purpose of this focused review is to summarize the obstacles to a comprehensive integration of simulation-based surgical skills training into surgical education and board certification and suggest potential solutions for those obstacles. First and foremost, validated simulators need to be rigorously assessed to ensure their feasibility and cost-effectiveness. All simulation-based courses should include clear objectives and outcome measures (with metrics) for the skills to be practiced by trainees. Furthermore, these courses should address a wide range of issues, including assessment of trainees' problem-solving and decision-making abilities and remediation of poor performance. Finally, which simulation-based surgical skills courses will become a standard part of the curriculum across training programs and which will be of value in board certification should be precisely defined. Sufficient progress in these areas will prevent excessive development of training and assessment tools with duplicative effort and large variability in quality.

1. Introduction

Simulation-based surgical skills training is widely recognized as a valuable method for improving trainees' performance and as an essential part of a comprehensive curriculum in surgical education [1–6]. Despite tremendous efforts to integrate simulation into orthopaedic surgical education, there is a continued need for simulation-based education to be a more substantial part of orthopaedic curricula. Rapidly growing orthopaedic techniques along with increasing subspecialization necessitate the wide and efficacious adaptation of simulators as basic educational tools in orthopaedic curricula. Evidence suggests that surgical simulation has positive effects on improving trainees' performance in the operating room (OR) [7–10]. As a result, there is currently a consensus among surgical specialties including the orthopaedic community that ideally the development of trainees' surgical skills should commence in a simulated training environment prior to progression to the OR. The purpose of the current review is to summarize the obstacles to, and provide recommendations for, a comprehensive integration of simulation-based surgical skills training into surgical education and board certification.

2. Overcoming Barriers to the Integration of Simulation-Based Surgical Skills Training into Surgical Education

2.1. Validation of Simulation-Based Surgical Skills Training. Although trainees from all levels—residents, fellows, and practicing surgeons—appreciate the introduction of simulation into surgical education, validation of simulation-based surgical skills training is the most important area that still needs further improvement. Simulators and curricula must be rigorously assessed and validated so that training can be proven to be valuable and performance can be reliably assessed.

Simulated surgical skills training should pass multiple validity tests prior to routine use in surgical curricula and competency assessment. Standard validity tests include face, content, construct, and concurrent validity. In the following paragraphs, we will define and elucidate the subtle differences between these key validity tests.

Face validity refers to a simulator's relevance as it appears to participants. In other words, a simulator platform can be said to have face validity if it "looks like" it correctly simulates the intended task/situation. Face validity is usually assessed subjectively via participants' responses to post-simulation questionnaires. Arikatla et al. assessed the face validity of a virtual navigation task trainer developed to simulate laparoscopic surgery tasks. After performing the tasks, the participants were asked to rate the simulator's face validity from 1 (not realistic/useful) to 5 (very realistic/useful) on a 10-item questionnaire. The subjects rated the simulator as highly useful by responding to 90% (9 out of 10) of the questions with a score of three or above [11].

Content validity refers to the extent to which a simulator measures the relevant aspects of the surgical task under study. For example, a simulator may lack content validity if it only assesses the accuracy of the reduction and hardware used in a simulated fracture fixation but fails to account for the correctness in the stepwise performance of the procedure. Alsalamah et al. studied the content validity of a virtual reality simulator reflecting real transvaginal ultrasound (TVUS) scanning [12]. The content validity assessment statements aimed to include all the aspects of TVUS scanning, such as the simulator's ability to test normal gynaecological anatomy and early pregnancy structures, and also the simulator's realism in providing measurements of endometrial thickness, ovaries, and crown-rump length. Participants scored the simulator on a visual analog scale based on their subjective perceptions of the simulator's accuracy in assessing the items included in the content validity scoring list. The median scores demonstrated strong agreement with the content validity statements.

Construct validity defines the degree to which the simulator measures the specific surgical skills that it was designed for. Construct validity can be described as the appropriateness of inferences made on the basis of test scores. In surgical simulation research, experience levels of subjects testing on a simulator are often used to asses construct validity. For example, if a simulator correctly detects expected variations in the proficiency levels between the expert and novice subjects—in other words, if it correctly identifies quantifiable aspects of a surgical skill—construct validity has been achieved. Lopez et al. studied the construct validity of an arthroscopy simulator in a group of participants that included medical students, residents, and attending physicians [13]. The arthroscopic surgical simulator objectively demonstrated that the attending physicians and senior residents performed at a higher level than the junior residents and novice medical students.

Concurrent validity refers to the correspondence between trainees' performance on a tested simulator and a previously validated measure. Researchers often assess the concurrent validity of surgical simulators by comparing participants' simulator scores with their objective structured assessment of technical skill (OSATS) scores. However, comparison with another previously validated simulator can also be used to endorse concurrent validity. In a study including three groups of participants with different levels of expertise (novice, intermediate, and expert) in pedicle screw insertion, Fürst et al. [14] assessed the face, content, construct, and concurrent validity of a novel simulator for minimally invasive spine surgery . The authors used questionnaires with a 5-point Likert scale to assess face and content validity. They evaluated the construct validity using a simulation-based performance score that they calculated for pedicle screw insertion and compared among the three groups. To establish concurrent validity, the performance of each participant was assessed by a specialist using a task-specific checklist and OSATS, and the association between the specialist rating and the simulation-based performance score was evaluated. Their results demonstrated significantly better simulation-based performance scores in the expert group (construct validity) compared with the novices ($P = 0.001$) and intermediates ($P = 0.01$). The association between the specialist's ratings and the simulation-based performance score (concurrent validity) was strong ($R = 0.86$, $P = 0.01$).

Although it is essential to prove face, content, construct, and concurrent validity for a simulation-based training platform to be considered for integration into educational curricula, *transferability* of the skills practiced on a simulator to the OR to perform on patients should also be achieved. In a randomized study, Howells et al. investigated the effect of laboratory-based simulator training on surgical trainees' ability to perform diagnostic arthroscopy of the knee in the OR [15]. The simulator-trained group performed significantly better than the control, demonstrating the transferability of psychomotor skills from simulator training to arthroscopy in the OR.

Arguably, the correlation between performance on the simulator with OR performance on patients provides the most convincing evidence to move forward. The reliability of both the simulated measurement of skills and the measures obtained from actual practice along with good-to-excellent correlation between these two assessments is an absolute necessity for a simulation-based surgical skills course to become part of a standardized educational curriculum. Unfortunately, demonstrating transferability of surgical skills requires fairly sophisticated research methodology, a sufficient number of learners to have the power to demonstrate important differences, and patient consent for the operating room portion of the trial. These issues provide substantial challenges to this type of validation of a simulation course.

2.2. Toward Evaluating Surgical Skills in the OR. Evaluating learners' surgical skills in the OR environment after simulation-based training in laboratories requires objective and standard measurement techniques that are also sensitive enough to differentiate various levels of expertise [16]. A fundamental challenge preventing the movement toward competency-based education is establishing objective criteria for when a resident is ready to advance to the next level. It is possible that the main reason for not being able to establish such criteria is the lack of standard, objective, reliable, and sensitive surgical skill measurement methods. Szasz et al. reviewed 6,814 publications and defined 85 surgical simulator studies that assessed trainees' technical competence [17]. The authors noted that "Very few studies identify standard-setting approaches that differentiate competent versus noncompetent performers; subsequently, this has been identified as an area with great research potential."

Specific surgical skills for various types of procedures can be hard to define, making it even more difficult to precisely measure them. For example, an individual skill such as navigating a surgical wire into a specific location in a bone is a complex interplay of task-specific knowledge, general knowledge of the anatomy and tools, hand-eye coordination, team communication, dexterity, self-control, experience, and a bit of luck. Hence, defining the essential elements (tasks) of the procedure-specific and surgical skills to be measured is critically important for accurate assessments of competency in the OR.

By definition, all procedures are comprised of specific tasks, and all tasks are comprised of specific skills. The most common method is to perform "task deconstruction," which accurately defines each task (e.g., anastomosis) and breaks that task into each of its elemental skills (e.g., tissue alignment, needle driving, suturing, and knot tying). It is true that subspecialties need to develop skills that are unique to their specialty; however, basic skills such as suturing, knot tying, developing dissection planes, and anastomosis are truly applicable to all orthopaedic (and other surgical) subspecialities as well.

One other, more global approach to assessing surgical skills in a clinical setting is to systematically observe the objective elements of a surgeon's behavior. Currently, surgical task-specific checklists and OSATS are two commonly used techniques for measuring surgical skills; however, studies demonstrated that OSATS scores do not always correlate well with the outcomes [18, 19]. In a study of simulated distal radius fracture fixation, Putnam et al. found that the participants' OSATS scores had no correlation with the actual mechanical strength of the fixation they performed [19]. Therefore, to be able to tie simulation-based surgical skills training to OR performance and surgical results, meticulously defined procedure-specific tasks should be assessed using standard measurement protocols that combine more than one objective technique, such as OSATS, motion analysis, and direct objective metrics, such as the accuracy of reduction, time to skill completion, and strength of a fracture fixation construct (Figure 1) [16].

2.3. Proficiency-Based Progression for Surgical Skills Training. Proficiency-based progression (PBP) is the next-generation approach to overcoming the challenge of defining the measurable criteria for technical performance proficiency in training with simulators. The outcome measures of technical skill performance in PBP are quantitative metrics, which can unambiguously quantify the performance of the learner. In this approach, benchmarks are defined by the performance scores of the experts who undergo the same course [6, 20]. Training with the simulator continues until students meet the benchmark scores for two consecutive trials, regardless of the number of trials or time it requires to meet proficiency benchmarks. PBP method provides quantitative evidence that the student is proficient: evidence-based medicine requires evidence-based education.

In order to build a standard nationwide curriculum for various specialties, benchmarks using multi-institutional experts can be developed for national-level courses. There are such courses accepted by the corresponding boards and recognized as national "standards" because they meet the requirements of the certifying boards of the specialty. Some examples include advanced trauma and life support (ATLS), fundamentals of laparoscopic surgery (FLS), and fundamentals of endoscopic surgery (FES). Orthopaedic surgery does not yet have a nationwide specialty course that the American Board of Orthopaedic Surgery (ABOS) recognizes as standard.

2.4. Addressing Problem Solving and Surgical Adversity. Most of the effort in teaching learners about surgery is spent on the knowledge base needed to arrive at an accurate diagnosis, applying the guidelines from the literature regarding the indications for a surgical procedure, and the experiential learning of the mechanics of conducting the procedure on a human. However, problem-solving and decision-making are not explicitly taught in orthopaedic surgery education [21]. Learning about problem-solving in surgery is often a matter of having to deal with a problem as it arises during a procedure or in the perioperative timeframe [22].

Although much of what is required for a successful surgical result comprises the knowledge and skills to perform a routine procedure, the ability to deal with adversity is another skill that can be taught during residency. Theoretically, if trainees can be taught to anticipate and handle certain potential problems, solving such problems in real-life situations can become a learned behavior. In addition to using technical skills in such challenging

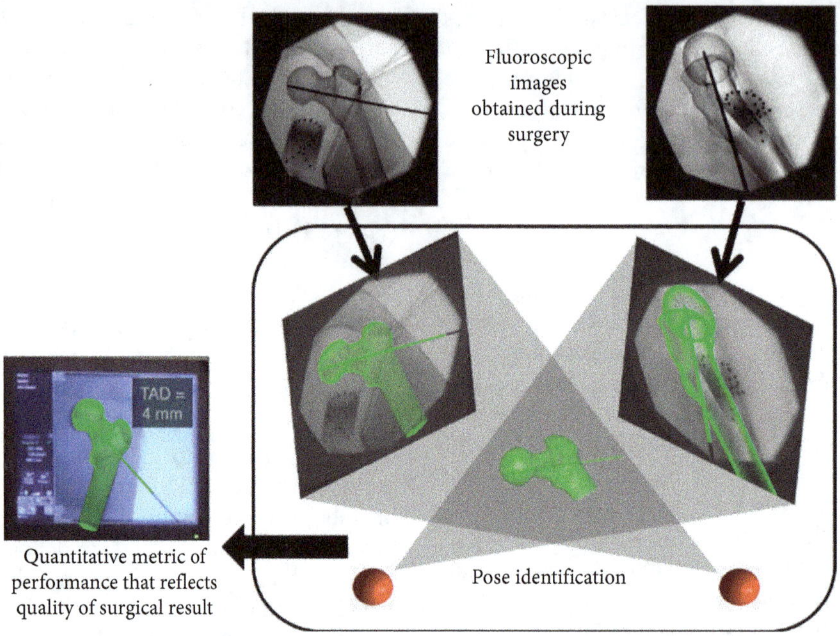

Figure 1: Image analysis software can be used to quantify the metrics for the quality of the surgical result (courtesy of Donald Anderson from the University of Iowa, Department of Orthopedics and Rehabilitation, Iowa City, IA, USA).

situations, nontechnical skills such as communication, situational awareness, ability to handle high stress, and decision-making can be equally important [23]. Simulators that are equipped with and programmed for certain intraoperative challenges can be beneficial in teaching problem-solving and decision-making skills. Currently, there is a need for high-fidelity models that can add intraoperative challenges to the routine performance of a procedure, such as excessive bleeding, dural tears, and iatrogenic fractures.

2.5. Remediation of Poor Performance. Another important aspect of simulation-based training is the remediation of poor surgical skills. Those trainees who perform poorly in the laboratory setting should be entered into a remediation program that includes more time and supervision in the skills lab and personal input from supervising faculty. The orthopaedic literature lacks studies that outline the remediation of struggling trainees. In a report summarizing the Council of Emergency Medicine Residency Directors' (CORD) recommendations for resident remediation, Katz et al. indicated that "Early identification of poor performance is key to successful remediation [24]." In the context of simulation-based orthopaedic skills training, early detection of poor performance can only be achieved by using validated simulators and objective, reliable, and sensitive measurement techniques. Gas et al. [25] tested general surgery residents' knowledge and surgical skills in an objective structured clinical examination-style assessment. Participants who scored poorly at any given task were required to remediate those tasks by practicing the simulated stations with staff surgeons and by using online instructional videos. Residents that required remediation were evaluated again in person by an instructor or sent in self-made videos of their performance that was then graded by an instructor.

2.6. Choosing the Right Simulator. There are three important criteria that educators should consider when choosing a simulator for surgical skills training: fidelity, cost, and feasibility.

Fidelity is defined as "the degree of association, resemblance, or correspondence with the original; exactness" [26]. In other words, fidelity does not define the "prettiness" or "genuineness" of the images or the model. In simulation for technical skills, which are the psychomotor skills and tasks that a learner must acquire, fidelity is about the motions that the learner must perform. The hand motions in the simulation should match the complexity of the motions in the corresponding real procedure. Although fidelity is an important criterion in choosing a simulator in health care, there is not enough literature to prove that high-fidelity simulators are better in terms of achieving skill proficiency or transfer of learned skills to the OR [27–30]. In a prospective randomized crossover study, Tan et al. [27] investigated whether there were any differences in the learning outcomes of participants who had trained to proficiency on low- or high-filaparoscopic surgical simulators. The participants were randomized to either high-fidelity (LapSim, Surgical Science) or low-fidelity (FLS, SAGES) laparoscopic simulators and trained to proficiency in a defined number of tasks. They then crossed over to the other fidelity simulator and were tested. The results demonstrated similar increases in participant scores from the baseline for both the high- and low-fidelity groups. However, FLS-trained participants demonstrated a greater ability to translate their skills to successfully complete LapSim tasks. The authors concluded

"... the FLS simulator is superior to the LapSim when teaching basic laparoscopic skills to participants." In a review article, Norman et al. [28] compared learning from high-fidelity simulation with learning from low-fidelity simulation based on measures of clinical performance. Although both high- and low-fidelity simulation learning resulted in consistent improvements in performance in comparison with no-simulation control groups, nearly all the studies showed no significant advantage of high-fidelity over low-fidelity simulation, with average differences ranging from 1 to 2%.

Complex high-fidelity simulators may cost up to 80,000–90,000 United States Dollars (USD). With further expenses such as maintenance and software upgrades, simulator-based training can become very costly. Although the ultimate goal of simulation-based training is to enhance learning, if the cost associated with implementing effective simulators is prohibitively high, it may not be a viable option [31]. Despite the consistent focus on the high costs of simulation, the literature does not include sufficient research regarding simulators' cost-effectiveness [31]. Berg et al. demonstrated that startup costs and operational expenses of a surgical skills laboratory decreased from 1,151 to 982 USD per resident over a three-year period [32]. It is sensible to assume that the initial expenses of building a simulation-based surgical skills laboratory will be a lot higher compared with the expenses of an established laboratory. Moreover, surgical skills training before residents enter the OR may bring additional savings of increased OR turnover in teaching hospitals.

Choosing the best simulator also depends upon the procedure or specific task that needs to be trained. Simulating full procedures is usually more difficult because the surrogates used for full procedure simulations, such as cadavers and live animal models, are not very feasible options due to procurement, cost, and logistics. Partial manikins with replaceable organs or tissues can be used repeatedly and are more feasible and cost-effective for training of specific simple tasks such as central line placements [33]. Virtual reality (VR) simulators, such as laparoscopic or arthroscopic simulators, have been developed with the addition of haptic properties and replica legs for increased fidelity. These VR simulators are very feasible due to their easy accessibility for trainees, the small space they occupy, the possibility to train with them repeatedly, and their resemblance to real laparoscopic or arthroscopic procedures. However, the cost is still considered as a drawback, especially for high-fidelity haptic arthroscopy simulators [6]. When considering the feasibility of implementing simulator-based training into a surgical educational curriculum, time spent in education and thus away from clinical practice should also be taken into account. Although more simulation-based surgical skills training may result in better learning for residents, conducting lab-based training for extended periods, especially early on in a residency, might not be feasible. As a generalization, the measure of value for a simulator should be as follows: "the fidelity of a simulator should match the complexity of the task or procedure to be trained and/or assessed." Simple models should be used for basic skills training and more sophisticated computer-based simulators for complex procedures.

3. Skills Assessment for Board Certification: What Are the Issues and Areas That Need to Be Improved?

Certifying boards' mission is to set standards for education and practice. Although many competencies are required to meet these standards, for surgical boards, technical skills in performing procedures is a particularly important competency. Since assessing technical skills in the OR is challenging, simulation should play an important role in assessing a skill during the training and certification process. Surgical boards have the opportunity to advance simulation by requiring its use during the steps toward initial and ongoing certification. Some surgical boards have taken initiatives to incorporate simulation into their certification process, but others have encountered barriers that have prevented the wide adoption of board-required simulation-based surgical skills training. In addition to the conservative attitude of opposing any new technology before there are sufficient evidence and validation to prove its efficacy, value, and utility, there is also the natural resistance to change, and the threat and fear of those who risk adverse consequences from the new change. From a practical aspect, there is the issue below of difficulty of transfer from simulation to the OR in order to provide the unequivocal evidence necessary to convince the boards of the value of simulation. Although the ABOS has required simulation-based training as part of residency in postgraduate year one since 2013, the standards of such training and of residents' performance have not been well defined.

One of the challenges for boards implementing simulation-based skills training is the fundamental need for both the simulation course and associated assessments to be rigorously validated prior to implementation. Unfortunately, there is not sufficient high-level evidence in orthopaedic surgery to prove that simulated skills training courses improve performance in the OR or that the associated assessments are reliable and valid. Another important point is that the surgical outcome is not completely determined by the success of the surgical procedure; rather, there are many confounding factors such as whether the surgeon has chosen the right treatment (or procedure) for the patient, the preoperative health of the patient, appropriate prepping before entering the OR, postoperative nonsurgical complications, and patient compliance with postoperative instructions. However, the closest evidence would be, subsequent to training to proficiency on a simulator, if the learner is able to demonstrate proficiency in an animal model that is nearly identical with a given patient procedure. The ABOS has recently sponsored grants through the Orthopaedic Research and Education Foundation to assist investigators in obtaining high-level evidence on certain simulation-based surgical skills training courses. These grants hold promise for the future of simulation in orthopaedic surgery.

Unfortunately, challenges in simulation-based skills training in orthopaedic surgery are not limited to a lack of sufficient evidence. Even when high-level scientific evidence proves the value of simulation in orthopaedic surgery, implementing simulation-based skills training courses across residency programs can be very expensive. Furthermore, a standard simulation-based skills training course and the associated assessments the board requires must be available locally or at regional testing centers—the logistics of building such a network can be extremely challenging.

4. Summary

Simulation-based skills training is becoming increasingly integrated into surgical education as an important teaching method across surgical specialties. There are challenges waiting to be addressed prior to further implementation of simulation in residency curriculum and board certification. These challenges can be summarized as the validation of simulation-based courses; proving that simulation-based surgical training improves trainees' performance in the OR; addressing the issues of expense, fidelity, feasibility, and standardizing assessment techniques; and boards' involvement in implementing simulation as a requirement for board eligibility or certification. Advancing simulation-based skills training will accelerate after the recognition and systematic solution of the challenges outlined in this article.

References

[1] K. Atesok, J. D. Mabrey, L. M. Jazrawi, and K. A. Egol, "Surgical simulation in orthopaedic skills training," *Journal of the American Academy of Orthopaedic Surgeons*, vol. 20, no. 7, pp. 410–422, 2012.

[2] M. D. Karam, B. Westerlind, D. D. Anderson, J. L. Marsh, and UI Orthopaedic Surgical Skills Training Committee Corresponding, "Development of an orthopaedic surgical skills curriculum for post-graduate year one resident learners—the University of Iowa experience," *Iowa Orthopedic Journal*, vol. 33, pp. 178–184, 2013.

[3] A. G. Gallagher, N. E. Seymour, J.-A. Jordan-Black, B. P. Bunting, K. McGlade, and R. M. Satava, "Prospective, randomized assessment of transfer of training (ToT) and transfer effectiveness ratio (TER) of virtual reality simulation training for laparoscopic skill acquisition," *Annals of Surgery*, vol. 257, no. 6, pp. 1025–1031, 2013.

[4] N. N. Khamis, R. M. Satava, S. A. Alnassar, and D. E. Kern, "A stepwise model for simulation-based curriculum development for clinical skills, a modification of the six-step approach," *Surgical Endoscopy*, vol. 30, no. 1, pp. 279–287, 2016 Jan.

[5] G. W. Thomas, B. D. Johns, J. L. Marsh, and D. D. Anderson, "A review of the role of simulation in developing and assessing orthopaedic surgical skills," *Iowa Orthopedic Journal*, vol. 34, pp. 181–189, 2014.

[6] K. Atesok, P. MacDonald, J. Leiter et al., "Orthopaedic education in the era of surgical simulation: still at the crawling stage," *World Journal of Orthopedics*, vol. 8, no. 4, pp. 290–294, 2017.

[7] B. A. Butler, C. D. Lawton, J. Burgess, E. S. Balderama, K. A. Barsness, and J. F. Sarwark, "Simulation-based educational module improves intern and medical student performance of closed reduction and percutaneous pinning of pediatric supracondylar humeral fractures," *The Journal of Bone and Joint Surgery*, vol. 99, no. 23, p. e128, 2017.

[8] H. Maertens, R. Aggarwal, N. Moreels, F. Vermassen, and I. Van Herzeele, "A proficiency based stepwise endovascular curricular training (PROSPECT) program enhances operative performance in real life: a randomised controlled trial," *European Journal of Vascular and Endovascular Surgery*, vol. 54, no. 3, pp. 387–396, 2017.

[9] A. S. S. Thomsen, D. Bach-Holm, H. Kjærbo et al., "Operating room performance improves after proficiency-based virtual reality cataract surgery training," *Ophthalmology*, vol. 124, no. 4, pp. 524–531, 2017.

[10] Y. Kurashima, L. S. Feldman, P. A. Kaneva et al., "Simulation-based training improves the operative performance of totally extraperitoneal (TEP) laparoscopic inguinal hernia repair: a prospective randomized controlled trial," *Surgical Endoscopy*, vol. 28, no. 3, pp. 783–788, 2014.

[11] V. Arikatla, S. Horvath, Y. Fu et al., "Development and face validation of a virtual camera navigation task trainer," *Surgical Endoscopy*, vol. 33, no. 6 , Article ID 30324462, 2018.

[12] A. Alsalamah, R. Campo, V. Tanos et al., "Face and content validity of the virtual reality simulator "ScanTrainer®"," *Gynecological Surgery*, vol. 14, no. 1, p. 18, 2017.

[13] G. Lopez, D. F. Martin, R. Wright et al., "Construct validity for a cost-effective arthroscopic surgery simulator for resident education," *Journal of the American Academy of Orthopaedic Surgeons*, vol. 24, no. 12, pp. 886–894, 2016.

[14] D. Fürst, M. Hollensteiner, S. Gabauer et al., "Transpedicular approach on a novel spine simulator: a validation study," *Journal of Surgical Education*, vol. 75, no. 4, pp. 1127–1134, 2018.

[15] N. R. Howells, H. S. Gill, A. J. Carr, A. J. Price, and J. L. Rees, "Transferring simulated arthroscopic skills to the operating theatre," *The Journal of Bone and Joint Surgery. British Volume*, vol. 90-B, no. 4, pp. 494–499, 2008.

[16] K. Atesok, R. M. Satava, J. L. Marsh, and S. R. Hurwitz, "Measuring surgical skills in simulation-based training," *Journal of the American Academy of Orthopaedic Surgeons*, vol. 25, no. 10, pp. 665–672, 2017.

[17] P. Szasz, M. Louridas, K. A. Harris, R. Aggarwal, and T. P. Grantcharov, "Assessing technical competence in surgical trainees," *Annals of Surgery*, vol. 261, no. 6, pp. 1046–1055, 2015.

[18] D. D. Anderson, S. Long, G. W. Thomas, M. D. Putnam, J. E. Bechtold, and M. D. Karam, "Objective structured assessments of technical skills (OSATS) does not assess the quality of the surgical result effectively," *Clinical Orthopaedics and Related Research®*, vol. 474, no. 4, pp. 874–881, 2016.

[19] M. D. Putnam, E. Kinnucan, J. E. Adams, A. E. Van Heest, D. J. Nuckley, and J. Shanedling, "On orthopedic surgical skill prediction-the limited value of traditional testing," *Journal of Surgical Education*, vol. 72, no. 3, pp. 458–470, 2015.

[20] A. G. Gallagher, E. M. Ritter, H. Champion et al., "Virtual reality simulation for the operating room," *Annals of Surgery*, vol. 241, no. 2, pp. 364–372, 2005.

[21] M. D. Timberlake, D. Stefanidis, and A. K. Gardner, "Examining the impact of surgical coaching on trainee physiologic response and basic skill acquisition," *Surgical Endoscopy*, vol. 32, no. 10, pp. 4183–4190, 2018.

[22] C. Braddock III, P. L. Hudak, J. J. Feldman, S. Bereknyei,

R. M. Frankel, and W. Levinson, ""Surgery is certainly one good option": quality and time-efficiency of informed decision-making in surgery," *The Journal of Bone and Joint Surgery-American Volume*, vol. 90, no. 9, pp. 1830–1838, 2008.

[23] O. Brunckhorst, M. S. Khan, P. Dasgupta, and K. Ahmed, "Nontechnical skill training and the use of scenarios in modern surgical education," *Current Opinion in Urology*, vol. 27, no. 4, pp. 330–336, 2017.

[24] E. D. Katz, R. Dahms, A. T. Sadosty, S. A. Stahmer, and D. Goyal, "Guiding principles for resident remediation: recommendations of the CORD remediation task force," *Academic Emergency Medicine*, vol. 17, no. 2, pp. S95–S103, 2010.

[25] B. L. Gas, E. H. Buckarma, M. Mohan, T. K. Pandian, and D. R. Farley, "Objective assessment of general surgery residents followed by remediation," *Journal of Surgical Education*, vol. 73, no. 6, pp. e71–e76, 2016.

[26] Oxford University Press, *The Oxford English Dictionary*, Oxford University Press, Oxford, UK, 2018, http://www.oed.com.

[27] S. C. Tan, N. Marlow, J. Field et al., "A randomized crossover trial examining low- versus high-fidelity simulation in basic laparoscopic skills training," *Surgical Endoscopy*, vol. 26, no. 11, pp. 3207–3214, 2012.

[28] G. Norman, K. Dore, and L. Grierson, "The minimal relationship between simulation fidelity and transfer of learning," *Medical Education*, vol. 46, no. 7, pp. 636–647, 2012.

[29] J. Kim, J. H. Park, and S. Shin, "Effectiveness of simulation-based nursing education depending on fidelity: a meta-analysis," *BMC Medical Education*, vol. 16, p. 152, 2016.

[30] D. Hart, J. Nelson, J. Moore, E. Gross, A. Oni, and J. Miner, "Shoulder dystocia delivery by emergency medicine residents: a high-fidelity versus a novel low-fidelity simulation model-A pilot study," *AEM Education and Training*, vol. 1, no. 4, pp. 357–362, 2017.

[31] W. Isaranuwatchai, R. Brydges, H. Carnahan, D. Backstein, and A. Dubrowski, "Comparing the cost-effectiveness of simulation modalities: a case study of peripheral intravenous catheterization training," *Advances in Health Sciences Education*, vol. 19, no. 2, pp. 219–232, 2014.

[32] D. A. Berg, R. E. Milner, C. A. Fisher, A. J. Goldberg, D. T. Dempsey, and H. Grewal, "A cost-effective approach to establishing a surgical skills laboratory," *Surgery*, vol. 142, no. 5, pp. 712–721, 2007.

[33] A. A. Alsaad, V. Y. Bhide, J. L. Moss Jr., S. M. Silvers, M. M. Johnson, and M. J. Maniaci, "Central line proficiency test outcomes after simulation training versus traditional training to competence," *Annals of the American Thoracic Society*, vol. 14, no. 4, pp. 550–554, 2017.

7

Role of Platelet-Rich Plasma in Spinal Fusion Surgery

Daudi R. Manini,[1,2] Frank D. Shega,[1,3] ChaoFeng Guo,[1] and YuXiang Wang[1]

[1]*Department of Spine Surgery, Xiangya Hospital of Central South University, Changsha 410008, Hunan Province, China*
[2]*Department of Orthopedic Surgery, Mwananyamala Regional Referral Hospital, P.O. Box 61665, Dar-es-Salaam, Tanzania*
[3]*Department of Orthopedic Surgery, Mount Meru Regional Referral Hospital, P.O. Box 3092, Arusha, Tanzania*

Correspondence should be addressed to ChaoFeng Guo; 343942471@qq.com

Academic Editor: Hiroshi Hashizume

Background. Platelet-rich plasma (PRP) has been used very successfully in enhancing bone fusion in animal experiments. Also, the efficaciousness of PRP in other specialties of medicine such as dentistry, dermatology ophthalmology, and sports medicine is well documented. But the use of PRP to augment bone fusion after spinal surgery in humans is still controversial. We conducted a meta-analysis to determine the role of PRP in enhancing spinal fusion by fastening the rate of new bone formation and decreasing pain after spinal surgery in humans. *Methods.* We searched PubMed, EMBASE, and the Cochrane Library studies that compared PRP versus control in enhancing spinal fusion after deformity correction. *Results.* Five retrospective studies with 253 participants and nine prospective cohort studies with 460 participants were identified. The bone fusion rate was excellent for studies that used a high platelet concentration in PRP relative to control (odds ratio (OR) = 4.35, 95% confidence interval (CI) (2.13, 8.83), and $P < 0.05$) while bone fusion was poor to studies that used a low concentrate of platelet in PRP relative to control. The rate of new bone formation was high in the PRP group compared to the control group with the mean difference in Hounsfield unit (HU) 144.91 (95% CI (80.63, 209.18), $P < 0.05$). Time to bone fusion was short in the PRP group during the first six months of surgery relative to the control group with a mean difference of −2.03 (95% CI (−2.35, −1.7); $P < 0.05$). No difference was found in pain reduction by visual analog score (VAS) between the PRP group and control. *Conclusion.* PRP facilitates new bone formation and bone fusion with a minimum concentration of the growth factor 5 times that of the peripheral blood. PRP stimulatory effects are not continuous and are very effective within six months of implantation.

1. Introduction

Platelet-rich plasma (PRP) is blood plasma with concentrated autologous platelets and various growth factors as well as cytokines above the normal baseline level. PRP is believed to contain several growth factors including platelet-derived growth factor (PDGF), transforming growth factor (TGF), insulin-like growth factor (IGF), epidermal growth factor (EGF), epithelial cell growth factor (EGR), and hepatocyte growth factor (HGF). These growth factors can promote the healing of bone and soft tissues [1–3]. Spinal fusion is a commonly performed procedure in the treatment of spinal instability due to different spinal pathologies. Despite the current advanced techniques in spinal fusion, failure of fusion and pseudarthrosis are still the main challenges. Therefore, additional materials such as bone graft extenders and biologics such as PRP are employed during spinal fusion surgery to enhance fusion [4, 5].

The use of PRP has been very successful in enhancing spinal fusion in an animal model [6, 7]. Also, PRP has been broadly and efficaciously used in other specialties of medicine such as oral dentistry, dermatology, ophthalmology, and sports medicine [8]. But the use of PRP to augment bone fusion after spinal deformity correction in humans is still controversial; Kubota et al. [9] in their prospective randomized control trial of posterolateral lumbar fusion surgery found a high fusion rate in the PRP group compared to control. Tarantino et al. [10] in their prospective cohort study of 21 patients who underwent posterolateral arthrodesis with implantation of cancellous bone substitute soaked with PRP found that PRP increases the rate of fusion and bone density adding osteoinductive and osteoconductive effect. Also, Hartmann et al. [11] in their 15 controlled cohort patients who underwent anterior spinal fusion after suffering lumbar or spinal injury found that PRP increased the rate of fusion and high-density value within the region of fusion compared to control. On the other hand, Feiz-Erfan et al. [12] in their double-blind randomized study with platelet-gel concentrate or control group of 50 patients undergoing anterior cervical microdiscectomy, allograft fusion, and plating found that platelet-gel concentrate had no consistent effect in promoting early fusion in cervical disc disease relative to control. Carreon et al. [13] in their retrospective cohort study of 76 patients who underwent posterolateral lumbar fusion with autologous iliac crest bone graft mixed with autologous growth factor (AGF) and control found a high nonunion rate in the AGF group compared to control. Also, Jenis et al. [14] in their prospective study of patients undergoing lumbar spinal fusion using iliac crest autograft and allograft combined with autogenous growth factors (AGF) found a similar outcome in terms of bone fusion, pain, and functional improvement between the two groups.

Therefore, the aim of this study is to investigate the role of PRP in promoting bone fusion after spinal surgery in humans, by using available published studies through meta-analysis.

2. Methods

2.1. Eligibility Criteria. Included articles had the following inclusion criteria: (1) studies conducted in humans evaluating spinal fusion; (2) studies comparing the outcome between PRP and control subject; (3) studies evaluating spinal fusion by either radiograph or computed tomography (CT); (4) the sample size was bigger than 10; (5) only retrospective/prospective studies published in English; and (6) no geographic restriction was set.

Exclusion criteria are as follows: (1) case reports and review studies; (2) studies based on animal research or cadaveric research; (3) studies that did not evaluate spinal fusion; and (4) studies that did have control subjects.

2.2. Information Sources. Three online databases, PubMed, EMBASE, and the Cochrane Library, were searched to come up with the list of eligible included studies. No date range customization of searches was set. Corresponding authors of articles searched could be contacted to provide further information or settle unclear explanations. Secondary referencing of eligible studies was done to extend the scope of the searches. The online databases were accessed via the Central South University Library's website: http://lib.csu.edu.cn/.

2.3. Study Search. To generate a set of citations that are relevant to our study's search question, an advanced search tool was used in all of the three databases previously mentioned. Free text words, as well as MeSH terms, were used to search. Using PubMed, advanced search builder was customized to "Title," "*human species*," and different combinations of free text words were run for search: "*cervical vertebrae*," "*thoracic vertebrae*," "*lumbar vertebrae*," "*platelet-rich plasma*," and "*spinal fusion*" connected by "AND." The searches were independently performed by two authors; differences of thought were settled through discussion with the third author. Results were exported to computer software, EndNote X9 (Bld 12062), which was used to manage and keep track of references throughout the study.

2.4. Study Selection Process. All studies resulting from online database search independently conducted by two authors were screened by their titles and abstracts to initially assess their relevance to our study question and grossly irrelevant articles were discarded. This was level-one screening and was done by the same two authors: Daudi Manini and Frank Shega. Compiled search results of level-one screening were then searched for their full-text articles from which eligibility for inclusion or exclusion was sought. Any differences of thoughts in the search process were settled by Wang YuXiang. The study search and selection process are summarized in Figure 1.

2.5. Data Extraction. Data from included articles were extracted by Daudi and Frank independently. Disagreements were solved through discussion with Wangyuxiang. Data extracted from each of the included studies were as follows: study title, author, and year of publication, the number of participants, study design, the region of spinal fusion, the material used for bone fusion, follow-up time, and tools used to assess bone fusion between PRP and control group; the number of bone fusion and the time to bone fusion between PRP and control; and means and standard deviation of the newly formed bone within the region of interest (ROI) in terms of density expressed as Hounsfield unit (HU) and visual analog score (VAS) for pain between PRP and control groups.

2.6. Quality Assessment. The quality assessment of the 14 included studies was done independently by two authors, and disagreement was solved through discussion with the 3rd author. All included studies scored more than 8 stars on the Newcastle–Ottawa scale (NOS). This means the quality of all included studies was high. The results for the NOS score for each study are summarized in Table 1.

2.7. Statistical Analysis. The Review Manager software (RevMan 5.3, The Cochrane Collaboration, Oxford, UK) was used to perform statistical analysis. Continuous variables were reported as mean difference (MD) and 95% confidence interval (95% CI), while dichotomous data were presented as odds ratio (OR) and 95% CI. A random-effects model was used for heterogeneous data ($I^2 \geq 50\%$ for heterogeneity

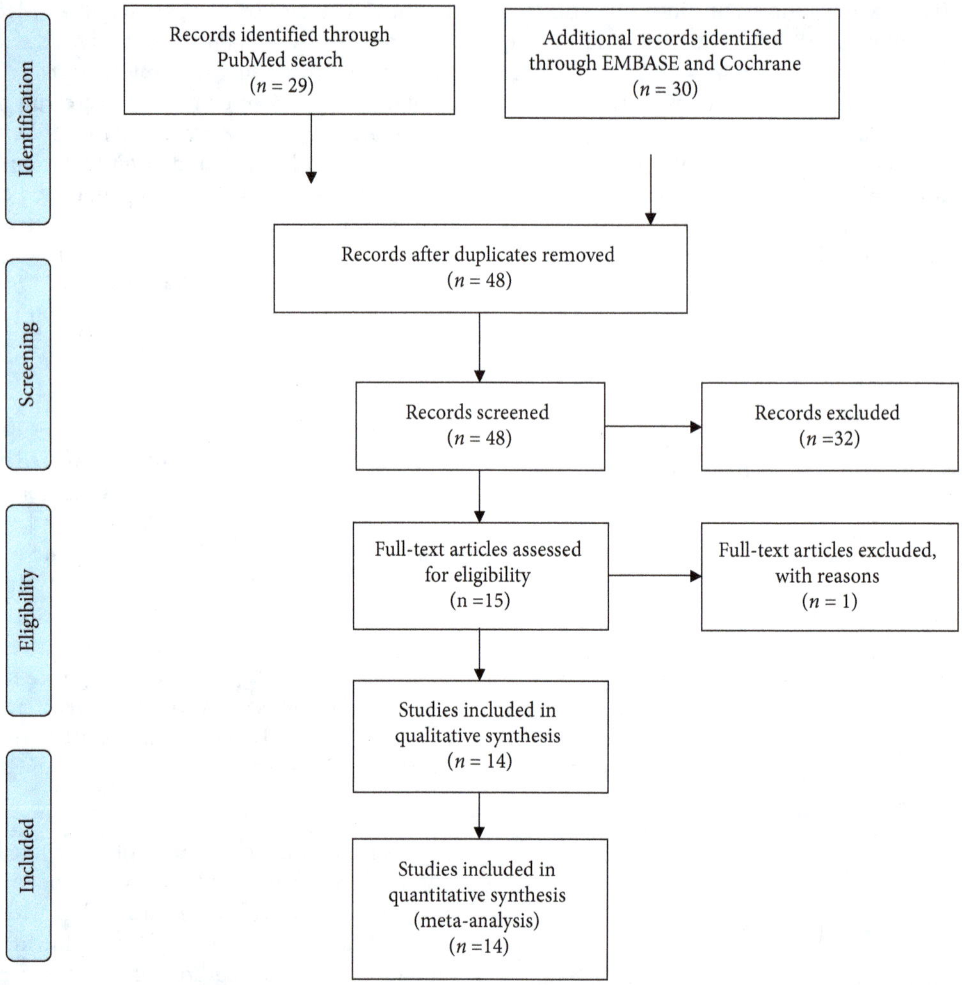

FIGURE 1: Study selection process according to PRISMA guidelines.

TABLE 1: Quality assessment of the included studies according to the Newcastle–Ottawa scale.

References	Selection	Comparability	Outcome	Total
Kubota et al. [15]	3	2	4	9
Kubota et al. [9]	3	2	4	9
Tarantino et al. [10]	3	1	4	8
Sys et al. [16]	3	1	4	8
Land et al. [17]	4	1	4	9
Tsai et al. [18]	4	1	3	8
Hartmann et al. [11]	4	2	3	9
Feiz-Erfan et al. [12]	4	2	3	9
Jenis et al. [14]	4	1	3	8
Carreon et al. [13]	4	2	3	9
Castro[19]	4	2	3	9
Hee et al. [20]	4	2	3	9
Weiner and walker [21]	4	2	3	9
Imagama et al. [2]	4	2	3	9

test). Collected data were entered into the computer and rechecked by two authors.

Some articles did not provide the change values and their standard deviation (SD) from preoperation to postoperation, but reported data before and after surgery, respectively. To get the data we needed, we consulted the authors for the data. And in articles that gave raw data, we computed the mean and standard deviation by IBM SPSS statistic 21 version software.

2.8. Assumptions and Simplifications. All participants, despite study countries' economic status and technological differences, were considered to have received standard surgical care.

3. Results

3.1. Study Selection. Eligible included studies were prospective and retrospective cohort comparing mean differences between PRP and control by measuring the rate of new bone formation in terms of HU and pain reduction in terms of VAS and also, the number of bone fusion and the time to bone fusion in terms of OR between the two groups at the final follow-up.

A total of 59 studies were obtained from 3 online databases. Study search from PubMed resulted in 29 studies, EMBASE resulted in 22 studies, and COCHRANE resulted in 8 studies. After the removal of 11 studies which were

Table 2: Characteristics of included studies.

Studies	Study design	Fusion type	Conc of PLT in PRP	Preparation of PRP	Material used	Sex (m/f)	Follow-up time (months)	Evaluation
1. Kubota et al. [15]	Retrospective case series	Lumbar PLF	8.7	400 mL of peripheral blood centrifuged. Buffy coat isolated. The second centrifugation done. 22 mL mixed with calcium chloride.	Local bone, CA, PRP ($n=11$) Local bone CA ($n=9$)	10/10	24	CT
2. Kubota et al. [9]	Prospective	Lumbar PLF	7.7	400 mL of peripheral blood centrifuged. Buffy-coat isolated. The second centrifugation done. 22 mL mixed with calcium chloride.	ABG lamina, PRP ($n=25$) ABG lamina ($n=25$)	29/21	24	Radiograph, CT
3.Tarantino et al. [10]	Prospective cohort	Lumbar PLF	Not measured	Venous blood centrifuged at 3100 rpm for 8 minutes. Buff coat removed. Platelets were suspended in plasma while shaking the tubes and were ready for use.	Heterologous bone, PRP ($n=20$) Heterologous bone ($n=20$)	8/12	6	CT
4. Sys et al. [16]	Prospective	Lumbar IF	Not measured	54 mL of peripheral blood put in SymphonyTM Platelet Concentration System (DePuy, Johnson & Johnson).	CA, ABG iliac, PRP ($n=19$) CA, ABG iliac ($n=19$)	24/14	12	Radiograph, CT
5. Land et al. [17]	Retrospective	Thoracic or lumbar IF	5	16 mL of peripheral blood in REGEN-THT_ (thrombocyte harvesting tube) followed by the addition of Ca gluconate and ethanol.	ABG local bone, PRP ($n=14$) ABG local bone ($n=14$)	9/5	6	Radiograph CT
6. Tsai et al. [18]	Prospective	Lumbar PLF	Not measured	10 mL of FFP mixed with calcium chloride. Mixture shaken for 30 minutes and ready for use.	ABG lamina PRP ($n=33$) ABG lamina ($n=34$)	17/50	24	Radiograph, CT
7. Hartmann et al. [11]	Prospective	Lumbar or thoracic PLF	Not measured	110 mL PVB in Gravitational Platelet Separation (GPS™) System mixed with thrombin.	CA, ABG fracture, PRP ($n=15$) CA, ABG fracture ($n=20$)	23/12	8	CT
8. Feiz-Erfan et al. [12]	Prospective	Cervical IF	Not measured	Anticoagulated blood put in Symphony (DePuy, Johnson & Johnson).	Cortical allograft bone, PRP ($n=42$) Cortical allograft bone alone ($n=39$)	21/29	24	Radiograph
9. Jenis et al. [14]	Prospective	Lumbar PLF	Not measured	450 mL PVB in centrifuge. Buffy coat mixed with thrombin.	Allograft bone, PRP($n=15$) ABG iliac bone ($n=22$)	24/13	24	Radiographic CT

Table 2: Continued.

Studies	Study design	Fusion type	Conc of PLT in PRP	Preparation of PRP	Material used	Sex (m/f)	Follow-up time (months)	Evaluation
10. Carreon et al. [13]	Retrospective cohort study	Lumbar PLF	Not measured	500 mL PVB, in a centrifuge. A buffy coat mixed with calcium chloride.	ABG iliac, PRP ($n = 76$) ABG iliac alone ($n = 76$)	40/36	24	Radiographic CT
11. Castro et al. [19]	Retrospective	TLIF	3.5	1 unit of PVB in centrifuge. A buffy coat mixed thrombin	AGF, iliac bone ($n = 22$) iliac bone ($n = 62$)	27/57	41	Radiograph
12. Hee et al. [20]	Prospective	Lumbar PLF	4.89	450 cc of WB in centrifuge buffy coat mixed with thrombin	CA, ABG iliac ($n = 23$) ABG iliac ($n = 111$)	50/84	24	Radiograph
13. Weiner and Walker [21]	Retrospective	Lumbar PLF	Not measured	From 1 unit of arterial blood, buffy coat collected and put in ultraconcentrator. Thrombin was added and the PRP was ready for use.	ABG iliac PRP($n = 32$) ABG iliac ($n = 27$)	24/35	12	Radiograph
14. Imagama et al. [2]	Prospective	Lumbar PLF	7.74	400 mL of WB put in centrifuge for 15 minutes, buffy coat collected. Buffy coat put in centrifuge again for 15 minutes followed by the addition of thrombin.	ABG local bone and PRP($n = 29$) ABG local bone ($n = 29$)	11/18	120	CT

CA = cage; PRP = platelet-rich plasma; ABG = autogenous bone graft; CT = computed tomography; IF = interbody fusion; PLF = posterolateral fusion; TLIF = transforaminal lumbar interbody fusion; PVB = peripheral venous blood; WB = whole blood; PLT = platelet; Conc = concentration.

duplicates, 48 studies were identified for screening. After reading abstract and title, 32 studies were irrelevant, and thus, 15 studies were sought for their full texts. After reading full texts of 15 studies, 1 study did not meet the eligibility criteria for our study. 14 studies were selected and included in our meta-analysis. The characteristics of the included studies are summarized in Table 2.

3.2. Study Bias. Bias in the included studies was assessed by NOS. NOS is approved by Cochrane Handbook version 5.1 to assess bias in observational studies.

In terms of study design, 5 studies were retrospective cohort [13, 15, 17, 19, 21] and 9 studies [2, 9, 11, 12, 14, 16–18, 20] were prospective. Generally, prospective studies have less bias compared to retrospective studies. The sample size from all included studies was small and none of them calculated the sample size before the conduction of the study. The smaller the sample size, the lesser the representative of the general population. Different techniques and fusion materials were used in spinal fusion surgery. Some surgeons employed PLF, TLIF, or IF as shown in Table 2.

3.3. Bone Fusion. The data for bone fusion were available in 10 studies as shown in Figure 2 from which one study [19] used a low platelet concentration in PRP (3.5 higher than the peripheral blood) and the 6 studies did not report the platelet concentration in their PRP [11–14, 18, 21]. The bone fusion in these seven studies was poor in the PRP group compared to control (odds ratio (OR): 0.55 at 95% CI (0.36, 0.83) and $P = 0.005$). Three studies [9, 15, 20] used a high platelet concentration in the PRP, 5 times higher than peripheral blood. The rate of bone fusion in the PRP group was excellent relative to the control group (OR = 4.35, 95% CI (2.15, 8.85), and $P = 0.0001$).

But the total effect of PRP on bone fusion in all 10 studies was poor compared to the control group (OR = 0.96, 95% CI (0.48, 1.96), and $I^2 = 95.9$) with high heterogeneity.

3.4. The Density of the Newly Formed Bone in ROI. The data for the density of the newly formed bone in ROI in HU between PRP and control groups were available in 4 studies [2, 10, 11, 17] as shown in Figure 3. The rate of newly formed bone mass was high in the PRP group compared to the control group, and the results are statistically significant with the mean difference of 144.91 (95% CI (80.63–209.18), $I^2 = 77\%$, and $P < 0.05$)

3.5. Time to Bone Fusion. The data for time to the bone fusion between PRP and control groups were available in 3 studies [9, 11, 15] as shown in Figure 4. There was less time for a bone fusion in the PRP group compared to control. The results are statistically significant with a mean difference of −2.05 (95% CI (−2.35–1.70); $P < 0.05$).

3.6. Pain. The data for the analysis of pain in terms of VAS were available in 3 studies [14–16] as shown in Figure 5. There was no statistical difference in pain reduction between the PRP and the control groups at the final follow-up. The mean VAS score was −0.64 (95% CI (−1.87–0.59), $I^2 = 75\%$, and $P = 0.31$).

4. Discussion

The use of PRP has been very successful in enhancing spinal fusion in an animal model [6, 7]. Also, PRP has been broadly and efficaciously used in other specialties of medicine such as oral dentistry, dermatology, ophthalmology, and sports medicine [8]. But the use of PRP to augment bone fusion after spinal deformity correction in humans is still controversial. Some scholars advocate the use of PRP to facilitate bone fusion during spinal surgery while other scholars are against the use of PRP to facilitate spinal fusion.

In our meta-analysis, we found that PRP promotes bone fusion when the concentration of platelet is very high. All researchers [2, 9, 15, 20], who used high platelet concentration in PRP, 5 times higher in the peripheral blood, found superior bone fusion in PRP compared to control. But the researcher in [19] who used a low platelet concentration in PRP found no difference in bone fusion rate between the PRP and control groups. The bone fusion rate in the PRP group was also poor in studies [11, 12, 14, 18, 20, 21] which did not measure the concentration of platelet in PRP relative to that of the baseline. Probably, the concentration of platelet in their PRP was not higher than 4- to 5-fold above the peripheral blood which has been reported in the literature to cause a stimulatory effect [5]. Kubota et al. [9] in their prospective study of 31 patients in both PRP and control groups, who underwent posterolateral lumbar fusion with local bone graft and PRP or local bone graft alone, used platelet concentration 7.7 times high in PRP and growth factor concentration 50 times higher than that of the plasma, and they found excellent bone fusion in PRP relative to the control group. Both the positive and negative effects of PRP in promoting bone fusion in animal and clinical research have been reported. Furthermore, it was argued that PRP had stimulating effects if the concentration of the platelet counts and that of the growth factor in PRP are extremely higher than those in the peripheral blood. Also, PRP does not continue to provide stimulatory effects for a long period of time. Hence, the amount and concentration of platelet in PRP in large-sized animals like humans being or to the tissue that takes a long time to regenerate like bone must be increased [22, 23]. This hypothesis has been proved in this meta-analysis.

In this study, we found that PRP is superior in promoting new bone formation compared to control. The data of new bone formation in the ROI were available in four studies [2, 10, 11, 17]. There was a statistically significant difference between the two groups ($P < 0.05$). Heterogeneity was high probably because of the different surgical techniques and material used during surgical fusion. This result is similar to what has been reported by other scholars. Imagama et al. [2] in their prospective clinical study of 29 patients in both experimental and control, who underwent PLF with both local bone and PRP in experimental and local bone only in control, found that the rate of bone formation in control was higher in the experiment group at 3 and 6 months of follow-up than control. The authors found no differences in bone formation between the two groups during the 12 months of follow-up. Also, in Hee et al.'s retrospective study [20], 23 patients who underwent transforaminal lumbar interbody fusion (TLIF) with AGF and autograft were compared with 111 control patients, who underwent TLIF with autograft alone. Radiographic assessment for bone fusion was done at 4, 6, and 24 months of follow-up time; more rapid incorporation of bone fusion was observed at 4 and 6 months in AGF patients; and during 24 months of assessment, no significant differences in bone fusion rate were found between the two groups. And the authors concluded that AGF was able to promote graft incorporation, hence speeding up faster fusion.

In this study, we also found that time to bone fusion was short in the PRP group compared to the control group. This finding is similar to what has been reported by other scholars. Tarantino et al. [10] found that PRP fastens bone fusion in PLF surgery by measuring bone density in the fusion area using CT scan on 20 patients who underwent PLF surgery with cancellous bone soaked with PRP and saline on right and left sides, respectively. Also, Imagama et al. [2] observed a fast bone fusion rate at 3 and 6 months after surgery, and authors found no difference in the bone fusion between PRP and control groups during 12 months of follow-up. On long-time follow-up, there was no difference in bone fusion between PRP and control groups, possibly because PRP does not continue to provide stimulatory effect for a long period of time [22, 24].

Our meta-analysis did not find any statistically significant difference in pain score during the final follow-up between the PRP and control groups. This is similar to what has been reported by other scholars. Kubota et al. [15] in their retrospective case series of 20 patients who underwent TLIF with local bone graft with PRP and local bone graft alone in the control group found no significant difference in lower back pain, leg pain, and leg numbness between the two groups at the final follow-up. Also, Sys et al. [16] in their retrospective study of 38 patients who underwent posterior stabilization with autograft addition to PRP and autograft alone in the control group found improvement of VAS in both groups, but the difference was not statistically significant between the groups at the final follow-up.

Our meta-analysis has several limitations, the sample space and the number of the included articles were few, and none of them calculated the sample size prior to the conduction of the study. There was variability among studies

Study or subgroup	PRP group Events	PRP group Total	Control group Events	Control group Total	Weight (%)	Odds ratio M-H, random, 95% CI
3.2.1 unknown concentration of platelet in PRP or low platelet concentration in PRP relative to peripheral blood						
Carreon et al 2005	57	76	63	76	12.9	0.55 [0.04, 0.57]
Castro 2004	10	28	42	76	12.3	0.45 [0.18, 1.10]
Feiz-erfan et al 2007	23	42	25	39	12.3	0.68 [0.28, 1.66]
Hartmann et al 2009	6	15	8	20	9.6	1.00 [0.25, 3.92]
jenis et al 2006	13	15	19	22	7.0	1.03 [0.15, 7.02]
Tsai et al 2009	29	34	30	33	8.8	0.58 [0.13, 2.65]
Weiner and Walker 2003	17	32	24	27	9.5	0.14 [0.04, 0.57]
Subtotal (95% CI)		*242*		*293*	*72.4*	*0.55 [0.04, 0.57]*
Total events	155		211			
Heterogeneity: $tau^2 = 0.00$; $Chi^2 = 5.33$, $df = 6$ ($P = 0.50$); $I^2 = 0\%$						
Test for overall effect: $Z = 2.83$ ($P = 0.005$)						
3.2.2 High platelet concentration in PRP, more than 5 times that of peripherial blood						
Heel et al 2003	13	23	40	111	11.9	4.06 [1.54, 10.69]
Kubota et al 2017	60	64	52	70	10.8	5.19 [1.65, 16.32]
Kubota et al 2018	10	11	7	9	4.9	2.86 [0.21, 37.99]
Subtotal (95% CI)		*98*		*190*	*27.6*	*4.35 [2.31, 8.85]*
Total events	86		99			
Heterogeneity: $tau^2 = 0.00$; $Chi^2 = 0.21$, $df = 2$ ($P = 0.90$); $I^2 = 0\%$						
Test for overall effect: $Z = 4.05$ ($P < 0.0001$)						
Total (95% CI)		*340*		*483*	*100.0*	*0.96 [0.48, 1.91]*
Total events	241		310			
Heterogeneity: $tau^2 = 0.80$; $Chi^2 = 29.79$, $df = 9$ ($P = 0.0005$); $I^2 = 70\%$						
Test for overall effect: $Z = 0.13$ ($P = 0.90$)						
Test for subgroup differences: $Chi^2 = 24.23$, $df = 1$ ($P < 0.00001$), $I^2 = 95.9\%$						

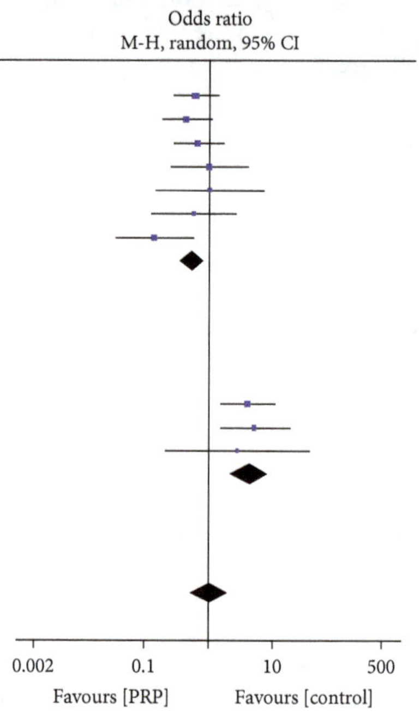

FIGURE 2: Forest plot for bone fusion between the PRP and control groups at the final follow-up.

Study or subgroup	PRP Mean	PRP SD	PRP Total	Control Mean	Control SD	Control Total	Weight (%)	Mean difference IV, random, 95% CI
Hartmann et al 2009	63.9	40	12	514.2	32.2	14	38.9	125.50 [97.27, 153.73]
Imagama et al 2017	88.7	266.5	29	73	268.1	29	14.4	15.70 [−121.88, 153.28]
Land et al 2011	558.19	238.35	14	345.7	238.88	14	10.1	212.49 [35.72, 389.26]
Tarantinol et al 2014	830.353	61.8	20	632.89	59.5	20	36.7	197.46 [159.87, 235.06]
Total (95% CI)			*75*			*77*	*100.0*	*144.91 [80.63, 209.18]*
Heterogeneity: $tau^2 = 2560$; $Chi^2 = 13.15$, $df = 3$ ($P = 0.004$); $I^2 = 77\%$								
Test for overall effect: $Z = 4.42$ ($P < 0.00001$)								

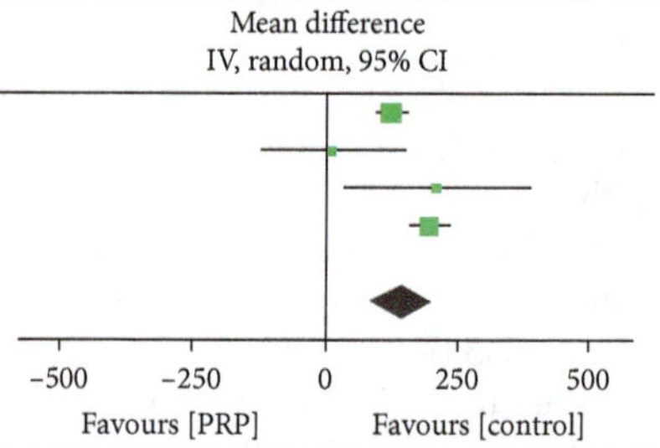

FIGURE 3: Forest plot for analysis of the newly formed bone in (HU) in ROI between the PRP and control groups.

Study or subgroup	PRP Mean	PRP SD	PRP Total	Control Mean	Control SD	Control Total	Weight (%)	Mean difference IV, random, 95% CI
Hartmann et al 2009	8.31	3.63	17	12	8.7	20	0.6	−3.69 [−7.88, 0.50]
Kubota et al 2017	7.8	0.6	25	9.58	0.6	25	93.9	−2.00 [−2.33, −1.67]
Kubota et al 2018	7.7	0.74	11	10	2	9	5.5	−2.30 [−3.68, −0.92]
Total (95% CI)			*53*			*54*	*100.0*	*−2.30 [−2.35, −1.70]*
Heterogeneity: $tau^2 = 0.00$; $Chi^2 = 0.78$, $df = 2$ ($P = 0.68$); $I^2 = 0\%$								
Test for overall effect: $Z = 12.32$ ($P < 0.00001$)								

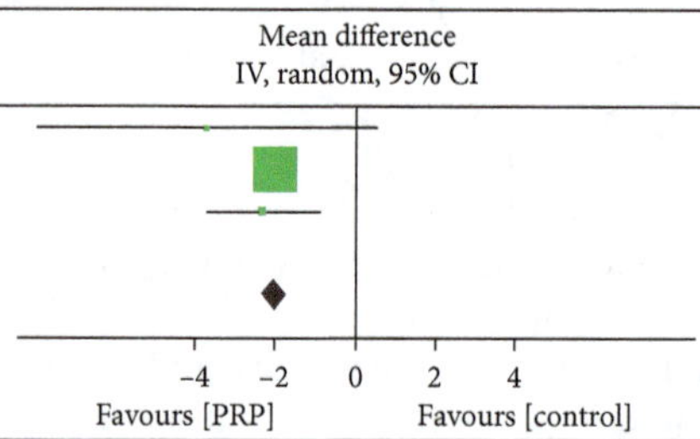

FIGURE 4: Forest plot for time to bone fusion in months between the PRP and control groups.

Study or subgroup	PRP Mean	PRP SD	PRP Total	Control Mean	Control SD	Control Total	Weight (%)	Mean difference IV, random, 95% CI
Jenis et al 2006	4.8	3.2	15	4.7	3	22	20.5	0.10 [−1.95, 2.15]
Kubota et al 2018	2	0.5	11	3.5	0.6	9	44.3	−1.50 [−1.99, −1.01]
Sys et al 2011	7.4	1.9	19	7.4	1.4	19	35.2	0.00 [−1.06, 1.06]
Total (95% CI)			*45*			*50*	*100.0*	*−0.64 [−1.87, 0.59]*
Heterogeneity: $tau^2 = 0.83$; $Chi^2 = 7.88$, $df = 2$ ($P = 0.02$); $I^2 = 75\%$								
Test for overall effect: $Z = 1.03$ ($P = 0.31$)								

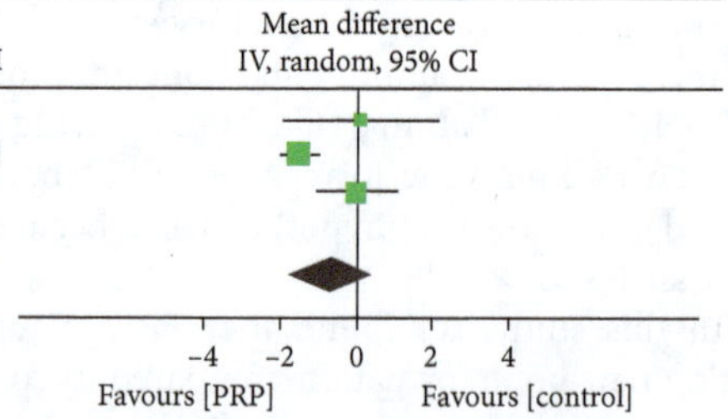

FIGURE 5: Forest plot for analysis of pain at the final follow-up in terms of VAS between the PRP and control groups.

with respect to surgical technique, methods of preparation of PRP, concentration of platelet in PRP, and dosage as well as the carrier of PRP. Furthermore, there was variability in terms of follow-up time among the included study. All these reduce the overall quality of its evidence.

The main finding of this meta-analysis is as follows: PRP promotes bone fusion and new bone formation well within 6 months of implantation, and after 6 months, the effect normalizes. Also, a minimum concentration of platelet in PRP, 5 times higher than that in the peripheral blood, has a stimulatory effect on bone fusion. This is clinically significant because it advocates that PRP could be employed to fasten postoperative recovery and hence shorten the time for rehabilitation and the use of orthopedic devices. Also, PRP is less expensive and easy to prepare and has no risk of disease transmission. We suggest future studies to focus much on the stable carrier of PRP which allows the continuous release of growth factor to the local tissue for a long period, optimal implantation time, frequency of implantation, and bioavailability of the growth factors.

5. Conclusion

PRP facilitates new bone formation and bone fusion with a minimum concentration of the growth factor 5 times that of the peripheral blood. PRP stimulatory effects are well effective within 6 months of implantation.

References

[1] G. Weibrich, W. K. G. Kleis, G. Hafner, and W. E. Hitzler, "Growth factor levels in platelet-rich plasma and correlations with donor age, sex, and platelet count," *Journal of Cranio-Maxillofacial Surgery*, vol. 30, no. 2, pp. 97–102, 2002.

[2] S. Imagama, K. Ando, K. Kobayashi et al., "Efficacy of early fusion with local bone graft and platelet-rich plasma in lumbar spinal fusion surgery followed over 10 years," *Global Spine Journal*, vol. 7, no. 8, pp. 749–755, 2017.

[3] B. D. Elder, C. Holmes, C. R. Goodwin et al., "A systematic assessment of the use of platelet-rich plasma in spinal fusion," *Annals of Biomedical Engineering*, vol. 43, no. 5, pp. 1057–1070, 2015.

[4] W. K. Hsu, R. E. Hashimoto, S. H. Berven, and A. Nassr, "Biological substitutes/extenders for spinal arthrodesis," *Spine (Phila Pa 1976)*, vol. 39, no. 22, pp. S86–98, 2014.

[5] R. E. Marx, E. R. Carlson, R. M. Eichstaedt, S. R. Schimmele, J. E. Strauss, and K. R. Georgeff, "Platelet-rich plasma," *Oral Surgery, Oral Medicine, Oral Pathology, Oral Radiology, and Endodontology*, vol. 85, no. 6, pp. 638–646, 1998.

[6] H. Kamoda, S. Ohtori, T. Ishikawa et al., "The effect of platelet-rich plasma on posterolateral lumbar fusion in a rat model," *The Journal of Bone and Joint Surgery-American Volume*, vol. 95, no. 12, pp. 1109–1116, 2013.

[7] H. Kamoda, "Platelet-rich plasma combined with hydroxyapatite for lumbar interbody fusion promoted bone formation and decreased an inflammatory pain neuropeptide in rats," *Spine (Phila Pa 1976)*, vol. 37, no. 20, pp. 1727–1733, 2012.

[8] I. Andia and M. Abate, "Platelet-rich plasma: underlying biology and clinical correlates," *Regenerative Medicine*, vol. 8, no. 5, pp. 645–658, 2013.

[9] G. Kubota, H. Kamoda, S. Orita et al., "Platelet-rich plasma enhances bone union in posterolateral lumbar fusion: a prospective randomized controlled trial," *The Spine Journal*, vol. 19, no. 2, pp. e34–e40, 2019.

[10] R. Tarantino, P. Donnarumma, C. Mancarella et al., "Posterolateral arthrodesis in lumbar spine surgery using autologous platelet-rich plasma and cancellous bone substitute: an osteoinductive and osteoconductive effect," *Global Spine Journal*, vol. 4, no. 3, pp. 137–141, 2014.

[11] E. K. Hartmann, T. Heintel, R. H. Morrison, and A. Weckbach, "Influence of platelet-rich plasma on the anterior fusion in spinal injuries: a qualitative and quantitative analysis using computer tomography," *Archives of Orthopaedic and Trauma Surgery*, vol. 130, no. 7, pp. 909–914, 2010.

[12] I. Feiz-Erfan, M. Harrigan, V. K. H. Sonntag, and T. R. Harrington, "Effect of autologous platelet gel on early and late graft fusion in anterior cervical spine surgery," *Journal of Neurosurgery: Spine*, vol. 7, no. 5, pp. 496–502, 2007.

[13] L. Y. Carreon, S. D. Glassman, Y. Anekstein, and R. M. Puno, "Platelet gel (AGF) fails to increase fusion rates in instrumented posterolateral fusions," *Spine*, vol. 30, no. 9, pp. E243–E246, 2005.

[14] L. G. Jenis, R. J. Banco, and B. Kwon, "A prospective study of autologous growth factors (AGF) in lumbar interbody fusion," *The Spine Journal*, vol. 6, no. 1, pp. 14–20, 2006.

[15] G. Kubota, H. Kamoda, S. Orita et al., "Efficacy of platelet-rich plasma for bone fusion in transforaminal lumbar interbody fusion," *Asian Spine Journal*, vol. 12, no. 1, pp. 112–118, 2018.

[16] J. Sys, J. Weyler, T. Van Der Zijden, P. Parizel, and J. Michielsen, "Platelet-rich plasma in mono-segmental posterior lumbar interbody fusion," *European Spine Journal*, vol. 20, no. 10, pp. 1650–1657, 2011.

[17] A. Landi, R. Tarantino, N. Marotta et al., "The use of platelet gel in postero-lateral fusion: preliminary results in a series of 14 cases," *European Spine Journal*, vol. 20, no. 1, pp. S61–S67, 2011.

[18] C.-H. Tsai, H.-C. Hsu, Y.-J. Chen, M.-J. Lin, and H.-T. Chen, "Using the growth factors-enriched platelet glue in spinal fusion and its efficiency," *Journal of Spinal Disorders & Techniques*, vol. 22, no. 4, pp. 246–250, 2009.

[19] F. P. Castro Jr., "Role of activated growth factors in lumbar spinal fusions," *Journal of Spinal Disorders & Techniques*, vol. 17, no. 5, pp. 380–384, 2004.

[20] H. T. Hee, M. E. Majd, R. T. Holt, and L. Myers, "Do autologous growth factors enhance transforaminal lumbar interbody fusion?" *European Spine Journal*, vol. 12, no. 4, pp. 400–407, 2003.

[21] B. K. Weiner and M. Walker, "Efficacy of autologous growth factors in lumbar intertransverse fusions," *Spine (Phila Pa 1976)*, vol. 28, no. 17, pp. 1968–1970, 2003.

[22] M. S. Park, "Platelet-rich plasma for the spinal fusion," *Journal of Orthopaedic Surgery (Hong Kong)*, vol. 26, no. 1, p. 2309499018755772, 2018.

[23] A. Grassi, F. Napoli, I. Romandini et al., "Is platelet-rich plasma (PRP) effective in the treatment of acute muscle injuries? A systematic review and meta-analysis," *Sports Medicine*, vol. 48, no. 4, pp. 971–989, 2018.

[24] M. Formica, L. Cavagnaro, C. Formica, M. Mastrogiacomo, M. Basso, and A. Di Martino, "What is the preclinical evidence on platelet rich plasma and intervertebral disc degeneration?" *European Spine Journal*, vol. 24, no. 11, pp. 2377–2386, 2015.

8

A Novel Spine Fixation System Made Entirely of Carbon-Fiber-Reinforced PEEK Composite: An In Vitro Mechanical Evaluation

Ofir Uri, Yoram Folman, Gil Laufer, and Eyal Behrbalk

Department of Orthopedic Surgery, Hillel Yaffe Medical Center, Hadera, Israel

Correspondence should be addressed to Ofir Uri; ofiruri@gmail.com

Academic Editor: Andreas K. Demetriades

Background. Semirigid spine fixation systems utilizing nonmetallic materials have emerged as a promising innovation to overcome the inherent disadvantages of metal instrumentation in spine surgery. This study tests the mechanical properties of a novel spine fixation system made entirely of carbon-fiber-reinforced PEEK (CFR-PEEK) composite material (CarboClear System, CarboFix Orthopedics Ltd., Israel). *Methods.* An in vitro mechanical evaluation of the CFR-PEEK CarboClear system was conducted in compliance with the American Society for Testing and Materials (ASTM) F1717, F2193, and F543 standards. *Results.* The mean bending yield load, bending ultimate load, and bending stiffness of the construct were 322 N, 363 N, and 45 N/mm, respectively. All tested samples completed 5×10^6 dynamic cycles successfully, with no evidence of fatigue failure at increasing load levels, up to 83% of ultimate bending load. The mean torsional stiffness was 1.0 Nm/deg and the mean screw axial pull-out strength was 2,037 N. *Conclusion.* The CarboClear Pedicle Screw System has mechanical properties comparable to those of other commonly used titanium-made systems, with superior fatigue properties. The fatigue resistance, modulus of elasticity which is very similar to that of bone, radiolucency, and CT/MRI artifact-free feature of this spine fixation system made entirely of CFR-PEEK may offer advantages over traditional spine fixation systems made of metal alloys.

1. Introduction

The use of rigid metal instrumentation in spine surgery has become common practice over recent decades [1]. Although such instrumentation has dramatically increased the union rate in spinal fusion [2, 3], evidence suggests that the stiffness of the metallic implants used far exceeds the requirements for successful fusion and may lead to postoperative complications such as adjacent level degeneration [4, 5], vertebral body osteopenia related to the load bearing effect of rigid instrumentation [6], and screw loosening, especially in osteoporotic patients [7]. Moreover, metal-induced scattering associated with the use of metal alloys in spinal fusion reduces the reliability of imaging modalities such as CT, MRI in the postoperative follow-up, and treatment [8].

Semirigid fixation systems that utilize nonmetallic materials were developed to address these inherent disadvantages of metal instrumentation [9]. One of the material alternatives is the thermoplastic polyetheretherketone (PEEK) biocompatible polymer. Biomechanical studies comparing rods of posterior spinal fusion systems made of Ti-alloy versus PEEK demonstrated that the PEEK-rod system provides increased load sharing along the anterior column and lower stress at the bone-screw interface. This potentially reduces the risk of adjacent level degeneration, vertebral body bone loss, and screw loosening [9, 10]. Being radiographically translucent, spinal instrumentation with rods made of PEEK interferes less with postoperative imaging, thus enabling easier radiographic follow-up at the rod area [9, 10].

A remaining disadvantage of the semirigid PEEK-rod systems is its inability to provide sufficient primary stability to allow spinal fusion due to micromovements attributed to the lower strength and modulus of elasticity of the PEEK compared to metals [8–10]. In order to provide PEEK with more strength and stiffness, a composite of PEEK-based matrix reinforced by carbon fibers (CFR-PEEK) has been introduced in orthopedic and spine surgery over the past years. It has been shown that orthopedic implants made of CFR-PEEK composite, with carbon fibers fraction of approximately 60% by volume, have mechanical properties (e.g., modulus of elasticity and fatigue strain) equivalent to that of cortical bone with promising results in spine surgery [11–14].

The CarboClear Pedicle Screw System (CarboFix Orthopedics Ltd., Herzliya, Israel) is a novel spine fixation system composed entirely of CFR-PEEK composite (i.e., rods and pedicle screws).

Preliminary reports of the CarboClear system for the treatment of spine tumors were recently published and showed outcomes comparable to the standard titanium system in terms of complications, stability, and functional scores [13, 14].

This study investigates the mechanical properties of the CarboClear system. To our knowledge, no previous study has evaluated the mechanical properties of the spine fixation system made entirely of CFR-PEEK composite. (Figure 1).

2. Materials and Methods

The study was conducted at the manufacturer's laboratories, CarboFix Orthopedics Ltd. (Herzliya, Israel), who provided financial support for the study, but was not involved in the manuscript writing and editing. All experiments were conducted under the strict protocols of the American Society for Testing and Materials (ASTM).

The CFR-PEEK specimens tested comprised 6.5 mm polyaxial pedicle screws with 6.0 mm straight rods and their locking elements. The manufacturer instructions were strictly kept throughout implant assembly.

The following mechanical tests were performed:

(1) Static axial compression bending test: the test was performed according to the ASTM F1717 standard [15], simulating a vertebrectomy model via a large gap between two ultrahigh-molecular weight polyethylene (UHMWPE) blocks simulating two vertebrae. Six CFR-PEEK constructs were tested, each comprising four pedicle screws and two rods. The apparatus included two UHMWPE blocks (with tensile breaking strength of 40 ± 3 MPa), mounted by metal hinge pins to side supports on the test machine (Testometric M350-10 kN, Testometric Ltd., UK) and attached to the actuator and to the load cell. The upper side support-upper UHMWPE block construct and the lower side support-UHMWPE block construct were aligned. The center axis of each hinge pin was perpendicular to and aligned with the load axis of the test machine. As per ASTM F1717 recommendation, the active length of the longitudinal element (rod) was set at 76 mm and the block moment arm at 40 mm (Figure 2). Loading rate was 5 mm/min. Test plots of load versus displacement were generated for each assembly tested and the mode of failure of each construct was documented.

(2) Fatigue axial compression bending test: the test was performed according to the ASTM F1717 protocol. Six CFR-PEEK constructs were tested, each comprising four pedicle screws and two rods. A similar apparatus as for the static axial compression bending test was utilized. The samples were tested using an Instron 8871 fatigue system. The samples were evaluated at a number of increased load levels (defined as a percentage of the average ultimate axial compression bending load found at the static axial compression bending test described above, i.e., 50%, 75%). The constructs were tested in phosphate-buffered saline solution at a temperature of 37°C. The cycle rate was set at 2 Hz. The endpoint of the test was defined as construct failure or completion of 5×10^6 cycles without failure. Plots of load vs. number of cycles and displacement vs. number of cycles were generated (Figure 3).

(3) Static torsion test: again, the test was performed according to the ASTM F1717 protocol, using a similar apparatus with the addition of aluminum blocks between the UHMWPE blocks and the base plate to stop rotation around the hinge pin. Four CFR-PEEK constructs were tested, each comprising four pedicle screws and two rods. The samples were tested using a tension/compression testing machine (Testometric M350-10 kN) at a rate of 6 deg/min. Plots of torque vs. angular displacement were generated for each assembly tested (Figure 4).

(4) Screw axial pull-out strength test: this test was designed to measure the axial pull-out strength of the CFR-PEEK pedicle screw and was performed according to ASTM F2193 and ASTM F543 standards [15, 16]. Four CFR-PEEK polyaxial pedicle screws (6.5 mm diameter, 35 mm length) were inserted into a rigid polyurethane foam block (density of 0.32 g/cm3), a widely used substitute to cadaveric bone with more uniform material properties [17]. The construct was mounted onto the Testometric M350-10 kN test machine. A constant tensile load was applied at a rate of 5 mm/min along the axis of the screw until the screw was released from the test block or broke (Figure 5).

3. Results

(1) Static axial compression bending test: a total of six CFR-PEEK construct samples, with 6.5 mm pedicle screws and 6.0 mm rods, were tested according to the ASTM F1717 protocol. The test results are summarized in Table 1. The failure mode for all the CFR-PEEK samples tested was rotational slip of the rod-screw link.

(2) Fatigue axial compression bending test: a total of six CFR-PEEK construct samples with 6.5 mm pedicle screws and 6.0 mm rods were tested according to the

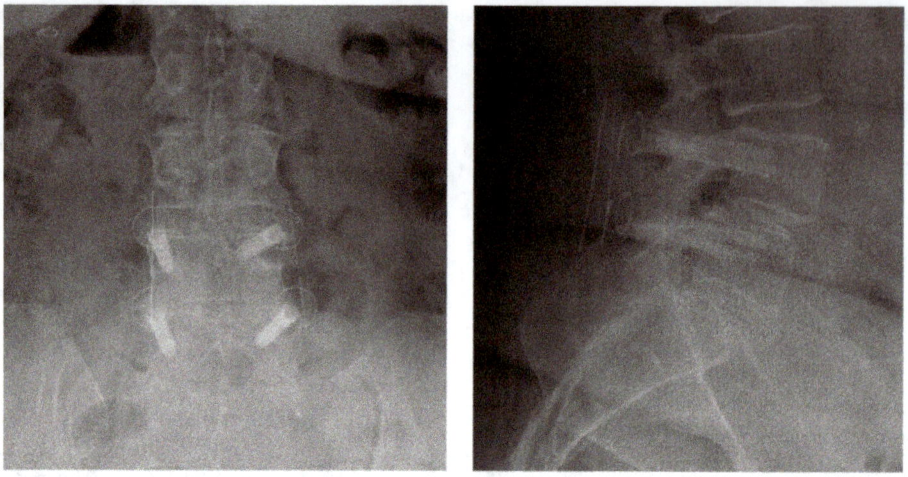

(a) (b)

Figure 1: The CarboClear spine fixation system. (a) Anterior-posterior and (b) lateral lumbar spine radiographs of a 64-year-old female at 3-year follow-up after spinal fusion with the radiolucent carbon-fiber-reinforced PEEK composite CarboClear system.

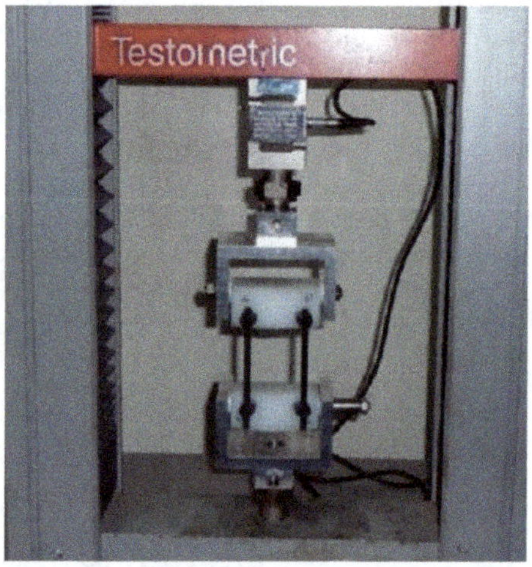

Figure 2: Static axial compression bending test performed in compliance with the ASTM F1717 standard, using a Testometric M350-10 kN testing machine, and simulating a vertebrectomy model via a large gap between two UHMWPE blocks simulating two vertebrae.

ASTM F1717 protocol. The test results are summarized in Table 2. No failure occurred at increasing load levels up to (and including) 300 N (83% of ultimate axial compression bending load) and the tested samples completed 5×10^6 cycles successfully with no evidence of fractures, loosening of interconnections, plastic deformation of components or the construct, or other signs of failure. Microscopic examination of the components surface using a digital microscope, with a magnification range of x20 to x200 (Keyence VHX-700F series, Keyence Co., IL, USA), did not reveal damage, such as cracks, delamination, or scratches. Construct measurements taken at the completion of 5×10^6 cycles revealed no change in the effective length of the rods (the center-to-center distance between two longitudinally connected locking elements remained as 76 mm), indicating that no permanent bending of the rods occurred. In all constructs, the four connections were intact, with no notable damage or loosening. The distance between the superior surface of the tulip and the rod was measured for all four interconnections in each construct and was found to be within the required range, indicating that no loosening/disassembly of the components occurred during the test. Also, the distances between the UHMWPE blocks at various points were measured for each construct, demonstrating that the blocks remained parallel to each other (i.e., indicating no slippage of the screw heads or bending of the rods has occurred). At a load level of 343 N (95% of ultimate axial compression bending load), the tested specimen failed after 150 cycles by slippage of the polyaxial screw head within the screw tulip.

(3) Static torsion test: a total of four CFR-PEEK construct samples, with 6.5 mm pedicle screws and 6.0 mm rods, were evaluated according to the ASTM F1717 standard. The results are presented in Table 3. The failure mode was slippage of the spherical screw head relative to the rod (slippage of the spherical screw head within the tulip).

(4) Screw axial pull-out strength test: a total of four samples of CFR-PEEK polyaxial pedicle screws (6.5 mm diameter, 35 mm length) were tested according to ASTM F2193 and ASTM F543 standards as applicable. Table 4 summarizes the test results. Failure in all the cases involved the polyurethane foam. No failure was detected in any of the screws.

4. Discussion

Spine fixation systems made of composite materials such as CFR-PEEK have emerged recently as promising innovations

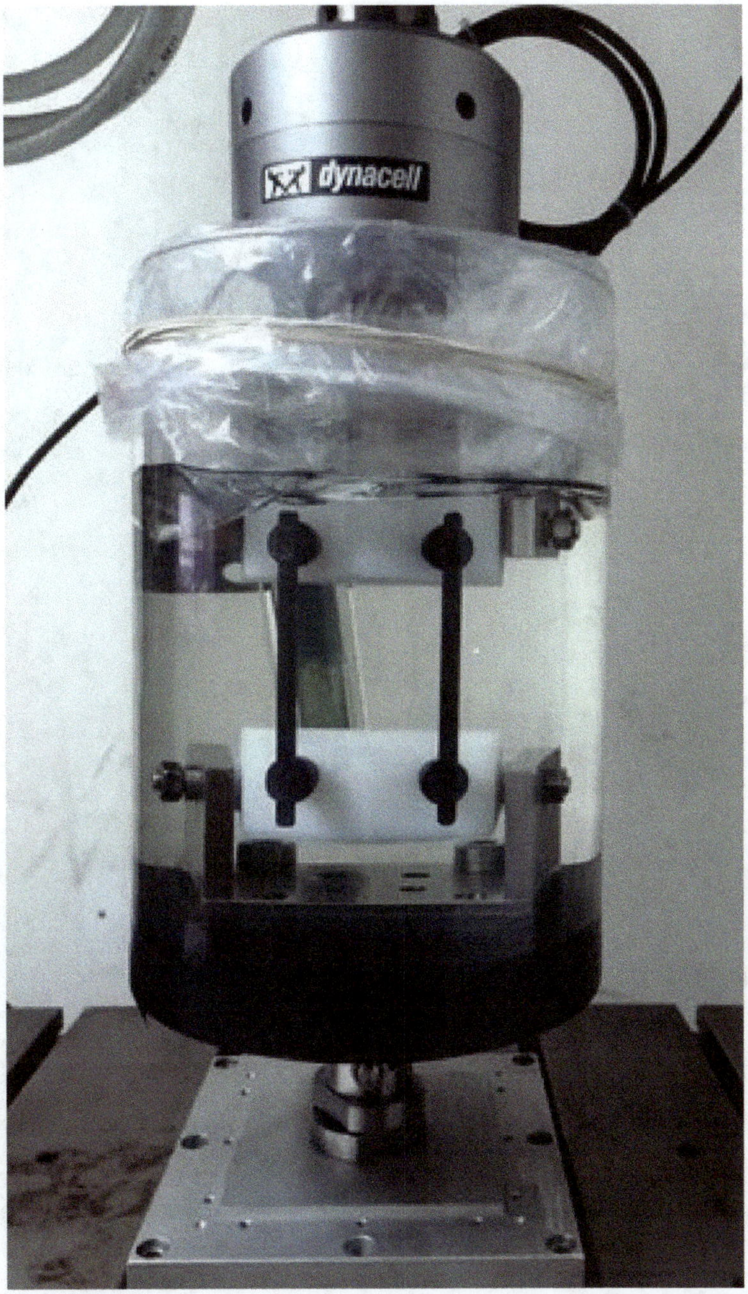

FIGURE 3: Fatigue axial compression bending test performed in compliance with the ASTM F1717 standard, using an Instron 8871 fatigue system testing machine, in phosphate-buffered saline solution setup at 37°C.

in spine surgery. This study is the first to test the mechanical properties of the CarboClear system, a novel spine fixation system made entirely (screws and rods) of CRF-PEEK composite material.

We tested the CFR-PEEK pedicle screw system using various mechanical tests according to the ASTM standards in order to assess whether its mechanical properties are comparable with published data on other commonly used metal spine fixation systems.

The mean bending yield load and bending ultimate load of the CFR-PEEK system were 322 N and 363 N, respectively, which are comparable to the values reported for the Moss Miami Ti system (DePuy, Warsaw, IN, USA) (299 N and 499 N, respectively) and superior to those reported for the Synergy VLS Open system (Biomet Spine, Broomfield, CO, USA) (214 N and 292 N, respectively) [18]. Bending stiffness of the CarboClear system was greater than the values reported for the titanium systems (CarboClear bending stiffness of 45 N/mm compared to 24 N/m and 33 N/mm for the Moss Miami Ti and the Synergy VLS Open systems, respectively). This is an unexpected and less favorable finding, considering that one of the known advantages of CFR-PEEK implants is their semirigidity compared to metal implants that should enable more load sharing and avoid disadvantages of rigid instrumentation. A higher fraction of carbon fibers dispersed in the PEEK

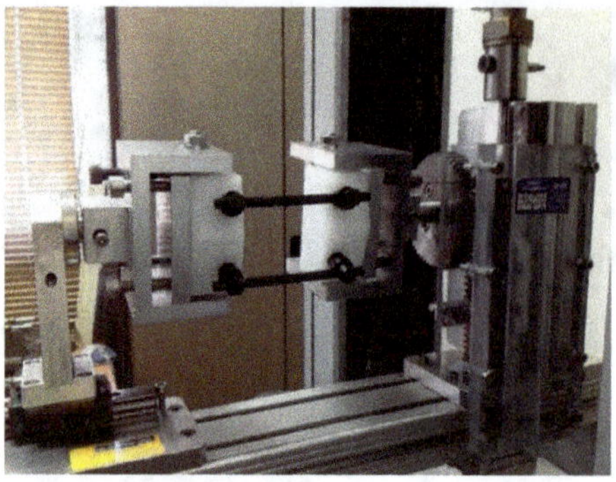

Figure 4: Static torsion test performed in compliance with the ASTM F1717 standard using a Testometric M350-10 kN testing machine at a rate of 6 deg/min.

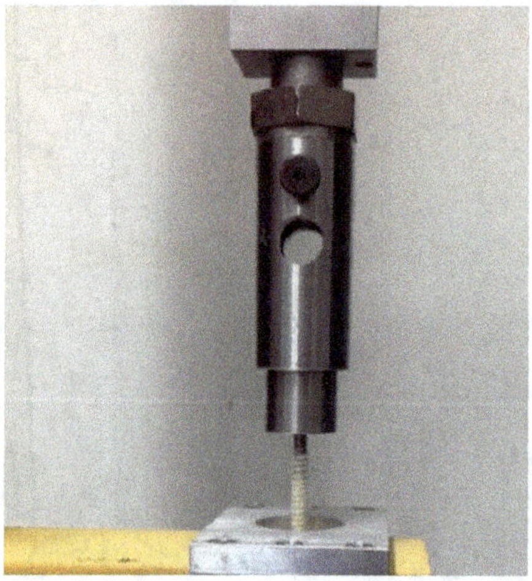

Figure 5: Screw axial pull-out strength test performed in compliance with ASTM F 2193 and ASTM F 543 standards using a Testometric M350-10 kN testing machine.

Table 1: Static axial compression bending test results of the CarboClear system.

Sample	Bending yield load (N)	Bending ultimate load (N)	Bending stiffness (N/mm)	Displacement at 2% offset yield (mm)	Elastic displacement (mm)	Bending ultimate displacement (mm)
1	302	312	42	9.5	8.0	11.0
2	310	325	50	7.7	6.5	8.3
3	312	351	48	8.0	6.5	9.5
4	350	401	44	9.4	7.9	11.8
5	325	408	42	9.3	7.8	13.4
6	335	381	46	8.8	7.3	12.2
Mean ± SD	322 ± 18	363 ± 40	45 ± 3.2	8.8 ± 0.8	7.3 ± 0.7	11 ± 1.8

Table 2: Fatigue axial compression bending test results of the CarboClear system.

Sample	Load (N)	Percentage of ultimate bending load (%)	No. of cycles to failure	Mode of failure
1	200	55	5×10^6	No failure, test terminated voluntarily
2	210	58	7.7×10^6	No failure, test terminated voluntarily
3	230	63	5×10^6	No failure, test terminated voluntarily
4	277	76	5×10^6	No failure, test terminated voluntarily
5	300	83	6×10^6	No failure, test terminated voluntarily
6	343	95	150	Slippage of the polyaxial screw head within the screw tulip

TABLE 3: Static torsion test results of the CarboClear system.

Sample	Yield torque (Nm)	Torsional stiffness (Nm/deg)	Angular displacement at 2% offset yield (deg)	Elastic angular displacement (deg)
1	12.4	0.9	16.1	14.2
2	10.4	1.1	11.1	9.2
3	12.4	1.2	12.4	10.2
4	15.1	0.9	18.3	16.2
Mean ± SD	12.6 ± 1.9	1.0 ± 0.1	14.4 ± 3.3	12.4 ± 3.3

TABLE 4: Screw axial pull-out test results of CarboClear pedicle screws (6.5 mm diameter, 35 mm length).

Sample	Axial pull-out strength (N)
1	2151
2	1901
3	2041
4	2057
Mean ± SD	2037 ± 103

matrix may explain this greater bending stiffness; however, this explanation is unlikely since the CarboClear system is designed to contain approximately 60% of carbon fibers by volume, which should yield stiffness similar to that of bone [11, 12] and not greater compared to metal implants. Further research may be required in order to clarify the nature of this finding.

The CFR-PEEK system showed no signs of fatigue at increasing cyclic axial compression loads up to 300 N (83% of its bending ultimate load) and successfully completed at least 5×10^6 cycles, with no evidence of mechanical failure. This meets the test acceptance criteria, which specifies that all samples tested at loads below 75% of the bending ultimate load should complete 5×10^6 cycles without failure. Both Moss Miami Ti and Synergy VLS Open systems showed inferior fatigue endurance and failed at 75% ultimate load after 0.04×10^6 and 0.98×10^6 cycles, respectively [18]. The superior fatigue endurance of the CFR-PEEK system may be attributed to the higher elasticity of the CFR-PEEK, as well as to the intrinsic properties of the composite material.

The torsional stiffness of the CFR-PEEK system (1.0 Nm/deg) was inferior to the values reported for several titanium systems, e.g., Globus Revolve polyaxial system (Globus Medical, Audubon, USA) (1.3 Nm/deg) [19], USS spine system (DePuy Synthes, Zuchwil, Switzerland) (2.2 Nm/deg) [19], and Moss Miami Ti system (1.8 Nm/deg) [20]. The failure mode of the CFR-PEEK specimens that we tested was a slippage of the spherical screw head relative to the rod (i.e., slippage of the spherical screw within screw tulip). A similar failure pattern, attributed to the coupling mechanism between the polyaxial screw head and its shaft, was found also in the Revolve and USS systems mentioned above [19, 20].

The axial pull-out strength of the CFR-PEEK 6.5 mm pedicle screws observed in our testing (2,037 N) is comparable to the pull-out strength of the Moss Miami 6.9 mm pedicle screw (1,888 N) and the Cotrel-Dubousset 6.5 mm pedicle screw (Medtronic Sofamor Danek, Memphis, TN) (1,895 N) [17]. All screw systems failed at the screw-polyurethane foam interface, with no structural damage to the screw itself.

Our adherence to the ASTM F1717 vertebrectomy model protocol may be considered as a limitation of the study, since the F1717 protocol has been shown to be a worst-case loading condition that may not actually represent loading within activities of daily living [21].

5. Conclusion

We demonstrated that the composite material spine fixation system, comprising CFR-PEEK pedicle screws and rods, has mechanical properties comparable to those of other commonly used titanium-made systems, with superior fatigue properties. The fatigue resistance, modulus of elasticity which is very similar to that of bone, radiolucency, and CT/MRI artifact-free feature of spine fixation systems made entirely of CFR-PEEK may offer advantages over traditional spine fixation systems made of metal alloys. Continued clinical research with large patient cohort, variety of surgical indications, and long-term follow-up is required in order to evaluate the performance of the CarboClear system over time.

Disclosure

The funders had no role in manuscript writing and editing.

Acknowledgments

The study was conducted at the manufacturer's laboratories, CarboFix Orthopedics Ltd. (Herzliya, Israel), who provided financial support for the study.

References

[1] H. Yoshihara, "Rods in spinal surgery: a review of the literature," *The Spine Journal*, vol. 13, no. 10, pp. 1350–1358, 2013.

[2] C. M. Bono and C. K. Lee, "Critical analysis of trends in fusion for degenerative disc disease over the past 20 years," *Spine*, vol. 29, pp. 455–463, 2004.

[3] N. Boos and J. Webb, "Pedicle screw fixation in spinal disorders: a European view," *European Spine Journal*, vol. 6, pp. 2–18, 1997.

[4] J. M. Highsmith, L. M. Tumialan, and G. E. Rodts Jr, "Flexible

rods and the case for dynamic stabilization," *Neurosurgical Focus*, vol. 22, pp. 1-5, 2007.

[5] M. D. Rahm and B. B. Hall, "Adjacent-segment degeneration after lumbar fusion with instrumentation: a retrospective study," *Journal of Spinal Disorders*, vol. 9, pp. 392–400, 1996.

[6] T. G. Craven, W. L. Carson, M. A. Asher et al., "The effects of implant stiffness on the bypassed bone mineral density and facet fusion stiffness of the canine spine," *Spine*, vol. 19, pp. 1664–1673, 1994.

[7] F. Galbusera, D. Volkheimer, S. Reitmaier, N. Berger-Roscher, A. Kienle, and H. J. Wilke, "Pedicle screw loosening: a clinically relevant complication?" *European Spine Journal*, vol. 24, no. 5, pp. 1005–1016, 2015.

[8] R. K. Ponnappan, H. Serhan, B. Zarda, R. Patel, T. Albert, and A. R. Vaccaro, "Biomechanical evaluation and comparison of polyetheretherketone rod system to traditional titanium rod fixation," *The Spine Journal*, vol. 9, no. 3, pp. 263–267, 2009.

[9] M. F. Gornet, F. W. Chan, J. C. Coleman et al., "Biomechanical assessment of a PEEK rod system for semi-rigid fixation of lumbar fusion constructs," *Journal of Biomechanical Engineering*, vol. 133, no. 8, 2011.

[10] F. Galbusera, C. M. Bellini, F. Anasetti, C. Ciavarro, A. Lovi, and M. Brayda-Bruno, "Rigid and flexible spinal stabilization devices: a biomechanical comparison," *Medical Engineering & Physics*, vol. 33, no. 4, pp. 490–496, 2011.

[11] C. S. Li, C. Vannabouathong, S. Sprague, and M. Bhandari, "The use of carbon-fiber-reinforced (cfr) PEEK material in orthopedic implants: a systematic review," *Clinical Medicine Insights: Arthritis and Musculoskeletal Disorders*, vol. 8, pp. 33–45, 2015.

[12] D. J. Hak, C. Mauffrey, D. Seligson, and B. Lindeque, "Use of carbon-fiber-reinforced composite implants in orthopedic surgery," *Orthopedics*, vol. 37, no. 12, pp. 825–830, 2014.

[13] G. Tedesco, A. Gasbarrini, S. Bandiera, R. Ghermandi, and S. Boriani, "Composite PEEK/Carbon fiber implants can increase the effectiveness of radiotherapy in the management of spine tumors," *Journal of Spine Surgery*, vol. 3, no. 3, pp. 323–329, 2017.

[14] S. Boriani, G. Tedesco, L. Ming et al., "Carbon-fiber-reinforced PEEK fixation system in the treatment of spine tumors: a preliminary report," *European Spine Journal*, vol. 27, no. 4, pp. 874–881, 2018.

[15] V. K. Goel, M. M. Panjabi, A. G. Patwardhan, A. P. Dooris, and H. Serhan, "American Society for Testing and Materials. Test protocols for evaluation of spinal implants," *The Journal of Bone and Joint Surgery (American)*, vol. 88, no. 2, pp. 103–109, 2006.

[16] A. Koistinen, S. Santavirta, and R. Lappalainen, "Apparatus to test insertion and removal torque of bone screws," *Proceedings of the Institution of Mechanical Engineers, Part H: Journal of Engineering in Medicine*, vol. 217, no. 6, pp. 503–508, 2003.

[17] C. C. Hsu, C. K. Chao, J. L. Wang, S. M. Hou, Y. T. Tsai, and J. Lin, "Increase of pullout strength of spinal pedicle screws with conical core: biomechanical tests and finite element analyses," *Journal of Orthopaedic Research*, vol. 23, no. 4, pp. 788–794, 2005.

[18] R. E. Stanford, A. H. Loefler, P. M. Stanford, and W. R. Walsh, "Multiaxial pedicle screw designs: static and dynamic mechanical testing," *Spine*, vol. 29, no. 4, pp. 367–375, 2004.

[19] D. Kubosch, E. J. Kubosch, B. Gueorguiev et al., "Biomechanical investigation of a minimally invasive posterior spine stabilization system in comparison to the Universal Spinal System (USS)," *BMC Musculoskelet Disord*, vol. 17, p. 134, 2016.

[20] D. Kok, P. J. Firkins, F. H. Wapstra, and A. G. Veldhuizen, "A new lumbar posterior fixation system, the memory metal spinal system: an in-vitro mechanical evaluation," *BMC Musculoskelet Disord*, vol. 14, p. 269, 2013.

[21] L. La Barbera, F. Galbusera, H. J. Wilke, and T. Villa, "Preclinical evaluation of posterior spine stabilization devices: can the current standards represent basic everyday life activities?" *European Spine Journal*, vol. 25, no. 9, pp. 2909–2918, 2016.

9

Radiographic and Functional Results following Subtalar Arthroereisis in Pediatric Flexible Flatfoot

David Ruiz-Picazo, Plácido Jiménez-Ortega, Francisco Doñate-Pérez, Natalia Gaspar-Aparicio, Victor García-Martín, José Ramírez-Villaescusa, and Sergio Losa-Palacios

Department of Pediatric Orthopaedics Surgery, Complejo Hospitalario Universitario de Albacete, Spain

Correspondence should be addressed to David Ruiz-Picazo; davidcop85@gmail.com

Academic Editor: Allen L. Carl

Introduction. Flexible flatfoot (FFF) is one of the most common skeletal disorders in children. In symptomatic patients who do not respond to conservative measures, surgery may be an option. Subtalar arthroereisis consists of limiting excessive eversion of the subtalar joint through different types of implants. *Materials and Methods.* We carried out a retrospective study of 16 patients (32 feet) intervened for FFF with a subtalar device (arthroereisis), across the period of 2008-2015 with a minimum follow-up period of one year. Pre- and postoperative measures of the Moreau-Costa-Bartani angle, dorsoplantar (DP) and lateral (L) talocalcaneal angle, talonavicular coverage angle, and naviculocuboid overlap were used to evaluate correction of the deformity. Two expert surgeons from the Pediatric Orthopedics Unit took separate measurements of these angles for subsequent analysis purposes and to obtain the interobserver correlation coefficient for quantitative variables. Pre- and postoperative differences in the measurement of angles were ascertained using Student's t-test for paired samples; and a functional evaluation of the patients intervened was carried out pre- and postoperatively by administering the parent version of the Oxford Ankle Foot Questionnaire for Children (OxAFQ-C) during a clinical interview. All statistical analyses were performed using the SPSS v. 19.0 program (SPSS, Chicago, IL), with values being deemed statistically significant at $p<0.05$. *Results.* A breakdown of the study population showed 81.25% (13 patients) males and 18.75% (3 patients) females, with mean age of 9 years (7-11). The interobserver coefficient for quantitative variables displayed a very high degree of concordance (0.7-0.9), indicating that the validity of the measures was adequate. Pre- and postoperative analysis of differences in the measurement of angles was statistically significant (p<0.005). In terms of functional evaluation, the postoperative results were positive, with statistical significance for the "school and play", "emotional", and "footwear" domains of the OxAFQ-C scale and no differences in the "physical" domain. *Conclusion.* Subtalar arthroereisis is a valid option for the treatment of symptomatic pediatric flatfoot, with good postoperative functional and radiographic results.

1. Introduction

Although flexible flatfoot (FFF) is one of the most common skeletal disorders among children, controversy surrounds the definition of pathological flexible flatfoot [1]. A habitual criterion of this condition is a very reduced or absent arch, excessive heal eversion during weight bearing, and forefoot abduction that causes a collapse of the foot. In children with FFF, the longitudinal arch is reconstructed when the child is standing on tiptoe or there is hyperextension of the hallux due to the fascia plantar windlass mechanism [2–4].

FFF seldom causes pain or disability in childhood [1]. Evaluation of these children at the physician's office is often due to parents' concern about the foot's appearance and/or excessive asymmetric shoe wear [5]. In a study of 242 children with FFF across a 3-year follow-up period, Coll Bosch et al. observed that pediatric FFF resolves spontaneously with growth, that the optimal age for diagnosis is from 5 to 6 years, and that treatment does not influence the natural evolution of flatfoot in the child [6].

Staheli et al. [7] describe a "typical" case of FFF as any asymptomatic pediatric patient who needs no specific treatment other than "wait and see" [1, 3]. If the clinical examination reveals an apparent shortening of the Achilles tendon, stretching exercises are indicated [1, 3]. Nonetheless, there have been reports that FFF, which leads to a retraction of the Achilles tendon, will inevitably worsen in adult life and become symptomatic [3]. MacKenzie et al. found very limited evidence of the effectiveness of conservative treatments in symptomatic patients [8].

Hence, in patients presenting with symptomatic FFF, which proves nonresponsive to conservative measures, surgical treatment may be considered.

The arthroereisis procedure has been described as a valid treatment option, which enables the internal plantar arch to be restored with few complications. Several procedures have been described, including subtalar extra-articular screw arthroereisis, the calcaneo-stop technique, and the subtalar implant [9–11]. This paper focuses on the last-mentioned procedure, which consists of placing a cylindrical device in the subtalar joint, with the aim of limiting eversion of the foot. Accordingly, this study sought to analyze any improvement, both radiologic and functional, seen in patients treated by means of this procedure.

2. Materials and Methods

We conducted a retrospective study of patients treated for symptomatic FFF with the arthroereisis technique, across the period of 2008-2015. Treated patients were intervened using a cannulated titanium subtalar device.

The inclusion criteria were defined as any child who (1) had idiopathic symptomatic FFF; (2) was aged 7 to 12 years; (3) had been intervened using subtalar arthroereisis without an associated surgical procedure (Achilles tendon lengthening or accessory navicular removal); (4) presented with no neuromuscular, neurogenic, or osseous anomalies; (5) had an appropriate pre- and postoperative radiologic study; and (6) had undergone a minimum of one-year follow-up. Patients with no valid radiologic study and/or a follow-up of less than one year were excluded.

All patients were intervened by general anaesthesia using lateral approach to subtalar joint. A curved 2 cm skin incision was made on the lateral side of the hindfoot over the sinus tarsi. A K-wire was placed on the subtalar joint and was checked with fluoroscopy. Then the trial implants (with increasing diameters) were inserted until the appropriate implant size was determined. The authors chose the smallest implant that corrected the deformity and remained stable in the sinus tarsi while moving the subtalar joint. Lastly, the definitive cannulated titanium device was placed in the subtalar joint.

Based on the parent version of the Oxford Ankle Foot Questionnaire for Children (OxAFQ-C) administered during a clinical interview, the clinical variables of age, sex, and functional status were evaluated preoperatively and again at the end of follow-up.

Radiologic study was performed in upright position. Dorsoplantar radiography is performed with the X-ray tube tilted 30 degrees from the vertical axis, in a distal-proximal (toe-to-heel) direction, at a distance of 90 cm from the foot. Lateral radiography was obtained by placing the X-ray tube parallel to the horizontal axis, at a distance of 90 cm from the foot. These angular and linear measurements were made with the aid of our institution's Radiologic Archive and Image Management (Raim-PC) computer software program.

To evaluate the degree of correction, the following angles were measured in pre- and postoperative study: (1) talonavicular coverage angle, (2) naviculocuboid overlap, (3) talocalcaneal angle in lateral radiography, (4) talocalcaneal angle in dorsoplantar (DP) radiography, and (5) the Moreau-Costa-Bartani angle (Figure 1).

The *talonavicular coverage angle* is the angle formed by the perpendicular to the line joining the medial and lateral edges of the articular surface of the talus bone and the perpendicular to the line joining the medial and lateral edges of the articular surface of the navicular bone. Davids et al. [12] established normal values for this angle, that is, 20° (±9.8) with a range of 5°-39°. High degrees of coverage are related to greater midfoot abduction. *Naviculocuboid overlap* is measured by dividing the product of the superior margin of the cuboid bones and inferior margin of the navicular bone by the product of the superior and inferior margins of the cuboids, expressed as a percentage. Naviculocuboid overlap indicates greater eversion, that is, collapse of the foot. In the study by Davids et al. [12], the normal values were 47% (±13.8) with a range of 22%-85%. In our study, the results were 66.43% (range: 52.37%-80.49%) in the right foot and 57.8% (range: 47.51%-68.11%) in the left foot. The *lateral talocalcaneal* angle is obtained from the intersection between the line drawn from the mid-talar axis and that joining the plantar prominence of the calcaneus to the calcaneocuboid surface, measured on lateral projection radiography. The normal values for this angle are 39° to 49° (range: 36°-61°) [13]. This angle evaluates hindfoot valgus and abduction (greater the angle, the greater the degree of hindfoot abduction and valgus). The *talocalcaneal angle* (Kite's angle) refers to the angle between lines drawn down the axis of the talus and calcaneus measured on a weight-bearing DP foot radiography. The talocalcaneal angle should measure between 25 and 40 degrees. Lastly, *the Moreau-Costa-Bartani* is the angle formed by the following lines: line formed from the lower point of the medial sesamoid to the lower point of the talonavicular joint and the line formed from the lower point of the talonavicular joint to the lower point of the posterior calcaneal tuberosity. The normal values for this angle are 115°-125°.

The statistical analysis consisted of describing the variables and analyzing the clinical (OxAFQ-C) and radiologic differences, both preoperatively and at the end of follow-up, using Student's t-test for paired samples. To establish the degree of reliability of their measurements, two expert surgeons from the Pediatric Orthopedics Unit took separate measurements of the angles and then used the intraclass correlation coefficient of quantitative variables to establish the degree of interobserver correlation according to the Fleiss scale [14].

All statistical analyses were performed using the SPSS v. 19.0 (SPSS, Chicago, IL) computer software program, with values being deemed statistically significant at $p<0.05$.

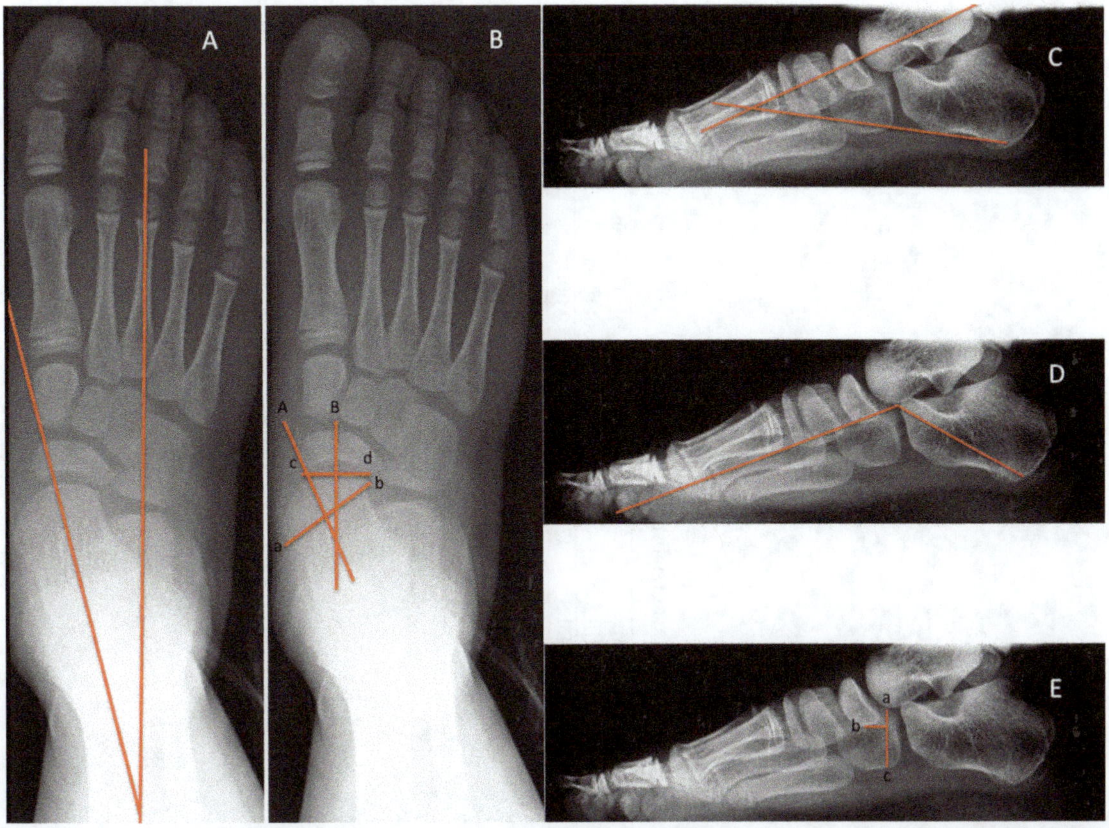

FIGURE 1: The graphical representation of angles measures used in the study. A: DP talocalcaneal angle. B: talonavicular coverage angle. Points a and b = medial and lateral edges (resp.) of the articular surface of the talus bone. Points c and d = medial and lateral edges (resp.) of the articular surface of the navicular bone. Line A is perpendicular to ab, and line B is perpendicular to cd. Talonavicular coverage is the angle created by the intersection of lines A and B. C: talocalcaneal angle in lateral radiography. D: Moreau-Costa-Bartani angle. E: naviculocuboid overlap. Points a and b = superior and inferior margins (resp.) of the cuboids. Point c = inferior margin of the navicular. Naviculocuboid overlap = ac/ab X 100.

3. Results

Of the initial 22 patients (44 feet), 16 (32 feet) were included in the study, with 6 patients being excluded due to the absence of a valid radiologic study. A breakdown of the study population showed 81.25% males (13 patients) and 18.75% females (3 patients), with mean age of 9 years (range: 7 to 11 years).

The preoperative clinical study evaluated with Student's t-test indicated significant differences in OxAFQ-C scale scores in the "school and play", "emotional", and "footwear" domains ($p<0.05$) but no differences in the "physical" domain (Table 1).

The radiologic study showed significant differences, evaluated preoperatively and again during follow-up (minimum one year), in the degree of correction of all angles in the dorsoplantar and lateral planes ($p<0.05$) (Table 2).

The degree of interobserver correlation for radiologic measurements was substantial or almost perfect, both preoperatively and at the end of follow-up (Table 3). In terms of functional evaluation (Table 3), the postoperative results were positive, displaying statistical significance for the "school and play", "emotional", and "footwear" domains of the OxAFQ-C (parent version) scale.

The implants were not removed because the patients had not yet achieved bone maturity.

Lastly, there were 4 cases of complications related with overcorrection of the foot and expulsion of the implant due to erroneous measurement.

4. Discussion

FFF is a common disorder characterized by plantar flexion and medial rotation of the talus, calcaneal eversion, medial longitudinal arch collapse, and abduction of the forefoot [5, 6, 15]. Its incidence is unknown but is estimated to be close on 5% among children and adults [16].

Pediatric FFF is often asymptomatic, and conservative treatment begins by using new footwear and ortheses. In cases where FFF is symptomatic and conservative modalities have failed, surgical intervention is indicated and in some patients arthroereisis may be considered.

Subtalar arthroereisis is a surgical procedure aimed at placing an implant in the sinus tarsi to limit excessive eversion of the subtalar joint. In 1946, Chambers et al. discussed this technique by describing the placement of a bone graft in the posterior subtalar joint to restrict hindfoot eversion [17].

TABLE 1: Pre- and postoperative differences in the measurement of angles. All values are statistically significant.

	Preoperative				Postoperative				Difference in means	
	Left foot	95% CI	Right foot	95% CI	Left foot	95% CI	Right foot	95% CI	Left foot (p value)	Right foot (p value)
Costa-Bartani angle	144.43	138.84 - 150.03	143.31	139.29 - 147.34	133.62	129.13 - 138.11	131.5	127.61 - 135.39	<0.001	<0.001
AP talocalcaneal angle	28.69	25.05 - 32.32	29.06	26.6 - 31.52	17.43	13.89 - 20.98	16.06	13.54 - 18.58	<0.001	<0.001
Lateral talocalcaneal angle	44.68	41.12 - 48.25	40.5	37.04 - 43.95	35	32.18 - 37.81	34.56	31.53 - 37.59	<0.001	0.002
Talonavicular coverage angle	31.18	25.77 - 36.6	34.12	29.71 - 38.53	14.37	8.78 - 19.96	16.12	11.18 - 21.06	<0.001	<0.001
Naviculocuboid overlap (%)	66.43	52.37 - 80.49	57.81	47.51 - 68.11	40.31	28.8 - 51.82	32.37	23.06 - 41.69	0.003	<0.001

TABLE 2: Degree of interobserver correlation. It will be noted that measurements range from 0.8 to close on 1, indicating a very high degree of correlation.

	Preoperative		Postoperative	
	Right foot	Left foot	Right foot	Left foot
Costa-Bartani angle	0.97	0.975	0.82	0.93
AP talocalcaneal angle	0.745	0.859	0.928	0.836
Lateral talocalcaneal angle	0.876	0.860	0.849	0.869
Talonavicular coverage angle	0.759	0.9	0.97	0.991
Naviculocuboid overlap	0.934	0.994	0.973	0.968

TABLE 3: Mean pre- and postoperative differences in the parent version of the Oxford Ankle Foot Questionnaire for Children (OxAFQ-C).

	Parent version of the OxAFQ-C score (mean)		
OxAFQ-C domains	Preoperative	Postoperative	*P* value
Physical	63.5	71.2	0.2
School and play	87.6	91.7	<0.05
Emotional	90.5	92.6	<0.05
Footwear	68.3	81.1	<0.05

Even so, subtalar arthroereisis continues to be controversial, especially in terms of indications, age at date of surgery, and adjunct procedures [18, 19].

Subtalar implants have been classified by reference to their biomechanical properties, for example, self-locking wedge, axis-altering, and impact-blocking devices [20]. Currently, most subtalar implants are of the self-locking wedge type, aimed at restricting hindfoot valgus. All our patients were intervened by placement of a titanium self-locking wedge device.

Patient age is a very important factor when it comes to the precise timing of the intervention [21]. It is recommended that surgery be performed between the ages of 8 and 12 years: all our patients were intervened at ages of 7 to 11 years. This is justified because, before the age of 8, many children may experience spontaneous correction. On the other hand, the performance of surgery beyond the age of 12 years tends to be exceptional, given that the aim of arthroereisis is to reposition the talus correctly on the calcaneus to enable remodeling of these bones and the subtalar joint during growth. Since at least 2 years are thought to be required for the purpose, this means that, after 12 years of age, there is insufficient time for the bones and ligaments of the hindfoot to be remodeled [22] (Figure 2).

Most studies that evaluate the functional outcomes of intervened patients classify such patients according to whether or not they present with postoperative symptoms. On observing the variability of symptoms among patients, Benedetti et al. stated that binary classification was inadequate [23]. An alternative approach is to carry out a continuous evaluation of the effect that symptoms have on these children's quality of life. The OxAFQ-C is a validated questionnaire that was drawn up to evaluate quality of life in this population [24]. This instrument not only evaluates disease burden but can also be used to record clinical change over time. In our study, parents perceived a significant improvement in the "school and play", "emotional", and "footwear" domains. The "physical" domain scores did not prove to be statistically significant. Morris et al. found that children with FFF had a worse quality of life than did children with normal feet [24]. The principal differences between groups were found to be in the dorsoplantar plane, where children with FFF presented with greater midfoot eversion and supination of the forefoot during gait. Both factors correlated with worsening of their quality of life. In addition, a recent OxAFQ-C-based study published by Martinelli et al., with more than 10 years of follow-up, evaluated other tests designed to ascertain the effect of subtalar implants on children's physical activity [25]. These authors observed that while surgery did not alter the duration, frequency, or type of sports activities engaged in by children, it did alter their participation in such activities, emotional state, and footwear problems. Given the time of follow-up, the authors attributed the above findings to changes in growth stage (child to adolescent) and priorities of life. In addition, Faldini et al. used self-reported questionnaires to evaluate patient-perceived quality of life after subtalar arthroereisis with a bioabsorbable implant. Patients reported a high degree of satisfaction, without perceiving their quality of life as being compromised [26]. Our findings are consistent with most of the literature on subtalar arthroereisis outcomes [27, 28].

The Moreau-Costa-Bartani angles and talocalcaneal or Kite angle (Figure 1) has been used in the past to evaluate the presence of flatfoot in lateral and dorsoplantar projections. In our study, these angles improved significantly after intervention to the point where they came to lie within their physiologic range. More recently, the talonavicular coverage angles [12] (Figure 1), previously described by Sangeorzan et al. [29], naviculocuboid overlap [12] (Figure 1), expressed in percentage terms, and the talocalcaneal angle in lateral radiography have been proposed for obtaining an overall evaluation of pediatric flatfoot. A significant postoperative improvement in talonavicular coverage angle ($p<0.001$) has been related to a reduction in midfoot abduction.

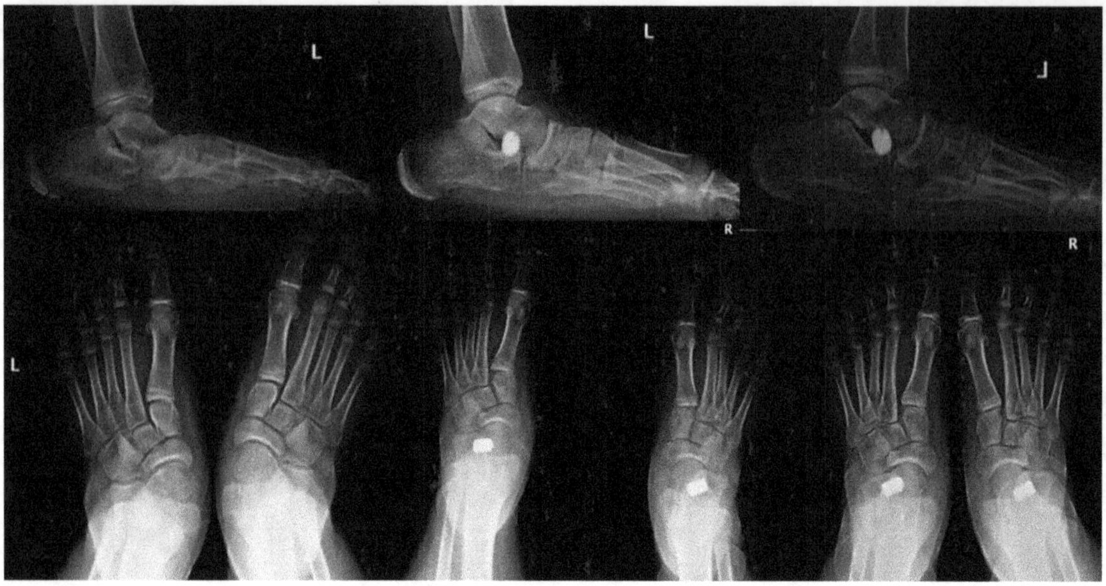

FIGURE 2: Male patient aged 11 years with bilateral flatfoot, showing foot remodeling trends after subtalar implant. The images in the centre were taken two months after operation; the images on the right correspond to two years after operation.

Naviculocuboid overlap has been linked by Davids et al. to midfoot eversion [12]. In this latter study, normal values were 47 ± 13.8. In our study, the preoperative values of this angle were high and were related to greater midfoot eversion. With respect to the lateral talocalcaneal angle, the greater the angle, the greater the degree of hindfoot valgus and abduction. The literature shows that normal values range from 49 (±6.9) (36–61) [10] to 39 (±7) [1]. The values registered in our study are similar to those reported in the literature (left foot: 44.68 (41.12 - 48.25); right foot: 40.5 (37.04 - 43.95)), with the postoperative results proving significant.

Insofar as complications are concerned, mention might be made of the more general types of complications, such as persistent pain in the sinus tarsi, overcorrection or undercorrection, and incorrect choice of size of implant, which may lead to its extrusion [30]. In our study, there were two cases (6.25%) in which extrusion of the implant due to incorrect choice of size was detected (Figure 3). In their study, Cook et al. established that a reduced postoperative talocalcaneal angle on AP X-ray protected against extrusion of the implant [31]. In addition, overcorrection was observed in two of the patients in the sample (6.25%). In these cases, the implant was changed with good results. There have been reports of implant-related complications closely linked to the materials used in their design, for example, wear, reaction to foreign bodies, and fracture [12, 13, 20, 21, 29, 30]. Furthermore, the following have also been documented in the literature: presence of intraosseous cysts in the talus bone, osteonecrosis of the talus, contraction of the peroneal muscles, and fractures of the calcaneus or talus [32–34].

The radiographic data on and subjective results of subtalar arthroereisis in FFF have been promising for children and adults alike. A review of data in the last decade showed a satisfaction rate of 81% to 90% among pediatric patients [17, 19, 22, 27].

5. Conclusion

Subtalar arthroereisis is a valid option for treatment of symptomatic pediatric flatfoot, with good postoperative radiographic results. We introduced measures for some angles which, though not commonly used, are nonetheless helpful when it comes to obtaining a more accurate preoperative evaluation of candidate patients. The talonavicular coverage angle furnished information on midfoot abduction; naviculocuboid overlap made it possible to assess eversion of the foot; that is, the greater the overlap, the greater the collapse of the foot; and the talocalcaneal angle in lateral radiography furnishes information on hindfoot valgus. Lastly, functional analysis of patients shows that surgery improves their participation in school and physical activities, emotional state, and footwear problems.

Consent

Informed consent was obtained from all individual participants included in the study.

Authors' Contributions

David Ruiz-Picazo, Plácido Jiménez-Ortega, Francisco Doñate-Pérez, and José Ramírez-Villaescusa contributed to conception and design. David Ruiz-Picazo, Francisco Doñate-Pérez, Natalia Gaspar-Aparicio, Victor García-Martín, and Sergio Losa-Palacios contributed to acquisition of data. All authors contributed to analysis and interpretation of data. David Ruiz-Picazo, Victor García-Martín, and José Ramírez-Villaescusa drafted the article. Plácido Jiménez-Ortega, Francisco Doñate-Pérez, José Ramírez-Villaescusa, Natalia Gaspar-Aparicio, Sergio Losa-Palacios, and David Ruiz-Picazo critically revised the article. All authors reviewed submitted version of manuscript. José Ramírez-

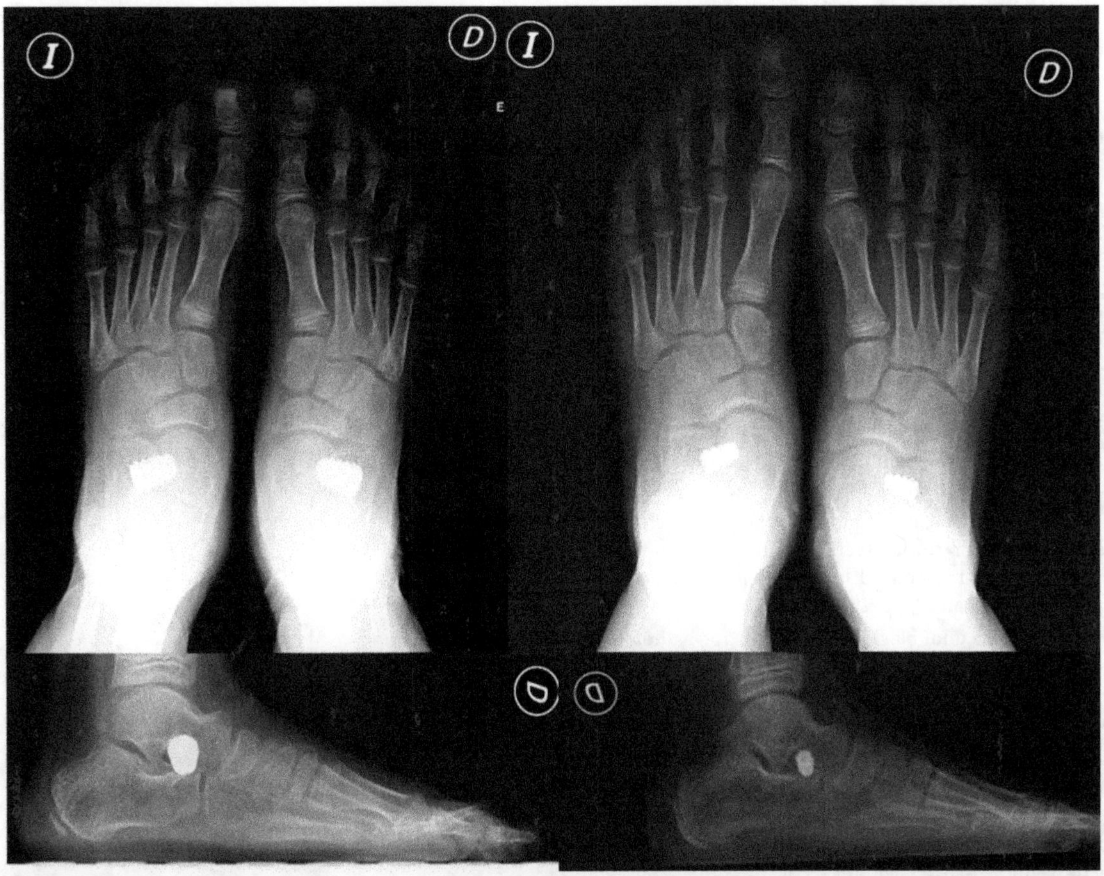

FIGURE 3: Example of overcorrection and expulsion of the implant. Revision surgery and placement of smaller-sized implants were necessary.

Villaescusa, Sergio Losa-Palacios, and David Ruiz-Picazo approved the final version of the manuscript on behalf of all authors. David Ruiz-Picazo, Francisco Doñate-Pérez, Plácido Jiménez-Ortega, Victor García-Martín, and José Ramírez-Villaescusa supervised the study.

References

[1] V. S. Mosca, "Flexible flatfoot in children and adolescents," *Journal of Children's Orthopaedics*, vol. 4, no. 2, pp. 107–121, 2010.

[2] A. M. Sheikh Taha and D. S. Feldman, "Painful flexible flatfoot," *Foot and Ankle Clinics*, vol. 20, no. 4, pp. 693–704, 2015.

[3] E. J. Harris, "The natural history and pathophysiology of flexible flatfoot," *Clinics in Podiatric Medicine and Surgery*, vol. 27, no. 1, pp. 1–23, 2010.

[4] J. A. Sullivan, "Pediatric flatfoot: evaluation and management," *Journal of the American Academy of Orthopaedic Surgeons*, vol. 7, no. 1, pp. 44–53, 1999.

[5] U. Bhaskara Rao and B. Joseph, "The influence of footwear on the prevalence of flat foot. A survey of 2300 children," *The Journal of Bone & Joint Surgery (British Volume)*, vol. 74, no. 4, pp. 525–527, 1992.

[6] C. D. M. Bosch, A. Viladot Perice, and A. Suso Vergara, "Estudio evolutivo del pie plano infantil," *Revista Española de Cirugía Ortopédica y Traumatología*, vol. 43, no. 3, pp. 167–241, 1999.

[7] L. T Staheli, D. E Chew, and M. Corbett, "The longitudinal arch. A survey of eight hundred and eighty-two feet in normal children and adults," *The Journal of Bone & Joint Surgery*, vol. 69, no. 3, pp. 426–428, 1987.

[8] M. De Pellegrin, D. Moharamzadeh, W. M. Strobl, R. Biedermann, C. Tschauner, and T. Wirth, "Subtalar extra-articular screw arthroereisis (SESA) for the treatment of flexible flatfoot in children," *Journal of Children's Orthopaedics*, vol. 8, no. 6, pp. 479–487, 2014.

[9] V. Pavone, L. Costarella, G. Testa, G. Conte, M. Riccioli, and G. Sessa, "Calcaneo-stop procedure in the treatment of the juvenile symptomatic flatfoot," *The Journal of Foot & Ankle Surgery*, vol. 52, no. 4, pp. 444–447, 2013.

[10] S. Giannini, M. Cadossi, A. Mazzotti et al., "Bioabsorbable calcaneo-stop implant for the treatment of flexible flatfoot: a retrospective cohort study at a minimum follow-up of 4 years," *Journal of Foot and Ankle Surgery*, vol. 56, no. 4, pp. 776–782, 2017.

[11] A. Jane MacKenzie, K. Rome, and A. M. Evans, "The efficacy of nonsurgical interventions for pediatric flexible flat foot: A critical review," *Journal of Pediatric Orthopaedics*, vol. 32, no. 8, pp. 830–834, 2012.

[12] J. R. Davids, T. W. Gibson, and L. I. Pugh, "Quantitative segmental analysis of weight-bearing radiographs of the foot and ankle for children: normal alignment," *Journal of Pediatric Orthopaedics*, vol. 25, no. 6, pp. 769–776, 2005.

[13] R. Vanderwilde, L. T. Staheli, D. E. Chew, and V. Malagon, "Measurements on radiographs of the foot in normal infants and children," *The Journal of Bone & Joint Surgery*, vol. 70, no. 3, pp. 407–415, 1988.

[14] J. L. Fleiss, "Measuring nominal scale agreement among many raters," *Psychological Bulletin*, vol. 76, no. 5, pp. 378–382, 1971.

[15] A. Gracia-Rodriguez, F. Martin-Jimenez, and M. Carnero-Varo, "Flexible flat feet in children: a real problem?" *Pediatrics*, vol. 103, no. 6, p. e84, 1999.

[16] J. Christensen, N. Campbell, and K. DiNucci, "Closed kinetic chain tarsal mechanics of subtalar joint arthroereisis," *Journal of the American Podiatric Medical Association*, vol. 86, no. 10, pp. 467–473, 1996.

[17] P. Highlander, W. Sung, and L. Weil, "Subtalar arthroereisis," *Clinics in Podiatric Medicine and Surgery*, vol. 28, no. 4, pp. 745–754, 2011.

[18] L. D. Cicchinelli, J. P. Huerta, F. J. G. Carmona, and D. F. Morato, "Analysis of gastrocnemius recession and medial column procedures as adjuncts in arthroereisis for the correction of pediatric pes planovalgus: a radiographic retrospective study," *Journal of Foot and Ankle Surgery*, vol. 47, no. 5, pp. 385–391, 2008.

[19] R. Vedantam, A. M. Capelli, and P. L. Schoenecker, "Subtalar arthroereisis for the correction of planovalgus foot in children with neuromuscular disorders," *Journal of Pediatric Orthopaedics*, vol. 18, no. 3, pp. 294–298, 1998.

[20] H. Vogler, "Subtalar joint blocking operations for pathological pronation syndromes," in *Comprehensive Textbook of Foot Surgery*, E. D. McGlamery, Ed., pp. 466–482, William & Wilkins, Baltimore, MD, USA, 1987.

[21] S. Giannini and A. Kenneth, "Johnson memorial lecture. operative treatment of the flatfoot: why and how," *Foot & Ankle International*, vol. 19, no. 1, pp. 52–56, 2016.

[22] P. Fernández de Retana, F. Álvarez, and R. Viladot, "Subtalar arthroereisis in pediatric flatfoot reconstruction," *Foot and Ankle Clinics*, vol. 15, no. 2, pp. 323–335, 2010.

[23] M. G. Benedetti, F. Ceccarelli, L. Berti et al., "Diagnosis of flexible flatfoot in children: a systematic clinical approach," *Orthopedics*, vol. 34, no. 2, pp. 94-94, 2011.

[24] C. Morris, H. A. Doll, A. Wainwright, T. Theologis, and R. Fitzpatrick, "The Oxford ankle foot questionnaire for children," *The Journal of Bone & Joint Surgery (British Volume)*, vol. 90-B, no. 11, pp. 1451–1456, 2008.

[25] N. Martinelli, A. Bianchi, P. Martinkevich et al., "Return to sport activities after subtalar arthroereisis for correction of pediatric flexible flatfoot," *Journal of Pediatric Orthopaedics B*, vol. 27, no. 1, pp. 82–87, 2018.

[26] C. Faldini, A. Mazzotti, A. Panciera et al., "Patient-perceived outcomes after subtalar arthroereisis with bioabsorbable implants for flexible flatfoot in growing age: a 4-year follow-up study," *European Journal of Orthopaedic Surgery & Traumatology*, vol. 28, no. 4, pp. 707–712, 2018.

[27] P. M. Koning, P. J. Heesterbeek, and E. de Visser, "Subtalar arthroereisis for pediatric flexible pes planovalgus," *Journal of the American Podiatric Medical Association*, vol. 99, no. 5, pp. 447–453, 2009.

[28] S. C. Nelson, D. M. Haycock, and E. R. Little, "Flexible flatfoot treatment with arthroereisis: radiographic improvement and child health survey analysis," *The Journal of Foot & Ankle Surgery*, vol. 43, no. 3, pp. 144–155, 2004.

[29] B. J. Sangeorzan, V. Mosca, and S. T. Hansen, "Effect of calcaneal lengthening on relationships among the hindfoot, midfoot, and forefoot," *Foot & Ankle*, vol. 14, no. 3, pp. 136–141, 2016.

[30] R. L. Needleman, "Current topic review: subtalar arthroereisis for the correction of flexible flatfoot," *Foot & Ankle International*, vol. 26, no. 4, pp. 336–346, 2016.

[31] E. A. Cook, J. J. Cook, and P. Basile, "Identifying risk factors in subtalar arthroereisis explantation: a propensity-matched analysis," *The Journal of Foot & Ankle Surgery*, vol. 50, no. 4, pp. 395–401, 2011.

[32] T. E. Siff and W. M. Granberry, "Avascular necrosis of the talus following subtalar arthrorisis with a polyethylene endoprosthesis: A case report," *Foot & Ankle International*, vol. 21, no. 3, pp. 247–249, 2000.

[33] A. K. Rockett, G. Mangum, and S. S. Mendicino, "Bilateral intraosseous cystic formation in the talus: A complication of subtalar arthroeresis," *The Journal of Foot & Ankle Surgery*, vol. 37, no. 5, pp. 421–425, 1998.

[34] G. T. Kuwada and G. L. Dockery, "Complications following traumatic incidents with STA-peg procedures," *Journal of Foot Surgery*, vol. 27, no. 3, pp. 236–239, 1988.

10

Optimal Correction of Adult Spinal Deformities Requires Restoration of Distal Lumbar Lordosis

S. Pesenti, S. Prost, A. Muñoz McCausland, K. Farah, P. Tropiano, S. Fuentes, and B. Blondel

Aix-Marseille Université, APHM, CNRS, ISM, Hôpital de La Timone, Spine Unit 264 Rue Saint Pierre, Marseille 13005, France

Correspondence should be addressed to B. Blondel; benjamin.blondel@ap-hm.fr

Academic Editor: Hiroshi Hashizume

Purpose. The aim of this study is to analyze results according to postoperative pelvic incidence-lumbar lordosis (PI-LL) mismatch in the management of adult spine deformity (ASD) patients. Recently, it has been reported that in addition to lumbar lordosis amount, lordosis repartition between its proximal and distal parts was crucial. *Methods.* We enrolled 77 consecutive ASD patients who underwent posterior spinal fusion and deformity correction between 2015 and 2018. On preoperative and 1-year follow-up radiographs, we analyzed different parameters such as L1-S1 lumbar lordosis, L1-L4 proximal lordosis (PLL), L4-S1 distal lordosis (DLL), pelvic tilt (PT), sagittal vertical axis (SVA), and PI-LL mismatch. Comparisons were performed according to postoperative PI-LL mismatch (defined as "aligned" when PI-LL was <10°). The relationship between lordosis distribution and postoperative alignment status was investigated. *Results.* On the whole series, average lumbar lordosis, SVA, and PI-LL improved (28.2° vs.43.5°, 82 vs. 51 mm, and 26°vs. 14°, all $p < 0.001$, respectively). On the other hand, PT remained unchanged (30° vs. 28°, $p > 0.05$). 35 patients were classified as "aligned" and 42 as "not aligned." Patients from the "aligned" group had a significantly lower PI than patients from the "not aligned" group (52° vs. 61°, $p = 0.009$). Postoperative PLL was not different between groups (18° vs. 16° $p > 0.05$), whereas DLL was significantly higher in the "aligned" group (31° vs. 22°, $p = 0.003$). PI-LL was significantly correlated to DLL (rho = 0.407, $p < 0.001$) but not with PLL (rho = 0.110, $p = 0.342$). *Conclusions.* Our results revealed that in ASD patients, postoperative malalignment was associated with a lack of DLL restoration. "Not aligned" patients had also a significantly higher pelvic incidence. Specific attention must be paid to restore optimal distal lumbar lordosis in order to set the amount and the distribution of optimal postoperative lumbar lordosis.

1. Introduction

Adult spinal deformity covers a broad range of pathologies and can be responsible for disability and altered quality of life [1]. When a surgical procedure is indicated, the aim is to restore sagittal and coronal alignment. Since the last decade, it has been largely reported that correction of sagittal alignment was of primary importance and associated with better outcomes [2–4].

ASD is commonly described with the SRS-Schwab classification [5] that also serves as guideline for sagittal correction (SVA < 50 mm, PI-LL < 10°, and PT < 20°). However, despite recent advances such as age-related spinopelvic alignment thresholds [6], postoperative sagittal objectives are reached in less than 50% of the cases [7].

The key parameter to evaluate postoperative alignment is the PI-LL mismatch. This parameter has been reported as a predictor of success and is correlated with health-related quality of life scores [8]. However, taking into account only the L1-S1 lumbar lordosis (LL) can be misleading for two reasons [8]:

The L4-S1 DLL was reported to be almost constant

Pelvic incidence is significantly related to the L1-L4 PLL

It seems therefore crucial to evaluate not only the global amount of LL restoration but also the PI-LL mismatch according to PLL and DLL.

This study aimed to analyze the results of ASD surgical management according to postoperative PI-LL mismatch with the hypothesis that aligned patients had a better restoration of the DLL.

2. Methods

2.1. Study Design and Patient Population. After institutional review board approval (IRB 00009118), we conducted a retrospective analysis of a prospectively maintained database of ASD patients operated between 2015 and 2018. Prior to inclusion, every patient signed an informed consent.

Inclusion criteria were as follows: all adult patients managed surgically for ASD with a posterior fixation that included all the lumbar spine (upper level instrumented vertebra L1 or above, lower instrumented vertebra S1 or below), primary surgery or revision case, pre and postoperative full spine X-rays available, and one-year minimal follow-up (including full spine X-rays).

For each patient, demographic data, clinical scores (lumbar VAS and Oswestry Disability Index), and full spine X-rays (AP and lateral) were obtained preoperatively, in the immediate postoperative period, and at one-year of follow-up. Complications during the follow-up period were systematically noted.

The surgical procedure consisted of a posterior fusion and bone resection if required (Grade 2 or 3 of the Schwab classification [9]).

2.2. Radiographic Parameters. On lateral radiographs, the following parameters were measured: T4-T12 thoracic kyphosis (TK), L1-S1 lumbar lordosis, L1-L4 PLL, L4-S1 DLL, SVA, pelvic parameters (PI and PT), and mismatch between pelvic incidence and lumbar lordosis (PI-LL).

2.3. Statistical Analysis. Data were formulated as means and standard deviations. Comparisons were carried out using Student's *t*-test for normally distributed variables. The population was analyzed as a whole and then stratified according to the 1-year postoperative PI-LL mismatch. Patients were classified as the "aligned" group when postoperative PI-LL was below 10° and "not aligned" otherwise. The two groups were compared with regards to radiographic parameters and mechanical complications. The relationship between PI-LL mismatch and lumbar lordosis distribution was investigated using Spearman correlation tests. The significance level was set at 95% (i.e., $p < 0.05$).

3. Results

3.1. Population and Surgical Data. Among the 97 patients who underwent ASD surgical correction in our institution during the inclusion period, 77 patients met inclusion criteria for the present study. Fifty-six women and 21 men with a mean age of 66.5 years old (SD = 8.8) were included. On average, 14 levels were fused during the procedure (SD = 3), and lower instrumented level included iliac screws for 43 patients and S1 screws for 34 patients.

3.2. Global Radiographic Analysis. On the whole series, the mean preoperative PI was 54.3° SD = 13 and did not change during follow-up.

With regards to regional parameters, a significant improvement of LL and TK was noted between preoperative and last follow-up evaluation (28.2° vs. 43.5°, $p < 0.001$ and 30.2° vs. 43.9°, $p < 0.001$, respectively).

SVA and PI-LL mismatch were significantly reduced (81.9 mm vs. 50.9 mm, $p < 0.001$ and 26° vs. 13.5°, $p < 0.001$, respectively). On the other hand, PT remained unchanged between pre and 1-year assessment (29.9° vs. 28.1°, $p > 0.05$).

3.3. Aligned vs. Nonaligned Group Analysis. Thirty-five patients were classified as "aligned" (PI-LL <10°) and 42 were classified as "not aligned" (PI-LL >10°). Of the 42 "not aligned" patients, 17 were revision cases, 10 requiring a grade 3 osteotomy (8 in L3 and 2 in L4). Among the 35 "aligned" patients, 19 were revision cases, 7 requiring a grade 3 osteotomy (5 in L3 and 2 in L4) (Figures 1 and 2).

Preoperatively, "not aligned" patients had a significantly higher pelvic incidence, higher pelvic tilt, smaller lumbar lordosis, and thoracic kyphosis, despite a nonsignificantly different sagittal vertical axis (Table 1).

With regards to preoperative LL distribution, the L1-L4 PLL (1.5° vs. 08°, $p = 0.9$) and the L4-S1 DLL (33.3° vs. 28.3°, $p = 0.254$) were not significantly different between groups (Table 1).

Postoperatively, "aligned" patients showed a significantly higher improvement of LL, TK, and SVA (Table 2).

With regards to postoperative LL distribution, the L1-L4 PLL was not significantly different between groups (18° vs. 16° $p > 0.05$), but the L4-S1 DLL was significantly higher in the "aligned" group (31° vs. 22°, $p = 0.003$).

The PI-LL mismatch was significantly correlated with the L4-S1 DLL (rho = 0.407, $p < 0.001$) but not with the L1-L4 PLL (rho = 0.110, $p = 0.342$). This significant correlation revealed that restoration of the PI-LL mismatch was significantly related to the correction of the distal lumbar lordosis.

3.4. Postoperative Complications and Clinical Evaluation. During the follow-up period, 7 postoperative infections were noted (4 in the "not aligned" group and 3 in the "aligned" group) that required surgical debridement and adapted antibiotics.

At last follow-up, 1 patient out of 35 (3%) in the aligned group had a mechanical complication (rod breakage) that required revision surgery. Six patients out of 42 (14%) of the "not aligned" group had a mechanical complication that required revision surgery (4 rod breakage and 2 proximal junctional failure).

With regards to final follow-up clinical scores, patients from the "aligned" group had a significantly lower lumbar

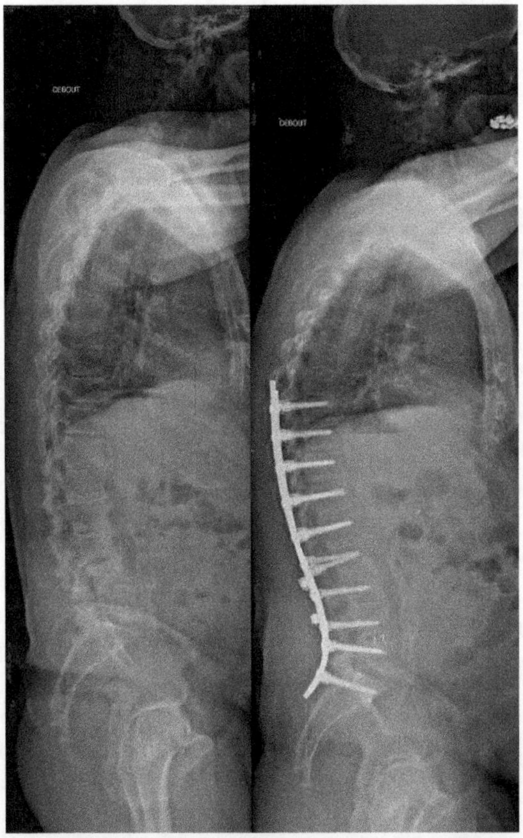

FIGURE 1: Clinical example of a patient from the “aligned group” with a low PI. Primary case, T9-S1 posterior fixation, multiples grade 2 osteotomies. Preoperative measurements (left) were PI = 41°, PT = 21°, PI-LL = 21, LL = -20°, TK = 22°, and SVA = 42 mm. One-year measurements (right) were PT = 17°, PI-LL = 0, LL = −41°, PLL = −8°, DLL = −33°, TK = 41°, and SVA = 41 mm.

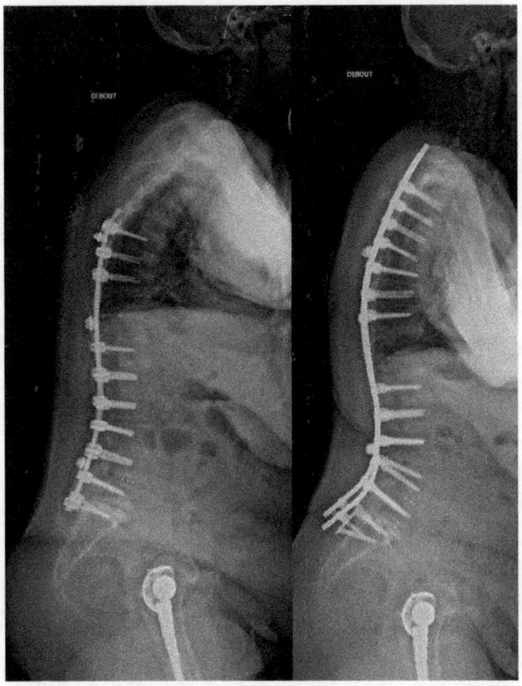

FIGURE 2: Clinical example of a patient form the “not aligned” group with a high PI. Revision case, T3-S2 posterior fixation, L3 grade 3 osteotomy. Preoperative measurements (left) were PI = 59°, PT = 34°, PI-LL = 32°, LL = −27°, TK = 3°, and SVA = 93 mm. One-year measurements (right) were PT = 25°, PI-LL = 15°, LL = −44°, PLL = −29°, DLL = −15°, TK = 36°, and SVA = 91 mm.

TABLE 1: Preoperative values of radiographic parameters between "aligned" and "not aligned" groups.

Preoperative	Aligned	Not aligned	p value
Pelvic incidence (°)	52	61	0.009
Pelvic tilt (°)	26	33	0.001
L1-S1 lumbar lordosis (°)	34	23	0.004
L1-L4 PLL (°)	1.5	0.8	0.9
L4-S1 DLL (°)	33.3	28.3	0.254
PI-LL (°)	16	34	<0.001
T4-T12 thoracic kyphosis (°)	37	25	0.008
Sagittal vertical axis (mm)	71	91	>0.05

TABLE 2: Postoperative values of radiographic parameters between "aligned" and "not aligned" groups.

Postoperative	Aligned	Not aligned	p value
Pelvic incidence (°)	52	61	0.009
Pelvic tilt (°)	24	33	<0.001
L1-S1 lumbar lordosis (°)	49	37	<0.001
L1-L4 PLL (°)	18	16	0.39
L4-S1 DLL (°)	31	22	0.003
PI-LL (°)	4	23	<0.001
T4-T12 thoracic kyphosis (°)	48	40	0.002
Sagittal vertical axis (mm)	23	63	<0.001

VAS (2.8/10 vs. 4.8/10, $p = 0.028$). ODI scores were not significantly different between groups ("aligned" 29% vs. "not aligned" 37%, $p = 0.095$).

4. Discussion

Surgical management of ASD remains challenging, and optimal management is still under debate. The complication rate after realignment procedures has been reported around 16.5% at 2 years of follow-up and 50% at 10 years of follow-up [10, 11].

According to the literature, a large proportion (up to 50%) of patients remains undercorrected after surgery [7]. Perfect understanding of this undercorrection is difficult especially, as alignment can still change postoperatively. According to McDowell et al. [12], a significant improvement of SVA can be seen during the first postoperative year without further modifications. However, this progressive correction of the SVA was also associated with an increase of pelvic tilt which can be considered as a compensatory mechanism in undercorrected patients.

Restoration of pelvic tilt might therefore be a crucial point for sagittal realignment procedures, especially in patients with a high pelvic incidence. Lafage et al. [13] suggested that patients with a high preoperative pelvic retroversion (related to a high pelvic incidence) require larger lumbar osteotomy procedures. In our series, pelvic tilt was the most difficult parameter to restore, with a nonsignificant postoperative correction. This lack of correction can be related to an insufficient bone resection, but it can also be associated with the level of the osteotomy. Mainly, L3 grade 3 osteotomies have been performed in our experience, and in order to achieve a proper spinopelvic alignment, performing osteotomy at a lower lumbar level (L4 or L5) can increase pelvic tilt correction with an average of 2° per level [14, 15].

Another important parameter for realignment procedures is the postoperative location of the LL apex. Based on Roussouly classification, Pizones et al. recently reported a decrease in mechanical complications with an adapted postoperative lumbar apex position and lumbar shape restoration [16, 17]. Of note, besides sagittal alignment goals, the use of multiple rods constructs has also been reported as a safe and effective method to reduce implant failures [18, 19], but this strategy was not used in our experience.

In our study, the choice was made to stratify patients according to postoperative PI-LL mismatch. Our results revealed that postoperatively "aligned" patients had a preservation of L4-S1 DLL and a higher pelvic incidence when compared to "not aligned" patients. These results are consistent with the study of Ylgor et al. who suggested taking into account lumbar lordosis distribution [20]. While L4-S1 DLL represents around 2/3 of global lordosis, it has been reported that the amount of this L4-S1 DLL was constant and independent from pelvic incidence. However, pelvic incidence is significantly correlated to the L1-L4 PLL [8]. As a whole, these results suggest that the loss of lumbar lordosis mainly occurs in the L4-S1 DLL. As a consequence, failure to restore DLL is correlated with an increased risk of proximal junctional failure [21], and DLL should be preserved or restored around 36° [8].

Results of this study confirm that restoration of L4-S1 DLL is a crucial objective for ASD patients as recently reported by Lafage et al. [22] as 1° of L4-S1 DLL correction produces 10 mm change in SVA and 0.5° in PT. Two strategies can therefore be advocated to reach this goal. First option is based on an anterior approach with intersomatic lordotic cages prior to the posterior fixation. According to recent studies [23–25], this technique can eliminate the need for a grade 3 osteotomy during the posterior approach, especially in primary cases. The second option is to perform L4 or even L5 grade 3 osteotomy [11].

This study presents several limitations such as the one-year follow-up and a limited number of patients included. Further studies will be needed to confirm these results.

5. Conclusion

Adult spinal deformity is a frequent and challenging condition for spine physicians. Based on postoperative PI-LL mismatch, the results of this study revealed that maintenance or restoration of L4-S1 DLL is crucial for postoperative alignment. Specific attention must be paid to restore optimal distal lumbar lordosis in order to decrease the rate of undercorrected patients and to improve outcomes.

Consent

Each patient signed an informed consent prior to inclusion.

References

[1] F. J. Schwab, B. Blondel, S. Bess et al., "Radiographical spinopelvic parameters and disability in the setting of adult spinal deformity," *Spine*, vol. 38, no. 13, pp. E803–E812, 2013.

[2] B. Blondel, F. Schwab, B. Ungar et al., "Impact of magnitude and percentage of global sagittal plane correction on health-related quality of life at 2-years follow-up," *Neurosurgery*, vol. 71, no. 2, pp. 341–348, 2012, discussion 348.

[3] J. S. Smith, C. I. Shaffrey, V. Lafage et al., "Comparison of best versus worst clinical outcomes for adult spinal deformity surgery: a retrospective review of a prospectively collected, multicenter database with 2-year follow-up," *Journal of Neurosurgery: Spine*, vol. 23, no. 3, pp. 349–359, 2015.

[4] J. Simon, P.-M. Longis, and N. Passuti, "Correlation between radiographic parameters and functional scores in degenerative lumbar and thoracolumbar scoliosis," *Orthopaedics & Traumatology: Surgery & Research*, vol. 103, no. 2, pp. 285–290, 2017.

[5] F. Schwab, B. Ungar, B. Blondel et al., "Scoliosis research society-schwab adult spinal deformity classification," *Spine*, vol. 37, no. 12, pp. 1077–1082, 2012.

[6] R. Lafage, F. Schwab, V. Challier et al., "Defining spino-pelvic alignment thresholds," *Spine*, vol. 41, no. 1, pp. 62–68, 2016.

[7] B. Moal, F. Schwab, C. P. Ames et al., "Radiographic outcomes of adult spinal deformity correction: a critical analysis of variability and failures across deformity patterns," *Spine Deformity*, vol. 2, no. 3, pp. 219–225, 2014.

[8] S. Pesenti, R. Lafage, D. Stein et al., "The amount of proximal lumbar lordosis is related to pelvic incidence," *Clinical Orthopaedics & Related Research*, vol. 476, no. 8, pp. 1603–1611, 2018.

[9] F. Schwab, B. Blondel, E. Chay et al., "The comprehensive anatomical spinal osteotomy classification," *Neurosurgery*, vol. 74, no. 1, pp. 112–120, 2014, discussion 120.

[10] P. G. Passias, A. Soroceanu, S. Yang et al., "Predictors of revision surgical procedure excluding wound complications in adult spinal deformity and impact on patient-reported outcomes and satisfaction," *Journal of Bone and Joint Surgery*, vol. 98, no. 7, pp. 536–543, 2016.

[11] A. Sebaaly, M. Gehrchen, C. Silvestre et al., "Mechanical complications in adult spinal deformity and the effect of restoring the spinal shapes according to the Roussouly classification: a multicentric study," *European Spine Journal*, vol. 29, no. 4, pp. 904–913, 2020.

[12] M. M. McDowell, Z. J. Tempel, G. S. Gandhoke et al., "Evolution of sagittal imbalance following corrective surgery for sagittal plane deformity," *Neurosurgery*, vol. 81, no. 1, pp. 129–134, 2017.

[13] V. Lafage, B. Blondel, J. S. Smith et al., "Preoperative planning for pedicle subtraction osteotomy: does pelvic tilt matter?" *Spine Deformity*, vol. 2, no. 5, pp. 358–366, 2014.

[14] V. Lafage, F. Schwab, S. Vira et al., "Does vertebral level of pedicle subtraction osteotomy correlate with degree of spinopelvic parameter correction?" *Journal of Neurosurgery: Spine*, vol. 14, no. 2, pp. 184–191, 2011.

[15] E. Ferrero, B. Liabaud, J. K. Henry et al., "Sagittal alignment and complications following lumbar 3-column osteotomy: does the level of resection matter?" *Journal of Neurosurgery: Spine*, vol. 27, no. 5, pp. 560–569, 2017.

[16] J. Pizones, L. Moreno-Manzanaro, L. Moreno-Manzanaro et al., "Restoring the ideal Roussouly sagittal profile in adult scoliosis surgery decreases the risk of mechanical complications," *European Spine Journal*, vol. 29, no. 1, pp. 54–62, 2020.

[17] J. Pizones, F. J. S. Perez-Grueso, F. J. S. Perez-Grueso et al., "Ideal sagittal profile restoration and ideal lumbar apex positioning play an important role in postoperative mechanical complications after a lumbar PSO," *Spine Deformity*, vol. 8, no. 3, pp. 491–498, 2020.

[18] F. Guevara-Villazón, L. Boissiere, K. Hayashi et al., "Multiple-rod constructs in adult spinal deformity surgery for pelvic-fixated long instrumentations: an integral matched cohort analysis," *European Spine Journal*, vol. 29, no. 4, pp. 886–895, 2020.

[19] S.-J. Hyun, L. G. Lenke, Y.-C. Kim, L. A. Koester, and K. M. Blanke, "Comparison of standard 2-rod constructs to multiple-rod constructs for fixation across 3-column spinal osteotomies," *Spine*, vol. 39, no. 22, pp. 1899–1904, 2014.

[20] C. Yilgor, N. Sogunmez, Y. Yavuz et al., "Relative lumbar lordosis and lordosis distribution index: individualized pelvic incidence-based proportional parameters that quantify lumbar lordosis more precisely than the concept of pelvic incidence minus lumbar lordosis," *Neurosurgical Focus*, vol. 43, no. 6, p. E5, 2017.

[21] R. Lafage, I. Obeid, B. Liabaud et al., "Location of correction within the lumbar spine impacts acute adjacent-segment kyphosis," *Journal of Neurosurgery: Spine*, vol. 30, no. 1, pp. 69–77, 2019.

[22] R. Lafage, F. Schwab, J. Elysee et al., "Surgical planning for adult spinal deformity: anticipated sagittal alignment corrections according to the surgical level," *Global Spine Journal*, vol. 11, Article ID 219256822098850, 2021.

[23] P. Hosseini, G. M. Mundis, R. K. Eastlack et al., "Preliminary results of anterior lumbar interbody fusion, anterior column realignment for the treatment of sagittal malalignment," *Neurosurgical Focus*, vol. 43, no. 6, p. E6, 2017.

[24] J.-C. Leveque, V. Yanamadala, Q. D. Buchlak, and R. K. Sethi, "Correction of severe spinopelvic mismatch: decreased blood loss with lateral hyperlordotic interbody grafts as compared with pedicle subtraction osteotomy," *Neurosurgical Focus*, vol. 43, no. 2, p. E15, 2017.

[25] A. A. Theologis, G. M. Mundis, S. Nguyen et al., "Utility of multilevel lateral interbody fusion of the thoracolumbar coronal curve apex in adult deformity surgery in combination with open posterior instrumentation and L5-S1 interbody fusion: a case-matched evaluation of 32 patients," *Journal of Neurosurgery: Spine*, vol. 26, no. 2, pp. 208–219, 2017.

11

Analysis of Proximal Femoral Parameters in Adolescent Idiopathic Scoliosis

Máté Burkus, Ádám T. Schlégl, Kristóf József, Ian O'Sullivan, István Márkus, and Miklós Tunyogi-Csapó

Department of Orthopedics, Medical School, University of Pécs, H-7623 Pécs, Akác St. 1., Hungary

Correspondence should be addressed to Máté Burkus; burkusmate@gmail.com

Academic Editor: Thorsten M. Seyler

Background. Assessment of the proximal femoral parameters in adolescent idiopathic scoliosis using three-dimensional radiological image reconstructions may allow better characterization than conventional techniques. *Methods.* EOS 3D reconstructions of spines and femurs of 320 scoliotic patients (10-18 years old) and 350 control children lacking spinal abnormality were performed and 6 proximal femoral parameters measured. *Results.* Individuals with adolescent idiopathic scoliosis showed a small but statistically significant decrease in neck shaft angle (average difference=2.58°) and a higher (0.22°) femoral mechanical axis–femoral shaft angle. When the two sides were compared based on curve direction, greater changes in the neck shaft angle and femoral mechanical axis–femoral shaft angle were found on the side of the convexity. *Conclusions.* Patients with adolescent idiopathic scoliosis were found to have a small but significantly lower neck shaft angle and higher femoral mechanical axis–femoral shaft angle, which related to the curve direction. This is postulated to be due to mechanical compensation for altered balance and centre of gravity associated with a scoliosis deformity, although the observed difference likely has negligible clinical effect.

1. Introduction

Adolescent idiopathic scoliosis (AIS) is one of the most common spinal deformities and may affect as many as 1-4% of adolescents [1]. While scoliosis primarily causes deformity in the frontal plane it is a complex three-dimensional disorder affecting the entire body, including also the lower extremities. Compensatory changes in the pelvis have been previously described by several authors [2–4], and further studies have found increased asymmetry of limb length and other body parts in addition to the spine deformity. For example, Burwell et al. found the upper arm on the convex side to be longer in thoracic scoliosis, whereas the right lower extremity was longer in lumbar and thoracolumbar scoliosis [5, 6]. Normelli et al. compared 18 normal and 15 scoliotic cadavers and observed a significant difference in the length of the ribs [7]. Pelvic changes have been described with changes observed in hip rotation [8], abduction and range of motion [9], and proximal femoral bone density [10]. Observed abnormalities in the pelvis, however, are believed by some to be due to rotation rather than bony deformity [11].

On reviewing the literature, studies assessing the proximal femur appear to be scarce, with just one publication evaluating the femoral parameters in AIS found in the English language. In this paper Saji et al. found abnormalities associated with the deformity, as the neck shaft angle appeared to be on average 8° higher in patients with scoliosis [12].

Accurate description of the anatomical parameters of the lower extremities is of importance as altered bony structures can affect the biomechanics of the whole limb. Changes in the mechanical axis, even if minimal, may alter joint loading and small changes have been linked to increased knee arthritis [13], and abnormal neck shaft angles and femoral torsion specifically are independent risk factors for hip osteoarthritis [14].

However, assessing the parameters of the lower limb in children accurately can pose some difficulties. While conventional full-leg, full-spine radiographs allow us to see the extremities during active weight-bearing, they suffer from magnification artifacts and only allow measurements in two dimensions at a time. CT and MRI, while allowing more accurate, three-dimensional imaging, generally require the patient to lie supine and entail higher costs and radiation burden (in the case of CT). Since 2007 our department has been using the EOS 2D/3D system for evaluation of many patients. This bidirectional X-ray scanner takes simultaneous anteroposterior and lateral images of standing patients and uses a slit collimator to prevent vertical magnification and drastically reduce dose exposure. With the EOS scanner 3D reconstructions can also be made that have been found to be similar or superior to those of CT scout-based reconstructions, while delivering a radiation dose 800-1000 times lower [15]. The feasibility and accuracy of the equipment and the sterEOS software for assessing the vertebral column, the lower extremities, and the entire lumbar-pelvic-femoral complex in routine orthopedic practice have been confirmed in several studies [15–20].

2. Materials and Methods

The present study aimed to identify and characterize the changes of anatomical parameters of the proximal femur using a large sample of AIS patients from 10 to 18 years old, using high accuracy 3D EOS reconstructions. We hypothesized that the asymmetrical loading due to scoliosis affects the bony anatomy of the proximal femur.

Medical records from 879 children with scoliosis were reviewed from our outpatient radiological database between 2007 and 2018. All cases with spinal deformities due to other etiologies (therefore not AIS), previous surgical intervention on the spine, and lower limb abnormality were excluded. Any images of lower quality, in which reconstruction was not reliable due to movements on recording, missing reference points, etc., were also excluded. From the remaining patients, 320 cases were selected at random (79 males and 241 females) with an age range of 10-18 years (mean age at scan 14.71±2.31). All images were recorded with the EOS 2D/3D system during routine clinical work with orthopedic indication. Prior to imaging written consent was obtained from the patients or their legal guardians, which included consent to use of the images for later clinical research. Our retrospective case-control study was permitted by the Institutional Ethical Committee.

The control group consisted of sample cases without prior spinal abnormality from the database of our department. 1024 such examinations were performed during routine work in our clinic with suspicion of orthopedic disease including suspected scoliosis (though scoliosis was not found), muscular pain of unknown origin, or follow-up scans for benign bone lesions. From this population we randomly selected a control group of patients matching our scoliosis cases in age and sex, to form the basis of this comparative study. Finally, the control group comprised 350 individuals (85 males, 265 females), with a mean age of 14.81±2.43.

Reconstructions were made using sterEOS software EOS 3D V1.4.4.5297 (EOS Imaging, Paris, France), Cobb angles measured, and superficial 3D models of both femurs made and assessed (Figure 1).

The procedure was performed by 2 postgraduate student medical residents with considerable experience with the modality and software.

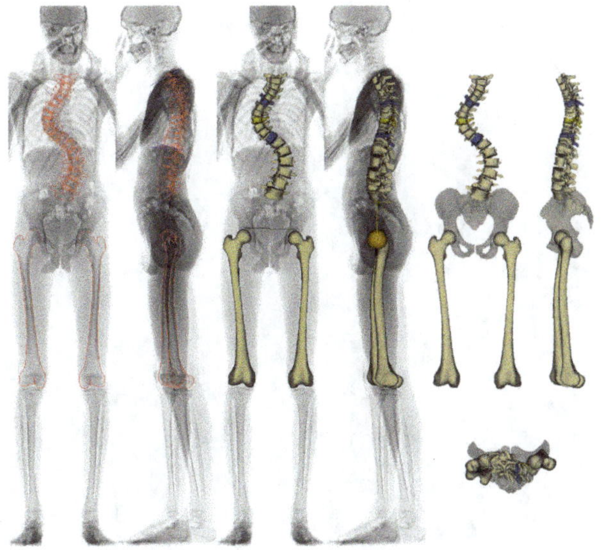

FIGURE 1: SterEOS 2D/3D spine, pelvis, and femur 3D reconstruction (from our database).

During remodeling, 30 randomly selected samples were used to assess interobserver error and intraobserver reliability of the spine reconstructions, and another 30 randomly selected 3D models of both femurs were used to assess the lower extremities on three different occasions. Intraclass coefficient was evaluated according to Winer's criteria: 0-0.24 indicating 'absent-to-poor' reliability, 0.25-0.49 'low', 0.50-0.69 'fair to moderate', 0.7-0.89 'good', and 0.90-1.0 'excellent' [21].

Six parameters relating to the proximal femur, which are calculated during reconstruction by the sterEOS 3D software, were evaluated during the present study (neck shaft (NS) angle, femur mechanical axis-femur shaft (FM-FS) angle, femoral torsion, femoral offset, femoral head diameter, and femoral neck length) (Figure 2).

For some assessments the population was classified into four different severity groups based on the Cobb angle, using the 2011 SOSORT guidelines [22];

Group 1: 10-25 degrees; (low or mild), n=129 (37 boys, 92 girls);

Group 2: 25-45 degrees; (moderate), n=101 (22 boys, 79 girls);

Group 3: 45-60 degrees; (severe), n=49 (10 boys, 39 girls);

Group 4: over 60 degrees; (very severe), n=41 (10 boys, 31 girls).

The group distribution of sex and age is shown in Table 1.

To examine curve laterality, the population was divided into two groups based on the direction of the main scoliotic curve convexity, as the sterEOS program also defines curve direction. 151 patients had right thoracic curves and 169 had left thoracolumbar or lumbar curvatures. In the case of double curves, the laterality of the main curve was taken.

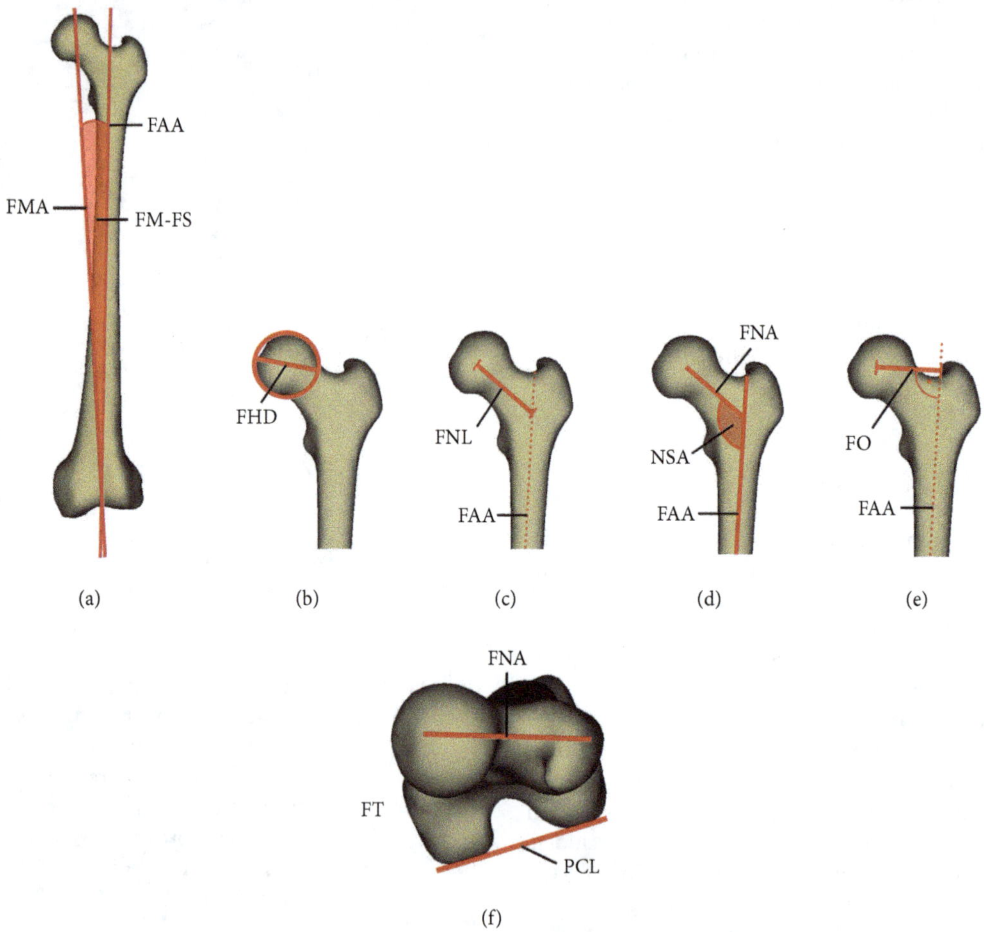

FIGURE 2: Measured parameters. (a) FM-FS: femoral mechanical axis-femoral shaft angle, FMA: femur mechanical axis, and FAA: femur anatomical axis; (b) FHD: femur head diameter; (c) FNL: femoral neck length; (d) NSA: neck shaft angle (FNA: femur neck axis); (e) FO: Femoral offset; (f) FT: femoral torsion (PCL: posterior condylar line).

TABLE 1: Age and gender distribution of the examined population.

Age (year)	Low		Moderate		Severe		Very severe		Sum
	Boy	Girl	Boy	Girl	Boy	Girl	Boy	Girl	
10	5	11	1	5	1	1	0	1	*25*
11	4	10	2	4	0	3	0	2	*25*
12	3	13	1	11	0	4	0	3	*35*
13	3	9	2	11	1	6	2	6	*40*
14	6	4	4	6	1	8	1	10	*40*
15	6	9	3	9	0	6	2	5	*40*
16	1	13	3	12	4	2	4	1	*40*
17	5	14	3	9	1	5	1	2	*40*
18	4	9	3	12	2	4	0	1	*35*
	37	*92*	*22*	*79*	*10*	*39*	*10*	*31*	***320***

Correlation between the right and left parameters and curve direction were subsequently evaluated.

The normality of values was evaluated using the Kolmogorov-Smirnov test. Differences between the mean values of the six measured parameters between control and AIS groups were evaluated using an independent sample t-test, and a one-way ANOVA was performed to assess correlation between the SOSORT severity groups and the parameters. Cobb angle parameter correlation was performed using Spearman correlation. The differences in the two sides were compared using paired t-test and regression analysis. Post-hoc power analysis was performed to control the statistical

TABLE 2: Results of the intra- and interobserver reliability study, assessing reliability of EOS reconstructions. Evaluation is as per Winer's criteria.

Parameter	Intraobserver				Interobserver	
	ICC (obs 1)	ICC (obs 2)	ICC (obs 3)	Evaluation	ICC (interobs)	Evaluation
Femoral head diameter	0.95	0.93	0.97	Excellent	0.92	Excellent
Femur neck length	0.93	0.91	0.95	Excellent	0.91	Excellent
Neck shaft angle	0.96	0.96	0.95	Excellent	0.93	Excellent
Femoral offset	0.92	0.94	0.93	Excellent	0.92	Excellent
Femur mechanical axis-shaft angle	0.97	0.94	0.98	Excellent	0.94	Excellent
Femoral torsion	0.90	0.90	0.93	Excellent	0.91	Excellent
SterEOS Cobb angle	0.91	0.91	0.94	Excellent	0.90	Excellent

ICC: intraclass coefficient, obs: observer.

TABLE 3: Mean and standard deviation (SD) of the examined parameters and the results of *t*-test and ANOVA.

Parameter		Control	AIS	*t*-test (p)	Low	Moderate	Severe	Very severe	One-way Anova (p)
	n=	*350*	*320*	*350/320*	*129*	*101*	*49*	*41*	*320*
Age (year)	mean	14.81	14.71		14.51	15.12	15.09	14.68	
	SD	2.43	2.31		2.66	2.41	2.24	1.82	
Femoral head diam. (mm)	mean	41.89	41.66	*0.251*	41.96	41.10	41.54	41.19	*0.413*
	SD	3.76	3.62		3.65	3.79	4.02	3.56	
Femoral offset (mm)	mean	38.62	37.99	*0.098*	38.16	37.50	38.46	38.22	*0.607*
	SD	5.29	4.67		4.51	4.79	5.62	3.55	
Neck length (mm)	mean	48.51	48.11	*0.735*	49.01	47.99	48.74	47.70	*0.494*
	SD	4.67	4.76		4.68	4.95	5.36	4.23	
Neck shaft angle (degree)	mean	129.64	127.06	***>0.001***	127.49	127.09	126.61	126.09	***0.022***
	SD	4.50	3.85		3.65	4.37	3.52	3.25	
FM-FS (degree)	mean	4.28	4.50	***0.004***	4.33	4.54	4.62	4.84	***0.023***
	SD	1.11	0.95		0.92	0.93	0.98	0.99	
Femoral torsion (degree)	mean	20.71	20.36	*0.598*	20.39	20.89	20.35	19.56	*0.955*
	SD	9.70	9.88		9.65	9.36	11.09	7.81	

power of the t-tests. A value of $p<0.05$ was considered significant during our evaluation. All statistical data was processed by the SPSS v22 (IBM Corp., Armonk, NY, USA) and by the Microsoft Office Professional Plus v14.0.6112.5000 (Microsoft Corp., Redmond, WA, USA) software packages.

3. Results and Discussion

Intra- and interobserver reliability values for the different examiners were greater than 0.9 for each parameter, regarded as excellent as per Winer's criteria (Table 2), and proximal femur measurements were found to be normally distributed, based on the Kolmogorov-Smirnov test. The mean Cobb angle in our sample was 35.3±20.7°, with a range of 10-123 degrees.

Mean proximal femur values of the whole group of 320 scoliotic patients and 350 control sample individuals are listed in Table 3.

A higher mean FM-FS angle was found in those with AIS, whereas all other measured parameters were lower with AIS than in the control group; however most differences were not significant. The neck shaft angle was significantly lower in AIS (control 129.64±4.50°; AIS 127.06±3.85°, $p<0.001$, statistical power=100.0%), and the higher FM-FS angle seen was also significant (control 4.28±1.11°; AIS 4.50±0.95°, $p=0.004$, statistical power=78.9%). No statistically significant difference was confirmed with femoral torsion, femoral offset, femoral head diameter, and femoral neck length; however, the values were often widely spread (e.g., in femoral torsion control 20.71±9.70°; AIS 20.36±9.88°).

When scoliosis was stratified by severity, a significant difference was found between severity groups and the NS angle ($p=0.022$) and the femur mechanical-femur anatomical angle ($p=0.023$). Additionally, the means were compared and results are shown in Figure 3.

When the correlation between the proximal femoral parameters and curvature was performed using just the value of the Cobb angle as a continuous variable, a statistically significant value was detected in relation to the NS angle ($B=-0.295$, $R^2=0.87$, $p<0.01$) and FM-FS angle ($B=0.101$, $R^2=0.031$, $p=0.002$).

With regard to laterality, when Cobb angle values and curve direction were used, it was found that the NS angle had an inverse relationship with the Cobb angle (correlation

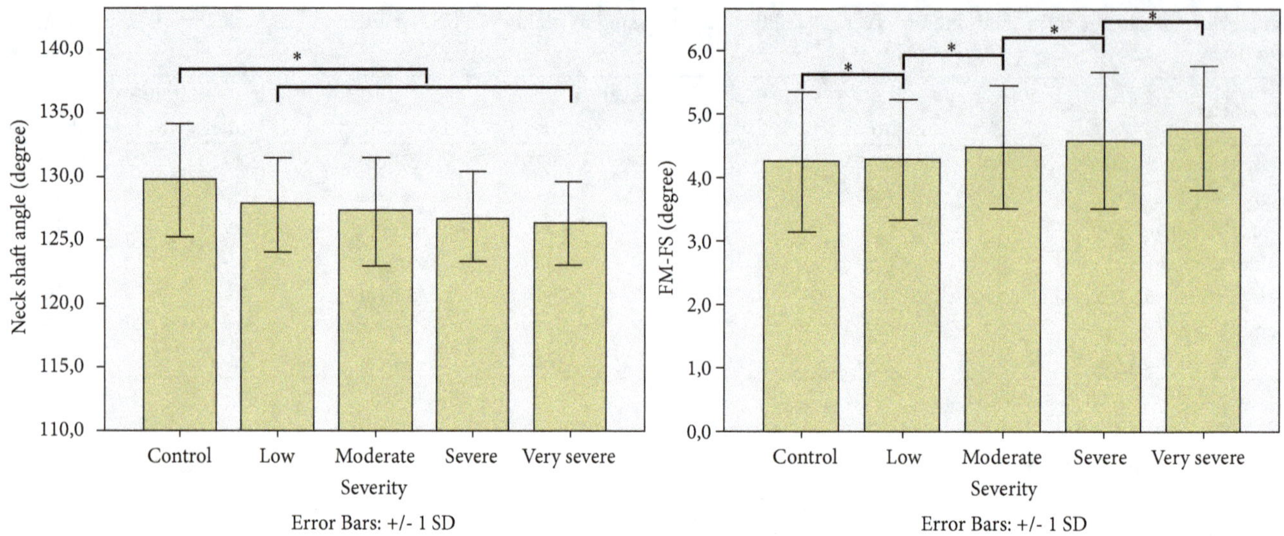

FIGURE 3: Mean values of the neck shaft angle (left) and FM-FS (right) based on the severity of the scoliosis. ∗: significant difference based on independent sample t-test (p<0.05).

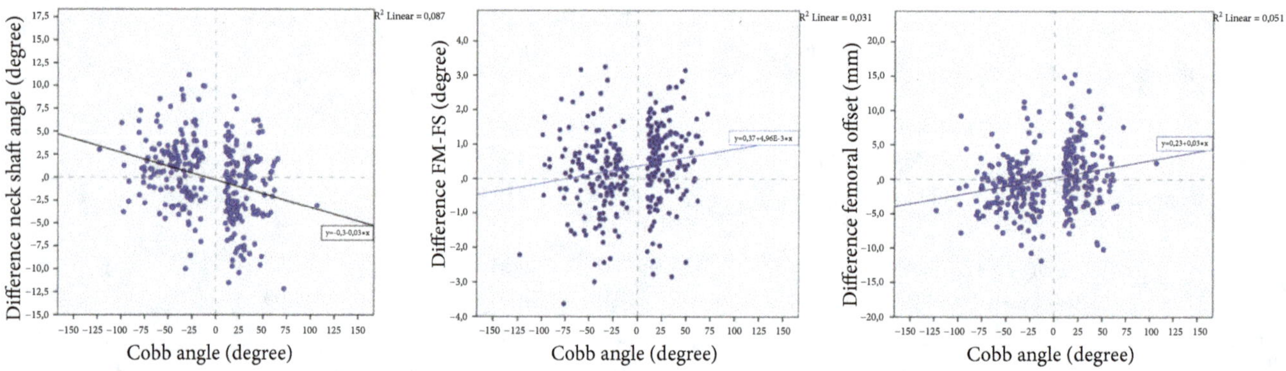

FIGURE 4: Side difference. Boxplot diagram presenting the correlation between the Cobb angle (positive values indicate a left main curve; negative values indicated right main curve) and the difference between the lower limb parameters (left side value-right side value).

coefficient=-0.290, p<0.001), and a positive correlation with both FM-FS angle (correlation coefficient=0.191, p=0.001) and femoral offset (correlation coefficient=0.237, p<0.001) (Figure 4).

Furthermore, when means were compared, the Cobb angle had a greater effect if the convexity was left facing, than if facing to the right. The mean neck shaft angle on the side of the convexity was 1.38° lower than that of the contralateral limb in the case of left-sided curves (p=0.017, statistical power=92.2%). In individuals with right-sided curves the NS angle was 1.27° lower on the side of the curve, than the contralateral limb (p<0.001, statistical power=80.9%). The mean FM-FS angle was 0.53° higher if left-sided (p<0.001, statistical power=69.2%) and 0.13° higher if right-sided (p= 0.049, statistical power=59.2%). No significant difference was observed in the femoral offset (correlation coefficient=0.061, p=0.147), or the other values. Differences between the left and right lower limbs are presented in Table 4.

This study aimed to find and evaluate proximal femur changes that may be associated with adolescent idiopathic scoliosis. To the best of our knowledge this is the only comparative study to simultaneously evaluate this number of parameters in weight-bearing position, and in so many patients. Therefore, we aimed to make a comprehensive evaluation of the proximal femoral region and its relationship with curve severity and direction.

The present study found a small, but statistically significant, decrease in neck shaft angle in our AIS group compared to the control. This clearly contradicts what Saji et al. found in their study of Chinese women in which they analyzed 94 anteroposterior conventional X-ray images (61 with AIS and 33 control women), detecting significantly higher NS angle values in the control group (129.5±3.7° left, and 129.9±3.7° right vs. scoliosis group: 137.5±6.6° on left, and 137.9±5.5° on the right side) [12]. Their results may be related to their imaging method, which does not compensate for individual variation of the femoral anteversion, in addition to their smaller sample size. Furthermore, ethnicity may play a role as pelvic parameters found in Chinese populations have been seen to differ from those in Caucasians [2, 23–27]. The

TABLE 4: Bilateral asymmetry. The presence of differences between patients limb sides are presented here with individuals divided into three groups based on the magnitude of difference between the two sides, irrespective of side.

Parameter / differences	Under 3 mm/degree (n=)	Between 3 and 5 mm/degree (n=)	More than 5 mm/degree (n=)
Femoral head diameter	319	1	0
Femoral offset	266	23	31
Neck length	274	20	26
Neck shaft angle	*252*	*39*	*29*
FM-FS	*318*	*2*	*0*
Femoral torsion	206	22	92

femur mechanical axis-femur shaft angle also saw a small but significant difference, with a higher value in scoliosis patients than in the control group, and this difference was seen at all severity groups and showed a significant correlation with the Cobb angle, increasing parallelly.

Interestingly the direction (convexity) of the curve was found to influence the magnitude of the change of the two parameters; if the curve is left-sided, the left NS angle was lower and FM-FS was higher, whereas if right-sided, similar changes were seen but not as great. This correlates somewhat with the findings of Chen et al. wherein the lumbar curve had significant effect on proximal femoral bone mineral density [10].

In general, both neck shaft angle and FM-FS angle exhibited similar changes that can be explained by their geometrical relationship. The axis of the neck shaft forms a triangle with the anatomical and mechanical axes of the femur, and so changes in the NS angle alter the FM-FS angle. It then becomes clear why a decrease in neck shaft angle was associated with an increase in FM-FS angle. The mean femoral offset was also elevated marginally, as would be expected from a fall in neck shaft angle without a change in femoral neck length (this marginal increase of femoral offset however was not statistically significant).

We found no statistical difference in femoral anteversion between the control group and the scoliosis group. The range of values was found to be high; however it was consistent with that of the control group findings. Previous findings for femoral anteversion by Szuper et al., obtained while studying anatomical parameters and growth factor effects, were very similar to those seen in the present study [16].

The changes seen in scoliosis patients are likely due to the altered biomechanical forces caused by a need for compensation of balance due to the deformity, or asymmetrical mechanical loading as a result of the deformity. Alterations were statistically significant, but rather small, and this minimal difference likely has no clinical effect.

AIS tends to develop during the later stages of adolescence, by which time the lower limb biomechanical parameters have been mostly established [16, 28] and hence alterations of a large magnitude are unlikely to develop. We assert that if scoliosis develops earlier, while the lower limb is undergoing more active growth, greater proximal femoral changes may be seen. However, the number of early-onset scoliosis patients is much lower than those with AIS, and even fewer among them are those who lack other systemic or generalized disorders, and so no significant group could be found in our clinical database during the period in question.

Potential limitations of this study include the control group used; individuals were not totally free of orthopedic complaints; however there are clear ethical difficulties with the exposure of 320 healthy children to ionizing radiation, even if low-dose scans are performed as with the EOS scanner. Furthermore, due to the natural incidence of AIS there was a much higher prevalence of girls in the scoliosis group, a limitation found in similar other AIS studies, and therefore we were unable to reliably evaluate sex differences in the different parameters.

4. Conclusions

Adolescent idiopathic scoliosis, in the absence of any other abnormalities, may have an effect on other parts of the skeleton including the proximal femur. Scoliosis patients were found to have significantly higher FM-FS angles, and significantly lower neck shaft angles, and changes exhibited a correlation with the magnitude and severity of the curve in the frontal plane. Interestingly, changes were greater if the curve convexity was left-sided. Although the observed differences were too small to conclude that AIS has an effect on the proximal femur that would be perceivable in the clinic, similar results have not been previously published.

Acknowledgments

The present scientific contribution is dedicated to the 650th anniversary of the foundation of the University of Pécs, Hungary. This work was supported by the *GINOP-2.3.3-15-2016-00031* grant of the Hungarian Government.

References

[1] J. C. Cheng, R. M. Castelein, W. C. Chu et al., "Adolescent idiopathic scoliosis," *Nature Reviews Disease Primers*, vol. 1, article no 15030, 2015.

[2] J.-M. Mac-Thiong, H. Labelle, M. Charlebois, M.-P. Huot, and J. A. De Guise, "Sagittal plane analysis of the spine and pelvis in adolescent idiopathic scoliosis according to the coronal curve type," *The Spine Journal*, vol. 28, no. 13, pp. 1404–1409, 2003.

[3] V. V. Upasani, J. Tis, T. Bastrom et al., "Analysis of sagittal alignment in thoracic and thoracolumbar curves in adolescent idiopathic scoliosis: how do these two curve types differ?" *The Spine Journal*, vol. 32, no. 12, pp. 1355–1359, 2007.

[4] J. Clément, A. Geoffray, F. Yagoubi et al., "Relationship between thoracic hypokyphosis, lumbar lordosis and sagittal pelvic parameters in adolescent idiopathic scoliosis," *European Spine Journal*, vol. 22, no. 11, pp. 2414–2420, 2013.

[5] R. G. Burwell, R. K. Aujla, B. J. C. Freeman et al., "Patterns of extra-spinal left-right skeletal asymmetries and proximo-distal disproportion in adolescent girls with lower spine scoliosis: Ilio-femoral length asymmetry & bilateral tibial/foot length disproportion," *Studies in Health Technology and Informatics*, vol. 123, pp. 101–108, 2006.

[6] R. G. Burwell, B. J. C. Freeman, P. H. Dangerfield et al., "Left-right upper arm length asymmetry associated with apical vertebral rotation in subjects with thoracic scoliosis: anomaly of bilateral symmetry affecting vertebral, costal and upper arm physes?" in *Proceedings of the 6th Biennial Meeting of the International Research Society of Spinal Deformities*, vol. 123, pp. 66–71, Belgium, June 2006.

[7] H. Normelli, J. Sevastik, and J. Akrivos, "The length and ash weight of the ribs of normal and scoliotic persons," *The Spine Journal*, vol. 10, no. 6, pp. 590–592, 1985.

[8] T. Kotwicki, A. Walczak, and A. Szulc, "Trunk rotation and hip joint range of rotation in adolescent girls with idiopathic scoliosis: Does the "dinner plate" turn asymmetrically?" *Scoliosis*, vol. 3, no. 1, 2008.

[9] K. M. Cheung, A. C. Cheng, W. Y. Cheung, Y. S. Chooi, Y. W. Wong, and K. D. Luk, "Right hip adduction deficit and adolescent idiopathic scoliosis," *Journal of Orthopaedic Surgery and Research*, vol. 16, pp. 24–26, 2008.

[10] R. Chen, K. Watanabe, N. Hosogane et al., "Spinal coronal profiles and proximal femur bone mineral density in adolescent idiopathic scoliosis," *European Spine Journal*, vol. 22, no. 11, pp. 2433–2437, 2013.

[11] X. Qiu, J. Zhang, S. Yang et al., "Anatomical study of the pelvis in patients with adolescent idiopathic scoliosis," *Journal of Anatomy*, vol. 220, no. 2, pp. 173–178, 2012.

[12] M. J. Saji, S. S. Upadhyay, and J. C. Leong, "Increased femoral neck-shaft angles in adolescent idiopathic scoliosis," *The Spine Journal*, vol. 20, no. 3, pp. 303–311, 1995.

[13] J. S. Schouten, F. A. van den Ouweland, and H. A. Valkenburg, "A 12 year follow up study in the general population on prognostic factors of cartilage loss in osteoarthritis of the knee.," *Annals of the Rheumatic Diseases*, vol. 51, no. 8, pp. 932–937, 1992.

[14] J. Chitnavis, "End-stage coxarthrosis and gonarthrosis. Aetiology, clinical patterns and radiological features of idiopathic osteoarthritis," *Rheumatology*, vol. 39, no. 6, pp. 612–619.

[15] T. Illés and S. Somoskeöy, "The EOS™ imaging system and its uses in daily orthopaedic practice," *International Orthopaedics*, vol. 36, no. 7, pp. 1325–1331, 2012.

[16] K. Szuper, Á. T. Schlégl, E. Leidecker, C. Vermes, S. Somoskeöy, and P. Than, "Three-dimensional quantitative analysis of the proximal femur and the pelvis in children and adolescents using an upright biplanar slot-scanning X-ray system," *Pediatric Radiology*, vol. 45, no. 3, pp. 411–421, 2015.

[17] A. T. Schlégl, K. Szuper, S. Somoskeöy, and P. Than, "Three dimensional radiological imaging of normal lower-limb alignment in children," *International Orthopaedics*, vol. 39, no. 10, pp. 2073–2080, 2015.

[18] Á. T. Schlégl, I. O'Sullivan, P. Varga, P. Than, and C. Vermes, "Determination and correlation of lower limb anatomical parameters and bone age during skeletal growth (based on 1005 cases)," *Journal of Orthopaedic Research*, vol. 35, no. 7, pp. 1431–1441, 2017.

[19] M. Wybier and P. Bossard, "Musculoskeletal imaging in progress: The EOS imaging system," *Joint Bone Spine*, vol. 80, no. 3, pp. 238–243, 2013.

[20] J. Y. Lazennec, A. Brusson, D. Folinais, A. Zhang, A. E. Pour, and M. A. Rousseau, "Measuring extension of the lumbar–pelvic–femoral complex with the EOS[5] system," *European Journal of Orthopaedic Surgery and Traumatology*, vol. 25, no. 6, pp. 1061–1068, 2015.

[21] B. J. Winer, *Statistical Principles in Experimental Design*, McGraw Hill, New York, NY, USA, 1st edition, 1971.

[22] S. Negrini, A. G. Aulisa, L. Aulisa et al., "2011 SOSORT guidelines: orthopaedic and rehabilitation treatment of idiopathic scoliosis during growth," *Scoliosis*, vol. 7, article no 3, 2012.

[23] J. Mac-Thiong, P. Roussouly, É. Berthonnaud, and P. Guigui, "Sagittal parameters of global spinal balance," *The Spine Journal*, vol. 35, no. 22, pp. E1193–E1198, 2010.

[24] P. Roussouly, S. Gollogly, E. Berthonnaud, and J. Dimnet, "Classification of the normal variation in the sagittal alignment of the human lumbar spine and pelvis in the standing position," *The Spine Journal*, vol. 30, no. 3, pp. 346–353, 2005.

[25] Z. Zhu, L. Xu, F. Zhu et al., "Sagittal alignment of spine and pelvis in asymptomatic adults," *The Spine Journal*, vol. 39, no. 1, pp. E1–E6, 2014.

[26] Q. Yong, L. Zhen, Z. Zezhang et al., "Comparison of sagittal spinopelvic alignment in Chinese adolescents With and Without Idiopathic Thoracic Scoliosis," *The Spine Journal*, vol. 37, no. 12, pp. 714–720, 2012.

[27] P. Hu, M. Yu, X. Liu, B. Zhu, X. Liu, and Z. Liu, "Analysis of the relationship between coronal and sagittal deformities in adolescent idiopathic scoliosis," *European Spine Journal*, vol. 25, no. 2, pp. 409–416, 2016.

[28] C. Birkenmaier, G. Jorysz, V. Jansson, and B. Heimkes, "Normal development of the hip: a geometrical analysis based on planimetric radiography," *Journal of Pediatric Orthopaedics B*, vol. 19, no. 1, pp. 1–8, 2010.

12

Postoperative Magnetic Resonance Imaging following Arthroscopic Primary Anterior Cruciate Ligament Repair

Jelle P. van der List,[1,2,3] Douglas N. Mintz,[4] and Gregory S. DiFelice[1]

[1] *Orthopaedic Trauma Service, Department of Orthopaedic Surgery, Hospital for Special Surgery, NewYork-Presbyterian, Weill Medical College of Cornell University, New York, NY, USA*
[2] *Spaarne Gasthuis Hospital, Department of Orthopaedic Surgery, Hoofddorp, Netherlands*
[3] *Amsterdam UMC, University of Amsterdam, Department of Orthopaedic Surgery, Amsterdam, Netherlands*
[4] *Department of Radiology, Hospital for Special Surgery, NewYork-Presbyterian, Weill Medical College of Cornell University, New York, NY, USA*

Correspondence should be addressed to Jelle P. van der List; jpjvanderlistmd@gmail.com

Academic Editor: Panagiotis Korovessis

Introduction. Recently, there has been a resurgence of interest in arthroscopic primary anterior cruciate ligament (ACL) repair. To date, no studies have assessed the role of postoperative magnetic resonance imaging (MRI) on the status and maturation of the repaired ligament. The goal of this study was therefore to assess (I) the accuracy of MRI on rerupture of the repaired ligament and (II) the maturation of the repaired ACL. *Methods.* All postoperative MRIs of patients that underwent arthroscopic primary ACL repair were included. A musculoskeletal radiologist, blinded for MRI indication, surgery-MRI time interval, and clinical stability, retrospectively assessed the ligament continuity and graded ligament maturation as hypointense (similar to intact PCL), isointense (>50% similar to PCL), or hyperintense (<50% similar to PCL). *Results.* Thirty-seven MRIs were included from 36 patients. Mean age was 30 years (range: 14–57 years), and mean surgery-MRI interval was 1.5 years (range: 0.1–4.9 years). The radiologist recognized 6 out of 8 reruptures and 26 out of 29 intact ligaments (sensitivity 75%, specificity 90%, and accuracy 86%). Ligaments in the first year were more often hyperintense than after one year (60% vs. 11%, p=0.02), most often isointense (60%) between one and two years, and more often hypointense after two years than before two years (56% vs. 10%, p=0.03). *Conclusion.* Postoperative MRI was found to accurately predict the rerupture of the primarily repaired ACL. Furthermore, it can be expected that the repaired ligament is hyperintense within the first year, while the signal becomes similar to the intact PCL after two years.

1. Introduction

Approximately 120 years ago, Mayo Robson was the first to surgically treat an anterior cruciate ligament (ACL) injury using open primary repair [1]. Over the following decades, Ivar Palmar and Don O'Donoghue further popularized this treatment and open primary repair became an important surgical treatment for ACL injuries in the 1970s and 1980s [1–6]. Although the short-term outcomes were promising [7–9], Feagin and Curl [10] and others [11–16] noted that the outcomes deteriorated at longer-term follow-up and as a result, the technique was abandoned and ACL reconstruction became the gold standard for all ACL injuries [6].

Several may have negatively influenced the early outcomes of primary repair [6]. Firstly, primary repair was historically used for patients with all tear types, while in hindsight better outcomes were found in patients with proximal tear types [16–19]. Secondly, primary repair was historically performed with an invasive open procedure (arthrotomy), while minimally invasive surgery (arthroscopy) decreases morbidity of the procedure [20]. Finally, patients were historically immobilized for four to six weeks postoperatively, while regaining early range of motion is now known to improve outcomes [21–23].

By applying several modern developments, such as magnetic resonance imaging (MRI) for appropriate patient

TABLE 1: Method of grading graft maturity in the ACL reconstruction literature.

MRI Appearance	Howell et al. [40]	Kanamiya et al. [41]	Figeroa et al. [39]
Part of graft evaluated	Complete graft	>50% of graft	>50% of graft
Reference	PCL	GM	SMT
Hypointense	Similar	< intense	< intense
Isointense	>50% similar	Similar	Similar
Hyperintense	<50% similar	> intense	> intense

ACL, anterior cruciate ligament; PCL, posterior cruciate ligament; GM, gastrocnemius muscle; SMT, semimembranosus tendon.

selection [24], arthroscopy for minimal invasive surgery [25], and early rehabilitation to prevent stiffness [23], better outcomes of primary repair can be expected. Indeed, DiFelice et al. showed excellent outcomes of primary repair of proximal ACL tears using minimally-invasive arthroscopy and focusing on early rehabilitation [26]. More recently, others have confirmed these promising outcomes [27–38]. In the reconstruction literature, many studies have assessed the role of postoperative MRI on graft maturation [39–42], but studies assessing the maturation of the repaired ACL following arthroscopic primary repair are currently lacking.

The goal of this study was therefore to assess the role of postoperative MRI following arthroscopic primary repair of proximal ACL tears. We hypothesized that postoperative MRI can be used to accurately assess (I) rerupture of the repaired ACL and (II) maturation of the repaired ACL.

2. Methods

2.1. Patient Selection. After Institutional Regional Board approval was obtained, a retrospective search was performed in the database of the senior author (GSD) for patients treated who had a postoperative MRI following arthroscopic primary repair between January 2008 and August 2018. The senior author has performed arthroscopic primary ACL repair in patients with proximal avulsion type tears using the pullout suture technique, suture anchor technique, or suture anchor technique with internal brace that have been previously described [25, 43, 44]. Out of 154 patients treated with arthroscopic primary repair, 37 MRIs of 36 patients could be identified.

2.2. MRI Grading. MRIs were performed at different institutions and therefore differed in quality and scanning details. However, all MRIs were minimum 1.5T scans and consisted of sagittal, coronal, and axial views. An experienced musculoskeletal radiologist reviewed all MRIs while blinded for the indication for the MRI, surgery-MRI time interval, and the clinical situation (i.e., stable or unstable knee). Using the sagittal, coronal, and axial views of both T1 and T2 sequences, the radiologist first graded the ligament in all patients as continuous or not continuous (reruptured). No additional sequences were used for this study to have similar MRI images for all patients. The maturation of the ligament was then graded similar to graft maturation in the ACL reconstruction literature [39–42, 45]: hypointense if the intensity of the repaired ligament was similar to the posterior cruciate ligament (PCL) and lower than posterior muscles (i.e., gastrocnemius muscle and semimembranosus), isointense if more than 50% of the ligament had the same intensity as the PCL and intensity was similar to posterior muscles, or hyperintense if less than 50% of the ligament had the same intensity as the PCL and more intensity than the posterior muscles. No computational software was used for this grading and the grading was performed on both T1 and T2 images and mainly based on the T1 images. An overview of the definitions of ligament intensity is provided in Table 1.

2.3. Data Collection. Data collected from the patients were data on the operative procedure, gender, age, BMI, time from surgery to MRI, reason for MRI, and clinical examination before and after MRI. Clinical examination was considered unstable if there was a minimum 2+ Lachman or 2+ pivot shift testing. All 37 MRIs were used to assess the accuracy of ACL rerupture, and all clinically stable and continuous ligaments were used to assess maturation in three time intervals based on ACL reconstruction literature [39–42, 45, 46]: MRI within one year of surgery, between one and two years of surgery, and after two years of surgery.

2.4. Statistical Analysis. Statistical analysis was performed using SPSS Version 24 (SPSS Inc., Armonk, NY, USA). Sensitivity, specificity, positive predictive value, negative predictive value, and accuracy were calculated using two by two tables. Fisher's exact test was used to compare the intensity of the ligament at different postoperative intervals. All tests were two-sided and differences with $p < 0.05$ were considered statistically significant.

3. Results

3.1. Baseline Characteristics. Thirty-seven MRIs from 36 patients were included in this study. Mean age of patients was 30 years (range: 14–57), 20 patients were male (57%), and mean time from operation to MRI was 1.5 years (range: 0.1–4.9 years). Eight MRIs (22%) were obtained in patients who suffered new trauma and had clinically unstable knees on clinical examination. Six of these eight unstable patients (75%) underwent arthroscopy in which the rerupture was confirmed. Of the 29 stable knees (78%), 10 (34%) were obtained within one year of surgery, 10 (34%) between one and two years of surgery, and 9 (30%) more than two years after surgery. Reasons for MRI were knee pain without trauma (n = 12; 32%), trauma with high suspicion for ACL re-injury (n = 9; 24%), evaluation of ligament healing (n = 8; 22%), trauma with low suspicion for ACL re-injury (n = 4;

TABLE 2: Baseline characteristics of all patients in this study cohort and the reasons for the postoperative MRI.

Baseline characteristics	
Number of patients (MRIs)	36 (37)
Male patients	20 (57%)
Right side	21 (60%)
Age (years; mean ± SD (range))	30 ± 12 (range 14–57)
BMI (kg/m^2; mean ± SD (range))	25 ± 4 (range 18–35)
Time from surgery to MRI (years; mean ± SD (range))	1.5 ± 1.1 (range 0.1–4.9)
Reasons for postoperative MRI	
Knee pain without trauma (n (%))	12 (32%)
Trauma with high suspicion for ACL re-injury (n (%))	9 (24%)
Evaluate ligament healing (n (%))	8 (22%)
Trauma with low suspicion for ACL re-injury (n (%))	4 (11%)
Superficial tenderness over suture anchor (n (%))	2 (5%)
Evaluate meniscal (root) repair (n (%))	2 (5%)
Postoperative MRI	
Unstable clinic examination (re-injury)	8 (22%)
Stable clinical examination (no re-injury)	29 (78%)
Within 1 year after primary repair	11 (38%)
Between 1 and 2 years after primary repair	10 (34%)
More than 2 years after primary repair	8 (28%)

MRI, magnetic resonance imaging; SD, standard deviation; BMI, body mass index; n, number.

TABLE 3: Assessment of intact ligament by the blinded radiologist.

		Clinical Stability on PE		
		Torn	Intact	Total
MRI	Torn	6	3	9
	Intact	2	26	28
		8	29	37

Sensitivity: 75%; specificity: 90%; positive predictive value: 67%; negative predictive value: 93%; accuracy: 86%; MRI, magnetic resonance imaging; PE, physical examination (consisting of Lachman, pivot, and anterior drawer examination).

11%), superficial tenderness over tibial internal brace suture anchor (n = 2; 5%), and evaluation of meniscal (root) repair (n=2; 5%) (Table 2).

3.2. Accuracy Rerupture of Repaired ACL. The radiologist graded 6 out of 8 unstable knees as not continuous (Figure 1) and graded 26 out of 29 stable knees as continuous. This corresponded to a sensitivity of 75%, specificity of 90%, positive predictive value of 67%, negative predictive value of 93%, and accuracy of 86% (Table 3).

3.3. Maturation of Repaired ACL. Within one year of surgery, ligaments were hyperintense (60%) or isointense (40%) and were more often hyperintense than after one year (60% vs. 11%, respectively, $p = 0.02$) (examples in Figure 2). Between one and two years postoperatively, majority of ligaments were isointense (60%) (examples in Figure 3). Minimum two years postoperatively, ligaments were hypointense (56%) or isointense (44%) and were more often hypointense than on MRIs within two years of surgery (56% vs. 10%, respectively, $p = 0.03$) (examples in Figure 4). Overview of the distribution of ligament intensity can be seen in Figure 5, and an early and a late MRI of the same patient can be seen in Figure 6.

4. Discussion

The goal of this study was to assess the role of postoperative MRI on the (I) accuracy of ACL rerupture and (II) ligament maturation following arthroscopic primary ACL repair. It was noted that postoperative MRI can accurately assess rerupture of the repaired ligament. Furthermore, it was noted that ligaments were generally hyperintense within one year of surgery, isointense between one and two years, and hypointense after more than two years.

This is the first study assessing the role of postoperative MRI following arthroscopic primary ACL repair and assessing maturation of the repaired ligament. It is therefore only possible to compare these findings with the reconstruction literature or experimental studies on primary repair. Howell et al. were one of the first to use MRI to assess graft maturation following hamstring autograft reconstruction and found that ligament intensity changed significantly during the first year after surgery [40]. More recently, Ntoulia et al. performed a prospective study in which they obtained MRIs at 3 days, 6 months, 12 months, and 24 months following autograft bone-patellar tendon-bone ACL reconstruction [46]. Interestingly, the patients underwent MRI before and after intravenous gadolinium contrast, which enabled them to look at the healing and remodeling of the graft. They noted similar findings as in our current study with significantly increased signal intensity in the intra-articular graft at 6 and 12 months and more homogeneous low signal at 24 months. With the gadolinium scans, they noted that the increased signal

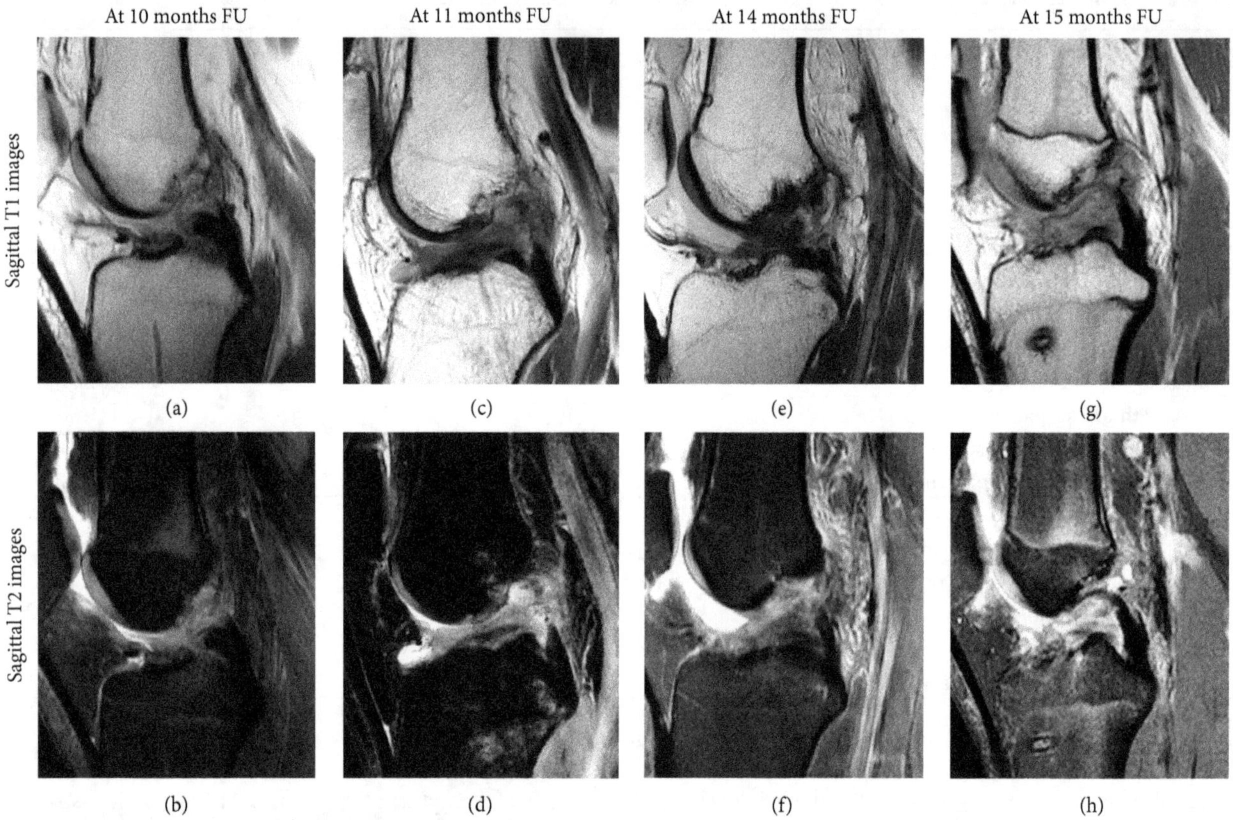

FIGURE 1: Sagittal T1 (upper row) and T2 (lower row) MR images of four patients are shown with a rerupture of the repaired ligament.

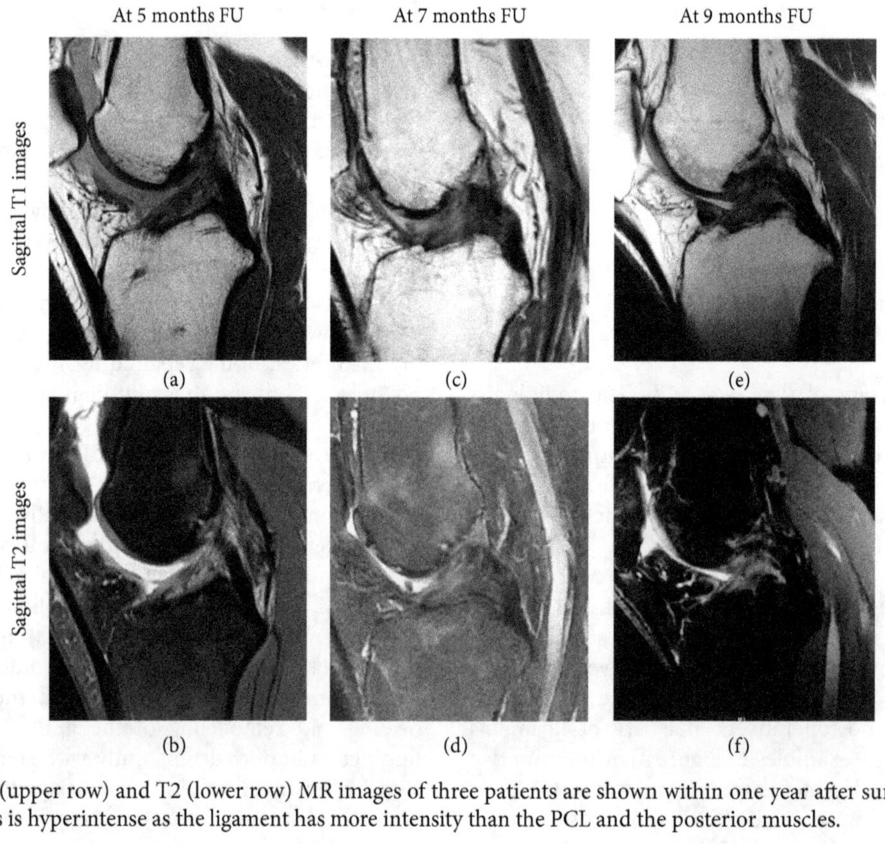

FIGURE 2: Sagittal T1 (upper row) and T2 (lower row) MR images of three patients are shown within one year after surgery. The ligament in most of these patients is hyperintense as the ligament has more intensity than the PCL and the posterior muscles.

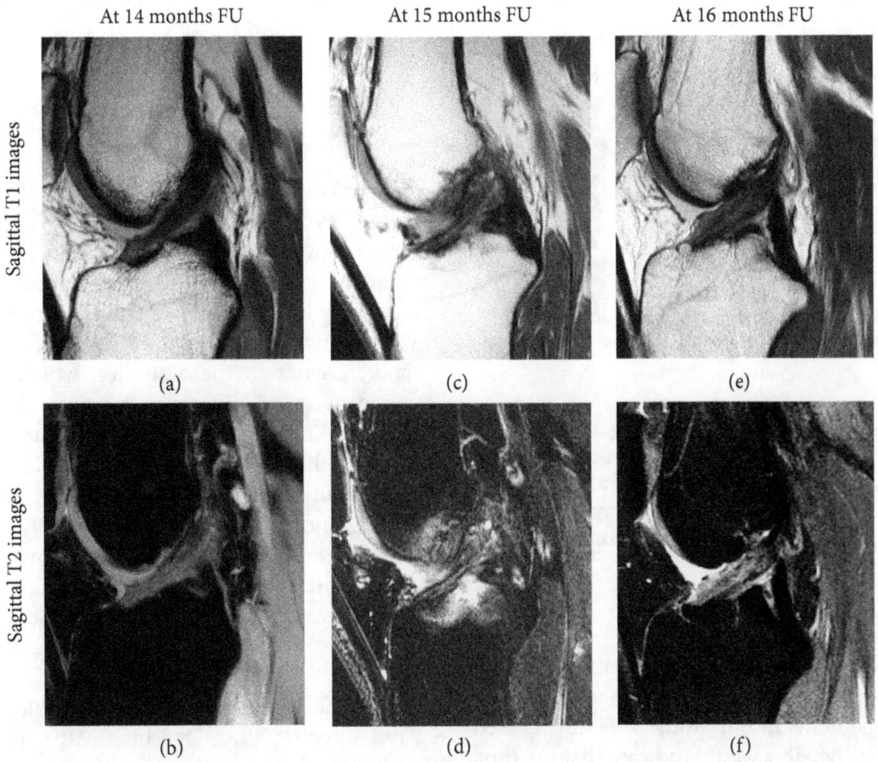

FIGURE 3: Sagittal T1 (upper row) and T2 (lower row) MR images of three patients are shown between one and two years after surgery. At this time interval, the ligament is often isointense as the ligament has more intensity than the PCL and similar intensity to the posterior muscles.

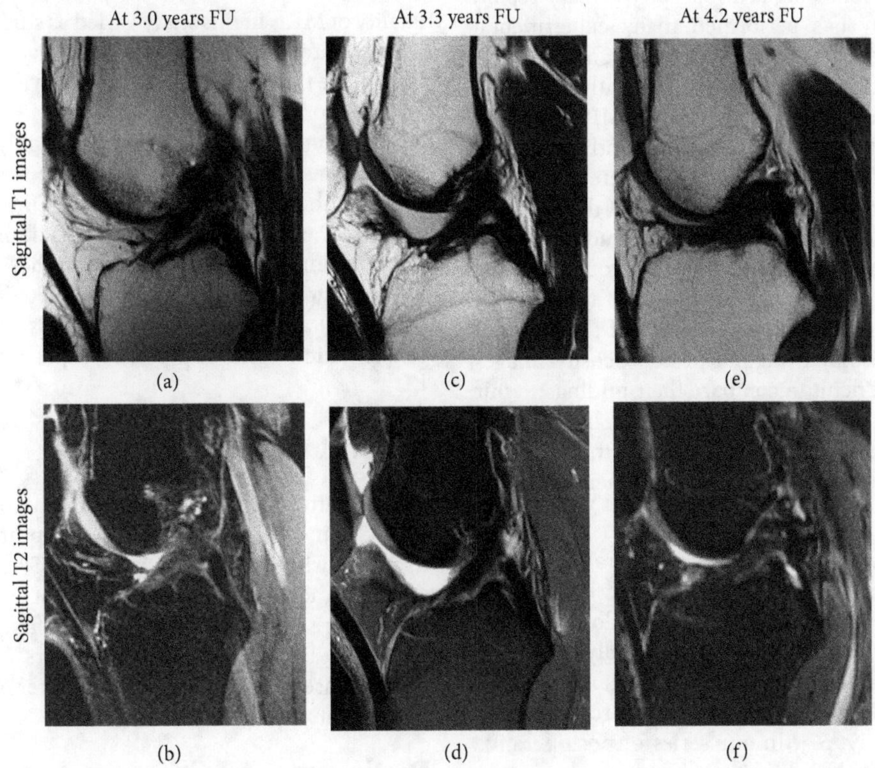

FIGURE 4: Sagittal T1 (upper row) and T2 (lower row) MR images of three patients are shown more than two years after surgery. The ligament is continuous and the intensity is similar to the PCL and lower than the posterior muscles.

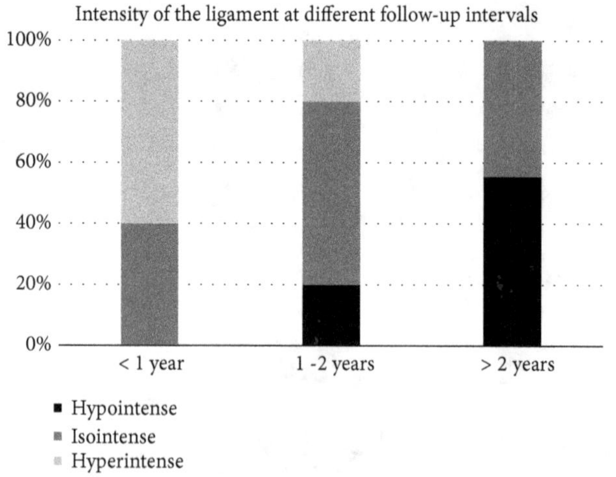

FIGURE 5: Graph displays the distribution of hypointense (black), isointense (dark gray), and hyperintense (light gray) at different follow-up intervals of the patients that had a functioning ACL (no rerupture).

intensity was caused by significant revascularization. Extrapolating these findings, it is possible that the hyperintense and isointense repaired ligaments in our study were also caused by healing and remodeling. This would indicate that the time to complete remodeling could take up to two years after arthroscopic primary ACL repair.

Although no clinical studies have assessed the postoperative MRI features following arthroscopic primary repair, the group of Murray has performed many experimental studies on primary repair with a biological scaffold [47, 48]. Biercevicz et al. performed primary repair with biological scaffold in Yucatan minipigs and performed MRI at 15 and 52 weeks of follow-up [47]. Similar to the findings of our study, they noted that the repaired ligaments were more often hypointense at longer follow-up, indicating that the ligament is healing and remodeling. In a first pilot study with ten human patients, Murray et al. assessed the outcomes at three months of follow-up and also obtained MRIs at this interval [49]. Since they did not grade the intensity of the repaired ligament and only displayed sagittal proton density images in their paper, it is difficult to compare their findings to our study. It can, however, be seen that the repaired ligaments in their study were grossly similar to the MRIs within one year of surgery in this current study (i.e., mostly hyperintense).

After the disappointing results of open primary repair in the historical literature, there has been a general consensus that primary repair of the ACL does not work, because the intra-articular synovial environment prevents clot formation and ligament healing [6, 50, 51]. When critically reviewing the literature, however, it seems proximal tears can heal when the ligament has sufficient length to be reapproximated to the femoral wall [17, 19, 52]. In our series of postoperative MRIs, the 29 patients without traumatic rerupture indeed had ligament continuity to the femoral insertion site and clinical stability. This finding, along several histological and clinical studies showing that the healing potential of the proximal ACL is similar to the MCL [52–56], indicates that primary ACL repair can result in healing of proximal tears and is therefore a good treatment for this select group of patients with proximal tears [26].

In this study, sensitivity of 75%, specificity of 90%, and accuracy of 86% were found for rerupture of the repaired ligament. Although it is not possible to compare these findings with other studies assessing this following primary repair, several studies have assessed these MRI characteristics following ACL reconstruction [57–59]. These studies found a sensitivity of 60–100%, accuracy of 85–87%, and specificity of 86–100% for a ruptured graft [57–59]. The MRI characteristics in our study were similar to the MRI characteristics in these studies, which can be expected as there was a clear difference in continuity between stable and unstable knees (Figure 1 versus Figures 2 and 3). In three patients, the radiologists graded a clinically stable ligament as not continuous, which can likely be explained by the early healing and fluid in the proximal part of the ligament that can be seen as a (high-grade) tear in the proximal part. It is therefore important to compare these findings with the clinical stability and that the radiologist is aware of the fact that there is a healing ligament rather than a reconstructed graft.

Limitations are present in this study. First of all, this is a retrospective study in which MRIs were made for several reasons and this was not a prospective study in which the same knees were followed at several time points. Nonetheless, we believe that the findings and MRI examples in this study are valuable for surgeons who perform arthroscopic primary ACL repair and obtain postoperative MRIs. Secondly, the quality of MRIs in this study varied as studies were performed at different institutions. Despite this lack of standardization, we believe this increases the external validity of the findings. Furthermore, the grading of the MRIs was a subjective grading, and although this is commonly performed in the ACL reconstruction literature, future studies with objective computational grading are needed. Finally, no arthroscopic validation of the findings was possible in the patients with stable examination. Prospective studies obtaining MRIs at regular intervals in the early rehabilitation phase (i.e., first 6 months) are therefore needed to assess healing and guide rehabilitation following arthroscopic primary ACL repair [23].

5. Conclusion

Postoperative MRI following arthroscopic primary ACL repair can be used to assess rerupture of the repaired ligament with excellent sensitivity (75%), specificity (90%), and accuracy (86%). Furthermore, it was noted that ligaments were often hyperintense in the first postoperative year, isointense between one and two years postoperatively, and hypointense and similar to the PCL after more than two years postoperatively.

Disclosure

This study has been presented in poster format in March at the 2018 Annual Meeting of the American Academy for Orthopaedic Surgeons (AAOS).

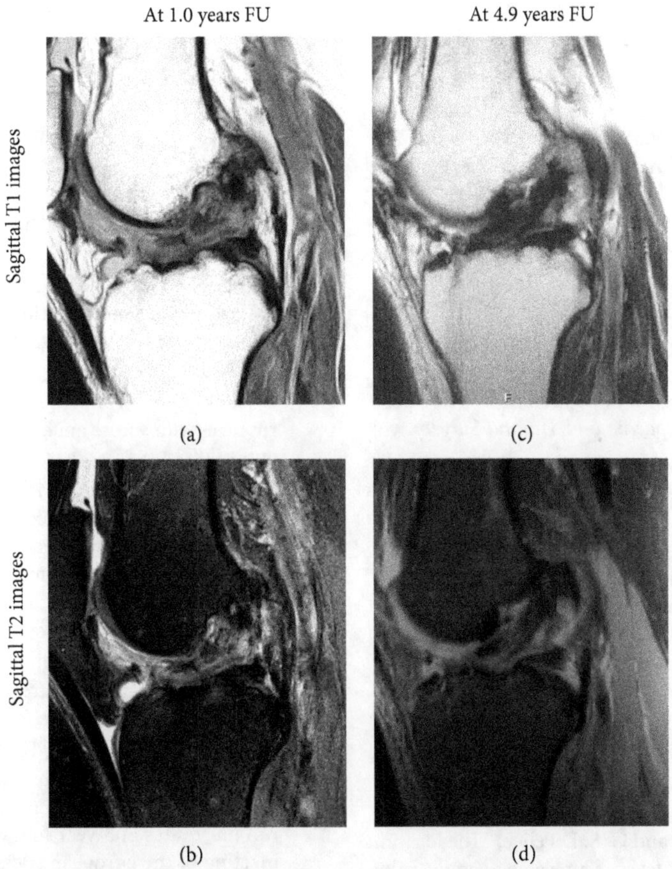

FIGURE 6: Sagittal T1 (upper row) and T2 (lower row) MR images are shown of the same patient at one and five years of follow-up. At one-year follow-up, the ligament is hyperintense and even appears to have a partial rupture of the ligament. This patient was clinically stable, and no intervention was undertaken. At five-year follow-up, the ligament on MRI was continuous and hypointense.

References

[1] A. W. Robson, "VI. Ruptured Crucial Ligaments and their Repair by Operation," *Annals of Surgery*, vol. 37, 1903.

[2] D. H. O'Donoghue, "Surgical treatment of fresh injuries to the major ligaments of the knee," *The Journal of Bone & Joint Surgery*, vol. 32, no. 4, pp. 721–738, 1950.

[3] D. H. O'Donoghue, "An analysis of end results of surgical treatment of major injuries to the ligaments of the knee," *The Journal of Bone & Joint Surgery*, vol. 37, no. 1, pp. 1–13, 1955.

[4] I. Palmer, "On the injuries to the ligaments of the knee joint," *Acta Orthopaedica*, p. 53, 1938.

[5] I. Palmer, "On the injuries to the ligaments of the knee joint: a clinical study. 1938," *Clinical Orthopaedics and Related Research*, vol. 454, pp. 17–22, 2007.

[6] J. P. van der List and G. S. DiFelice, "Primary repair of the anterior cruciate ligament: a paradigm shift," *The Surgeon*, vol. 15, no. 3, pp. 161–168, 2017.

[7] R. L. England, "Repair of the ligaments about the knee," *Orthopedic Clinics of North America*, vol. 7, no. 1, pp. 195–204, 1976.

[8] J. A. Feagin, H. G. Abbott, and Rokous. J. R., "The isolated tear of the anterior cruciate ligament," *Journal of Bone and Joint Surgery*, vol. 54, no. 6, pp. 1340-1341, 1972.

[9] S. O. Liljedahl, N. Lindvall, and J. Wetterfors, "Early diagnosis and treatment of acute ruptures of the anterior cruciate ligament; a clinical and arthrographic study of forty-eight cases.," *The Journal of Bone & Joint Surgery*, vol. 47, no. 8, pp. 1503–1513, 1965.

[10] J. A. Feagin Jr. and W. W. Curl, "Isolated tear of the anterior cruciate ligament: 5 year follow up study," *The American Journal of Sports Medicine*, vol. 4, no. 3, pp. 95–100, 1976.

[11] L. Engebretsen, P. Benum, and S. Sundalsvoll, "Primary suture of the anterior cruciate ligament a 6-year follow-up of 74 cases," *Acta Orthopaedica*, vol. 60, no. 5, pp. 561–564, 1989.

[12] N. Kaplan, T. L. Wickiewicz, and R. F. Warren, "Primary surgical treatment of anterior cruciate ligament ruptures: a long-term follow-up study," *The American Journal of Sports Medicine*, vol. 18, no. 4, pp. 354–358, 1990.

[13] J. Lysholm, J. Gillquist, and S. O. Liljedahl, "Long-term results after early treatment of knee injuries," *Acta Orthopaedica Scandinavica*, vol. 53, no. 1, pp. 109–118, 1982.

[14] J. Lysholm, J. Gjllquist, and S.-O. Liljedahl, "Long-term results after early treatment of knee injuries," *Acta Orthopaedica*, vol. 53, no. 1, pp. 109–118, 1982.

[15] M. Odensten, J. Lysholm, and J. Gillquist, "Suture of fresh ruptures of the anterior cruciate ligament: A 5-year follow-up," *Acta Orthopaedica*, vol. 55, no. 3, pp. 270–272, 1984.

[16] M. F. Sherman, L. Lieber, J. R. Bonamo, L. Podesta, and I. Reiter, "The long-term followup of primary anterior cruciate ligament repair: defining a rationale for augmentation," *The American Journal of Sports Medicine*, vol. 19, no. 3, pp. 243–255, 1991.

[17] F. Genelin, A. Trost, C. Primavesi, and P. Knoll, "Late results

following proximal reinsertion of isolated ruptured ACL ligaments," *Knee Surgery, Sports Traumatology, Arthroscopy*, vol. 1, no. 1, pp. 17–19, 1993.

[18] J. P. van der List and G. S. DiFelice, "Preservation of the Anterior Cruciate Ligament: A Treatment Algorithm Based on Tear Location and Tissue Quality," *American journal of orthopedics (Belle Mead, N.J.)*, vol. 45, no. 7, pp. E393–E405, 2016.

[19] J. P. van der List and G. S. DiFelice, "Role of tear location on outcomes of open primary repair of the anterior cruciate ligament: a systematic review of historical studies," *The Knee*, vol. 24, no. 5, pp. 898–908, 2017.

[20] T. Strand, A. Mølster, M. Hordvik, and Y. Krukhaug, "Long-term follow-up after primary repair of the anterior cruciate ligament: clinical and radiological evaluation 15-23 years postoperatively," *Archives of Orthopaedic and Trauma Surgery*, vol. 125, no. 4, pp. 217–221, 2005.

[21] P. J. Millett, T. L. Wickiewicz, and R. F. Warren, "Motion loss after ligament injuries to the knee: part i: Causes," *The American Journal of Sports Medicine*, vol. 29, no. 5, pp. 664–675, 2001.

[22] K. D. Shelbourne, J. H. Wilckens, A. Mollabashy, and M. Decarlo, "Arthrofibrosis in acute anterior cruciate ligament reconstruction: the effect of timing of reconstruction and rehabilitation," *The American Journal of Sports Medicine*, vol. 19, no. 4, pp. 332–336, 1991.

[23] J. P. van der List and G. S. DiFelice, "Range of motion and complications following primary repair versus reconstruction of the anterior cruciate ligament," *The Knee*, vol. 24, no. 4, pp. 798–807, 2017.

[24] J. P. van der List, D. N. Mintz, and G. S. DiFelice, "The location of anterior cruciate ligament tears: a prevalence study using magnetic resonance imaging," *Orthopaedic Journal of Sports Medicine*, vol. 5, no. 6, 2017.

[25] G. S. DiFelice and J. P. van der List, "Arthroscopic primary repair of proximal anterior cruciate ligament tears," *Arthroscopy Techniques*, vol. 5, no. 5, pp. e1057–e1061, 2016.

[26] G. S. DiFelice, C. Villegas, and S. Taylor, "Anterior cruciate ligament preservation: early results of a novel arthroscopic technique for suture anchor primary anterior cruciate ligament repair," *Journal of Arthroscopic and Related Surgery*, vol. 31, no. 11, pp. 2162–2171, 2015.

[27] A. Achtnich, E. Herbst, P. Forkel et al., "Acute proximal anterior cruciate ligament tears: outcomes after arthroscopic suture anchor repair versus anatomic single-bundle reconstruction," *Journal of Arthroscopic and Related Surgery*, vol. 32, no. 12, pp. 2562–2569, 2016.

[28] M. Bigoni, D. Gaddi, M. Gorla et al., "Arthroscopic anterior cruciate ligament repair for proximal anterior cruciate ligament tears in skeletally immature patients: Surgical technique and preliminary results," *The Knee*, vol. 24, no. 1, pp. 40–48, 2017.

[29] G. M. Mackay, M. J. G. Blyth, I. Anthony, G. P. Hopper, and W. J. Ribbans, "A review of ligament augmentation with the InternalBrace™: the surgical principle is described for the lateral ankle ligament and ACL repair in particular, and a comprehensive review of other surgical applications and techniques is presented," *Surgical Technology International*, vol. 26, pp. 239–255, 2015.

[30] J. O. Smith, S. K. Yasen, H. C. Palmer, B. R. Lord, E. M. Britton, and A. J. Wilson, "Paediatric ACL repair reinforced with temporary internal bracing," *Knee Surgery, Sports Traumatology, Arthroscopy*, vol. 24, no. 6, pp. 1845–1851, 2016.

[31] G. S. DiFelice and J. P. van der List, "Clinical outcomes of arthroscopic primary repair of proximal anterior cruciate ligament tears are maintained at mid-term follow-up," *Journal of Arthroscopic and Related Surgery*, vol. 34, no. 4, pp. 1085–1093, 2018.

[32] A. Jonkergouw, J. P. van der List, and G. S. DiFelice, "Arthroscopic primary repair of proximal anterior cruciate ligament tears: outcomes of the first 56 consecutive patients and the role of additional internal bracing," *Knee Surg Sports Traumatol Arthrosc*, 2018.

[33] G. Bucci, M. Begg, K. Pillifant, and S. B. Singleton, "Primary ACL repair vs reconstruction: investigating the current conventional wisdom," *Orthopaedic Journal of Sports Medicine*, vol. 6, no. 3, 2018.

[34] J. Hennings, "Primary anatomical repair of proximal ACL ruptures with suture anchors: 1 year follow-up," *Annual Meeting of the DKG*, 2018.

[35] C. Hoffmann, J. Friederichs, C. von Ruden, C. Schaller, V. Buhren, and C. Moessmer, "Primary single suture anchor re-fixation of anterior cruciate ligament proximal avulsion tears leads to good functional mid-term results: a preliminary study in 12 patients," *Journal of Orthopaedic Surgery and Research*, vol. 12, no. 1, p. 171, 2017.

[36] R. Mukhopadhyay, N. Shah, R. Vakta, and J. Bhatt, "ACL femoral avulsion repair using suture pull-out technique: a case series of thirteen patients," *Chinese Journal of Traumatology*, 2018.

[37] D. N. Caborn, J. Nyland, B. Wheeldon, and A. Kalloub, "ACL femoral avulsion reapproximation with internal bracing and prp augmentation: excellent return to sports outcomes and low re-injury rates at 3 year follow-up. paper presented at: annual meeting of the european society of sports traumatology," *Knee Surgery and Arthroscopy*, 2018.

[38] C. H. W. Heusdens, G. P. Hopper, L. Dossche, E. Roelant, and G. M. Mackay, "Anterior cruciate ligament repair with Independent Suture Tape Reinforcement: a case series with 2-year follow-up," *Knee Surg Sports Traumatol Arthrosc*, 2018.

[39] D. Figueroa, P. Melean, R. Calvo et al., "Magnetic resonance imaging evaluation of the integration and maturation of semitendinosus-gracilis graft in anterior cruciate ligament reconstruction using autologous platelet concentrate," *Arthroscopy: The Journal of Arthroscopic and Related Surgery*, vol. 26, no. 10, pp. 1318–1325, 2010.

[40] S. M. Howell, J. A. Clark, and R. D. Blasier, "Serial magnetic resonance imaging of hamstring anterior cruciate ligament autografts during the first year of implantation: a preliminary study," *The American Journal of Sports Medicine*, vol. 19, no. 1, pp. 42–47, 1991.

[41] T. Kanamiya, M. Hara, and M. Naito, "Magnetic resonance evaluation of remodeling process in patellar tendon graft," *Clinical Orthopaedics and Related Research*, no. 419, pp. 202–206, 2004.

[42] S. M. Lee, K. H. Yoon, S. H. Lee, and D. Hur, "The relationship between ACL femoral tunnel position and postoperative MRI signal intensity," *Journal of Bone and Joint Surgery - American Volume*, vol. 99, no. 5, pp. 379–387, 2017.

[43] J. P. van der List and G. S. DiFelice, "Preservation of the Anterior Cruciate Ligament: Surgical Techniques," *American journal of orthopedics*, vol. 45, no. 7, pp. E406–E414, 2016.

[44] J. P. van der List and G. S. DiFelice, "The role of ligament repair in anterior cruciate ligament surgery," in *Ligamentous Injuries of the Knee*, R. Mascarenhas, S. Bhatia, and W. R. Lowe, Eds., vol. 1, pp. 199–220, Nova Science Publishers, Houston, USA, 2016.

[45] T. Naraoka, Y. Kimura, E. Tsuda, Y. Yamamoto, and Y. Ishibashi, "Is remnant preservation truly beneficial to anterior cruciate ligament reconstruction healing? clinical and magnetic resonance imaging evaluations of remnant-preserved reconstruction," *The American Journal of Sports Medicine*, vol. 45, no. 5, pp. 1049–1058, 2017.

[46] A. Ntoulia, F. Papadopoulou, F. Zampeli, S. Ristanis, M. Argyropoulou, and A. Georgoulis, "Evaluation with contrast-enhanced magnetic resonance imaging of the anterior cruciate ligament graft during its healing process: a two-year prospective study," *Skeletal Radiology*, vol. 42, no. 4, pp. 541–552, 2013.

[47] A. M. Biercevicz, D. L. Miranda, J. T. MacHan, M. M. Murray, and B. C. Fleming, "In situ, noninvasive, T2*-weighted mri-derived parameters predict Ex vivo structural properties of an anterior cruciate ligament reconstruction or bioenhanced primary repair in a porcine model," *The American Journal of Sports Medicine*, vol. 41, no. 3, pp. 560–566, 2013.

[48] M. M. Murray and B. C. Fleming, "Use of a bioactive scaffold to stimulate anterior cruciate ligament healing also minimizes posttraumatic osteoarthritis after surgery," *The American Journal of Sports Medicine*, vol. 41, no. 8, pp. 1762–1770, 2013.

[49] M. M. Murray, B. M. Flutie, and L. A. Kalish, "The bridge-enhanced anterior cruciate ligament repair (bear) procedure: an early feasibility cohort study," *Orthopaedic Journal of Sports Medicine*, vol. 4, no. 11, Article ID 2325967116672176, 2016.

[50] M. M. Murray and B. C. Fleming, "Biology of anterior cruciate ligament injury and repair: kappa delta ann doner vaughn award paper 2013," *Journal of Orthopaedic Research*, vol. 31, no. 10, pp. 1501–1506, 2013.

[51] S. L. Woo, T. M. Vogrin, and S. D. Abramowitch, "Healing and repair of ligament injuries in the knee," *Journal of the American Academy of Orthopaedic Surgeons*, vol. 8, no. 6, pp. 364–372, 2000.

[52] E. H. Crain, D. C. Fithian, E. W. Paxton, and W. F. Luetzow, "Variation in anterior cruciate ligament scar pattern: does the scar pattern affect anterior laxity in anterior cruciate ligament-deficient knees?" *Arthroscopy - Journal of Arthroscopic and Related Surgery*, vol. 21, no. 1, pp. 19–24, 2005.

[53] M. Costa-Paz, M. A. Ayerza, I. Tanoira, J. Astoul, and D. L. Muscolo, "Spontaneous healing in complete ACL ruptures: a clinical and MRI study," *Clinical Orthopaedics and Related Research*, vol. 470, no. 4, pp. 979–985, 2012.

[54] E. Fujimoto, Y. Sumen, M. Ochi, and Y. Ikuta, "Spontaneous healing of acute anterior cruciate ligament (ACL) injuries—conservative treatment using an extension block soft brace without anterior stabilization," *Archives of Orthopaedic and Trauma Surgery*, vol. 122, no. 4, pp. 212–216, 2002.

[55] I. Hetsroni, D. Delos, G. Fives, B. W. Boyle, K. Lillemoe, and R. G. Marx, "Nonoperative treatment for anterior cruciate ligament injury in recreational alpine skiers," *Knee Surgery, Sports Traumatology, Arthroscopy*, vol. 21, no. 8, pp. 1910–1914, 2013.

[56] D. T. Nguyen, T. H. Ramwadhdoebe, C. P. Van Der Hart, L. Blankevoort, P. P. Tak, and C. N. Van Dijk, "Intrinsic healing response of the human anterior cruciate ligament: an histological study of reattached ACL remnants," *Journal of Orthopaedic Research*, vol. 32, no. 2, pp. 296–301, 2014.

[57] M. S. Collins, K. P. Unruh, J. R. Bond, and J. N. Mandrekar, "Magnetic resonance imaging of surgically confirmed anterior cruciate ligament graft disruption," *Skeletal Radiology*, vol. 37, no. 3, pp. 233–243, 2008.

[58] Y. Nakayama, Y. Shirai, T. Narita, A. Mori, and K. Kobayashi, "The accuracy of MRI in assessing graft integrity after anterior cruciate ligament reconstruction," *Journal of Nippon Medical School*, vol. 68, no. 1, pp. 45–49, 2001.

[59] R. A. Waltz, D. J. Solomon, and M. T. Provencher, "A radiographic assessment of failed anterior cruciate ligament reconstruction: can magnetic resonance imaging predict graft integrity?" *The American Journal of Sports Medicine*, vol. 42, no. 7, pp. 1652–1660, 2014.

13

Adult Spinal Deformities: Can Patient-Specific Rods Change the Preoperative Planning into Clinical Reality? Feasibility Study and Preliminary Results about 77 Cases

S. Prost, S. Pesenti, K. Farah, P. Tropiano, S. Fuentes, and B. Blondel

Aix-Marseille Université, APHM, CNRS, ISM, Hôpital de la Timone, Unité de Chirurgie Rachidienne, 264 Rue Saint Pierre, Marseille 13005, France

Correspondence should be addressed to B. Blondel; benjamin.blondel@ap-hm.fr

Academic Editor: Panagiotis Korovessis

Surgical management of adult spinal deformities remains challenging, and one of the major goals is to restore sagittal alignment. Spinal rods used for posterior fixation are usually delivered straight and bended manually during surgery. This manual bending can be responsible for undercorrection of the deformity. In the last years, prebended patient-specific rods have been developed and might be a valuable tool in order to optimize surgical results. The objective is therefore to use the time between surgical decision and operative room in order to realize a precise surgical planning and obtain patient-specific rods. We describe here the planning process and our preliminary experience with patient-specific rods in the management of adult deformity about 77 cases. On the 77 cases, PSR were used without further modifications of the shape. Based on 3-month postoperative evaluation, a significant decrease of sagittal vertical axis (−41%, $p < 0.0001$) and pelvic incidence-lumbar lordosis (−62%, $p < 0.0001$) was reported. Pelvic tilt was not significantly corrected, except in patients with Parkinson's disease. In this subgroup of patients, measurements revealed a significant correction of SVA and PI-LL (−53%, $p = 0.005$, and −81%, $p < 0.0001$, respectively) but also of PT (−23%, $p < 0.001$). The use of PSR, in our experience, was feasible and provided satisfactory short-term results. It can be a valuable tool in the management of adult spinal deformities. Further studies will be needed in order to confirm these preliminary results.

1. Introduction

Prevalence of adult spinal deformity (ASD) has been reported as high as 32% of the population and up to 68% of patients over 60 years old or patients with Parkinson's disease [1, 2]. These deformities can be responsible for various disability and increasing healthcare costs with respect to global population aging [1].

In some cases, when spinal deformity leads to high level of disability, surgical management may be warranted. If so, common strategy includes a posterior fixation and a sagittal realignment procedure (osteotomy). Data from the literature have widely reported the positive impact of sagittal realignment in terms of health-related quality of life scores [3].

Despite the development in the last decades of specific tools (rods, screws, and intervertebral cages) and surgical techniques (osteotomies), a large proportion of patients remain undercorrected after surgery [4]. One of the surgical steps that remains unchanged is related to the manual bending of spinal rods, which is probably nor precise or reproducible.

It can therefore seem logical to develop patient-specific rods (PSR) based on a preoperative surgical planning, in order to obtain rods that would provide a frame for each patient correction individually. Potential results of this strategy will be associated to a better correction of the deformity, a lower risk of rod breakage, and a reduction of operative time [5, 6].

The aim of this study was to describe the surgical planning used in order to obtain PSR and to report our preliminary experience using PSR in the management of ASD.

2. Methods

Surgical management of ASD usually requires a posterior vertebral fixation in association to a posterior bone resection for sagittal realignment. In daily practice, the surgeon will preoperatively decide levels of fixation, type of osteotomy, need for intervertebral graft, and sagittal alignment objectives. However, so far, rod bending is performed manually during surgery (Figure 1) using straight rods provided by the manufacturer. This step is therefore not always reproducible (Figure 2) and is associated with a risk of postoperative undercorrection. It can also be theoretically with an increased risk of rod breakage due to the use of the French bender (Figure 3).

Recently, a company offered the possibility to obtain PSR based on a preoperative planning for each patient, using calibrated full-spine radiographs. The surgical planning can be done directly by the surgeon or by the company (Medicrea International, Rillieux-la-Pape, France) according to various parameters: levels of fixation, level and type of osteotomy, sagittal correction objectives, and rod material (titanium or cobalt-chrome).

Using dedicated software and based on a calibrated lateral full-spine X-ray, a simulation of postoperative alignment is obtained in the sagittal plane, and PSR is designed according to the planning (Figure 4). When a coronal deformity is also present, the calibrated anteroposterior full-spine X-ray will help to anticipate the length of PSR according to the amount of coronal correction planned. Once the planning is achieved, the surgeon will validate the design of PSR and can therefore obtain a pair of rods specifically for each patient.

We report here the feasibility and preliminary results of our experience with the use of PSR in the management of ASD about 77 cases. Parameters of the SRS-Schwab classification were measured preoperatively and at 3 months of follow-up (sagittal vertical axis (SVA), pelvic incidence and lumbar lordosis (PI-LL) mismatch, and pelvic tilt (PT)). Pre- and postoperative measurements were compared using a Student test (level of significance 5%).

3. Results

On the whole series, all surgeries were planned as described and all PSRs were used without further rod bending. Surgical indications included 43 ASD cases, 24 adolescent idiopathic scoliosis cases, and 10 deformity cases related to Parkinson's disease. Mean age was 59.1 years old ±18.6, and 71% of the patients were women.

Based on 3-month postoperative evaluation (Table 1), a significant decrease of SVA (−41%, $p < 0.0001$) and PI-LL (−62%, $p < 0.0001$) was reported. PT was not significantly corrected (−7%, $p = 0.154$) (Figure 5).

For patients diagnosed with AIS, 15 levels were fused on average and a pedicle subtraction osteotomy (PSO) was done in 4 cases (17%). This subgroup of patients were aligned preoperatively and remained aligned postoperatively (postoperative SVA = 27 mm, PI-LL = 5°, and PT = 20°). Four

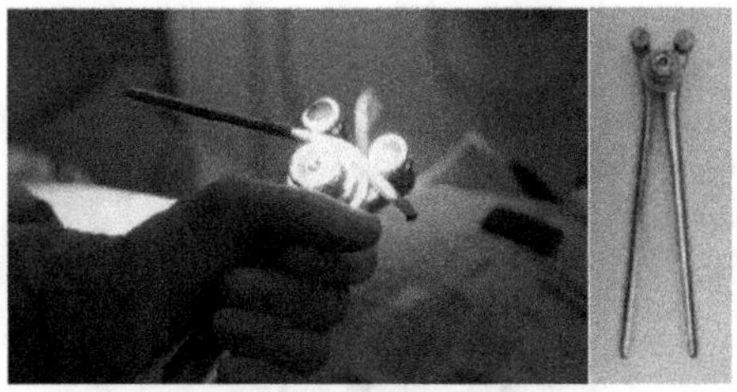

FIGURE 1: classic French bender use to shape rods.

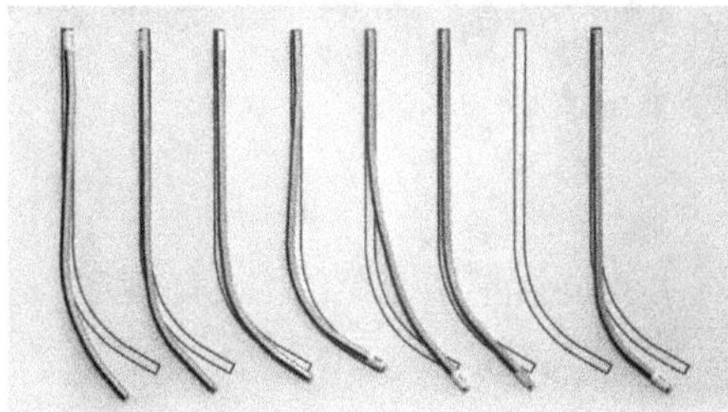

FIGURE 2: Example of rod bending by 7 surgeons showing the difficulty of reproducibility.

patients had a preoperative hypokyphosis (<20°) and were corrected postoperatively.

For patients diagnosed with ASD, 14 levels were fused on average and a PSO was done in 12 cases (28%). A significant correction of SVA (77 vs. 42 mm, $p < 0.001$) and PI-LL (21 vs. 8°, $p < 0.001$) was noted. Pelvic tilt was not significantly modified (29 vs. 27°, $p = 0.437$).

For patients diagnosed with Parkinson's disease, 17 levels were fused on average and a PSO was done in 7 cases (70%). In this subgroup of patients, measurements revealed a significant correction of SVA (100 vs. 47 mm, $p = 0.005$) and PI-LL (29 vs. 6°, $p < 0.001$) but also of PT (32 vs. 25°, $p < 0.001$).

No intraoperative complications were reported; however, during the follow-up period, 7 patients (9%) presented a postoperative infection that required a revision surgery without implant removal and adapted antibiotic treatment. Mechanical complication rate at 3 months was reported at 4% (3 patients with proximal junctional kyphosis).

4. Discussion

Results from this preliminary study support the use of PSR for different reasons. Firstly, there is a crucial impact of preoperative surgical planning in order to reach postoperative alignment objectives. As reported by El Rahal et al. [7], risk for adjacent failures can be related to a lack of surgical planning or a problem during execution of the surgical procedure. This planning will allow simulations of various postoperative sagittal alignments according different types of surgery. It can also help to understand compensatory mechanisms related to the deformity and those that can occur after surgical correction and therefore help to establish the theoretical most appropriate surgical procedure taking into account Schwab's classification, Roussouly's types, theoretical lumbar lordosis, and age of the patient [7].

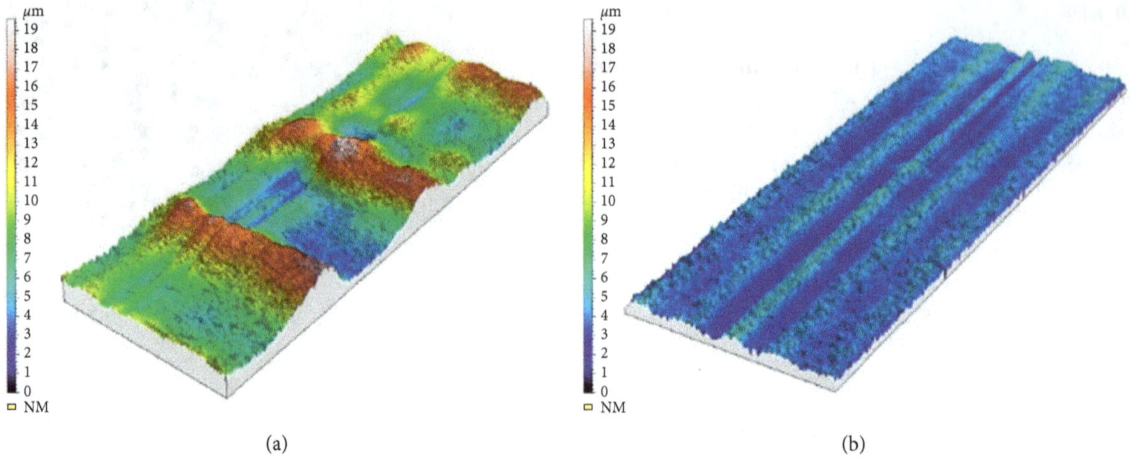

FIGURE 3: 3D high-resolution surface view of titanium rods bended manually (a) and industrially (b). Notches are visible on the surface of manually bended rods.

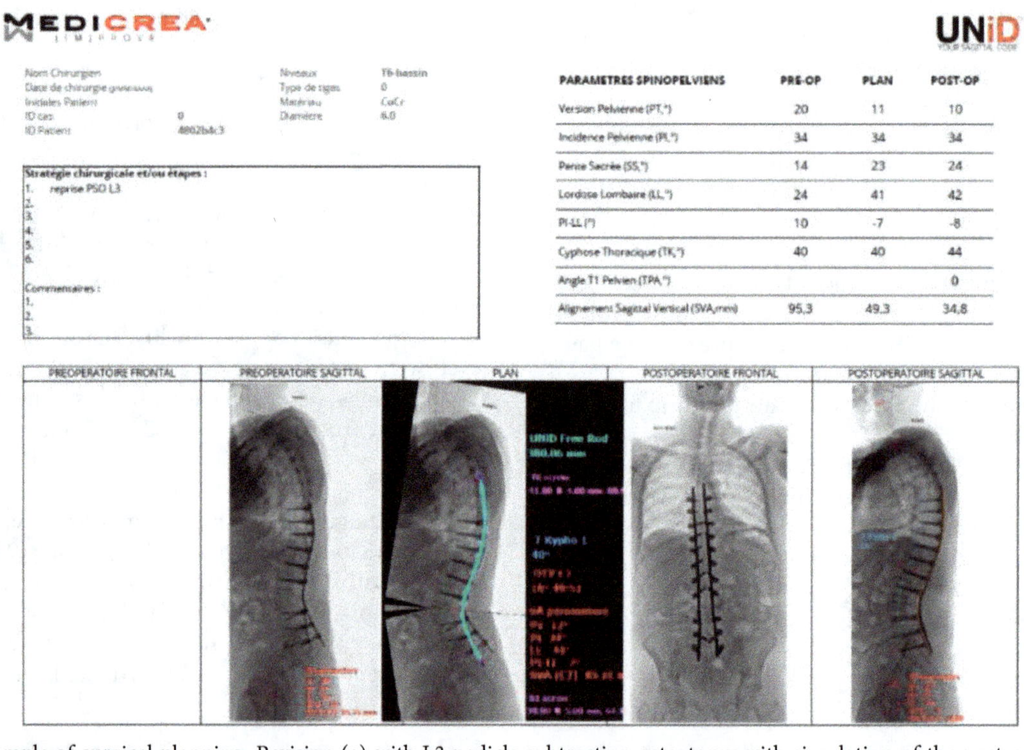

FIGURE 4: Example of surgical planning. Revision (a) with L3 pedicle subtraction osteotomy with simulation of the postoperative result, shape of the PSR, and postoperative results (b).

Secondly, with regards to sagittal correction, PSR can be a helpful tool in order to reduce the rate of undercorrected patients postoperatively, related to the lack of planning or suboptimal bending of rods during surgery [4]. The results presented here are in line with the study of Barton et al. [8] who also reported significant improvement of sagittal parameters using PSR. More recently, Solla et al. [9] reported their experience about 60 patients managed using PSR with a correction of PI-LL mismatch in 66% of the cases, a correction of SVA in 38% of the cases, and a correction of PT in 29% of the cases. According to their results, postoperative PI-LL mismatch was correlated with preoperative PI-LL and performing a PSO; postoperative SVA was correlated with preoperative SVA, performing a PSO, and age of the patient, and postoperative PT was correlated with preoperative PT. With regards to Parkinson's disease patients, a better correction was reported, especially for pelvic tilt. One reason for these findings might be related to the importance of initial deformity. In this subgroup of patients, preoperative malalignment was more important than in other groups, and as a consequence, a PSO was performed more frequently (70% of the cases) leading to a better restoration of lumbar lordosis and pelvic tilt [10].

Table 1: Radiographic results.

		Total ($n = 77$)	ASD ($n = 43$)	AIS ($n = 24$)	Parkinson ($n = 10$)
Age		59.1	66.7	42.0	68.1
Sex		$F = 71\%$	$F = 72\%$	$F = 83\%$	$F = 40\%$
Number of levels fused		14.5 ± 3.0	14.0 ± 3.4	14.8 ± 2.3	16.6 ± 1.3
PSO		24 PSO (31%)	12 PSO (28%)	4 PSO (17%)	7 PSO (70%)
	Baseline	65.6 ± 65.7	77.3 ± 60.6	27.2 ± 58.0	100.3 ± 68.3
SVA (mm)	3M	38.5 ± 36.6	41.9 ± 38.0	27.3 ± 32.1	47.3 ± 38.5
	Δ (p value)	−41% ($p < 0.0001$)	−46% ($p < 0.0001$)	0% ($p = 0.997$)	−53% ($p = 0.005$)
	Baseline	18.1 ± 20.3	20.8 ± 17.8	7.8 ± 23.7	28.8 ± 10.9
PI-LL (°)	3M	6.9 ± 11.8	8.3 ± 12.8	5 ± 10.9	5.5 ± 10.3
	Δ (p value)	−62% ($p < 0.0001$)	−60% ($p < 0.0001$)	−35% ($p = 0.458$)	−81% ($p < 0.0001$)
	Baseline	26.3 ± 11.3	28.6 ± 9.9	19.7 ± 11.8	31.7 ± 9.9
PT (°)	3M	24.6 ± 11.9	27.1 ± 12.9	20.4 ± 11.0	24.5 ± 6.7
	Δ (p value)	−7% ($p = 0.154$)	−5% ($p = 0.437$)	+4% ($p = 0.663$)	−23% ($p < 0.001$)

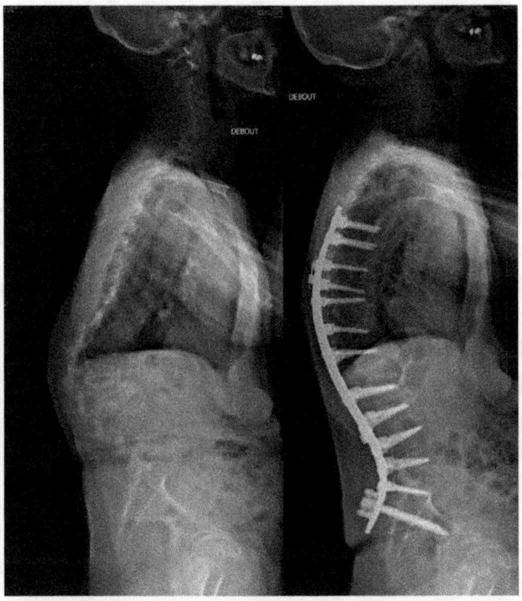

Figure 5: Example of sagittal realignment procedure using PSR in a patient with fixed thoracolumbar junction kyphosis (a). Surgical planning included a T6-ileum fixation with a L1 osteotomy and 3-month postoperative result (b).

With regards to AIS patients, a recent study by Solla et al. [11] reported the results of 37 patients managed using PSR. Their strategy involved an over bending of the rod in the concavity of the deformity which led to a correction of thoracic kyphosis for hypokyphotic patients underlining the interest of PSR in the management of AIS.

Finally, results from our study revealed a low rate of mechanical complications (4%) without rod breakage which is comparable with previous report [9]; however, our mechanical results must be taken into account cautiously due to the short follow-up (3 months).

Of course, this study presents also limits related to its design, the short-term follow-up, and the lack of clinical scores. It is also important to note that an initial learning curve is needed in order to plan and anticipate the surgical procedure in order to obtain PSR that will not require further modifications. When PSR is used, the strategy is to use the rods as a template for correction of the spine and not to adapt the rods to the spine. This point seems particularly important in our experience as it pushes the surgeon to follow the preoperative planning and avoid intraoperative changes (levels of fusion or osteotomy) that may actually be necessary in order to obtain optimal sagittal realignment.

While further studies will be needed in order to confirm these preliminary results, the use of PSR can be a turning point in the management of ASD. The exact knowledge of rod shape preoperatively will allow further postoperative analyses. It will therefore be possible to measure precisely the flattening effect of the rods, to anticipate further compensatory mechanisms in ASD and may be a way to decrease postoperative mechanical complications (proximal junctional failure or rod breakage).

5. Conclusion

Results from this preliminary study confirm the clinical feasibility of the use of PSR in the management of ASD. Three-month results are encouraging with regards to sagittal alignment. PSR can be valuable tools in order to optimize postoperative radiographic results even if further studies will be needed in order to confirm these results.

Authors' Contributions

S. Prost, S. Pesenti, and K. Farah extracted data and wrote the manuscript. B. Blondel, S. Fuentes, and P. Tropiano coordinated the research and revised the manuscript.

Acknowledgments

The authors thank Medicrea International.

References

[1] C. P. Ames, J. K. Scheer, V. Lafage et al., "Adult spinal deformity: epidemiology, health impact, evaluation, and management," *Spine Deformity*, vol. 4, no. 4, pp. 310–322, 2016.

[2] B. Bouyer, C. Scemama, P. Roussouly et al., "Evolution and complications after surgery for spine deformation in patients

with Parkinson's disease," *Orthopaedics & Traumatology: Surgery & Research*, vol. 103, no. 4, pp. 517–522, 2017.

[3] S. D. Glassman, S. Berven, K. Bridwell, W. Horton, and J. R. Dimar, "Correlation of radiographic parameters and clinical symptoms in adult scoliosis," *Spine*, vol. 30, no. 6, pp. 682–688, 2005.

[4] B. Moal, F. Schwab, C. P. Ames et al., "Radiographic outcomes of adult spinal deformity correction: a critical analysis of variability and failures across deformity patterns," *Spine Deformity*, vol. 2, no. 3, pp. 219–225, 2014.

[5] C. Lindsey, V. Deviren, Z. Xu, R.-F. Yeh, and C. M. Puttlitz, "The effects of rod contouring on spinal construct fatigue strength," *Spine*, vol. 31, no. 15, pp. 1680–1687, 2006.

[6] H. Yoshihara, "Rods in spinal surgery: a review of the literature," *The Spine Journal*, vol. 13, no. 10, pp. 1350–1358, 2013.

[7] A. El Rahal, F. Solla, V. Fière, A. Toquart, and C. Y. Barrey, "Sagittal balance and preoperative planning," *Spine Surgery. Case-Based Approach*, pp. 447–458, Springer Nature, Berlin, Germany, 2019.

[8] C. Barton, A. Noshchenko, V. Patel, C. Kleck, and E. Burger, "Early experience and initial outcomes with patient-specific spine rods for adult spinal deformity," *Orthopedics*, vol. 39, no. 2, pp. 79–86, 2016.

[9] F. Solla, C. Y. Barrey, E. Burger, C. J. Kleck, and V. Fière, "Patient-specific rods for surgical correction of sagittal imbalance in adults," *Clinical Spine Surgery*, vol. 32, no. 2, pp. 80–86, 2019.

[10] V. Lafage, F. Schwab, S. Vira et al., "Does vertebral level of pedicle subtraction osteotomy correlate with degree of spinopelvic parameter correction?" *Journal of Neurosurgery: Spine*, vol. 14, no. 2, pp. 184–191, 2011.

[11] F. Solla, J.-L. Clément, V. Cunin, C. M. Bertoncelli, V. Fière, and V. Rampal, "Patient-specific rods for thoracic kyphosis correction in adolescent idiopathic scoliosis surgery: preliminary results," *Orthopaedics & Traumatology: Surgery & Research*, vol. 106, no. 1, pp. 159–165, 2020.

14

Long-Term Effectiveness of Polymerized-Type I Collagen Intra-Articular Injections in Patients with Symptomatic Knee Osteoarthritis: Clinical and Radiographic Evaluation in a Cohort Study

Adrián Borja-Flores,[1] Salvador I. Macías-Hernández,[2] Gabriela Hernández-Molina,[3] Andric Perez-Ortiz,[4] Eloy Reyes-Martínez,[1] José Belzazar-Castillo de la Torre,[1] Laura Ávila-Jiménez,[5] María Cristina Vázquez-Bello,[5] Marco Antonio León-Mazón,[6] Janette Furuzawa-Carballeda,[3] Gonzalo Torres-Villalobos,[7] Fernanda Romero-Hernández,[7] Cidronio Albavera-Hernández,[6] Jesús Pérez-Correa,[8] and Hilda A. Castro-Rocha[9]

[1]*HGZ 5 Con MF, Delegación Estatal Morelos, Zacatepec, Morelos, Mexico*
[2]*Orthopedic Rehabilitation Division, Instituto Nacional de Rehabilitación Luis Guillermo Ibarra, Mexico City, Mexico*
[3]*Department of Immunology and Rheumatology, Instituto Nacional de Ciencias Médicas y Nutrición Salvador Zubirán, Mexico City, Mexico*
[4]*Escuela de Medicina, Universidad Panamericana, Donatello 59, Insurgentes Mixcoac, Benito Juárez, Mexico City 03920, Mexico*
[5]*Coordinación de Planeación y Enlace Institucional, Jefatura de Servicios de Prestaciones Médicas, Delegación Estatal Morelos, Cuernavaca, Morelos, Mexico*
[6]*Centro de Investigación Educativa y Formación Docente, Coordinación de Planeación y Enlace Institucional, Jefatura de Servicios de Prestaciones Médicas, Delegación Estatal Morelos, Cuernavaca, Morelos, Mexico*
[7]*Departments of Experimental Surgery and Surgery, Instituto Nacional de Ciencias Médicas y Nutrición Salvador Zubirán, Mexico City, Mexico*
[8]*Department of Traumatology and Orthopedics, Hospital "Dr. Victorio de la Fuente Narváez", Mexico City, Mexico*
[9]*Siracusa No. 51 Col. Lomas Estrella, Mexico City, Mexico*

Correspondence should be addressed to Janette Furuzawa-Carballeda; jfuruzawa@gmail.com and Gonzalo Torres-Villalobos; torresvgm@yahoo.com.mx

Academic Editor: Benjamin Blondel

Objective. Polymerized-type I collagen (polymerized-collagen) is a downregulator of inflammation and a tissue regenerator. The aim was to evaluate the effect of intra-articular injections (IAIs) of polymerized-collagen among patients with symptomatic knee osteoarthritis (OA) in delaying or preventing joint replacement surgery. *Patients and Methods.* This was a cohort study of 309 patients with knee OA. Patients with mild-to-moderate disease were treated weekly with IAIs of 2 mL of polymerized-collagen for six weeks ($n = 309$). Follow-up was for 6–60 months. The primary endpoints included the following determinations: (1) therapeutic effect; (2) survival from total knee replacement surgery (TKR); (3) Western Ontario and McMaster University Osteoarthritis Index (WOMAC) and pain (visual analogue scale, VAS). Clinical improvement was defined as a decrease in pain exceeding 20 mm on the VAS and the achievement of at least 20% improvement from baseline with respect to the WOMAC score. Radiographic analysis was performed at baseline and 60 months. The joint space width in the medial, lateral, and patellofemoral compartments was calculated. *Results.* Patients who received IAIs of polymerized-collagen had a statistically significant improvement in the primary criteria ($p < 0.05$). Kaplan–Meier survival analysis of the therapeutic effect demonstrated 98.8% survival at 60 months with TKR as the endpoint. There was no significant reduction in joint space in any compartment based on the analyzed radiographs. No serious adverse events were recorded. *Conclusion.* Polymerized-collagen increased the time to TKR by at least 60 months, modifying the disease course, improving functional disability, and decreasing pain.

1. Introduction

Osteoarthritis (OA) is a disease entity that is characterized by alterations in the articular cartilage, subchondral bone, ligaments, capsule, and synovial membrane. In Latin America, according to the Community Oriented Program for the Control of Rheumatic Diseases (COPCORD), the prevalence of OA ranges from 2.3 to 20.4%, and the global burden of disease in individuals between 50 and 69 years is 679.55 years lived with disability per 100,000 habitants (http://www.healthdata.org) [1–4]. Nonsteroidal anti-inflammatory drugs (NSAIDs) and analgesics are the predominant modality of OA treatments, which at long-term or high-dose use may cause significant side effects, such as gastrointestinal bleeding, nephrotoxicity, and cardiovascular disease. However, intra-articular (IA) therapies employing diverse active drugs, such as corticosteroids and viscosupplementation, are also used [3, 4].

OA is considered an inflammatory disease [5–9], and interleukin (IL)-1β, tumor necrosis factor (TNF)-α, and IL-6 are the main proinflammatory cytokines involved in its pathogenesis. Moreover, IL-15, IL-18, IL-21, leukemia inhibitory factor 2 (LIF), chemokines (IL-8, MCP-1, RANTES), and adipokines have also been implicated [10]. Studies suggest that there is a window of opportunity early in OA's inflammatory process; thus, new therapeutic strategies to modify the structural progression of OA (disease-modifying OA drugs [DMOADs]) are needed. DMOADs in phase II/III/IV clinical development include oral salmon calcitonin, SD-6010, vitamin D3 (cholecalciferol), collagen hydrolysate, recombinant human fibroblast growth factor (FGF)-18, bone morphogenetic protein-7 (BMP-7), and avocado-soybean unsaponifiables (ASU) [11, 12].

For some years, our research group has focused on the effect of modified extracellular matrix proteins on the regulation of inflammation [13–23]. Particularly, polymerized-type I collagen is a γ-irradiated mixture of pepsinized porcine type I collagen and polyvinylpyrrolidone. The addition of 1% polymerized-type I collagen to cocultures of OA cartilage and synovial tissue induces cartilage regeneration due to a 3- to 6-fold increase in chondrocyte proliferation (Ki-67), proteoglycans, cartilage oligomeric matrix protein (COMP), and type II collagen [18]. Polymerized-type I collagen induces the downregulation of inflammation-inhibiting proinflammatory cytokine expression (IL-1β and TNF-α) through the modulation of NF-kB activation [15, 20]. In addition, polymerized-type I collagen downregulates the circulating number of Th22, Th17, and Th1 cells and upregulates IL-10 expression and the circulating number of regulatory T, B, and plasmacytoid dendritic cells [15, 18, 20], *unpublished observations*.

Previously, the effect on cartilage repair of four intra-articular injections (IAIs) of polymerized-type I collagen was evaluated in a rat model of early and long-term OA. The biodrug induced chondroprotection and high-quality cartilage repair (hyaline cartilage) and reduced degenerative damage in the cartilage structure [21]. In addition, the IA administration of 2 mL of polymerized-type I collagen to the knees of OA patients showed improvement in the Lequesne Index, Western Ontario and McMaster University Osteoarthritis Index (WOMAC) score, pain intensity according to the visual analogue scale (VAS), and patient global score at 6 months of follow-up, as well as 75% decreased daily consumption of NSAIDs. In addition, the patients who received this treatment had a threefold decrease in urinary CTX-II [19, 20]. Its clinical effect seems to be related to a decrease in proinflammatory cytokine- (IL-1β- and TNF-α-) expressing cells and an increase in IL-10-producing cells and CD4 T-regulatory cells [20].

The aims of the study were the following: (1) evaluating the long-term effectiveness and safety of polymerized-type I collagen IAIs in patients with knee OA; (2) determining the five-year therapeutic effect on knee survival, taking knee arthroplasty and arthroscopic knee surgery as endpoints; and (3) assessing whether polymerized-type I collagen improves the clinical and radiographic conditions of OA and delays and/or prevents joint replacement.

2. Patients and Methods

2.1. Study Design. This was an open-label, single-center study.

2.2. Patients. From March 2010 to June 2016, a total of 335 consecutive patients from Hospital General de Zona Número 5 con Unidad de Medicina Familiar, IMSS, received polymerized-type I collagen. All the patients were recruited from the IMSS National Program for deferral of total knee replacement surgery (institutional program to implement institutional strategies for nonsurgical treatment of knee OA).

2.3. Inclusion and Exclusion Criteria. All the patients fulfilled the American College of Rheumatology classification criteria for knee OA (knee pain with a duration of at least 3 months and at least five of the following: age >50 years; stiffness <30 min; crepitus; bony tenderness; bony enlargement; no palpable warmth; erythrocyte sedimentation rate (ESR) $<40\,mmh^{-1}$; RF <1 : 40; and synovial fluid signs of OA (e.g., clear, viscous, or white blood cell count $<2000/mm^3$)) [22]. In addition, to be included, the patients had to have a body mass index (BMI) $<40\,kg/m^2$, a stable therapeutic regimen with NSAIDs, and a negative standard forearm skin test result for polymerized-collagen (evaluated 72 h after the administration of 0.2 mL of polymerized-collagen) [23].

We excluded patients undergoing treatment with oral, IA, or parenteral corticosteroids, as well as IA injections of any hyaluronic substance into the knee in the 3 months prior to the basal visit. In addition, we excluded patients with concurrent medical or arthritic conditions that could interfere with the evaluation of the knee joint, including fibromyalgia, Reiter's syndrome, rheumatoid arthritis, psoriatic arthritis, ankylosing spondylitis, lymphoma, arthritis associated with inflammatory bowel disease, sarcoidosis, amyloidosis, septic arthritis, crystal disease,

Maquet high tibial osteotomy (HTO), bone–patellar tendon–bone (B–PT–B) reconstruction, anterior cruciate ligament (ACL) reconstruction, and cancer, as well as patients with disabling back or hip pain (Figure 1).

2.4. Intra-Articular Injections. IA injections were administered by either a lateral or medial approach after the instillation of 1 mL of 1% xylocaine solution at weeks 1, 2, 3, 4, 5, and 6 in the same knee. The most symptomatic knee was selected by the physician for treatment.

In case the patients had similar pain intensity in both knees, they were eligible to receive injections in both knees. The treating physician was board-certified orthopedic surgeon highly trained in IA injection techniques.

2.5. Clinical Evaluation and Efficacy Assessment. Patients' clinical records were carefully reviewed according to a pre-established protocol. The following data were collected for each study participant: demographic features and WOMAC score [24]. Pain intensity was evaluated on a 100 mm VAS (patient and physician). Each patient's and investigator's global assessment of disease activity on a 5-point rating scale, global assessment of disease activity change at the end of the treatment (Likert score), and assessment of therapy response were also determined. A clinical evaluation and efficacy assessment were performed at baseline and at 6, 12, 36, and 60 months during the study.

The primary endpoints were the WOMAC score, the pain on a VAS (patient and physician), and the need for total knee replacement (TKR) or arthroscopy of the knee due to OA. Secondary outcome measures included each patient's and investigator's global assessment of disease activity on a 5-point rating scale and global assessment of change in disease activity at the end of the treatment (Likert score: 0 = very poor; 1 = poor; 2 = fair; 3 = well; 4 = very well). The patient and physician assessments of therapy response were also determined (evaluation of medication: 0 = none: no good at all, ineffective drug; 1 = poor: some effect, but unsatisfactory; 2 = fair: reasonable effect, but could be better; 3 = good: satisfactory effect with occasional episodes of pain or stiffness; 4 = excellent: ideal response, virtually pain-free) [25]. Clinically significant improvement was defined as the decrease in pain exceeding 20 mm on the 0–100 mm VAS [22] and the achievement of at least 20% improvement from baseline with respect to the WOMAC score [24, 26–28].

2.6. Safety Assessment. Adverse events (AEs) were assessed at each visit. AEs were defined as any unwanted event occurring during the trial related to administration of the study biodrug. The assessment of each AE (local or systemic) was performed by the treating physician. At each visit, AEs were registered from a self-reported questionnaire as well as from clinical records.

2.7. Radiographic Analysis. Standard standing weight-bearing knee radiographic images were randomly obtained at baseline and 60 months after treatment. Measurement of the joint space in the anteroposterior and lateral compartments of the tibiofemoral and patellofemoral joints of the treated knee was performed. Radiographs were analyzed using a DICOM viewer (Poznan, Poland), which includes tools for radiological distance measurement. The radiological evaluation was carried out by two trained experts in musculoskeletal radiology. The intraclass correlation coefficients for the inter- and intraobserver evaluations were calculated (intra- and interobserver reliability were measured using the weighted kappa statistic and intraclass correlation coefficient [ICC]). *Kappa* <0.20 indicated slight agreement, 0.21–0.40 fair, 0.41–0.60 moderate, 0.61–0.80 substantial, and 0.81–1.0 almost perfect agreement [24]. The progression of OA was defined as a decrease in joint space width (JSW) of 0.48 to 0.50 mm [29]. The radiological staging was performed on the KL scale.

2.8. Treatment Failures. Patients treated with polymerized-type I collagen who received oral or parenteral corticosteroids or IA injection of steroids, glucosamine/chondroitin sulphate products, or any hyaluronic substance during the follow-up were considered as treatment failures. Patients who underwent TKR, arthroscopy, high tibial osteotomy (HTO), bone-patellar tendon-bone (B-PT-B) reconstruction, or anterior cruciate ligament (ACL) reconstruction were also considered as failures.

2.9. Ethical Considerations. The protocol was approved by the National Commission for Scientific Research (IMSS Ref No. 09-B5-61-2800/201700/1336). The study was conducted in accordance with the principles of good clinical practice and the revised Declaration of Helsinki, 1989. All the participants provided written informed consent.

2.10. Statistical Analysis. We used descriptive statistics. For the primary analysis, the means of the scores between the two treatment groups were compared using an intention to treat (ITT) analysis. Multiple regression analysis was performed to assess associations between baseline characteristics and clinical outcomes. p values ≤0.05 were considered significant. Statistical analysis was performed using SPSS v.21 (SPSS Inc., Chicago, IL). For our survival approach, we estimated the unadjusted survival from TKR, arthroscopic surgery, or osteotomy by the Kaplan–Meier method and curves in SAS v.9.4 (Figure 2). We then performed Cox-regression modeling between baseline patient characteristics and outcome-free survival. For the clinical efficacy assessments (e.g., WOMAC, 100 mm VAS) at different time points, we implemented an extended Cox regression model with time-varying covariates. Finally, we reestimated the survival from endpoints using the Cox model (Figure 3). We assessed the proportionality of the hazards of all our models with the ASSESS statement in SAS.

3. Results

3.1. Patient Characteristics. At the beginning of the study, the national program for deferral of total knee replacement

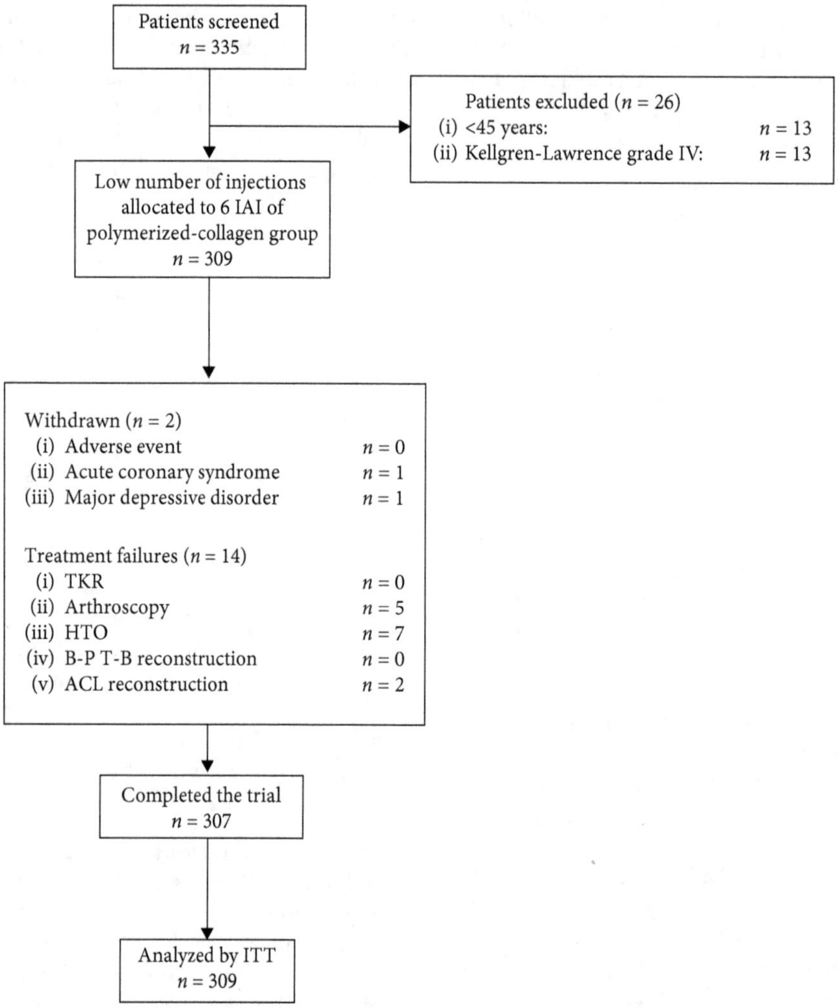

FIGURE 1: Enrolment and Outcomes. Course of the 60-month trial. ACL: anterior cruciate ligament reconstruction; B-P-T-B: bone-patellar tendon-bone reconstruction; IAI: intra-articular injections; ITT: intention to treat; HTO: high tibial osteotomy; TKR: total knee replacement.

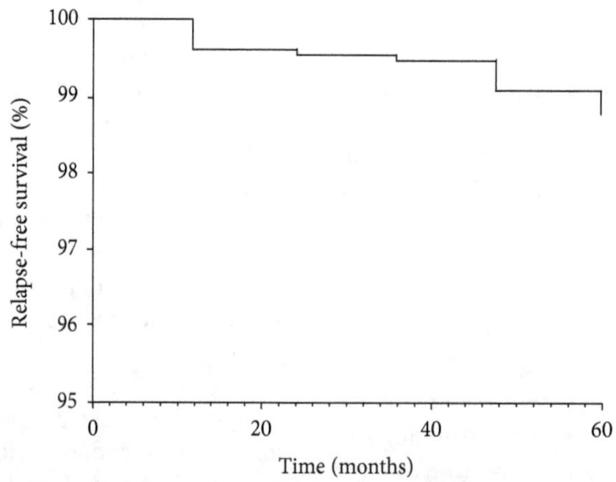

FIGURE 2: Covariate-adjusted relapse-free survival during the follow-up period ($n = 309$).

surgery included 335 patients. We excluded 26 patients as follows: 13 patients younger than 45 years and 13 patients with Kellgren-Lawrence (KL) grade IV.

Sixty-seven percent of all patients were women. The mean age at the time of intervention was 64.0 ± 8.7 years. Most of the patients had Kellgren-Lawrence (KL) grade II

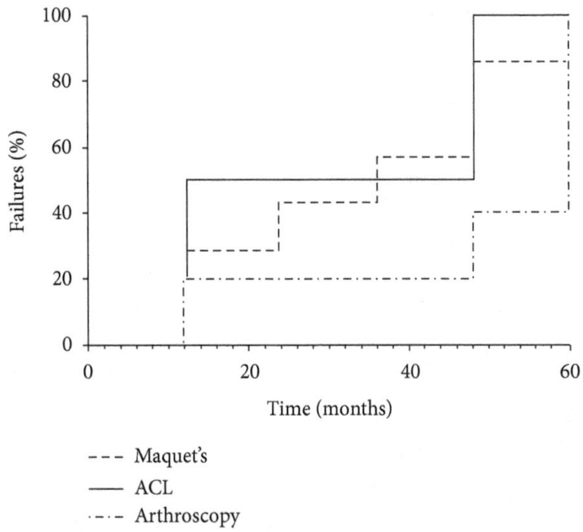

Figure 3: Failure function stratified by endpoint ($n = 309$).

($n = 160$, 52%), followed by KG III ($n = 149$, 48%). The demographic and clinical characteristics of the patients are presented in Table 1.

During the follow-up, 2 (0.6%) patients withdrew from the study (Figure 1).

3.2. Primary Clinical Outcomes. The WOMAC pain subscale score, WOMAC disability subscale score, WOMAC stiffness subscale score, patient pain on the VAS, and pain evaluated by a physician decreased significantly from baseline to 60 months (Table 1).

At 60 months, 295 (95.5%) patients who received the intervention responded to treatment, and none underwent TKR due to the persistence of symptoms. Five (1.6%) patients underwent arthroscopic surgery; 7 (2.3%) patients underwent HTO; and 2 (0.6%) patients underwent ACL reconstruction (Figure 1).

3.3. Secondary Clinical Outcomes. The measures of efficacy included each patient's and investigator's global assessment of disease activity on a 5-point rating scale (Likert Score) and their assessments of therapy response (Table 1). The Likert score improved considerably during the follow-up, reaching a significant difference ($p < 0.05$) between baseline and the posttreatment period (Table 1). The patients' and physicians' drug evaluations showed statistically significant differences after only 12 months following treatment (Table 1).

3.4. Radiological Evaluation. Radiographs of forty-one knees were analyzed, 21 of which were right knees. Patients were evaluated for KL grading before and 60 months after treatment. There was a significant difference between baseline and follow-up ($p < 0.014$) (Table 2). However, there was no significant decline in minimum joint space width in any compartment (Table 2).

3.5. Adverse Events. Throughout the five-year study period, there were no records of serious adverse reactions or long-term complications related to the IAIs of polymerized-type I collagen except for injection site pain lasting <24 h in all patients.

3.6. Concomitant Medication. Patients received stable doses of NSAIDs during the administration of polymerized-type I collagen. Thus, during first week of treatment phase, all patients received 1600 mg per day of ibuprofen. Then, during the follow-up, NSAIDs were taken as needed. Patients took on average 1-2 tablets per month of ibuprofen. None of the patients received corticosteroids, glucosamine/chondroitin sulphate products, or viscosupplementation during the study period.

3.7. Survival Analysis. To estimate the freedom from TKR, HTO, ACL reconstruction, and arthroscopy surgery of our cohort, we performed a thorough survival analysis with the latter as endpoints. At 60 months, the survival from a surgical procedure was 98.8% (Figure 2). Males had 2.4-fold hazard failing compared to females (HR: $_{1.25}\,2.38\,_{4.52}$, $p < 0.0001$). Also, overweight, and obese in dividuals had a higher risk compared to normal weighted individuals (HR_{OW}: $_{1.17}\,2.37\,_{4.72}$, $p < 0.0159$; HR_{OB}: $_{1.46}\,3.45\,_{8.19}$, $p = 0.0047$) (Table 3). At baseline, an increase in the WOMAC score by one unit significantly increased the risk of failure by 5% (HR: $_{1.00}\,1.05\,_{1.10}$, $p = 0.0059$). However, the changes over time of our symptom assessments, WOMAC and 100 mm VAS, were not predictors of failure. Arthroscopy had the most considerable freedom from outcome compared to HTO and ACL reconstruction (Figure 3).

4. Discussion

OA of the knee is a common cause of chronic joint pain. It affects 35% of individuals >65 years and is the leading cause of disability in this group of patients. Several therapeutic

TABLE 1: Demographic and disease history at baseline and during follow-up of the study.

Demographics	Baseline ($n = 309$)	6–11 Mo ($n = 309$)	12–35 Mo ($n = 255$)	36–48 Mo ($n = 206$)	49–60 Mo ($n = 48$)
Gender					
Female; n (%)	208 (67)				
Male; n (%)	101 (33)				
Age (years); mean ± SD	64.0 ± 8.7				
(Range)	(45–82)				
Body mass index (kg/m^2); mean ± SD;	23.9 ± 3.2				
(Range)	(18.2–34.6)				
Kellgren-Lawrence grade					
II; n (%)	160 (52)				
III; n (%)	149 (48)				
Deformity					
Valgus; n (%)	7 (2)				
Varus; n (%)	302 (98)				
Clinical variables					
WOMAC pain subscale; mean ± SD	6.1 ± 3.4	4.4 ± 3.1	3.4 ± 2.4	4.3 ± 2.2	3.6 ± 2.1
(Range)	(2–16)	(0–14)	(0–14)	(2–10)	(2–12)
Δ (%)		**−27.8**	**−44.2**	**−29.5**	**−41.0**
WOMAC stiffness subscale; mean ± SD	4.2 ± 2.0	3.2 ± 1.7	2.5 ± 1.5	2.8 ± 1.5	2.4 ± 1.1
(Range)	(2–10)	(1–10)	(0–12)	(2–8)	(0–6)
Δ (%)		**−23.8**	**−40.47**	**−33.3**	**−42.9**
WOMAC disability; mean ± SD	21.0 ± 4.9	19.1 ± 4.8	16.3 ± 4.9	17.2 ± 5.4	15.9 ± 5.5
(Range)	(2–36)	(10–32)	(2–30)	(6–32)	(4–32)
Δ (%)		−9.0	**−22.4**	−18.1	**−24.3**
Patient pain (mm); mean ± SD	56.2 ± 13.5	32.1 ± 15	35.5 ± 13.6	29.4 ± 11.7	20.4 ± 10.6
(Range)	(30–100)	(0–80)	(20–70)	(0–70)	(0–60)
Δ (%)		**−42.9**	**−36.8**	**−47.7**	**−63.7**
Physician pain (mm); mean ± SD	54.0 ± 12.6	29.7 ± 13.2	30.4 ± 13.9	25.1 ± 12.1	20.1 ± 10.6
(Range)	(30–100)	(0–80)	(20–70)	(0–70)	(0–60)
Δ (%)		**−45.0**	**−43.7**	**−53.5**	**−62.8**
Patient Likert score (cm); mean ± SD	1.8 ± 0.9	2.1 ± 1.0	2.3 ± 0.9	2.5 ± 0.8	2.9 ± 0.7
(Range)	(0–3)	(0–8)	(0–6)	(0–6)	(1–6)
Δ (%)		18.3	**27.8**	**38.9**	**61.1**
Physician Likert score (cm); mean ± SD	1.8 ± 1.0	2.2 ± 1.0	2.3 ± 0.9	2.6 ± 0.9	3.0 ± 0.7
(Range)	(0–6)	(0–6)	(0–6)	(0–6)	(1–6)
Δ (%)		**22.0**	**27.8**	**44.4**	**66.7**
Patient drug evaluation (cm); mean ± SD		2.4 ± 0.9	2.0 ± 0.9	2.2 ±0.7	3.1 ± 0.5
(Range)		(0–4)	(0–4)	(1–4)	(2–4)
Δ (%)			6.0	9.1	**29.2**
Physician drug evaluation (cm); mean ± SD		2.1 ± 1.0	1.9 ± 0.9	2.1 ± 0.9	2.8 ± 0.7
(Range)		(0–4)	(0–3)	(0–4)	(1–4)
Δ (%)			8.0	0.0	**33.3**

Bold numbers depict clinically significant improvement.

TABLE 2: Kellgren–Lawrence grading scale. The intraclass correlation coefficient for interobserver was 0.778 ($p < 0.001$) and the intraobserver 0.80 ($p < 0.001$).

		Baseline	Follow-up	Δ (%)	CI95%	p
KL, n (%)	II	20 (48.8)	9 (21.9)	−26.9	16.5–42	0.001
	III	16 (39.0)	23 (56.0)	17.0	5–27.2	0.05

approaches have been used, including medication (oral, topical, intra-articular) and a core treatment program consisting of exercise, education, dietary advice, and biomechanical interventions, as well as surgery as the last resort [30].

Total knee replacement is an effective treatment for end-stage knee OA. However, this option is only suitable for a subset of patients with controlled comorbidities, patients who are older than 40 years, and patients who can afford the intervention [31]. Nevertheless, the number of total knee replacements is expected

Table 3: Extended Cox model of relapse-free survival during the follow-up period including time-varying covariates.

Characteristic	Adjusted HR (95% CI)	p value
Fixed effects		
Age (years)	**0.9190 (0.8850, 0.9530)**	**<0.0001**
Females (ref.) vs. males	**2.3790 (1.2510, 4.5220)**	**0.0008**
Baseline BMI (kg/m^2)		
Underweight	0.0000 (0.0000, 0.0000)	0.9872
Normal weight	Ref.	-
Overweight	**2.3560 (1.1740, 4.7270)**	**0.0159**
Obese	**3.4610 (1.4620, 8.1900)**	**0.0047**
Arthrosis grade		
II	Ref.	
III	**2.6460 (1.3230, 5.2900)**	**0.0059**
Baseline clinical scores (U)		
WOMAC	**1.0500 (1.0010, 1.1020)**	**0.0442**
100 mm VAS-MD	0.8790 (0.5850, 1.3190)	0.5327
100 mm VAS-PT	1.1080 (0.7480, 1.6410)	0.6090
Time covarying effects		
WOMAC	0.9990 (1.9980, 1.0010)	0.5449
100 mm VAS-MD	—	—
100 mm VAS-PT	—	—

"—" means model did not converge. Significant predictors at the 0.05 level are displayed in bold, and those at the 0.10 level (marginally significant) are displayed in italics.

to increase in parallel with the ageing of the population, which highlights the associated future economic burden. For example, in our institution, the number of total knee replacements increased dramatically from 3,200 to 4,250 during the period from 2006 to 2017 [*unpublished data*].

Herein, we evaluated the clinical benefit of intra-articular polymerized-type I collagen and found that the weekly application of six injections decreased pain as well as the need for TKR and arthroscopy at the five-year follow-up.

There are at least two previous clinical trials that have evaluated the effect of collagen in OA treatment. One of them has investigated a medical device, MD-Knee (Guna S.p.a., Milan, Italy), containing collagen of porcine origin of molecular weight equal to 300,000 dalton, produced through a process of tangential filtration. It is a pure product, contaminant-free, with standardized chemical and physical characteristics. The purpose of an in situ introduction of collagen is to provide an effective bioscaffold. On the other hand, its degradation in the constituent amino acids constitutes a nutritional support for tissues of the other joint structures. MD-Knee preparation is equally effective in knee OA symptoms over six months after a five-week injection course as the HA formulation (SUPARTZ®) [32]. Moreover, 3 mL IAI of porcine type I atelocollagen (BioCollagen group) has been also demonstrated to alleviate knee pain in OA patients at 24 weeks [33].

Nonetheless, our patients showed clinical improvement according to the WOMAC and VAS scores at all the follow-up visits. Indeed, polymerized-type I collagen also had a clinical benefit in the group with severe knee OA, defined as patients with a WOMAC subscale of functional disability score ≥20 and EVA ≥50.

According to a meta-analysis of 74 randomized clinical trials of IA hyaluronic acid products vs. placebo in knee OA, saline solution had a placebo effect characterized by an approximately 30% reduction in pain that persisted for at least 3 months, while hyaluronic acid improved pain by 40–50% [34]. In the present study, the improvement in the VAS pain score ranged from 43 to 62% during the 60 months of follow-up. In addition, a previous meta-analysis of randomized controlled trials demonstrated that the administration of a single IAI of saline significantly improved short-term (≤3 months) and long-term (6–12 months) knee pain. Our long-term study diminished the possibility of the placebo effect [35]. We also found that the use of polymerized-type I collagen prevented the use of any other intra-articular treatment during the study period.

The other main outcome of our study was the need for TKR or arthroscopy. We described a 98.8% covariate-adjusted knee survival rate at 60 months (characterized by the absence of TKR or arthroscopy). In comparison, a study that evaluated the IAI effect of a high-molecular-weight hyaluronic preparation in knee OA reported a 67% knee survival rate (absence of TKR) at 60 months [36]. Our results suggest that polymerized-type I collagen is able to control the relief of symptoms and may act as disease-modifying OA drug that could slow or halt the radiographic evolution of the disease and prevent tissue damage [18–21]. Further RCTs with specific clinical or radiological endpoints are necessary to confirm these data. Thus, polymerized-type I collagen may be a therapeutic option for patients considered too young for arthroplasty, patients whose occupation precludes them from having arthroplasty, or patients who, due to health complications, cannot undergo surgery despite having an orthopedic indication.

Regarding the radiological results, significant progress was observed when they were evaluated for KL grading. Most of the patients advanced from stage II to III, but not from III to IV. Nonetheless, reduction in radiographic joint space width is recognized as a standard for demonstrating structural benefits in knee OA [37].

In the present study, polymerized-type I collagen prevented any significant change in joint space narrowing in the medial, lateral, and patellofemoral compartments at five years of follow-up. This suggests that the patients had no radiological progression, implying preservation of the hyaline cartilage.

In addition, it is important to highlight the low incidence of local and systemic AEs of the drug. This result is in agreement with the low incidence of AEs attributable to IA therapies reported in clinical trials in knee OA, with the main AEs being postinjection pain and swelling, as in our study [38]. Moreover, we previously reported that polymerized-type I collagen was a dominant cost-benefit alternative compared with NSAIDs in the treatment of symptomatic knee OA [39].

The main limitation of our study was our open design. It is well known that a placebo is effective in the treatment of OA, especially with respect to pain, stiffness, and self-reported function [35, 40–43]. Nevertheless, our study included a nonnegligible number of patients with symptomatic knee OA who had a better clinical improvement than that described for placebo in the literature, as well as a long follow-up period. Another limitation includes the low number of radiographs analyzed. However, a reduction in radiographic joint space width was determined indicating a structural benefit in knee OA and no progression of the disease.

5. Conclusion

Polymerized-type I collagen has an excellent long-term clinical outcome and a safe profile. The obtained data show that polymerized-type I collagen improves functional disability, decreases pain, and increases the time of surgical deferral of TKR, suggesting that it could slow or halt the radiographic evolution of the disease. It is a nonsurgical treatment option that certainly deserves future research.

Consent

Informed consent was obtained from all enrolled participants.

Authors' Contributions

A. B-F., S. I. M-H., G. H-M., A. P-O., J. F-C., and G. T-V. contributed to conceptualization; data curation; formal analysis; investigation; methodology; original draft writing; and manuscript writing, reviewing, and editing. E. R-M., J. B-CdlT, L. A-J., M. C. V-B., M. A. L-M., F. R-H., C. A-H., J. P-C., and H. A. C-R. participated in clinical information collection; data curation; data analysis; and manuscript writing, reviewing, and editing. A.B.-F., S. I. M-H., G. H-M., and A. P-O. contributed equally to this work.

Acknowledgments

The authors would like to thank Dr. Andrea Martınez Pederzini (Matrícula: 20131006992) for her valuable assistance in organizing the database.

References

[1] I. Peláez-Ballestas, L. H. Sanin, J. Moreno-Montoya et al., "Epidemiology of the rheumatic diseases in mexico. a study of 5 regions based on the copcord methodology," *The Journal of Rheumatology Supplement*, vol. 86, no. 0, pp. 3–8, 2011.

[2] A. Obregón-Ponce, I. Iraheta, H. García-Ferrer, B. Mejia, and A. García-Kutzbach, "Prevalence of musculoskeletal diseases in Guatemala, Central America," *JCR: Journal of Clinical Rheumatology*, vol. 18, no. 4, pp. 170–174, 2012.

[3] R. Burgos-Vargas, M. H. Cardiel, A. Loyola-Sánchez et al., "Characterization of knee osteoarthritis in Latin America. a comparative analysis of clinical and health care utilization in Argentina, Brazil, and Mexico," *Reumatología Clínica*, vol. 10, no. 3, pp. 152–159, 2014.

[4] A. M. Reginato, H. Riera, M. Vera et al., "Osteoarthritis in Latin America," *JCR: Journal of Clinical Rheumatology*, vol. 21, no. 8, pp. 391–397, 2015.

[5] L. Haywood, D. McWilliams, C. Pearson et al., "Inflammation and angiogenesis in osteoarthritis," *Arthritis & Rheumatism*, vol. 48, no. 8, pp. 2173–2177, 2003.

[6] M. Benito, D. Veale, O. FitzGerald et al., "Synovial tissue inflammation in early and late osteoarthritis," *Annals of the Rheumatic Diseases*, vol. 64, no. 9, pp. 263–1267, 2005.

[7] C. R. Scanzello, A. Plaas, and M. K. Crow, "Innate immune system activation in osteoarthritis: is osteoarthritis a chronic wound?" *Current Opinion in Rheumatology*, vol. 20, no. 5, pp. 565–572, 2008.

[8] C. R. Crow, E. Umoh, F. Pessler et al., "Local cytokine profiles in knee osteoarthritis: elevated synovial fluid interleukin-15 differentiates early from end-stage disease," *Osteoarthritis and Cartilage*, vol. 17, no. 8, pp. 1040–1048, 2009.

[9] J. Sokolove and C. M. Lepus, "Role of inflammation in the pathogenesis of osteoarthritis: latest findings and interpretations," *Therapeutic Advances in Musculoskeletal Disease*, vol. 5, no. 2, pp. 77–94, 2013.

[10] D. Azamar-Llamas, G. Hernández-Molina, B. Ramos-Ávalos, and J. Furuzawa-Carballeda, "Adipokine contribution to the pathogenesis of osteoarthritis," *Mediators of Inflammation*, vol. 2017, pp. 1–26, 2017.

[11] M. Kapoor, J. Martel-Pelletier, D. Lajeunesse, J.-P. Pelletier, and H. Fahmi, "Role of proinflammatory cytokines in the pathophysiology of osteoarthritis," *Nature Reviews Rheumatology*, vol. 7, no. 1, pp. 33–42, 2011.

[12] J. Martel-Pelletier, A. J. Barr, F. M. Cicuttini et al., "Osteoarthritis," *Nature Reviews Disease Primers*, vol. 2, no. 1, p. 16072, 2016.

[13] J. Furuzawa-Carballeda, J. Alcocer-Varela, and L. Díaz de León, "Collagen-PVP decreases collagen turnover in synovial tissue cultures from rheumatoid arthritis patients," *Annals of the New York Academy of Sciences*, vol. 878, no. 1, pp. 508–602, 1999.

[14] J. Furuzawa-Carballeda, R. Rodriquez-calderon, L. D. D. Leon, and J. Alcocer-varela, "Mediators of inflammation are down-regulated while apoptosis is up-regulated in rheumatoid arthritis synovial tissue by polymerized collagen," *Clinical and Experimental Immunology*, vol. 130, no. 1, pp. 140–149, 2002.

[15] J. Furuzawa-Carballeda, P. Macip-Rodríguez, A. S. Galindo-Feria et al., "Polymerized-type I collagen induces upregulation of Foxp3-expressing CD4 regulatory T cells and down-regulation of IL-17-producing CD4$^+$ T cells (Th17) cells in collagen-induced arthritis," *Clinical and Developmental Immunology*, vol. 2012, p. 11, 2012.

[16] J. Furuzawa-Carballeda, A. R. Cabral, M. Zapata-Zuñiga, and J. Alcocer-Varela, "Subcutaneous administration of polymerized-type I collagen for the treatment of patients with rheumatoid arthritis," *The Journal of Rheumatology*, vol. 30, pp. 256–259, 2003.

[17] J. Furuzawa-Carballeda, R. Fenutria-Ausmequet, V. Gil-Espinosa et al., "Polymerized-type I Collagen for the treatment of patients with rheumatoid arthritis. Effect of intramuscular administration in a double blind placebo-controlled clinical trial," *Clinical and Experimental Rheumatology*, vol. 24, pp. 521–528, 2006.

[18] J. Furuzawa-Carballeda, O. A. Muñoz-Chablé, J. Barrios-Payán, and R. Hernández-Pando, "Effect of polymerized-type I collagen in knee osteoarthritis. I.In vitrostudy," *European Journal of Clinical Investigation*, vol. 39, no. 7, pp. 591–597, 2009.

[19] J. Furuzawa-Carballeda, O. A. Muñoz-Chablé, S. I. Macías-Hernández, and A. Agualimpia-Janning, "Effect of poly-

merized-type I collagen in knee osteoarthritis. II.in vivostudy," *European Journal of Clinical Investigation*, vol. 39, no. 7, pp. 598–606, 2009.

[20] J. Furuzawa-Carballeda, G. Lima, L. Llorente et al., "Polymerized-type I collagen downregulates inflammation and improves clinical outcomes in patients with symptomatic knee osteoarthritis following arthroscopic lavage: a randomized, double-blind, and placebo-controlled clinical trial," *The Scientific World Journal*, vol. 2012, p. 11, 2012.

[21] A.-B. M, A. B. Enríquez, and F.-C. J, "Polymerized-type I collagen induces a high quality cartilage repair in a rat model of osteoarthritis," *International Journal of Bone and Rheumatology Research*, vol. 4, no. 2, pp. 68–76, 2017.

[22] R. Altman, E. Asch, D. Bloch et al., "Development of criteria for the classification and reporting of osteoarthritis: classification of osteoarthritis of the knee," *Arthritis & Rheumatism*, vol. 29, no. 8, pp. 1039–1049, 1986.

[23] J. Furuzawa-Carballeda, E. Rojas, M. Valverde, I. Castillo, L. D. de León, and E. Krötzsch, "Cellular and humoral responses to collagen–polyvinylpyrrolidone administered during short and long periods in humans," *Canadian Journal of Physiology and Pharmacology*, vol. 81, no. 11, pp. 1029–1035, 2003.

[24] N. Bellamy, W. W. Buchanan, C. H. Goldsmith et al., "Validation study of WOMAC: a health status instrument for measuring clinically important patient relevant outcomes to antirheumatic drug therapy in patients with osteoarthritis of the hip and knee," *The Journal of Rheumatology*, vol. 15, no. 2, pp. 1833–1840, 1988.

[25] E. W. Ehrich, G. M. Davies, D. J. Watson, J. A Bolognese, B. C Seidenberg, and N Bellamy, "Minimal perceptible clinical improvement with the Western Ontario and mcmaster universities osteoarthritis index questionnaire and global assessments in patients with osteoarthritis," *The Journal of Rheumatology*, vol. 27, no. 11, pp. 2635–2641, 2000.

[26] J. W. J. Bijlsma, "Patient centred outcomes in osteoarthritis," *Annals of the Rheumatic Diseases*, vol. 64, no. 1, pp. 1-2, 2005.

[27] N. Bellamy, W. F. Kean, W. W. Buchanan et al., "Double blind randomised controlled trial of sodium meclofenamate (meclomen) and diclofenac sodium (voltaren): post validation reapplication of the WOMAC Osteoarthritis Index," *The Journal of Rheumatology*, vol. 19, no. 1, pp. 153–159, 1992.

[28] H. Iijima, T. Aoyama, K. Nishitani et al., "Coexisting lateral tibiofemoral osteoarthritis is associated with worse knee pain in patients with mild medial osteoarthritis," *Osteoarthritis and Cartilage*, vol. 25, no. 8, pp. 1274–1281, 2017.

[29] B. Gallager, F. P. Tjoumakaris, M. I. Harwood, R. P. Good, M. G. Ciccotti, and K. B. Freedman, "Chondroprotection and the prevention of osteoarthritis progression of the knee: a systematic review of treatment agents," *The American Journal of Sports Medicine*, vol. 43, no. 3, pp. 734–744, 2015.

[30] T. E. McAlindon, R. R. Bannuru, M. C. Sullivan et al., "OARSI guidelines for the non-surgical management of knee osteoarthritis," *Osteoarthritis and Cartilage*, vol. 22, no. 3, pp. 363–388, 2014.

[31] S. T. Skou, E. M. Roos, M. B. Laursen et al., "A randomized, controlled trial of total knee replacement," *New England Journal of Medicine*, vol. 373, no. 17, pp. 1597–1606, 2015.

[32] L. S. Martin Martin, U. Massafra, E. Bizzi, and A. Migliore, "A double blind randomized active controlled clinical trial on the intra-articular use of md-knee versus sodium hyaluronate in patients with knee osteoarthritis (joint)," *BMC Musculoskelet Disord*, vol. 17, no. 1, p. 94, 2016.

[33] H. S. Lee, K. J. Oh, Y. W. Moon, Y. In, H. J. Lee, and S. Y. Kwon, "Intra-articular injection of type I atelocollagen to alleviate knee pain: a double-blind, randomized controlled trial," *Cartilage*, 2019.

[34] S. Colen, M. P. J. van den Bekerom, M. Mulier, and D. Haverkamp, "Hyaluronic acid in the treatment of knee osteoarthritis," *BioDrugs*, vol. 26, no. 4, pp. 257–268, 2012.

[35] R. D. Altman, T. Devji, M. Bhandari, A. Fierlinger, F. Niazi, and R. Christensen, "Clinical benefit of intra-articular saline as a comparator in clinical trials of knee osteoarthritis treatments: a systematic review and meta-analysis of randomized trials," *Seminars in Arthritis and Rheumatism*, vol. 46, no. 2, pp. 151–159, 2016.

[36] T. Boutefnouchet, G. Puranik, E. Holmes, and K. M. Bell, "Hylan GF-20 viscosupplementation in the treatment of symptomatic osteoarthritis of the knee: clinical effect survivorship at 5 years," *Knee Surgery & Related Research*, vol. 29, no. 2, pp. 129–136, 2017.

[37] P. G. Conaghan, D. J. Hunter, J. F. Maillefert, W. M. Reichmann, and E. Losina, "Summary and recommendations of the OARSI FDA osteoarthritis assessment of structural change working group," *Osteoarthritis and Cartilage*, vol. 19, no. 5, pp. 606–610, 2011.

[38] C. Nguyen and F. Rannou, "The safety of intra-articular injections for the treatment of knee osteoarthritis: a critical narrative review," *Expert Opinion on Drug Safety*, vol. 16, no. 8, pp. 897–902, 2017.

[39] X. Burbano-Levy, D. Cardona, E. Palacios et al., "Costo utilidad de colágena polivinilpirrolidona en el tratamiento de osteoartrosis de rodilla en México," *Value in Health Regional Issues*, vol. 5, pp. 40–47, 2014.

[40] P. T. Dawes, C. Kirlew, and I. Haslock, "Saline washout for knee osteoarthritis: results of a controlled study," *Clinical Rheumatology*, vol. 6, no. 1, pp. 61–63, 1987.

[41] R. W. Ike, W. J. Arnold, E. W. Rothschild, and H. L. Shaw, "Tidal irrigation versus conservative medical management in patients with osteoarthritis of the knee: a prospective randomized study," *The Journal of Rheumatology*, vol. 19, no. 5, pp. 772–779, 1992.

[42] I. Uthman, J. P. Raynauld, and B. Haraoui, "Intra-articular therapy in osteoarthritis," *Postgraduate Medical Journal*, vol. 79, no. 934, pp. 449–453, 2003.

[43] W. Zhang, J. Robertson, A. C. Jones, P. A. Dieppe, and M. Doherty, "The placebo effect and its determinants in osteoarthritis: meta-analysis of randomised controlled trials," *Annals of the Rheumatic Diseases*, vol. 67, no. 12, pp. 1716–1723, 2008.

15

Ultrasound-Guided Peripheral Nerve Blocks Performed by Orthopedic Surgeons: A Retrospective, Multicenter Study in Akita Prefecture, Japan

Tatsuru Tomioka,[1,2] Seietsu Senma,[2] Yuichiro Narita,[2] Masakazu Urayama,[2] Satoshi Yumoto,[2] Hiroki Ito,[2] Toshiaki Aizawa,[2] Tsuyoshi Shirahata,[2] Hiroshi Aonuma,[2] Nozomi Kaga,[2] Norimitsu Masutani,[2] Yusuke Yuasa,[2] Hikaru Saito,[2,3] Kunio Ebata,[1] Kentaro Ouchi,[1] Naohisa Miyakoshi,[2,3] and Yoichi Shimada[2,3]

[1]*Department of Orthopedic Surgery, Yokote Municipal Hospital, Akita 013-8602, Japan*
[2]*Akita Hand Group, Akita 010-8543, Japan*
[3]*Department of Orthopedic Surgery, Akita University Graduate School of Medicine, Akita 010-8543, Japan*

Correspondence should be addressed to Tatsuru Tomioka; tomioka@sky.plala.or.jp

Academic Editor: Andreas K. Demetriades

The shortage of doctors is a societal problem, especially in rural areas such as Akita Prefecture, Japan. Therefore, it is not unusual in Akita for orthopedic surgeons to perform upper and lower limb surgeries under ultrasound-guided peripheral nerve blocks managed by the operators themselves. Multicenter studies of ultrasound-guided peripheral nerve blocks performed by orthopedic surgeons have not been reported. The purpose of this study was to clarify the safety and reliability of ultrasound-guided peripheral nerve blocks performed by orthopedic surgeons in Akita. A total of 1,674 upper extremity surgery cases operated under ultrasound-guided peripheral nerve blocks at 8 hospitals in Akita prefecture from April 2016 to April 2018 were investigated retrospectively. These blocks were performed by a total of 37 orthopedic surgeons, including senior surgeons and residents. In 321 of the 1,674 cases (19%), local anesthetics were added to the surgical field. Two cases with special factors were converted to general anesthesia. There were 2 cases of complications associated with the nerve block, but they were all transient and recovered promptly. The block site and the hospital where the block was performed showed a significant relationship with the addition of local anesthetics to the surgical site ($P < 0.001$). Surgery time, age at surgery, and surgical site showed no significant relationships with the addition of local anesthetics. The volume of the anesthetic used for the nerve block showed a significant inverse relationship with the addition of local anesthetics ($P = 0.040$). Many orthopedic surgeons in Akita prefecture began to perform ultrasound-guided peripheral nerve blocks, which had a reliable anesthesia effect with no noticeable complications, whether performed by residents or senior orthopedic surgeons, and this is a useful anesthetic technique for orthopedic surgeons.

1. Introduction

The shortage of doctors is a societal problem, especially in rural areas such as Akita Prefecture, Japan. There are many hospitals with no full-time anesthesiologists, and the number of operations performed under anesthesiologist management is limited. Therefore, it is not unusual that orthopedic surgeons perform upper and lower limb surgeries under ultrasound-guided peripheral nerve blocks managed by the operators themselves in Akita.

The usefulness and complications of ultrasound-guided peripheral nerve blocks performed by anesthesiologists have been reported [1–4], but no multicenter studies of ultrasound-guided peripheral nerve blocks performed by orthopedic surgeons have been reported. The purpose of this study was to clarify the safety and reliability of ultrasound-guided peripheral nerve blocks performed by orthopedic surgeons in Akita.

2. Materials and Methods

A total of 1,674 upper extremity surgery cases operated under ultrasound-guided peripheral nerve blocks at 8 hospitals in Akita prefecture from April 2016 to April 2018 were investigated retrospectively. All patients were preoperatively informed by an attending doctor and agreed to undergo surgery with a peripheral nerve block. The types of operations included distal radius fracture open reduction and internal fixation (ORIF) in 261 cases, finger or hand fracture ORIF in 111 cases, elbow joint fracture ORIF in 35 cases, extensor tendon repair in 59 cases, flexor tendon repair in 14 cases, and nerve repair in 58 cases (Figure 1).

The patients' average age at surgery was 58 years (range: 10–95 years). The average operation time was 67 minutes (range: 2–395 minutes). The type of block to be performed was determined by the visibility of patient's nerves, physical size, and the preference of each practitioner. Using a linear ultrasound probe, the needle was inserted across or parallel to the probe, and the needle was inserted near the nerve under ultrasound guidance. The syringe containing the anesthetics was connected to an extension tube line and 23 gauge sterile standard blunt needle (Figure 2).

The anesthetics were injected little by little about 0.5–2 ml, so as to be diffused the whole circumference of the outside epineurium and never injected intraneurally. Ultrasound-guided peripheral nerve blocks were always performed in the same image with landmark parts visualized. In the interscalene block, the C5–C7 nerves depicted as straight three circular hypoechoic images between the anterior and middle scalene muscles were visualized on the short-axis view, and each nerve was blocked (Figures 3(a) and 3(b)). In the supraclavicular block, the nerve trunks adjacent to the subclavian artery were blocked with the pleura visualized so as not to cause pneumothorax (Figure 4). In the axillary block, the triangle surrounded by the coracobrachialis and latissimus dorsi muscles was revealed. The median nerve, ulnar nerve, and radial nerve inside the triangle and the musculocutaneous nerve inside the coracobrachialis muscle were blocked (Figures 5(a) and 5(b)). In the forearm block, the median nerve, ulnar nerve, and radial nerve between the muscles were identified, and each nerve was blocked (Figures 6–8).

There were double-level blocks in some cases (17.1%). In the cases of double-level blocks, the most proximal block was considered the main block. The main blocks were the interscalene block in 86 cases, the supraclavicular block in 786 cases, the axillary block in 761 cases, and the forearm block in 41 cases. These blocks were performed by a total of 37 orthopedic surgeons, including senior surgeons and residents. In all cases, no intravenous anesthetic was used in combination. There were no cases using neurostimulators, sterile probe covers, or sterile gloves. The anesthetics used in the block were 0.25% bupivacaine, 0.75% ropivacaine, 1% mepivacaine, and 1% lidocaine, which were used alone or in combination. The volume of anesthetics in the block was 5–40 ml, with the majority of cases (87%) using less than 30 ml, depending on the weight and age of the patient. In all cases, the postoperative condition was examined by operators themselves during hospitalization and outpatient care. The operators examined for complications associated with peripheral nerve blocks.

The relationships between the addition of local anesthetics to the surgical field and the main block site, the hospital where the block was performed, and the surgical site were analyzed using the χ^2 test. The relationships between the addition of local anesthetics to the surgical field and operation time, patient's age at surgery, and the amount of anesthetic fluid volume used for nerve blocks were analyzed by logistic regression analysis. All statistical tests were performed using SPSS software (SPSS 16.0J for Windows Base System, SPSS Japan Inc., Tokyo, Japan). Significance was set at $P < 0.05$.

3. Results

In 321 of 1,674 cases (19%), local anesthetics were added to the surgical field. Lidocaine and mepivacaine were used, but the additional anesthetic volumes were low (approximately 3–10 ml). Two cases (0.1%) were converted to general anesthesia; one case was a reduction of elbow joint dislocation with severe obesity and poor visualization of the nerves by ultrasound, and the other was a radial fracture ORIF case that was considered unsuitable for surgery under a nerve block because of psychological factors. There were two cases of complications associated with nerve blocks, namely, nausea in one case and decreased oxygen saturation in another, but both patients recovered promptly. There were no cases of persistent neuropathy or infection of the nerve block injection sites. The rate of the additional local anesthetic to the surgical field was 35% in the interscalene block, 18% in the supraclavicular block, 20% in the axillary block, and 5% in the forearm block. There was a significant relationship between the addition of the local anesthetic to the surgical site and the main block site ($P < 0.001$). The rate of addition of the local anesthetic for each hospital ranged from 6% to 34%; it was significantly different depending on the hospital in which the block was performed ($P < 0.001$).

Surgery time, age at surgery, and surgical site showed no significant relationships with the addition of the local anesthetic. On the contrary, the volume of anesthetics used for the nerve block showed a significant inverse relationship with the addition of local anesthetics ($P = 0.040$).

4. Discussion

In a peripheral nerve block, high success rates have been reported even with conventional methods such as the transarterial technique [5] and the paresthesia technique [6], but they have the disadvantages of directly puncturing arteries and nerves. Although nerve puncture and intraneural injection were reported to, sometimes, produce temporary sensory disturbances, they did not lead to permanent neuropathy [7], whereas it was reported that neuropathy occurred in 2.8% of cases with the seeking paresthesia

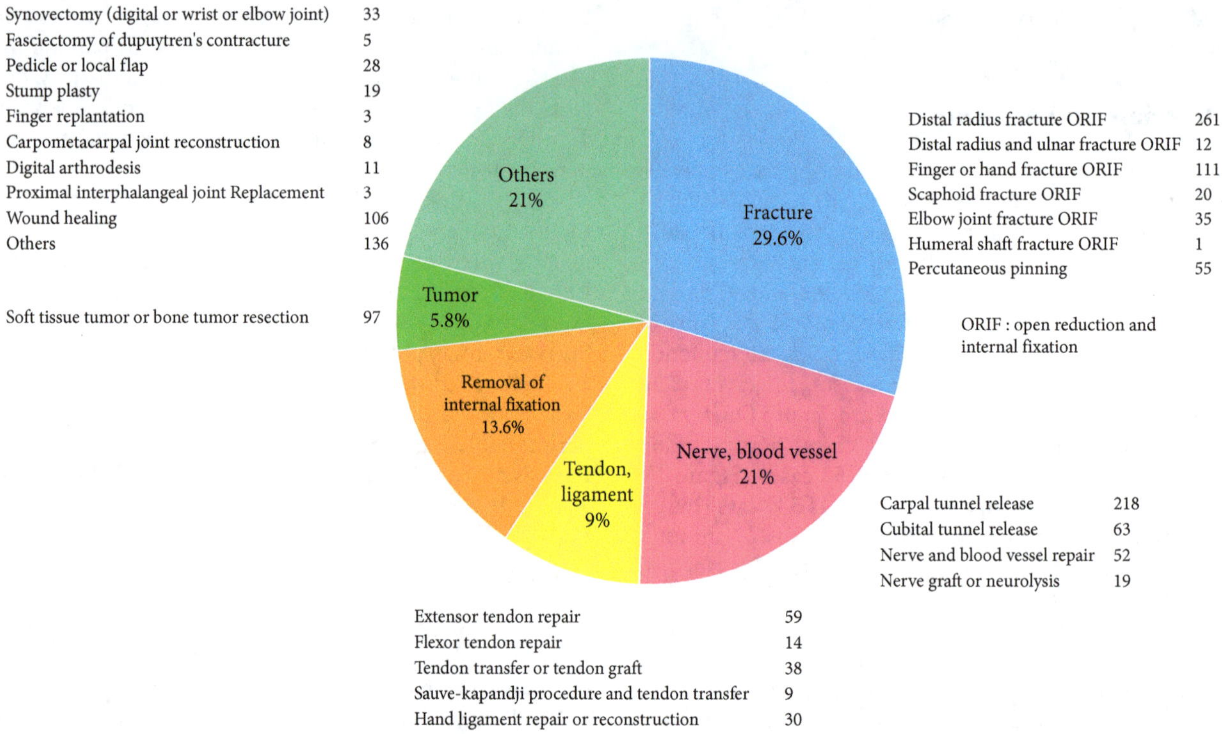

FIGURE 1: The types of 1,674 upper extremity surgery cases under ultrasound-guided peripheral nerve blocks.

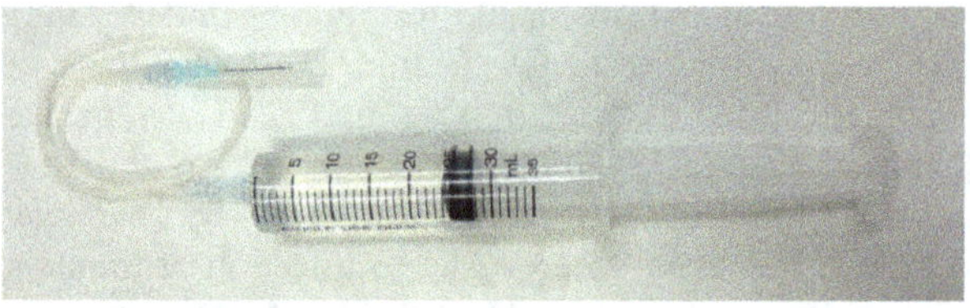

FIGURE 2: Syringe, extension tube, and needle.

technique [8]. Nerve puncture and intraneural injection should be avoided as much as possible to prevent neuropathy. In a report on multiple-injection technique comparing ultrasound guidance with nerve stimulation guidance, although ultrasound guidance showed shorter time to onset of the sensory block and fewer needle insertions than nerve stimulation guidance, success rates and complication rates were similar [1]. However, there were individual variations in the locations of the nerves, and it seems easier to perform peripheral nerve blocks by identifying nerves with ultrasound [9–11]. In fact, it has been reported that the ultrasound-guided technique had less vessel puncture [12], a significantly higher success rate [13, 14], and fewer complications than the nerve stimulation-guided technique [15, 16]. However, it is necessary to be careful because there are reports that pneumothorax and nerve palsy have occurred even under ultrasound guidance [17, 18], but in the present study, despite being performed by many orthopedic surgeons, complications were only transient and mild, affecting only 0.1% of cases. Ultrasound-guided peripheral nerve blocks were performed mainly by interscalene, supraclavicular, and axillary approaches. The rate of additional local anesthetic to the surgical field was higher with the interscalene block than with other blocks, and it was thought that it was difficult to block the C8 and Th1 nerves even under ultrasound guidance. Although the number of cases of forearm blocks was small, the rate of additional local anesthetic was the lowest.

Soberón et al. reported that forearm blocks might be used as the primary anesthetic in patients undergoing hand surgery [19]. In the future, the use of forearm blocks may increase in hand and finger surgeries. The volume of the anesthetic used for the blocks in the present study was mostly 30 ml or less depending on the patient's weight and age, which was substantially less than the maximum dose. A study of the Australian and New Zealand Registry of Regional Anaesthesia reported that ultrasound guidance reduced the incidence of local anesthetic toxicity [2]. It was reported that a higher dose and concentration of the anesthetic, but not a higher volume, were associated with longer block duration [20]. On the contrary, a higher volume of the anesthetic showed a lower rate of requiring additional local anesthetic to the surgical field in the present study. It was thought that the higher volume of the anesthetic used for the nerve block could be injected more easily all around the nerve. However, it was reported that 45% of the patients who underwent an ultrasound-guided interscalene block with only 5 ml of ropivacaine developed diaphragmatic paralysis [21]; thus, it is necessary to be careful when increasing the volume of the anesthetic, especially in interscalene blocks.

The Akita Hand Surgery Group has continued to hold skill practice workshops on ultrasound-guided peripheral nerve blocks free of charge for orthopedic surgeons in cooperation with the Akita University Department of

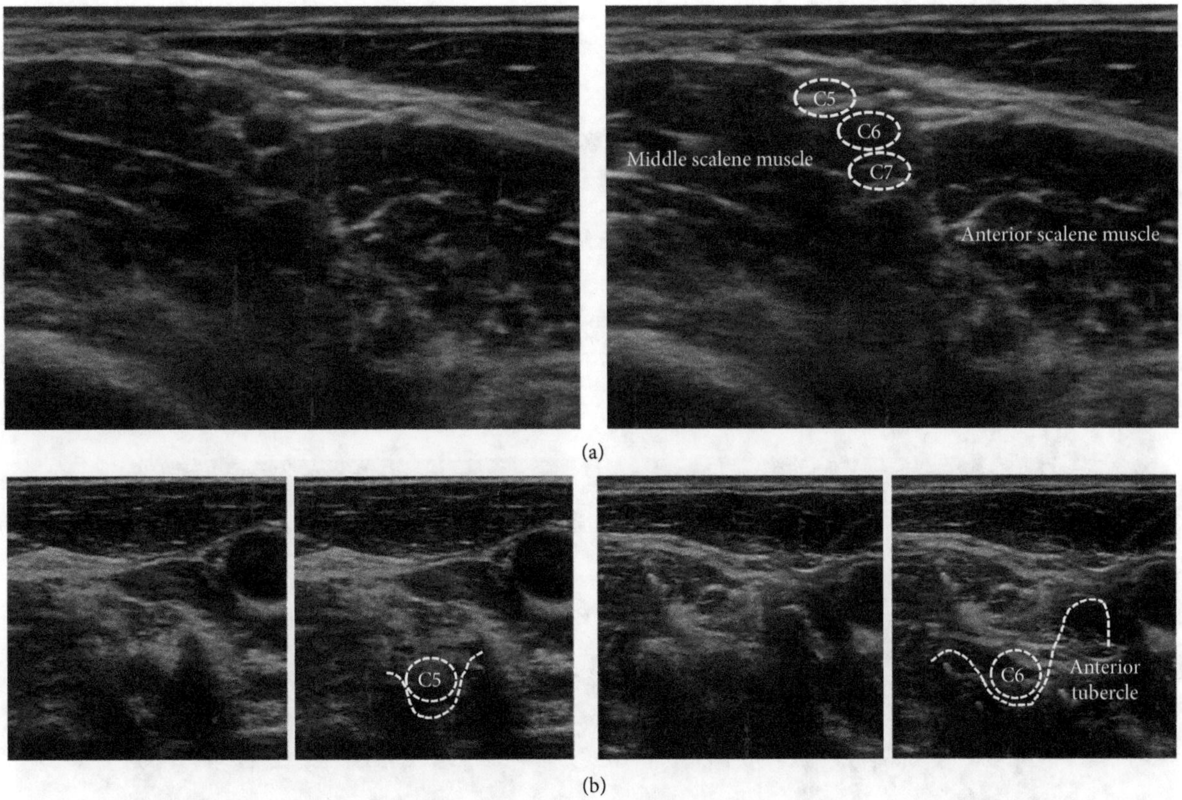

FIGURE 3: (a) In the short-axis view of the interscalene, the C5–C7 nerves depicted as straight three circular hypoechoic images between the anterior and middle scalene muscles are visualized. (b) The groove of the C5 transverse process between the anterior and posterior tubercles is U-shaped. The C6 anterior tubercle is large, so the groove of the C6 transverse process is J-shaped. The C5 and C6 nerves lead to the peripheral side through the groove of the transverse processes. Tracing the nerves depicted as circular hypoechoic images from the groove of the transverse processes to the peripheral side is useful for identifying the nerves at the interscalene.

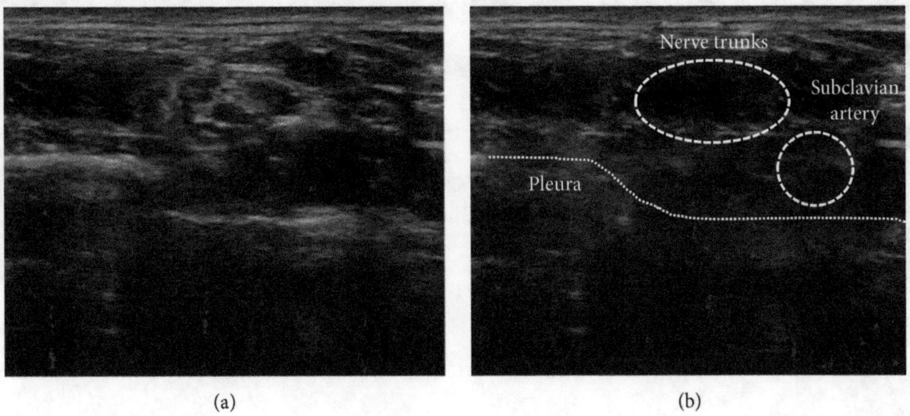

FIGURE 4: In the supraclavicular view, the linear hyperechoic pleura and hypoechoic lung are depicted, and the nerve trunks adjacent to the subclavian artery are visualized.

Orthopedic Surgery. As a result, ultrasound-guided peripheral nerve blocks, which were previously performed in only a few hospitals, are now performed in many hospitals throughout Akita.

However, the block site and the hospital where the block was performed showed a significant relationship with the addition of the local anesthetic to the surgical site. It may be due to the difference in the skills of the practitioners who performed the nerve block and the difference in the performance of the ultrasonic equipment used in each hospital. Therefore, in order to further improve the anesthesia success rate, it may be necessary to improve the workshop to be more accurate and comprehensible by teaching the tips and tricks for ultrasound-guided peripheral nerve blocks.

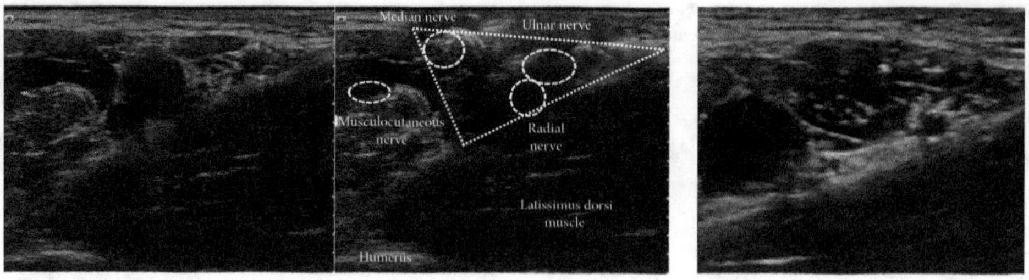

(a) (b)

FIGURE 5: (a) In the axillary view, finding the triangle surrounded by the coracobrachialis and latissimus dorsi muscles helps identify the nerves. The median, ulnar, and radial nerves pass through inside the triangle. (b) Hypoechoic anesthetics are injected all around the nerve.

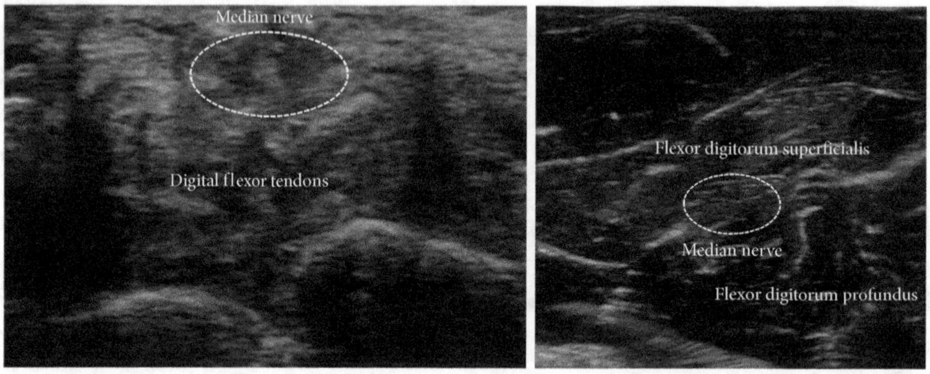

FIGURE 6: The median nerve depicted as a fascicular pattern can be identified on the superficial layer of the flexor tendons at the wrist joint level. Identifying the median nerve at the wrist level and then moving the probe to the forearm makes it easier to identify the median nerve between the flexor digitorum superficialis and flexor digitorum profundus. (a) Wrist. (b) Middle part of the forearm.

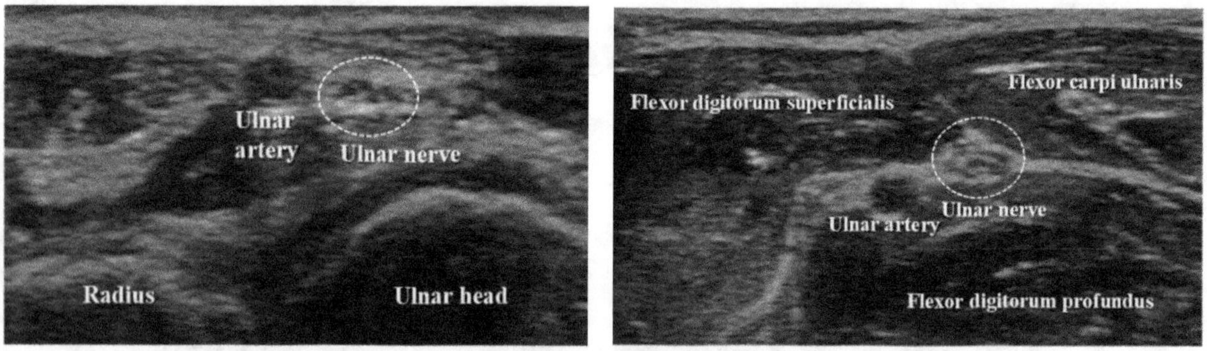

(a) (b)

FIGURE 7: The ulnar nerve is located near the ulnar side of the ulnar artery in the range from the wrist joint to the middle part of the forearm.

As of March 1, 2020, the total population of Akita prefecture was 960,271 and that of Akita city was 304,943; 2/3 of the population is outside of Akita city, but full-time anesthesiologists are concentrated in Akita city. Outside of Akita city, there are few emergency hospitals that have full-time anesthesiologists, and these hospitals provide surgical treatment with part-time anesthesiologists and have a manpower shortage. Under such circumstances, the number of operations that an anesthesiologist can manage for orthopedic surgery is not at all adequate. Therefore, it is not unusual that orthopedic surgeons perform upper limb and lower limb surgeries under ultrasound-guided peripheral nerve blocks performed by the operators themselves. Until now, it is unclear whether ultrasound-guided peripheral nerve blocks in Akita prefecture were performed reliably and safely.

The present study showed that cases of transition to general anesthesia were very rare, there were no noticeable complications, and the anesthesia success rate was acceptable in all hospitals.

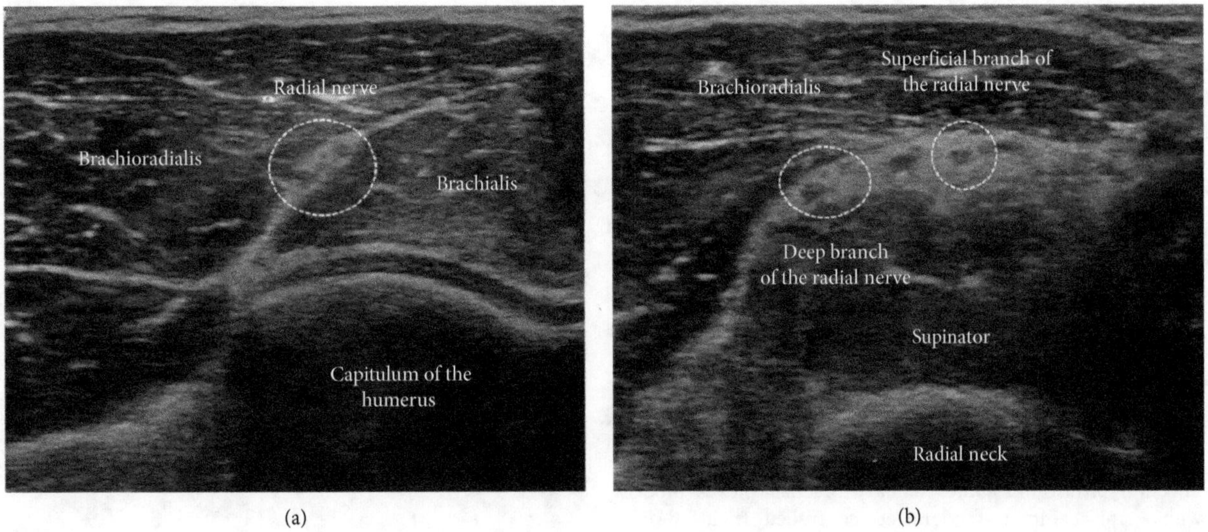

FIGURE 8: In the anterolateral short-axis view of the elbow joint level, the radial nerve is visible as a fascicular pattern between the brachioradialis and brachialis muscles. The radial nerve is divided into deep and superficial branches at the radial neck level. It is also possible to block only the superficial branch, which is the sensory branch.

5. Conclusion

As a result of continuing dissemination activities through skill practice workshops, many orthopedic surgeons in Akita prefecture began performing ultrasound-guided peripheral nerve blocks, which had a reliable anesthesia effect with no noticeable complications, whether performed by residents or senior orthopedic surgeons. This is a useful anesthetic technique for orthopedic surgeons to use.

References

[1] A. Casati, G. Danelli, M. Baciarello et al., "A prospective, randomized comparison between ultrasound and nerve stimulation guidance for multiple injection axillary brachial plexus block," *Anesthesiology*, vol. 106, no. 5, pp. 992–996, 2007.

[2] M. J. Barrington and R. Kluger, "Ultrasound guidance reduces the risk of local anesthetic systemic toxicity following peripheral nerve blockade," *Regional Anesthesia and Pain Medicine*, vol. 38, no. 4, pp. 289–297, 2013.

[3] S. Gili, A. Abreo, M. GóMez-Fernández, R. Solà, C. Morros, and X. Sala-Blanch, "Patterns of distribution of the nerves around the axillary artery evaluated by ultrasound and assessed by nerve stimulation during axillary block," *Clinical Anatomy*, vol. 32, no. 1, pp. 2–8, 2019.

[4] M. J. Fredrickson and D. H. Kilfoyle, "Neurological complication analysis of 1000 ultrasound guided peripheral nerve blocks for elective orthopaedic surgery: a prospective study," *Anaesthesia*, vol. 64, no. 8, pp. 836–844, 2009.

[5] T. C. Stan, M. A. Krantz, D. L. Solomon, J. G. Poulos, and K. Chaouki, "The incidence of neurovascular complications following axillary brachial plexus block using a transarterial approach. a prospective study of 1,000 consecutive patients," *Regional Anesthesia*, vol. 20, no. 6, pp. 486–492, 1995.

[6] L. E. Schroeder, T. T. Horlocker, and D. R. Schroeder, "The efficacy of axillary block for surgical procedures about the elbow," *Anesthesia & Analgesia*, vol. 83, no. 4, pp. 747–751, 1996.

[7] P. E. Bigeleisen, "Nerve puncture and apparent intraneural injection during ultrasound-guided axillary block does not invariably result in neurologic injury," *Anesthesiology*, vol. 105, no. 4, pp. 779–783, 2006.

[8] D. Selander, S. Edshage, and T. Wolff, "Paresthesiae or no paresthesiae? Nerve lesions after axillary blocks," *Acta Anaesthesiologica Scandinavica*, vol. 23, no. 1, pp. 27–33, 1979.

[9] E. E. Beheiry, "Anatomical variations of the median nerve distribution and communication in the arm," *Folia Morphologica*, vol. 63, no. 3, pp. 313–318, 2004.

[10] G. Retzl, S. Kapral, M. Greher, and W. Mauritz, "Ultrasonographic findings of the axillary part of the brachial plexus," *Anesthesia and Analgesia*, vol. 92, no. 5, pp. 1271–1275, 2001.

[11] C. F. Royse, S. Sha, P. F. Soeding, and A. G. Royse, "Anatomical study of the brachial plexus using surface ultrasound," *Anaesthesia and Intensive Care*, vol. 34, no. 2, pp. 203–210, 2006.

[12] D. B. Conceição, P. E. Helayel, and G. R. Oliveira Filho, "A comparative study between ultrasound and neurostimulation guided axillary brachial plexus block," *Rev Bras Anestesiol*, vol. 59, no. 5, pp. 585–591, 2009.

[13] V. W. S. Chan, A. Perlas, C. J. L. McCartney, R. Brull, D. Xu, and S. Abbas, "Ultrasound guidance improves success rate of axillary brachial plexus block," *Canadian Journal of Anesthesia/Journal Canadien D'anesthésie*, vol. 54, no. 3, pp. 176–182, 2007.

[14] S. R. Williams, P. Chouinard, G. V. Arcand et al., "Ultrasound guidance speeds execution and improves the quality of supraclavicular block," *Anesthesia & Analgesia*, vol. 97, no. 5, pp. 1518–1523, 2003.

[15] S. R. Lewis, A. Price, K. J. Walker, K. McGrattan, and A. F. Smith, "Ultrasound guidance for upper and lower limb blocks," *Cochrane Database Systematic Reviews*, vol. 11, no. 9, Article ID CD006459, 2015.

[16] P. F. Soeding, S. Sha, C. F. Royse, P. Marks, G. Hoy, and A. G. Royse, "A randomized trial of ultrasound-guided brachial plexus anaesthesia in upper limb surgery," *Anaesthesia and Intensive Care*, vol. 33, no. 6, pp. 719–725, 2005.

[17] A. Bhatia, J. Lai, V. W. Chan, and R. Brull, "Pneumothorax as a complication of the ultrasound-guided supraclavicular approach for brachial plexus block," *Anesthesia & Analgesia*, vol. 111, no. 3, pp. 817–819, 2010.

[18] J. M. Cohen and A. T. Gray, "Functional deficits after intraneural injection during interscalene block," *Regional Anesthesia and Pain Medicine*, vol. 35, no. 4, pp. 397–399, 2010.

[19] J. R. Soberón, J. W. Crookshank, B. D. Nossaman, C. E. Elliott, L. E. Sisco-Wise, and S. F. Duncan, "Distal peripheral nerve blocks in the forearm as an alternative to proximal brachial plexus blockade in patients undergoing hand surgery: a prospective and randomized pilot study," *The Journal of Hand Surgery*, vol. 41, no. 10, pp. 969–977, 2016.

[20] M. G. Fenten, K. P. Schoenmakers, P. J. Heesterbeek, G. J. Scheffer, and R. Stienstra, "Effect of local anesthetic concentration, dose and volume on the duration of single-injection ultrasound-guided axillary brachial plexus block with mepivacaine: a randomized controlled trial," *BMC Anesthesiol*, vol. 15, p. 130, 2015.

[21] S. Riazi, N. Carmichael, I. Awad, R. M. Holtby, and C. J. L. McCartney, "Effect of local anaesthetic volume (20 vs 5 ml) on the efficacy and respiratory consequences of ultrasound-guided interscalene brachial plexus block," *British Journal of Anaesthesia*, vol. 101, no. 4, pp. 549–556, 2008.

16

Correlation between Findings in Physical Examination, Magnetic Resonance Imaging and Nerve Conduction Studies in Lumbosacral Radiculopathy Caused by Lumbar Intervertebral Disc Herniation

Safa Yousif,[1] **Afraa Musa**,[1] **Ammar Ahmed**,[1] **and Ahmed Abdelhai**[2]

[1]*Department of Physiology, Faculty of Medicine, University of Khartoum, Khartoum, Sudan*
[2]*Department of Orthopaedics Surgery and Traumatology, Faculty of Medicine, University of Khartoum, Khartoum, Sudan*

Correspondence should be addressed to Safa Yousif; safaayousif27@yahoo.com

Academic Editor: Hiroshi Hashizume

Purpose. The aim of this study was to find out the correlation between magnetic resonance imaging (MRI) and nerve conduction studies' (NCS) findings in patients with lumbosacral radiculopathy caused by lumbar intervertebral disc herniation. In addition, the study aimed at finding the correlation between the clinical manifestations of lumbosacral radiculopathy and both MRI and NCS. *Patients and Methods.* The study was a cross-sectional analytic study which included thirty patients with a history suggestive of lumbosacral radiculopathy. Inclusion criteria were as follows: patients who had an MRI confirmed L4/5 and/or L5/S1 intervertebral disc prolapse in addition to one or more of the following (dermatomal distribution of symptoms appropriate with MRI level, presence of motor weakness, sensory impairment, absent ankle jerk, or positive straight leg raising test). All patients underwent clinical assessment and NCS, and their MRI examination was reviewed. The Chi-Squared/Fisher's exact test was used to test the correlation. *Results.* There was a statistically significant correlation between abnormal physical findings and nerve root compression in MRI. Statistically significant correlation was neither found between abnormal physical examination findings and abnormal NCS nor between nerve root compression in MRI and abnormal NCS findings. *Conclusion.* Abnormal neurological examination findings can be used to predict nerve root compression in MRI examination. On the contrary, positive findings of physical examination do not predict abnormal NCS, as well as negative findings do not exclude abnormal NCS; therefore, it is useful to add NCS when MRI findings do not match clinical examination findings or when no neuroimaging abnormalities can be identified.

1. Introduction

Lumbar disc herniation is a common cause of low back pain in the third and fourth decade of life. Usually, pain is brought on by repetitive twisting, bending, or heavy lifting, and it starts in the lower back and radiates to the buttock and posterior thigh. The radicular pain usually extends below the knee following the involved nerve root dermatome [1]. Lumbosacral radiculopathy due to disc herniation is defined as localized displacement of disc material beyond the normal margins of the intervertebral disc space resulting in pain, weakness, or numbness in a myotomal or dermatomal distribution [2]. Clinical manifestations of lumbosacral radiculopathy range from sensory symptoms (paresthesia) to motor weakness and sphincteric disturbance or even cauda equina syndrome.

Clinical assessment and imaging studies are used to evaluate the patient's symptoms, and magnetic resonance imaging (MRI), being the most diagnostic importance, is employed to identify the etiology and determine the level of the anatomical abnormality. The clinical significance of the MRI findings has been questioned, although being highly sensitive for identifying disc problems; not all of the identified lesions cause symptoms [3]. Neural foramen compromise and multiple disc lesions are the radiological findings that are most likely to cause clinical symptoms [4, 5]. In some patients, MRI findings do not coincide with clinical findings, or the lesion cannot be identified (e.g., far extraforaminal lesion); therefore, sometimes the need arises to use another test to reach the diagnosis.

Nerve conduction studies (NCS) are electrodiagnostic tests (EDX) used to evaluate peripheral nerve functions in patients with neuromuscular complaints and can be used to diagnose radiculopathy [6]. EDX are not regularly used in our practice to assess patients with clinical lumbosacral radiculopathy. When compared with MRI, nerve conduction studies assess the physiological integrity of the nerve function, while MRI identifies structural abnormalities. NCS cannot identify the exact etiology of impaired nerve root function (e.g., disc herniation and tumour), but in contrast to MRI, it can detect far extraforaminal lesions (e.g., piriform fossa syndrome). Anatomical abnormalities identified by MRI aids in surgical planning, while NCS can determine the severity of nerve root damage and can be used for post-operative follow-up [7].

We all agree that the clinical examination is the most important tool to assess the patients. Few studies were performed to test the correlation between clinical examination, nerve conduction studies, and magnetic resonance imaging findings in lumbosacral radiculopathy.

The objectives of our study were to find the correlation between magnetic resonance imaging findings and nerve conduction studies' findings and between each of the two tests (MRI and NCS) and the physical examination findings in patients with lumbosacral radiculopathy caused by lumbar intervertebral disc herniation.

2. Materials and Methods

2.1. Study Design and Study Sample. This was a cross-sectional analytic study. Sample size was calculated by a statistician using Chi-squared equation, and the results of study were conducted by Soltani et al. in 2014 [8]. Sample technique used was a convenient sample. Two study groups were included: patients and control group. Subjects of the control group were selected from volunteers among workers and students of Faculty of Medicine of Khartoum University. Patients were selected from referred clinics (Ibrahim Malik Teaching Hospital-referred clinic and Ribat University Hospital-referred clinic) and specialized clinic (Mr. Ahmed Abdelhai clinic in Royal Scan diagnostic center) in Khartoum city.

2.2. Participants

2.2.1. Patients Group. Thirty patients presented with a history suggestive of lumbosacral radiculopathy were included.

2.2.2. Inclusion Criteria

(1) Patients who had an MRI confirmed L4/5 and/or L5/S1 intervertebral disc prolapse

(2) In addition to one or more of the following:

  (a) Dermatomal distribution of symptoms appropriate with MRI level
  (b) Presence of motor weakness
  (c) Sensory impairment
  (d) Absent ankle jerk
  (e) Positive straight leg raising test.

2.2.3. Exclusion Criteria

(1) A history suggestive of polyneuropathy (e.g., diabetes)

(2) Radiculopathy due to other pathology (e.g., tumour and instability)

(3) Previous spinal surgery

2.2.4. Control Group. In order to obtain reference values for the NCS parameters, a control group was included and composed of twenty-five healthy volunteers with no history of radiculopathy, neuromuscular problems, or risk factors for having impaired nerve function besides normal neurological examination.

2.3. Data Collection Tools. Data collection was carried out from July to November, 2016. All patients underwent clinical assessment; their MRI films and reports were reviewed, and nerve conduction studies were performed at the Physiology department in the Faculty of Medicine of Khartoum University.

Clinical assessment included history taking and examination carried out by the principal investigator. The history included duration of symptoms, side affected, dermatomal distribution of symptoms, history of weakness or sphincteric disturbance, and previously received treatment. Symptoms considered to arise from L5 nerve root (L5 dermatomal distribution), if pain or numbness described by the patient radiates to the anterolateral leg, dorsum of the foot, or the great toe. S1 nerve root involvement is considered (S1 dermatomal distribution), if pain or numbness described by the patient radiates to the lateral malleolus, lateral, and planter surface of the foot or the heel. Physical examination included observation of the patient's gait, examination of lower limb tone and power, ankle jerk, pin prick sensation, and straight leg raising test.

All patients' MRI lumbosacral spine films (sagittal and axial T1- and T2-weighted sequences) were reported by a radiologist blinded to physical examination findings. MRI reports were used by the principal investigator to obtain the following information: the level of the involved intervertebral discs, extent, and localization of the disc prolapse, presence of nerve root compression, and neural canal compromise. Demographic data, history, clinical examination, and MRI findings were entered into special questionnaire.

Nerve conduction studies were performed by the principal investigator using the Digital Medelec Synergy machine and reviewed by a neurophysiologist blinded to the physical examination findings. Both lower limbs in all subjects were examined, and the tests performed include motor nerve conduction study of the tibial and common peroneal nerves. Tibial nerve compound motor action potential (CMAP) was recorded from abductor halluces muscle, two stimulation sites used: the distal one was posterior to the medial malleolus 10 cm proximal the recording electrode and a proximal stimulation site at the middle of the popliteal crease. Peroneal nerve CMAP was recorded from extensor digitorum brevis, and two stimulation sites were used: the distal one in dorsal lower leg between the tendons of tibialis anterior and extensor hallucis longus 9 cm proximal to active recording electrode and a proximal stimulation site about 3-4 cm distal to the proximal tip of fibular head. F-wave latencies of both nerves were recorded, using electrodes placement similar to that of motor studies. Ten subsequent stimuli were applied to the distal stimulation site, and F-waves recorded for latency measurements were the F-minimum, F-maximum, and F-mean latencies. H-reflex latency of the tibial nerve was recorded, posterior tibial nerve was stimulated in the centre of the popliteal crease and recorded over the soleus muscle, and the shortest latency recorded was the parameter studied. In addition, sensory nerve conduction study of the sural nerve was carried out to exclude patients with polyneuropathy. Machine setting for each test is illustrated in Table 1.

Table 1: Machine setting for nerve conduction studies.

Setting	Sweep velocity (msec/division)	Sensitivity (μv/division)	Filters high/low (kHz/Hz)	Stimulator duration/rate (msec/Hz)
Motor NCS	2	5000	10 kHz/2 Hz	0.2 msec/1 Hz
Sensory NCS	1	10	2 kHz/20 Hz	0.1 msec/2 Hz
H-reflex	10	500	10 kHz/20 Hz	1 msec/0.5 Hz
F-wave	10	500	10 kHz/20 Hz	0.2 msec/1 Hz

Table 2: Frequency of physical examination findings (number of patients: 30).

Positive sign	Number of cases
Antalgic gait	8 (26.7%)
Listing gait	7 (23.3%)
Weakness	0
Ankle jerk	9 (30%)
Impaired sensation	16 (53.3%)
Positive straight leg raising test	18 (60%)

2.4. Analysis. Data analysis was carried out using Statistical Package for the Social Sciences (IBM SPSS) version 20 software. Descriptive statistics presented as mean and standard deviation for continuous variables and frequencies for categorical variables. Association between physical examination findings, NCS findings, and MRI findings were examined by Chi-Squared/Fisher's exact test. *P* value ˂0.05 was considered significant. Nerve root compression on MRI was considered as radiological evidence of radiculopathy. Reduced amplitude or conduction velocity of compound motor action potential, prolonged mean F-wave latency, and prolonged H-reflex latency were considered NCS findings suggestive of radiculopathy.

3. Results

The total number of patients included in the study was 30, with a mean age of 41.07 ± 11.47 years, 70% were males, and 30% were females. The number of healthy subjects was 25, with a mean age of 37.24 ± 10.4 years, 60% were males, and 40% were females.

3.1. Clinical Assessment. The mean duration of patients' symptoms was 21.47 ± 26 months, 60% of the patients have symptoms for more than 6 months. The left limb was involved in two-third (66.7%) of patients, right limb in 26.7%, while bilateral involvement occurred in 6.7% only. L5 dermatomal distribution of parasthesia was encountered in 40% of patients compared with 56.7% patients with S1 dermatomal distribution, while 3.3% only showed involvement of both dermatomes. Physical examination findings are demonstrated in Table 2.

3.2. MRI. MRI of 9 (30%) patients showed isolated L4/5 disc involvement, 7 (23.3%) showed isolated L5/S1 disc involvement, while 14 (46.7%) showed both L4/5 and L5/S1 disc level involvement. Distribution of the MRI findings among the patient group is shown in Table 3.

3.3. NCS. Concerning the compound motor action potential (CMAP) parameters, 6 (20%) patients showed reduced amplitude of the common peroneal nerve, and 3 (10%) patients showed reduced velocity. Reduced amplitude of the tibial nerve was detected in 2 (6.7%) patients, while 5 (16.7%) patients showed reduced velocity. Study of the F-wave of the common peroneal nerve showed prolonged mean latency of the symptomatic side in 6 (20%) patients. The mean latency of the F-wave of the tibial nerve was prolonged in 3 (10%) of the symptomatic sides. The most prevalent abnormality prolonged H-reflex latency which was detected in 12 (40%) of the studied patients.

3.4. Correlation Tests. There was statistically significant association between L5 dermatomal distribution of symptoms and L4/5 nerve root compression on MRI, and also statistically significant association was found between L5/S1 nerve root compression and S1 dermatomal distribution of symptoms ($P < 0.05$). The test of the correlation between abnormal physical findings and MRI detected nerve root compression revealed statistically significant association ($P < 0.05$) as presented in Table 4. Statistically significant association was neither found between abnormal NCS and abnormal physical examination nor between abnormal NCS findings and the presence of nerve root compression in MRI ($P < 0.05$) as shown in Tables 5 and 6, respectively. Sensitivity, specificity, and positive and negative predictive values

Table 3: Frequency of MRI findings (number of patients: 30).

	L4/5 Number of levels = 23	L5/S1 Number of levels = 21
Axial localization *n* (%)	Diffuse: 9 (39.1%) Central disc: 7 (30.4%) Paracentral disc: 7 (30.40%)	Diffuse: 7 (33.3%) Central disc: 2 (9.5%) Paracentral: 12 (57.1%)
Extent *n* (%)	Herniation: 15 (65.2%) Migration: 1 (4.3%) Bulge: 7 (30.4%)	Herniation: 14 (66.7%) Migration: 2 (9.5%) Bulge: 5 (23.8%)
Nerve root compression *n* (%)	Left side: 9 (39.1%) Right side: 3 (13.04%) Bilateral: 3 (13.04%)	Left side: 7 (33.3%) Right side: 1 (4.7%) Bilateral: 5 (23.8%)
Central canal stenosis *n* (%)	10 (43.4%)	4 (19%)
Ligamentum flavum hypertrophy/facet joint arthropathy *n* (%)	2 (8.7%)	2 (9.5%)

Table 4: Association between abnormal physical examination and nerve root compression in MRI.

Physical examination	Nerve root compression in MRI			
	No compression	Compression	Total	*P* value
Normal	4 (13.3%)*	3 (10%)*	7	
Abnormal	3 (10%)*	20 (66.7%)*	23	0.033
Total	7	23	30	

*Percent calculated from the total number of patients.

Table 5: Association between abnormal physical examination and abnormal NCS.

Physical examination	NCS			
	Normal	Abnormal	Total	*P* value
Normal	2 (6.7%)*	5 (16.7%)*	7	
Abnormal	6 (20%)*	17 (56.7%)*	23	1.00
Total	8	22	30	

*Percent calculated from the total number of patients.

Table 6: Association between nerve root compression in MRI and abnormal NCSs.

Nerve root compression in MRI	NCSs			
	Normal	Abnormal	Total	*P* value
No compression	1 (3.3%)*	6 (20%)*	7	
Compression	7 (23.3%)*	16 (53.3%)*	23	0.638
Total	8	22	30	

*Percent calculated from the total number of patients.

of MRI and NCS in relation to physical examination findings are shown in Table 7.

4. Discussion

Magnetic resonance imaging is a sensitive tool in detecting structural lesion, while nerve conduction studies evaluate physiological changes in the nerve function. We conducted our study to find out the correlation between MRI findings and NCS findings in patients with clinical lumbosacral radiculopathy as well as their relation to the physical examination findings.

In our study, any degree of nerve root compression was considered as radiological findings of radiculopathy. There was no statistically significant association between abnormal physical examination findings (abnormal gait, absent ankle jerk, impaired sensation, and positive SLR test) and nerve root compression in MRI similar to previous studies [5, 8]. This would suggest that abnormal physical examination findings can predict nerve root compression in MRI. Soltani et al. conducted a study in 2014, and their results revealed a significant agreement between the clinical findings and relevant MRI; the results also showed that MRI had higher abnormalities than EDX in clinically irrelevant levels [8]. In our study, abnormal physical examination findings associated with the presence of nerve root compression is detected in 66.6% of patients (20 from total 30), compared with 71% and 58.6% in two previous studies [8, 9].

Prolonged H-reflex latency was the commonest encountered abnormality in NCS followed by prolonged F-wave latency. Other abnormalities detected include reduced amplitude and reduced conduction velocity. No statistically significant association was detected in the current study between physical examination and NCS findings; consequently, the physical examination is not a good predictor of abnormal nerve conduction studies. This agrees with the findings of many previous studies [10–13]. Our study results showed that 56.7% of patients had abnormal findings in physical examination as well as nerve conduction studies, compared with 58% and 89.5% in two previous studies [8, 9]. Electromyography (EMG) was used in conjunction with NCS to evaluate patients, and this might explain their higher figures. Lauder et al. concluded from their study that having at least one abnormal physical examination finding makes the probability of having an abnormal electrodiagnostic study more likely; however, having normal physical examination does not rule out the probability of finding abnormal EDX [11].

The current study failed to show a statistically significant correlation between MRI and NCS findings, and this corresponds with the findings of Soltani et al.'s study [8]. This can be explained by the fact that MRI concerned mainly with

TABLE 7: Sensitivity, specificity, and positive and negative predictive values of MRI and NCS in relation to physical examination findings.

Study	Sensitivity (%)	Specificity (%)	Positive predictive value (%)	Negative predictive value (%)
MRI	87.0	57.1	86.9	57.1
NCS	65.2	28.6	75	20

structural abnormalities, while NCS reflects the physiological integrity of the studied nerves [14]. Soltani et al. concluded from their study that MRI and EDX are complementary in general, and it is reasonable to add EDX when there is disagreement between MRI and clinical findings or when MRI neurologic findings are not detectable [8]. The current study showed that NCS has lower specificity compared with MRI in relation to the physical examination findings in contrast to previous studies [8, 9, 15]; this can be explained by inclusion of EMG in addition to NCS in the previous studies. MRI showed higher sensitivity compared with NCS, and this correlates with the findings of many previous studies [8, 9, 15]. The lower sensitivity and specificity of the NCS coincide with the findings of the correlation test (the presence or absence of positive findings in the physical examination does not predict positive or negative findings in the NCS). The lack of gold standard test to diagnose radiculopathy is one of limitation to the comparison between MRI and NCS diagnostic tests.

Our study supports the current practice of considering MRI as the gold standard investigation in diagnosing and detecting the cause of clinical radiculopathy, being very sensitive in detecting structural abnormalities and correlates with clinical findings. On the contrary, using NCS as an assessment tool has several limitations: one limitation is being not widely available in our settings and the other limitation is that specific root affected is difficult to be localized (each muscle supplied by several roots); adding EMG of lower limbs and paraspinal muscle would help to increase the specificity and determination of the specific root affected. Nevertheless, NCS has several advantages; the EDX is the only laboratory examination that directly assesses the physiologic integrity of the nerve root. In addition, EDX can identify changes when physical examinations are normal or inconclusive [16]. In certain cases, when neuroimaging studies cannot identify certain pathology, EDX may be abnormal (for example, patients with noncompressive radiculopathy) [16]. Another advantage is that imaging study cannot define the severity of axon loss; therefore, it cannot determine the prognosis in contrast to EDX [17]. Finally, nerve conduction studies are noninvasive tests and can be used to follow patients' progression over time or after operations [17, 18].

5. Conclusion

We can conclude from our study that abnormal neurological examination findings can be used to predict nerve root compression in MRI. On the contrary, positive findings of physical examination do not predict abnormal NCS, as well as negative findings do not exclude abnormal NCS. Furthermore, it is useful to add nerve conduction studies examination when clinical examination findings do not match MRI study findings or structural abnormalities cannot be identified by neuroimaging.

Consent

Informed written consent was obtained from all participants included in the study.

References

[1] S. T. Canale and J. H. Beaty, *Campbell's Operative Othopaedics*, Elsevier Health Sciences, Amsterdam, Netherlands, 12th edition, 2013.

[2] D. S. Kreiner, S. W. Hwang, J. E. Easa et al., "An evidence-based clinical guideline for the diagnosis and treatment of lumbar disc herniation with radiculopathy," *The Spine Journal*, vol. 14, no. 1, pp. 180–191, 2014.

[3] M. C. Jensen, M. N. Brant-Zawadzki, N. Obuchowski, M. T. Modic, D. Malkasian, and J. S. Ross, "Magnetic resonance imaging of the lumbar spine in people without back pain," *New England Journal of Medicine*, vol. 331, no. 2, pp. 69–73, 1994.

[4] D. G. Borenstein, J. W. O'Mara, S. D. Boden et al., "The value of magnetic resonance imaging of the lumbar spine to predict low-back pain in asymptomatic subjects," *The Journal of Bone and Joint Surgery-American Volume*, vol. 83, no. 9, pp. 1306–1311, 2001.

[5] A. Janardhana, S. R. Rajagopal, S. Rao, and A. Kamath, "Correlation between clinical features and magnetic resonance imaging findings in lumbar disc prolapse," *Indian Journal of Orthopaedics*, vol. 44, no. 3, pp. 263–269, 2010.

[6] H. Matsui, M. Kanamori, Y. Kawaguchi, H. Kitagawa, H. Nakamura, and H. Tsuji, "Clinical and electrophysiologic characteristics of compressed lumbar nerve roots," *Spine*, vol. 22, no. 18, pp. 2100–2105, 1997.

[7] M. Wojtysiak, J. Huber, A. Wiertel-Krawczuk, A. Szymankiewicz-Szukała, J. Moskal, and J. Janicki, "Pre- and postoperative evaluation of patients with lumbosacral disc herniation by neurophysiological and clinical assessment," *Spine*, vol. 39, no. 21, pp. 1792–1800, 2014.

[8] Z. R. Soltani, S. Sajadi, and B. Tavana, "A comparison of magnetic resonance imaging with electrodiagnostic findings in the evaluation of clinical radiculopathy: a cross-sectional study," *European Spine Journal*, vol. 23, no. 4, pp. 916–921, 2014.

[9] E. G. Hasankhani and F. Omidi-Kashani, "Magnetic resonance imaging versus electrophysiologic tests in clinical diagnosis of lower extremity radicular pain," *ISRN Neuroscience*, vol. 2013, Article ID 952570, 4 pages, 2013.

[10] T. D. Lauder, T. R. Dillingham, M. Andary et al., "Effect of history and exam in predicting electrodiagnostic outcome among patients with suspected lumbosacral radiculopathy," *American Journal of Physical Medicine & Rehabilitation*, vol. 79, no. 1, pp. 60–68, 2000.

[11] T. D. Lauder, "Physical examination signs, clinical symptoms,

and their relationship to electrodiagnostic findings and the presence of radiculopathy," *Physical Medicine and Rehabilitation Clinics of North America*, vol. 13, no. 3, pp. 451–467, 2002.

[12] S. Nafissi, S. Niknam, and S. S. Hosseini, "Electrophysiological evaluation in lumbosacral radiculopathy," *Iranian Journal of Neurology*, vol. 11, no. 3, pp. 83–86, 2012.

[13] E. E. İnal, F. Eser, L. A. Aktekin, E. Öksüz, and H. Bodur, "Comparison of clinical and electrophysiological findings in patients with suspected radiculopathies," *Journal of Back and Musculoskeletal Rehabilitation*, vol. 26, no. 2, pp. 169–173, 2013.

[14] R. A. Nardin, M. R. Patel, T. F. Gudas, S. B. Rutkove, and E. M. Raynor, "Electromyography and magnetic resonance imaging in the evaluation of radiculopathy," *Muscle & Nerve*, vol. 22, no. 2, pp. 151–155, 1999.

[15] J. Lee and S. Lee, "Physical examination, magnetic resonance image, and electrodiagnostic study in patients with lumbosacral disc herniation or spinal stenosis," *Journal of Rehabilitation Medicine*, vol. 44, no. 10, pp. 845–850, 2012.

[16] M. J. Albeck, G. Taher, M. Lauritzen, and W. Trojaborg, "Diagnostic value of electrophysiological tests in patients with sciatica," *Acta Neurologica Scandinavica*, vol. 101, no. 4, pp. 249–254, 2000.

[17] A. J. Wilbourn and M. J. Aminoff, "AAEM minimonograph 32: the electrodiagnostic examination in patients with radiculopathies," *Muscle & Nerve*, vol. 21, no. 12, pp. 1612–1631, 1998.

[18] M. Toyokura, A. Ishida, and K. Murakami, "Follow-up study on F-wave in patients with lumbosacral radiculopathy. Comparison between before and after surgery," *Electromyography and Clinical Neurophysiology*, vol. 36, no. 4, pp. 207–214, 1996.

17

Effects of Knee Osteoarthritis on Hip and Ankle Gait Mechanics

Du Hyun Ro, Joonhee Lee, Jangyun Lee, Jae-Young Park, Hyuk-Soo Han, and Myung Chul Lee

Department of Orthopaedic Surgery, Seoul National University College of Medicine, Seoul, Republic of Korea

Correspondence should be addressed to Myung Chul Lee; leemc@snu.ac.kr

Guest Editor: Yasushi Oshima

Introduction. Knee osteoarthritis (OA) can affect the hip and ankle joints, as these three joints operate as a kinetic/kinematic chain while walking. *Purpose.* This study was performed to compare (1) hip and ankle joint gait mechanics between knee OA and control groups and (2) to investigate the effects of knee gait mechanics on the ipsilateral hip and ankle joint. *Methods.* The study group included 89 patients with end-stage knee OA and 42 age- and sex-matched controls without knee pain or OA. Kinetic and kinematic parameters were evaluated using a commercial optoelectric gait analysis system. Range of motion (ROM) during gait, coronal motion arc, and peak joint moment of hip, knee, and ankle joints were investigated. *Results.* Ankle varus moment was 50% higher in the OA group ($p=0.005$) and was associated with higher knee adduction moment ($p<0.001$). The ROM of the hip and ankle joints were significantly smaller in the OA group and were associated with limited ROM of the knee joint (both $p<0.001$). The coronal motion arc of the hip was smaller in the OA group and was also associated with limited motion arc of the knee ($p<0.001$). *Conclusions.* Knee OA has a negative effect on the ROM, coronal motion arc, and joint moment of the ankle joint and hip joint. As knee OA is associated with increased moment of the ankle joint, attention should be paid to the ankle joint when treating patients with knee OA.

1. Introduction

Knee osteoarthritis (OA) is a leading cause of disability in the elderly population [1]. More than 250 million people suffer from knee OA worldwide, and 1%–2% of the gross national product is spent on OA [2, 3]. Knee OA causes pain and gait disturbances and has a characteristic gait pattern [4, 5].

Knee OA patients have reduced range of motion (ROM) and increased ground reaction force [4, 5]. Stride length and walking speed are decreased in OA [6]. Patients attempt to reduce pain by minimizing the impact on their knees [4, 5]. The gait of knee OA patients is also characterized by higher knee adduction moment (KAM), a marker of medial joint loading and known risk factor for progression of arthritis [7–9]. Such gait changes in knee OA can directly or indirectly affect adjacent weight-bearing joints, i.e., the hip and ankle joints [10–12].

In fact, we often encounter knee OA patients with ankle and hip joint pathology. The joint line orientation angle of the ankle changes and hip arthritis is often observed on X-ray examination [13]. Epidemiological studies also showed that significant numbers of patients have pathologies in more than two of the three weight-bearing joints, which may indicate that problems with one joint are biomechanically related to problems in the others [14, 15]. Many studies have focused on the gait mechanics of the knee in patients with knee arthritis. However, few studies have examined secondary gait changes in adjacent joints, i.e., the hip and ankle joints [10–12]. Theoretically, gait changes in the knee joint can cause gait changes in the hip and ankle joints, as these three joints operate as a kinetic/kinematic chain while walking. Investigation of secondary biomechanical changes in the ankle and hip joints in knee OA patients will provide a better understanding of the gait mechanics of knee OA patients.

In this study, we hypothesized that the gait mechanics of the knee joint would differ between the knee OA group and controls without knee OA, which would have different effects on the hip and ankle joints. This study was performed to compare (1) hip and ankle joint gait mechanics between knee

Table 1: Characteristics of knee OA and control groups.

	Knee OA group (n=89) Mean (SD)	Control group (n=42) Mean (SD)	p-value
Age, yr	65.8 (5.5)	64.5 (2.9)	0.224
Height, cm	151.7 (5.4)	153.7 (5.2)	0.304
Weight, kg	61 (8.6)	58.2 (7.2)	0.004
Body mass index, kg/m2	26.5 (3.5)	24.6 (2.9)	0.002
HKA axis (right side)	5.9 (3.8)	1.7 (1.8)	<0.001
Gait speed (cm/s)	88.7 (17.5)	111.2 (8.4)	<0.001
Stride length (cm)	97.9 (13.7)	115.7 (7)	<0.001
Step width (cm)	10.3 (3.2)	8.5 (1.8)	<0.001

SD: standard deviation, HKA axis: hip-knee-ankle mechanical axis

OA patients and controls and (2) to investigate the effects of knee gait mechanics on the ipsilateral hip and ankle joints.

2. Methods

2.1. Study Subjects. This study was approved by our Institutional Review Board. We retrospectively reviewed 143 patients with three-compartment end-stage OA. End-stage OA was defined as Kellgren–Lawrence (KL) grade 4 in anteroposterior (AP) and lateral knee radiography. We excluded 31 subjects according to the following criteria: (1) aged > 75 or < 55 years ($n = 26$); (2) spine disease, hip or ankle arthritis (KL grade > 2) on X-ray ($n = 15$); (3) male gender (n = 5); (4) inflammatory or traumatic arthritis of the knee ($n = 4$); or (5) any prior bone surgery in the lower extremities ($n = 4$). Consequently, 89 patients with end-stage knee OA were included in the final analysis. The study population had a mean age of 65.8 years, mean height of 151.7 cm, and mean weight of 61.0 kg (Table 1).

The control group consisted of a total of 42 asymptomatic sex- and age-matched volunteers. Gait analysis and X-ray evaluation were performed after receiving informed consent. None of the volunteers experienced concurrent knee pain, had a diagnosis of knee OA, or violated any other exclusion criterion. The controls had a mean age of 64.5 years, mean height of 153.7 cm, and mean weight of 58.2 kg (Table 1).

2.2. Gait Analysis Protocol. Gait data were collected from the Human Motion Analysis Lab at our institution. Participants were asked to perform an gentle 5-minute walk to warm up. After warming up, reflective markers were placed on the subjects [16], and they were asked to walk at a self-selected speed along a 9-m track.

Motion (kinematic) data were acquired at a sample rate of 120 Hz using 12 charge-coupled device cameras equipped with a three-dimensional optical motion capture system (Motion Analysis, Santa Rosa, CA, USA). Ground reaction force (kinetic) data were acquired at a sampling rate of 1,200 Hz using three AMTI (Advanced Mechanical Technology Inc., Watertown, MA, USA) force plates. The kinetic data were then normalized by height and weight (% body weight × height) [17].

We used Eva Real-Time software (Motion Analysis), Microsoft Excel 2016 (Microsoft Corp., Redmond, WA, USA), and MATLAB R2017a (MathWorks, Natick, MA, USA) for real-time motion capture, postprocessing, and marker data tracking. The average of three representative strides from five or six separate trials was used for the analysis of each session. Data for the right side of participants were used in the analysis.

Spatiotemporal data are shown in Table 1. The kinematic parameters investigated were the range of motion (ROM) of the hip, knee, and ankle joints, and the coronal motion arcs of the knee and hip joints. Coronal motion arc was defined as the difference in angle between the maximum valgus (or adduction) angle and the maximum varus (or abduction) angle during a stance phase. For kinetics, the peak moments of the sagittal and coronal planes were evaluated. The sagittal plane moment included internal knee extension moment, hip extension/flexion moment, and ankle plantar flexion moment, and the coronal plane moment included the KAM, hip abduction moment, and ankle varus moment.

2.3. Radiological Measurement. Radiographic evaluations were performed independently by two authors (both trained in arthroplasty) blinded to other patient information. The interobserver reliability of the radiological assessments was satisfactory (intraclass correlation coefficient, 0.87–0.93). The average values measured by the two observers were used in the analysis. Mechanical axis (hip-knee-ankle axis) was measured using standing full-limb radiography. All radiographic images were digitally acquired using a picture archiving and communication system (PACS) (Maroview 5.4; Infinitt, Seoul, Republic of Korea), and assessments were performed using the PACS software.

2.4. Statistical Analysis. Kinetic and kinematic variables were compared using independent Student's t test. The normality of the data was assessed using the Kolmogorov–Smirnov test. Correlations were assessed using Pearson's correlation coefficient. The partial correlation coefficient was calculated to control the effect of gait speed on ROM. For all analyses, $p<0.05$ was taken to indicate statistical significance. Statistical analyses were performed using SPSS® for Windows (ver. 19.0.1; SPSS Inc., Chicago, IL, USA).

TABLE 2: Range of motion and coronal motion arc of each joint.

		Knee OA group (n=89) Mean	Control group (n=42) Mean	p-value
Range of motion (°)	Knee	51	63	<0.001
	Hip	43	48	<0.001
	Ankle	26	28	0.004
Coronal motion arc (°)	Knee	4	9	<0.001
	Hip	8	12	<0.001

TABLE 3: Mean peak moment of each joint.

		Knee OA group (n=89) Mean (SD)	Control group (n=42) Mean (SD)	p-value
Sagittal	Knee extension	2.44 (1.16)	3.38 (1.03)	<0.001
	Hip flexion/extension	6.41 (1.19)	6.94 (0.89)	0.010
	Ankle plantar flexion	7.1 (1.15)	7.64 (0.61)	0.005
	Total sagittal moment	15.94 (2.43)	17.97 (1.59)	<0.001
Coronal	Knee adduction	3.27 (0.92)	2.76 (0.65)	0.002
	Hip abduction	4.93 (0.83)	5.34 (0.54)	0.005
	Ankle varus	0.69 (0.44)	0.46 (0.36)	0.005
	Total coronal moment	8.89 (1.58)	8.56 (1.13)	0.239

The unit of moment is %Bw∗Ht. SD: standard deviation

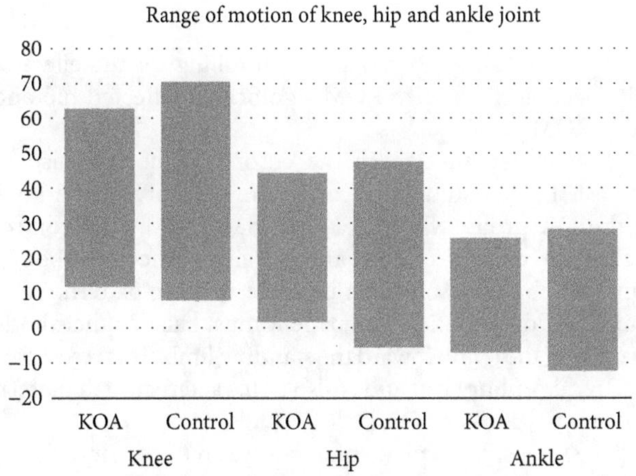

FIGURE 1: *Range of motion (ROM) of the knee, hip, and ankle joint.* The knee OA (KOA) group showed smaller ROM than the control group. In the knee joint, a negative value indicates hyperextension. In the hip joint, a negative value indicates extension. In the ankle joint, a negative value indicates plantar flexion.

3. Results

The hip and ankle ROM were significantly smaller in the OA group than the control group (Table 2, Figure 1). Knee ROM was also smaller in the OA group (p<0.001), and it was correlated with hip and ankle ROM (both p<0.001, Figure 2). Controlling the effect on gait speed did not change the fact that knee ROM affected hip and ankle ROM (both p<0.001); smaller knee ROM was associated with smaller hip ROM and angle (r^2 = 0.71–0.42).

The coronal motion arcs of the hip and knee were also smaller in the OA group than the control group (all p<0.001, Figure 3). The coronal motion arc of the knee joint was also correlated with that of the hip joint (r^2 = 0.36, p<0.001).

The sagittal moments of the hip and ankle were smaller in the OA group compared to the controls (Table 3). Sagittal knee moment was also smaller in the OA group than the control group (p<0.001).

The coronal moment of the hip was smaller, but the coronal moment of the ankle joint was higher, in the OA group compared to the control group (both p=0.005). The ankle varus moment was 50% higher in the OA group than the control group. KAM was also higher in the OA group than the controls (p<0.001). The coronal knee moment (KAM) was correlated with those of the hip (r^2 = 0.19, p=0.032) and ankle joints (r^2 = 0.32, p<0.001). Total sagittal moment was smaller in the knee OA group than the control group (p<0.001). However, total coronal moment was similar between the two groups (p=0.239).

4. Discussion

The results of this study showed that changes in gait mechanics in the knee joint have a strong effect on the ROM, coronal motion arc, and joint moment of the ankle and hip joints. ROM and sagittal moment were significantly limited and gait became stiffer in patients with OA. Interestingly, ankle varus moment was 50% higher and associated with an increase of KAM. Such changes are important as they can be risk factors for the subsequent development of secondary arthritis and result in increased pain [10, 13, 18]. Limited ROM of the lower extremities can cause joint stiffness and may result in significant disability [19]. Clinicians should keep these points in mind when planning treatments or in educating knee OA patients. In our knee OA patients, the ROM of the knee

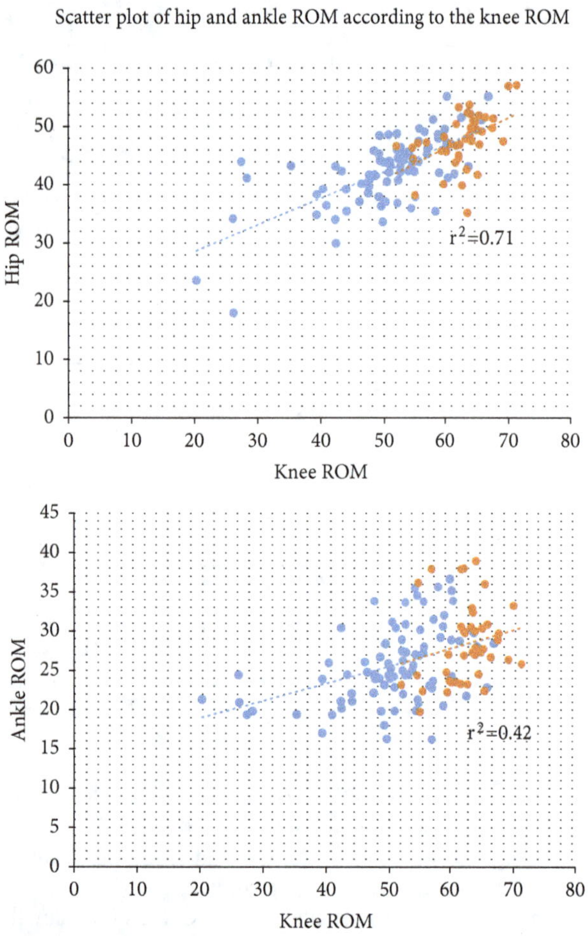

FIGURE 2: *Correlation between knee ROM and hip and ankle ROM.* Strong correlations were observed between knee ROM and the hip and ankle ROM. Blue dots indicate the knee OA group. Orange dots indicate the control group. Dotted lines indicate the trend lines. r^2: Pearson correlation coefficient.

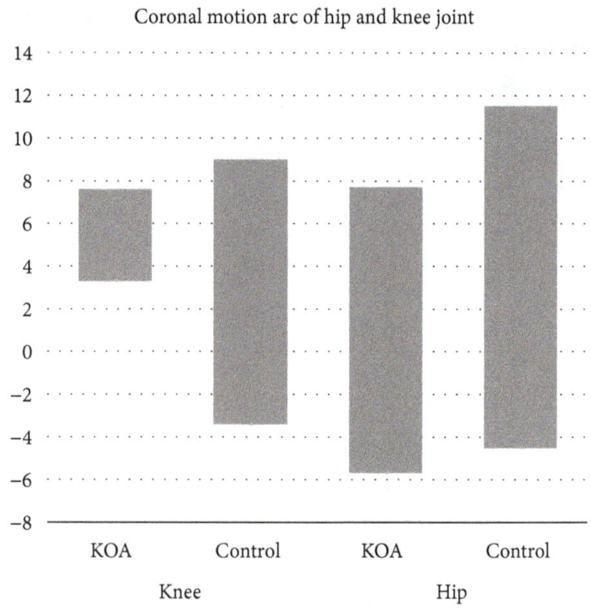

FIGURE 3: *Coronal motion arcs of the hip and knee joints.* The KOA group showed smaller coronal motion arcs compared to the control group. Negative values indicate valgus and abduction in the knee and hip joints, respectively. There was a significant correlation between the hip and knee joints.

was reduced in both the sagittal and coronal planes and was associated with limited ROM of the hip and ankle joints. The mean knee ROM in the OA group was 51°, which was 19% smaller than the knee ROM of 63° in the control group. This reduced the ROM of the hip and ankle joints by 10.4% and 7.1%, respectively. In the clinic, knee OA patients are often seen to walk with bending and stiffness of the hip, knee, and ankle joints. In particular, the extension angle of the hip joint was about 5° in the control group, but there was 2° of flexion contracture in knee OA patients, and these patients have a bent posture. This pattern was reported previously in knee OA patients [19]. Steultjens et al. measured the ROM using a goniometer and reported close relations between the ROM of the hip and knee joint [19]. Our observations were consistent with their results, and we showed that the relationship still exists during gait. As gait is coordinated by work of the muscle and joint, flexion contracture can cause constant contraction of the quadriceps femoris [20]. Thus, knee OA patients will suffer from pain as well as increased quadriceps load during gait [20]. The gait speed can also be reduced by limited ROM of each joint, similar to that in patients with total knee arthroplasty [6]. However, after controlling for the effect of gait speed, limited knee ROM significantly affected hip and ankle ROM.

The limited motion in the coronal plane was also of interest. In this study, the coronal motion arc of the knee in the OA group was 55.6% less than that in the control group. The coronal motion arc was also reduced in the hip joint, which can result in an unstable walking pattern. With limited coronal motion, the patient must balance their body by moving the trunk toward the standing limb. This resembles the Trendelenburg gait and is also a characteristic gait pattern of patients with knee OA [21].

The total sagittal plane moment was reduced in the knee OA group. As the sagittal moment is related to gait speed, it may be related to the slow gait speed of knee OA patients [6]. In contrast, the coronal moment was higher in the knee and ankle joints. Increased KAM has been described in knee OA patients in the literature; it is associated with increased medial joint loading and is a surrogate marker for future progression of arthritis [18]. However, it is interesting that ankle varus moment was increased and associated with KAM. Ankle varus moment was 50% higher in the knee OA group compared to the control group. This can be a risk factor for future progression of arthritis [10, 13, 18]. In fact, we often encounter ankle subluxation in patients with knee OA, and further studies are needed regarding this issue.

This study had some limitations. First, no definitive conclusions on causality can be drawn because of the cross-sectional nature of the study design. A further prospective longitudinal study is warranted to determine the nature of the bidirectional relationship. However, this problem was minimized in this study by excluding patients with KL grade

3 or higher arthritis of the hip and ankle joints. In fact, the incidence rates of hip and ankle joint arthritis are not as high as that for the knee joint, and there is no evidence that hip and ankle arthritis precede knee OA [15]. Therefore, knee OA was thought to influence the mechanics of the hip and ankle joints. Second, generalizability could be limited only to female patients, where this study excluded male patients as there is a significant difference in gait between males and females [22]. However, as only the KAM showed gender differences and there were no differences in joint range of motion or hip angle joint moment, generalization should also be possible to male patients.

5. Conclusions

Knee OA has a negative effect on the ROM, coronal motion arc, and joint moment of the ankle joint and hip joint. As knee OA is associated with increased moment of the ankle joint, attention should be paid to the ankle joint when treating patients with knee OA.

Authors' Contributions

Du Hyun Ro was responsible for design, data acquisition, data interpretation, and manuscript drafting. Joonhee Lee performed data acquisition, analysis, and manuscript drafting. Jangyun Lee and Jae-Young Park contributed to data acquisition, analysis, and interpretation. Hyuk-Soo Han made data acquisition and data interpretation. Myung Chul Lee was responsible for design, data acquisition, data interpretation, and manuscript revision.

References

[1] T. Neogi, "The epidemiology and impact of pain in osteoarthritis," *Osteoarthritis and Cartilage*, vol. 21, no. 9, pp. 1145–1153, 2013.

[2] T. Vos, R. M. Barber, and B. Bell, "Global, regional, and national incidence, prevalence, and years lived with disability for 301 acute and chronic diseases and injuries in 188 countries, 1990–2013: a systematic analysis for the Global Burden of Disease Study 2013," *The Lancet*, vol. 386, no. 9995, pp. 743–800, 2013.

[3] L. Murphy and C. G. Helmick, "The impact of osteoarthritis in the United States: a population-health perspective," *American Journal of Nursing*, vol. 112, no. 3, pp. S13–S19, 2012.

[4] J. Favre and B. M. Jolles, "Gait analysis of patients with knee osteoarthritis highlights a pathological mechanical pathway and provides a basis for therapeutic interventions," *EFORT Open Reviews*, vol. 1, no. 10, pp. 368–374, 2016.

[5] M. Henriksen, T. Graven-Nielsen, J. Aaboe, T. P. Andriacchi, and H. Bliddal, "Gait changes in patients with knee osteoarthritis are replicated by experimental knee pain," *Arthritis Care & Research*, vol. 62, no. 4, pp. 501–509, 2010.

[6] D. H. Ro, H.-S. Han, D. Y. Lee, S. H. Kim, Y.-H. Kwak, and M. C. Lee, "Slow gait speed after bilateral total knee arthroplasty is associated with suboptimal improvement of knee biomechanics," *Knee Surgery, Sports Traumatology, Arthroscopy*, vol. 26, no. 6, pp. 1671–1680, 2018.

[7] M. Hall, K. L. Bennell, T. V. Wrigley et al., "The knee adduction moment and knee osteoarthritis symptoms: relationships according to radiographic disease severity," *Osteoarthritis and Cartilage*, vol. 25, no. 1, pp. 34–41, 2017.

[8] N. Foroughi, R. Smith, and B. Vanwanseele, "The association of external knee adduction moment with biomechanical variables in osteoarthritis: a systematic review," *The Knee*, vol. 16, no. 5, pp. 303–309, 2009.

[9] D. H. Ro, H.-S. Han, S. H. Kim, Y.-H. Kwak, J.-Y. Park, and M. C. Lee, "Baseline varus deformity is associated with increased joint loading and pain of non-operated knee two years after unilateral total knee arthroplasty," *The Knee*, vol. 25, no. 2, pp. 249–255, 2018.

[10] A. Mündermann, C. O. Dyrby, and T. P. Andriacchi, "Secondary gait changes in patients with medial compartment knee osteoarthritis: Increased load at the ankle, knee, and hip during walking," *Arthritis & Rheumatology*, vol. 52, no. 9, pp. 2835–2844, 2005.

[11] D. Schmitt, A. Vap, and R. M. Queen, "Effect of end-stage hip, knee, and ankle osteoarthritis on walking mechanics," *Gait & Posture*, vol. 42, no. 3, pp. 373–379, 2015.

[12] J. L. Astephen, K. J. Deluzio, G. E. Caldwell, and M. J. Dunbar, "Biomechanical changes at the hip, knee, and ankle joints during gait are associated with knee osteoarthritis severity," *Journal of Orthopaedic Research*, vol. 26, no. 3, pp. 332–341, 2008.

[13] V. B. Kraus, T. W. Worrell, J. B. Renner, R. E. Coleman, and C. F. Pieper, "High prevalence of contralateral ankle abnormalities in association with knee osteoarthritis and malalignment," *Osteoarthritis and Cartilage*, vol. 21, no. 11, pp. 1693–1699, 2013.

[14] N. Arden and M. C. Nevitt, "Osteoarthritis: epidemiology," *Best Practice & Research Clinical Rheumatology*, vol. 20, no. 1, pp. 3–25, 2006.

[15] K. D. Allen and Y. M. Golightly, "State of the evidence," *Current Opinion in Rheumatology*, vol. 27, no. 3, pp. 276–283, 2015.

[16] M. P. Kadaba, H. K. Ramakrishnan, and M. E. Wootten, "Measurement of lower extremity kinematics during level walking," *Journal of Orthopaedic Research*, vol. 8, no. 3, pp. 383–392, 1990.

[17] J. W. Wannop, J. T. Worobets, and D. J. Stefanyshyn, "Normalization of ground reaction forces, joint moments, and free moments in human locomotion," *Journal of Applied Biomechanics*, vol. 28, no. 6, pp. 665–676, 2012.

[18] T. Miyazaki, M. Wada, H. Kawahara, M. Sato, H. Baba, and S. Shimada, "Dynamic load at baseline can predict radiographic disease progression in medial compartment knee osteoarthritis," *Annals of the Rheumatic Diseases*, vol. 61, no. 7, pp. 617–622, 2002.

[19] M. P. M. Steultjens, J. Dekker, M. E. Van Baar, R. A. B. Oostendorp, and J. W. J. Bijlsma, "Range of joint motion and disability in patients with osteoarthritis of the knee or hip," *Rheumatology*, vol. 39, no. 9, pp. 955–961, 2000.

[20] K. Harato, T. Nagura, H. Matsumoto, T. Otani, Y. Toyama, and Y. Suda, "Knee flexion contracture will lead to mechanical overload in both limbs: a simulation study using gait analysis," *The Knee*, vol. 15, no. 6, pp. 467–472, 2008.

[21] K. M. Song, S. Halliday, C. Reilly, and W. Keezel, "Gait abnormalities following slipped capital femoral epiphysis," *Journal of Pediatric Orthopaedics*, vol. 24, no. 2, pp. 148–155, 2004.

[22] D. H. Ro, D. Y. Lee, G. Moon et al., "Sex differences in knee joint loading: cross-sectional study in geriatric population," *Journal of Orthopaedic Research*, vol. 35, no. 6, pp. 1283–1289, 2017.

18

Double Endoprosthesis in the Management of Refractory Metastatic Primary Bone Tumors in Children and Young Adults

Anna Raciborska, Iwona Malesza, Katarzyna Bilska, Tomasz Koziński, and Bartosz Pachuta

Department of Oncology and Surgical Oncology for Children and Youth, Institute of Mother and Child, Warsaw, Poland

Correspondence should be addressed to Anna Raciborska; anna.raciborska@hoga.pl

Academic Editor: Francesco Liuzza

Background. Although not all children can be cured yet, much more emphasis is placed on the quality of life during and after cancer treatment. In the case of recurrence, mutilating treatment is still the prevalent option. In our study, we explored the role of limb salvage surgery for young patients with metastatic malignant bone tumors after endoprosthesis reconstruction during the first line of treatment and evaluated the impact of the local control modality in disease control and functional outcomes. *Materials and Methods*. Eleven patients with bone tumor treated between 2007 and 2018 were included in this study. Both during primary treatment and during recurrence, limb salvage surgery was performed using a modular or expandable custom-made replacement system. Peri- and postoperative care for both surgeries were similar. All patients were given chemotherapy before and after both surgeries, according to the oncological guidelines. *Results*. Seven patients (63.6%) are alive with a median follow-up of 6.5 years from diagnosis. None had local recurrence. Five-year estimates of event-free survival and overall survival were 36.27% and 79.55%, respectively. Median time between the first and second surgery was 2.7 years. Three patients presented with postoperative complications following both surgeries and required resurgical intervention. Three months following the second surgery, the Musculoskeletal Tumor Society Scale (MSTS) scores were 15–27 points (21 points on average—60%). *Conclusions*. Limb salvage surgery is feasible and offers good chance of cure with a reasonable rate of complications and good function in patients with recurrent bone sarcoma after endoprosthesis reconstruction during the first line of treatment.

1. Introduction

Over the years, there has been tremendous progress in the treatment of cancer in children and adolescents. Although not all children can be cured yet, much more emphasis is placed on the quality of life during and after cancer treatment [1–5].

Currently, methods used in anticancer treatment are as follows: chemotherapy (CHT), surgery, and radiotherapy (RTH). They are applied with different intensities in different combinations, depending on the kind of the disease and its stage. Radical surgery is the most significant prognostic factor in osteosarcoma and plays an important role in the treatment of Ewing sarcoma (ES). This refers to both primary disease treatment and subsequent recurrences [6].

Recurrent osteosarcoma occurs in 30–50% of patients with initially localized disease and 80% of patients presenting with metastatic disease. The recurrence rate in ES is comparable, with treatment failure seen in 50%–80% of patients depending on the site of metastases. The most common sites are the lungs. Factors influencing the results of treatment include the time of recurrence, response to CHT, and resectability of recurrence. The outcome was significantly better for patients who relapsed after having achieved complete remission than for patients who progressed to initial therapy. This highlights the importance of prior disease response in the outcome. Furthermore, patients with subsequent recurrences may be cured, as long as recurrences are resectable [7]. In the case of relapsed or refractory primary bone tumors, until a few years ago, conservative mutilation surgery was the most common choice (amputation and/or exarticulation).

As a result of research and improvement of the effectiveness of chemotherapy/radiotherapy, as well as the development of technology, organ-preserving surgical procedures can be used more often in these patients [6, 8]. However, in the case of relapse, mutilating treatment is still the prevalent option. Nonetheless, patients and their families often expect physicians to consider their quality of life while selecting treatment options, even in the most clinically difficult circumstances.

Therefore, in our study, we explored the role of limb salvage surgery (LSS) for young patients with recurrent malignant bone tumors after endoprosthesis reconstruction during the first line of treatment. Our aim was to evaluate the impact of the local control modality in disease control and functional outcomes.

2. Materials and Methods

2.1. Patients. The present study includes eleven patients (7 males and 4 females) treated between 2007 and 2018 due to primary malignant bone sarcoma (5 Ewing sarcomas and 6 osteosarcomas) followed by isolated distant bone metastases. Local control included double limb salvage surgery (Table 1). As per the oncological guidelines, all patients had standard diagnostic tests, both during first-line and metastatic treatments as clinically indicated, and all had a histological confirmation of the diagnosis. All patients had genetic test (NGS) to evaluate the development cancer predisposition. All patients underwent limb salvage surgery (LSS) using a modular or expandable custom-made replacement system twice, first during primary treatment as well as during recurrence. Surgical inclusion criteria to the second LSS were as follows: (1) minimum partial response to neoadjuvant chemotherapy according to the WHO criteria, (2) good or very good limb function after the first LSS according to Musculoskeletal Tumor Society Scale (MSTS), (3) lack of infiltration of neurovascular structures, and (4) lack of pathological fracture. Demographic, clinical, treatment, and outcome data were collected. Written informed consent was obtained from all patients or their guardians before each treatment. Approval for this retrospective study was obtained from all the relevant institutions in compliance with international regulations for the protection of human research subjects.

2.2. Treatment. All patients were treated in accordance with the following chemotherapy guidelines: (1) during the first-line treatment, Ewing sarcoma patients according to the Euro-EWING regimen and patients with osteosarcoma under the European Osteosarcoma Intergroup [9]; (2) systemic treatment of recurrences was individualized. ES patients received VIT (vincristine, irinotecan, and temozolomide) or PACE (cisplatin, doxorubicin, cyclophosphamide, and etoposide) regimen, and patients with osteosarcoma received ifosfamide and etoposide or gemcitabine and docetaxel depending on the previously applied treatment arm [9]. Both during primary treatment and during recurrence, LSS was performed following 2–6 cycles of CHT. In each case, chemotherapy was restarted no later than 2 weeks after surgery. In line with the ES protocol, as an additional local control, radiotherapy (45.0–54.0 Gy) was available to patients with Ewing sarcoma and microscopic residual after surgery or poor histologic response (<90% necrosis). RTH was also offered for bone metastasis control (40.0–45.0 Gy). For patients with complete tumor resection, with good response to chemotherapy (≥90% necrosis) and small tumor volume (≤200 mL), radiation was not recommended. All patients with lung metastases underwent metastasectomy. Additionally, those with ES were offered whole-lung radiation following the lung surgery. To the ES patient with bone marrow metastases, autologous bone marrow transplant was proposed.

All surgeries were performed at the Mother and Child Institute in Warsaw by our surgical team familiar with a wide range of surgical options. The aim was to completely excise the tumor and biopsy tract en bloc and perform the reconstruction using post-resection endoprosthesis while preserving the neurovascular bundle and tendons. All reconstructions were made using a custom-made bone replacement system. The biological age of patients was the most important factor while selecting the type of implant. For older patients (with bone growth completed), the preferred solution was the modular system and for younger (before growth plate fusion), the expandable one. Tumor removal and engraftment of the bone replacement systems were conducted in accordance with standard operating procedures. Peri- and postoperative care for both surgeries were similar. Intrasurgery histopathology test was performed in all patients. Intravenous antibiotics were administered one hour before and throughout surgery (including the second dose of cefazolin two hours after the start of surgery) [9]. Walker orthoses were recommended for the period of approximately 3 months after surgery. All patients were offered intensive individualized rehabilitation.

Surgical complications were treated as follows: (1) periprosthetic infections were treated in two stages; in the first stage, endoprosthesis was removed, and a spacer was inserted; in the second stage, a few months later, after normalizing the inflammation parameters, the spacer was removed, and the endoprosthesis was implemented again; (2) in the case of fracture, revision surgery was performed with clamp stabilization; (3) wound necrosis was treated using a vascularized skin graft.

2.3. Evaluation. Oncological evaluation was performed according to the standard protocols for osteosarcoma and Ewing sarcoma, at diagnosis, every two courses of chemotherapy, before surgery, at the end of therapy, every 3 months during the first 3 years of follow-up, and every 6 months up to 5 years or until death. Response to chemotherapy was evaluated using the WHO scale. Surgical assessment was performed every 3 weeks during therapy and in conjunction with oncological evaluation thereafter. Limb function was evaluated using the MSTS 3 months after each surgery. Functional rating was assessed as follows: outstanding (90% and more), good (85%–70%), average (70%–65%), and poor (less than 65%).

Table 1: Patient characteristics.

Pt no.	Gender	Type of disease	Age at diagnosis	Meta at diagnosis	Primary site	First treatment	Kind of recurrence	Site of bone recurrence	Age at the 2nd surgery	Second treatment	Outcome
1	M	ES	13.5	Lung	Femur L	CHT, loc S, met S, lung RT	Bone	Shoulder L	24.0	CHT, loc S	AWD
2	M	ES	12.2	Lung, bones, lymph nodes	Shoulder R	CHT, loc S, met S, lung RT	Bone, lung	Femur L	16.5	CHT, loc S, met S	AWD
3	M	ES	14.6	Lung, bones, lymph nodes	Shoulder R	CHT, loc S, met S, lung RT	Bone	Femur R	19.8	CHT, loc S	DOD
4	K	ES	14.1	No	Femur R	CHT, loc S	Bone	Femur L	16.3	CHT, loc S	AWD
5	M	ES	20.0	Lung, bone marrow	Femur L	CHT, loc S, met S, lung RT	Bone, lung	Femur R	22.8	CHT, loc S, met S	DOD
6	M	OS	13.6	Lung	Femur L	CHT, loc S, met S	Bone	Femur R	16.7	CHT, loc S	AWD
7	K	OS	17.4	No	Femur R	CHT, loc S	Bone, lung	Femur L	18.9	CHT, loc S, met S	DOD
8	K	OS	9.3	No	Femur R	CHT, loc S	Bone	Pelvic R	13.5	CHT, loc S	DOD
9	M	OS	21.8	No	Femur R	CHT, loc S	Bone	Tibia R	22.4	CHT, loc S	AWD
10	K	OS	15.3	No	Tibia L	CHT, loc S	Bone	Femur R	22.6	CHT, loc S	AWD
11	M	OS	12.1	No	Femur L	CHT, loc S	Bone	Femur R	14.6	CHT, loc S	AWD

No: number; M: male; F: female; ES: Ewing sarcoma; OS: osteosarcoma; L: left; R: right; CHT: chemotherapy; RT: radiation; loc S: surgery of bone lesion; met S: surgery of lung metastases; AWD: alive without the disease; DOD: death of disease.

2.4. Statistical Methods. Overall survival was defined as the time interval from the date of diagnosis to the date of death or the last follow-up. Event-free survival was defined as the time interval from the date of diagnosis to the date of disease progression, recurrence, second malignancy, or death or to the date of the last follow-up for patients without events. Result distributions were estimated using the method of Kaplan–Meier. $P \leq 0.05$ was regarded as significant. Statistical analysis was performed using Stata 13.3 for Windows.

3. Results

Five patients had metastatic disease at diagnosis (two of them only to the lung, another two to the lung, bones, and lymph nodes, and one to the lung and bone marrow). Median age at diagnosis was 14.1 years (range: 9.7 to 21.8 years). No predisposition changes were found in the NGS test. All patients were treated with neoadjuvant CHT followed by limb-sparing surgery and adjuvant CHT as part of the first-line treatment. All patients responded well to neoadjuvant CHT: lung nodules reduced in CT, clear bone marrow, and no pathological lymph nodes in the ultrasound test. All patients finished treatment in complete remission (CR).

All patients included in the study recurred, presenting with an isolated metastatic bone lesion. Additionally, three of them had lung metastases. All received systemic treatment followed by LSS. Due to clear margin and good histological response, local radiation was not offered. Median age at the second surgery was 18.9 years (range: 13.5 to 24 years). Median time between the first and second surgery was 2.7 years (range: 0.4 to 6.9 years). Patient characteristics are summarized in Table 1.

3.1. First Surgery. Expandable systems were used in three patients (Figure 1). All patients had microscopically complete resections. There were no major perioperative complications. Late surgery-related complications requiring resurgical intervention occurred in three patients: periprosthetic infection in two cases and iatrogenic fracture in one. Three months following the first surgery, the MSTS scores were 25–27 points (26 points on average—75%). Ten out of eleven patients were ambulatory without crutches at the end of the first oncological treatment (Table 2).

3.2. Second Surgery. Modular systems were used in all patients (Figure 2). Ten of them had microscopically complete resections, while the positive margin was recorded in one case. There were no major perioperative complications. As in the case of the first surgery, surgery-related complications requiring resurgical intervention occurred in three patients: wound necrosis in one case, posttraumatic fracture in one case, and periprosthetic infection in one (Table 2).

3.3. Function and Outcome. With a median follow-up of 6.5 years (range: 1.8 to 12.9 years), 7 out of 11 patients (63.63%) are alive. Median time to recurrence was 2.3 years (range: 1.1 to 10.3 years). No local recurrences were observed. Four out of eleven patients died due to disease progression (2 with

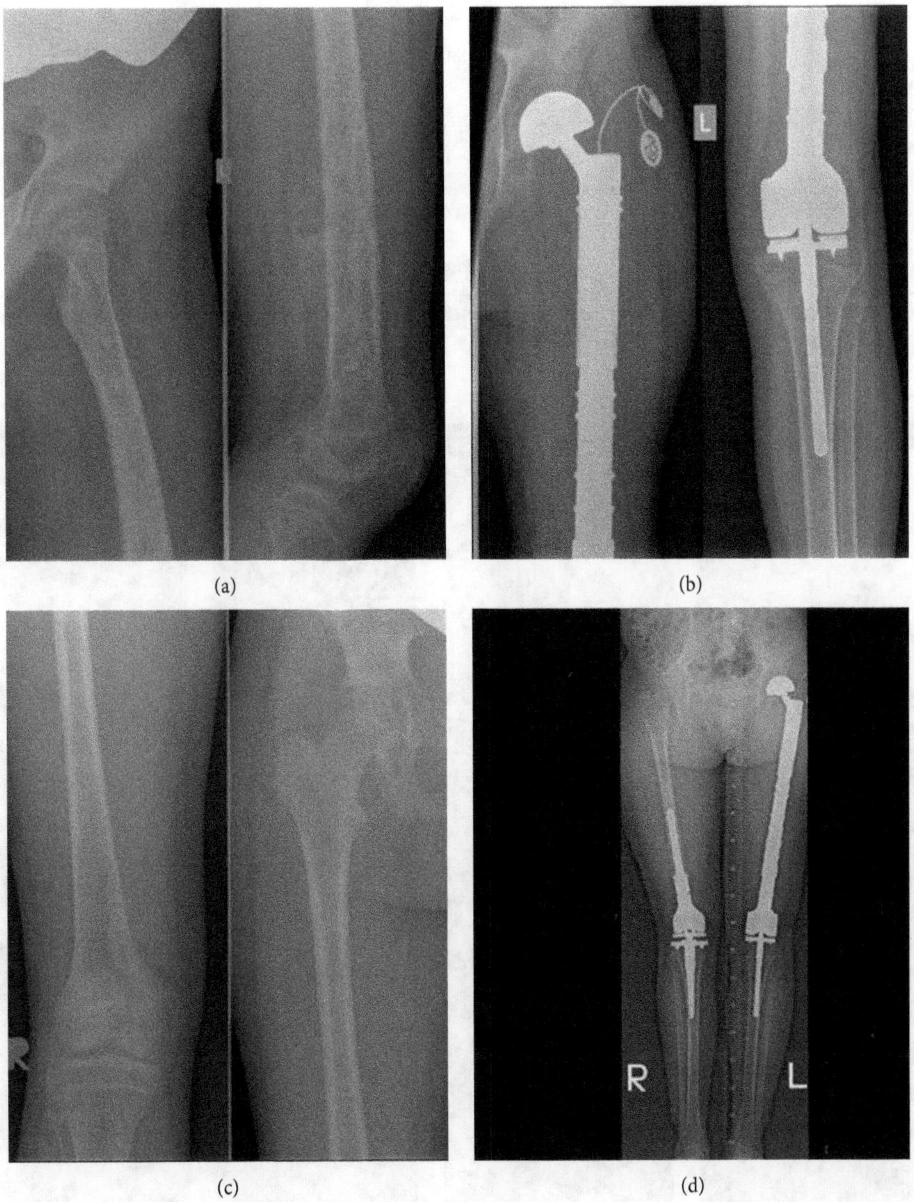

Figure 1: Patient with osteosarcoma where the expandable system was used followed by the modular one: (a) at diagnosis—left femur osteosarcoma, (b) after the first surgery with the expandable system, (c) at recurrence—right distal femur osteosarcoma, and (d) after the second surgery with the modular system.

Table 2: Patient characteristics at the first and second surgery, function, and outcome.

Pt no.	Site of the first surgery	Implant	Surgery-related complications	MSTS score (%)	Function	Site of the second surgery	Implant	Surgery-related complications	MSTS score (%)	Function	Outcome
1	Femur L	Modular	No	77	Ambulatory	Shoulder L	Modular	No	77	Ambulatory	AWD
2	Humerus R	Modular	No	80	Ambulatory	Femur L	Modular	No	77	Ambulatory	AWD
3	Humerus R	Modular	No	74	Ambulatory	Femur R	Modular	No	62	Ambulatory	DOD
4	Femur R	Modular	No	77	Ambulatory	Femur L	Modular	No	65	Ambulatory	AWD
5	Femur L	Modular	Periprosthetic infection	71	Ambulatory	Femur R	Modular	Periprosthetic infection	45	On crutches	DOD
6	Femur L	Expanded	No	71	On crutches	Femur R	Modular	No	42	On crutches	AWD
7	Femur R	Modular	No	77	Ambulatory	Femur L	Modular	No	62	Ambulatory	DOD
8	Femur R	Expanded	No	77	Ambulatory	Pelvic R	Modular	No	45	On crutches	DOD

TABLE 2: Continued.

Pt no.	Site of the first surgery	Implant	Surgery-related complications	MSTS score (%)	Function	Site of the second surgery	Implant	Surgery-related complications	MSTS score (%)	Function	Outcome
9	Femur R	Modular	No	71	Ambulatory	Tibia R	Modular	Posttraumatic fracture	60	Ambulatory	AWD
10	Tibia L	Modular	Iatrogenic fracture	77	Ambulatory	Femur R	Modular	Wound necrosis	65	Ambulatory	AWD
11	Femur L	Expanded	Periprosthetic infection	74	Ambulatory	Femur R	Modular	No	63	On crutches	AWD

No: number; M: male; F: female; ES: Ewing sarcoma; OS: osteosarcoma; L: left; R: right; AWD: alive without the disease; DOD: death of disease; MSTS: musculoskeletal tumor society scale.

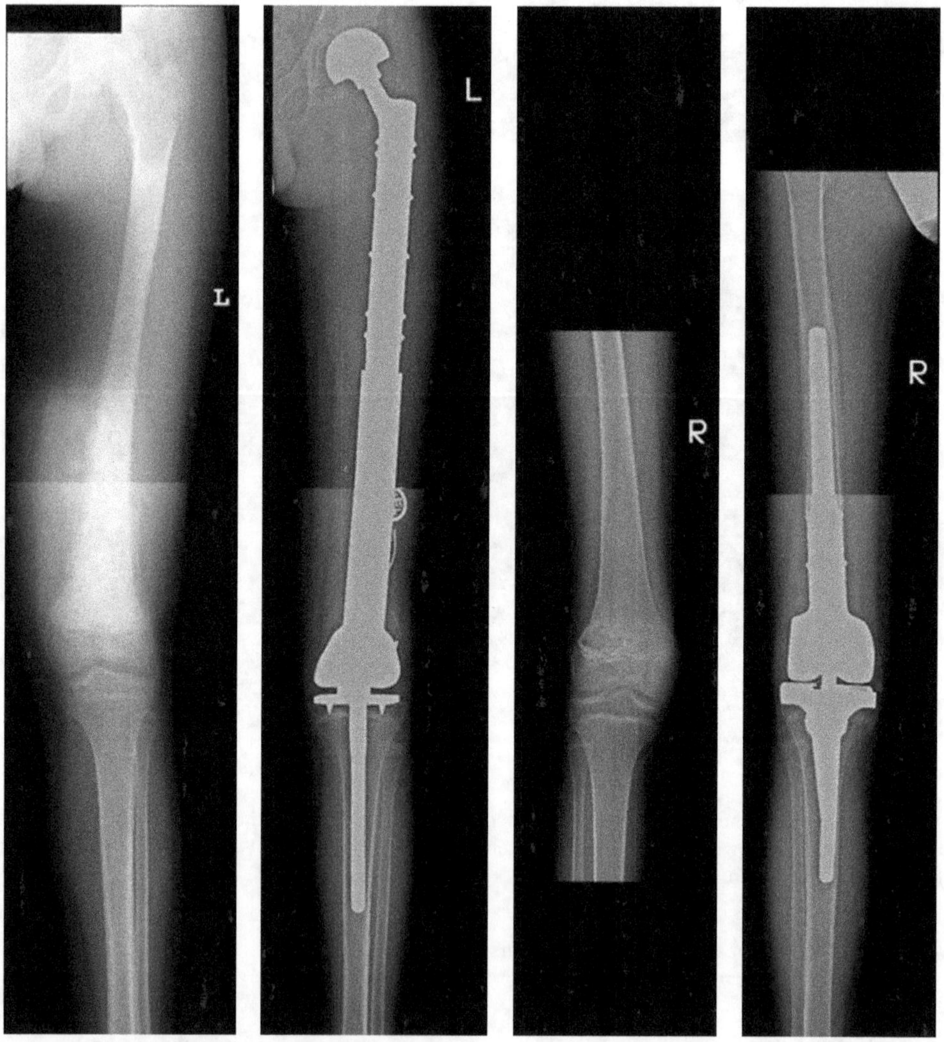

(a) (b) (c) (d)

FIGURE 2: Patient with osteosarcoma where two modular systems were used: (a) at diagnosis, (b) after the first surgery with the modular system, (c) at recurrence, and (d) after the second surgery with the modular system.

primary metastatic ES and 2 with osteosarcoma—1 of them had a positive surgical margin). Five-year estimates of event-free survival and overall survival were 36.27% and 79.55%, respectively. Limb function was satisfactory in all patients. Three months following the second surgery, the MSTS scores were 15–27 points (21 points on average—60%). At a median follow-up of 3.6 years (range: 0.7 to 6.8 years) after the second limb salvage surgery, all alive patients are ambulatory; two of them are still on crutches (Table 2).

4. Discussion

Primary malignant bone tumors constitute less than 10% of all malignant neoplasms diagnosed in children and adolescents [6]. In Poland, bone tumors account for 7%–8.2% [10]. Until recently, the prognosis in this group of patients was poor. The introduction of multimodal therapy including multiagent chemotherapy, radiation, and effective local control surgery significantly improved prognosis in this group. Recently, physicians have been reporting increasingly positive outcomes in low-grade (80–90%) and advanced high-grade localized tumors (60–80%) [6, 11, 12]. Similarly, even the most advanced cases can be expected to achieve good long-term results (up to 45%).

However, the outcome after relapse of bone sarcoma is still dismal. The management of recurrent bone sarcoma needs to take into account the timing of recurrences, the number of metastases, and the metastatic sites. Until recently, given the challenges for the LSS, as well as low survival rates, many of the patients underwent a mutilating procedure: amputation or exarticulation and/or only radiation therapy in the case of Ewing sarcoma. Nevertheless, in the case of good response to CHT and provided that the recurrences are resectable, the survival rate increases significantly [7].

In our study, we explored the role of limb salvage surgery for young patients with recurrent malignant bone tumors after endoprosthesis reconstruction during the first line of treatment. We believe that the existing body of literature could be enriched with more such studies (to our knowledge, this is the first such report). Our aim was to evaluate the impact of the local control modality in disease control and functional outcomes. Our experience shows that this approach is not only feasible but also can improve the quality of life in this poor prognosis population. Nevertheless, other surgeons hold the opposite view, arguing that amputation can lead to better disease control with long-term functional outcomes comparable to those achieved through limb-sparing surgery [4, 5, 13]. However, some studies have shown that the results of organ-preserving surgery are no worse than mutilating procedures. Sparing treatment does not deteriorate outcomes and brings good functional results [3, 8, 14, 15].

Moreover, although radiation therapy has been an integral component in the treatment of unresectable or metastatic Ewing sarcoma patients, its outcomes seem to remain inferior to surgery [16, 17]. For patients with small and localized tumors, radiation therapy can offer local control rates similar to surgery [18, 19].

Being aware of these opinions in our study, limb salvage surgery was still proposed as a local control modality. Arguments for this decision were as follows: our patients' life expectancy was better than average, they responded well to CHT, and their recurrence was resectable (there was a high probability of a clear margin nonmutilating procedure). Moreover, limb salvage surgery was much more acceptable to patients than mutilating surgery, and the results of the first LSS (measured by the patient's quality of life) were good (all our patients were ambulatory after the first surgery).

Unfortunately, malignant bone tumor patients are still at a much higher risk of poor quality of life compared to other childhood cancer survivors [2]. Marina et al. reported that even half of the bone cancer survivors may experience mobility limitations at various levels, affecting their social and professional life due to high-dose chemotherapy, aggressive surgical resection, and/or high-dose radiotherapy [20]. Currently, good quality of life (QQL) after cancer treatment is increasingly being considered. Quality of life assessment is part of holistic healthcare [1]. More resources are aimed at improving the patient's quality of life during and after anticancer treatment. Influenced by this trend, more and more researchers explore the impact of different treatment modalities on minimizing the rate of late side effects (e.g., comparing different surgical approaches or different CHT regimens) [20]. In our study, all survivors are ambulatory. Just two of them (28.5%) still need crutches. Then, this surgical approach could potentially provide an alternative to mutilation surgery.

The outcome of our patients undergoing second LSS despite the recurrence was good (5-year OS was 78.56%). Moreover, all patients had limited acute complications. Only three patients required surgical intervention due to late surgery-related complications. In one patient, periprosthetic infection was detected after both first and second LSS. Unfortunately, late complications, especially infection, can continue for a long time, which should be taken into account when selecting local therapy approaches [21, 22].

We acknowledge that small study groups may result in biased outcome data. While the present study did not include a control group as such, in previous years, patients of our hospital did undergo both mutilating procedures or only palliative radiotherapy. These have been associated with a worse outcome and a worse quality of life [23].

In recent years, many papers have been published to establish the place of surgery in bone tumor therapy. Currently, both in osteosarcoma and Ewing sarcoma, surgical resection with clear margin is an essential part of the curative treatment strategy [6, 24, 25]. Lack of complete surgical resection usually results in worse outcomes, also in relapsed patients [26–28]. Also, based on the developing technology, more and more patients are fighting not only for life but also for the quality of life. Modern patients are increasingly aware of the importance of informed consent and often want to be a part of the decision-making process. It is also not uncommon for patients and their families to put pressure on doctors to choose their preferred therapy. Therefore, we believe that it is very important for doctors to be able to evaluate available treatment options.

Additionally, it is worth mentioning that, in the case of patients requiring more than one endoprosthesis in the same limb, one needs to make sure that the second implant is compatible with the first. This is commonly not an issue if both replacement systems are provided by the same manufacturer. If using the same provider is not possible, a converter is needed to join the two systems.

5. Conclusion

In our opinion, advances in reconstructive surgery with good rehabilitation cooperation do have the potential to extend the role of radical surgery to the group of patients we studied. This study confirms that limb salvage surgery is feasible in patients with recurrent bone sarcoma after endoprosthesis reconstruction during the first line of treatment. Furthermore, it also has the potential to offer very good quality of life with good local control and functional outcomes. With appropriate patient selection and reconstructive surgery, the quality of life of these patients will continue to improve.

Authors' Contributions

AR and BP were responsible for the conception and design of the study, interpretation of the data, and preparation of the final manuscript for publication. AR, KB, TK, and IM contributed to patients' clinical data extraction and data analyses and were responsible for the acquisition of literature studies for the manuscript. The final manuscript was reviewed and approved by all authors.

References

[1] R. L. Jones and A. L. Cesne, "Quality of life and patients' expectations in soft tissue sarcoma," *Future Oncology*, vol. 14, no. 10s, pp. 51–62, 2018.

[2] J. Stokke, L. Sung, A. Gupta, A. Lindberg, and A. R. Rosenberg, "Systematic review and meta-analysis of objective and subjective quality of life among pediatric, adolescent, and young adult bone tumor survivors," *Pediatric Blood & Cancer*, vol. 62, no. 9, pp. 1616–1629, 2015.

[3] W. P. Bekkering, T. P. M. Vliet Vlieland, H. M. Koopman et al., "A prospective study on quality of life and functional outcome in children and adolescents after malignant bone tumor surgery," *Pediatric Blood & Cancer*, vol. 58, no. 6, pp. 978–985, 2012.

[4] J. Mei, X.-Z. Zhu, Z.-Y. Wang, and X.-S. Cai, "Functional outcomes and quality of life in patients with osteosarcoma treated with amputation versus limb-salvage surgery: a systematic review and meta-analysis," *Archives of Orthopaedic and Trauma Surgery*, vol. 134, no. 11, pp. 1507–1516, 2014.

[5] G. Ottaviani, R. S. Robert, W. W. Huh, and N. Jaffe, "Functional, psychosocial and professional outcomes in long-term survivors of lower-extremity osteosarcomas: amputation versus limb salvage," *Cancer Treatment and Research*, vol. 152, pp. 421–436, 2009.

[6] P. G. Casali, S. Bielack, N. Abecassis et al., "Bone sarcomas: ESMO-PaedCan-EURACAN clinical practice guidelines for diagnosis, treatment and follow-up," *Annals of Oncology: Official Journal of the European Society for Medical Oncology*, vol. 29, no. 4, pp. iv79–iv95, 2018.

[7] B. Kempf-Bielack, S. S. Bielack, H. Jürgens et al., "Osteosarcoma relapse after combined modality therapy: an analysis of unselected patients in the cooperative osteosarcoma study group (COSS)," *Journal of Clinical Oncology*, vol. 23, no. 3, pp. 559–568, 2005.

[8] J. Schrager, R. E. Patzer, P. J. Mink, K. C. Ward, and M. Goodman, "Survival outcomes of pediatric osteosarcoma and ewing's sarcoma: a comparison of surgery type within the SEER database, 1988–2007," *Journal of Registry Management*, vol. 38, no. 3, pp. 153–161, 2011.

[9] I. Babiak, A. Górecki, and P. Małdyk, "Zasady profilaktyki, rozpoznawania i leczenia nieswoistych zakażeń kości i stawów. (guidelines for prophylaxis, diagnosis and treatment of non-specific bone and joint infections)," *Ortopedia Traumatologia Rehabilitacja*, vol. 10, pp. 396–415, 2008.

[10] J. Kowalczyk, "Epidemiologia nowotworów dziecięcych. (epidemiology of cancer in children)," in *Wprowadzenie Do Onkologii I Hematologii Dziecięcej [Introduction to Paediatric Oncology and Haematology*, J. Kowalczyk, Ed., CMKP, Warszaw, Poland, 2011.

[11] S. S. Bielack, D. Carrle, J. Hardes, A. Schuck, and M. Paulussen, "Bone tumors in adolescents and young adults," *Current Treatment Options in Oncology*, vol. 9, no. 1, pp. 67–80, 2008.

[12] J. C. Wittig, J. Bickels, D Priebat et al., "Osteosarcoma: a multidisciplinary approach to diagnosis and treatment," *American Family Physician*, vol. 65, no. 6, pp. 1123–1132, 2002.

[13] G. R. Schirò, S. Sessa, A. Piccioli, and G. Maccauro, "Primary amputation vs limb salvage in mangled extremity: a systematic review of the current scoring system," *BMC Musculoskeletal Disorders*, vol. 16, no. 1, p. 372, 2015.

[14] X. He, Z. Gao, H. Xu, Z. Zhang, and P. Fu, "A meta-analysis of randomized control trials of surgical methods with osteosarcoma outcomes," *Journal of Orthopaedic Surgery and Research*, vol. 12, no. 1, p. 5, 2017.

[15] G. Han, W.-Z. Bi, M. Xu, J.-P. Jia, and Y. Wang, "Amputation versus limb-salvage surgery in patients with osteosarcoma: a meta-analysis," *World Journal of Surgery*, vol. 40, no. 8, pp. 2016–2027, 2016.

[16] C. Rodríguez-Galindo, F. Navid, T. Liu, C. A. Billups, B. N. Rao, and M. J. Krasin, "Prognostic factors for local and distant control in Ewing sarcoma family of tumors," *Annals of Oncology*, vol. 19, no. 4, pp. 814–820, 2008.

[17] A. Raciborska, K. Bilska, M. Rychlowska-Pruszynska et al., "Internal hemipelvectomy in the management of pelvic ewing sarcoma - are outcomes better than with radiation therapy?" *Journal of Pediatric Surgery*, vol. 49, no. 10, pp. 1500–1504, 2014.

[18] D. J. Indelicato, S. R. Keole, A. H. Shahlaee et al., "Impact of local management on long-term outcomes in ewing tumors of the pelvis and sacral bones: the University of Florida experience," *International Journal of Radiation Oncology*, vol. 72, no. 1, pp. 41–48, 2008.

[19] T. H. La, P. A. Meyers, L. H. Wexler et al., "Radiation therapy for Ewing's sarcoma: results from memorial sloan-kettering in the modern era," *International Journal of Radiation Oncology*, vol. 64, no. 2, pp. 544–550, 2006.

[20] N. Marina, M. M. Hudson, K. E. Jones et al., "Changes in health status among aging survivors of pediatric upper and lower extremity sarcoma: a report from the childhood cancer survivor study," *Archives of Physical Medicine and Rehabilitation*, vol. 94, no. 6, pp. 1062–1073, 2013.

[21] R. J. Grimer, B. K. Aydin, H. Wafa et al., "Very long-term outcomes after endoprosthetic replacement for malignant tumours of bone," *The Bone & Joint Journal*, vol. 98-B, no. 6, pp. 857–864, 2016.

[22] A. Angelini, D. Kotrych, G. Trovarelli, A. Szafrański, A. Bohatyrewicz, and P. Ruggieri, "Analysis of principles inspiring design of three-dimensional-printed custom-made prostheses in two referral centres," *International Orthopaedics*, vol. 44, no. 5, pp. 829–837, 2020.

[23] A. Raciborska, K. Bilska, K. Drabko et al., "Validation of a multi-modal treatment protocol for ewing sarcoma-a report from the polish pediatric oncology group," *Pediatric Blood & Cancer*, vol. 61, no. 12, pp. 2170–2174, 2014.

[24] B. R. Eaton, R. Schwarz, R. Vatner et al., "Osteosarcoma," *Pediatric Blood & Cancer*, vol. 68, no. S2, Article ID e28352, 2020.

[25] E. Palmerini, E. Torricelli, S. Cascinu et al., "Is there a role for chemotherapy after local relapse in high-grade osteosarcoma?" *Pediatric Blood & Cancer*, vol. 66, no. 8, Article ID e27792, 2019.

[26] C. Meazza and P. Scanagatta, "Metastatic osteosarcoma: a challenging multidisciplinary treatment," *Expert Review of Anticancer Therapy*, vol. 16, no. 5, pp. 543–556, 2016.

[27] C. Rodriguez-Galindo, N. Shah, M. B. McCarville et al., "Outcome after local recurrence of osteosarcoma," *Cancer*, vol. 100, no. 9, pp. 1928–1935, 2004.

[28] N. Vijayamurugan and S. Bakhshi, "Review of management issues in relapsed osteosarcoma," *Expert Review of Anticancer Therapy*, vol. 14, no. 2, pp. 151–161, 2014.

19

Clinical and Radiological Outcomes of Corrective Surgery on Adult Spinal Deformity Patients: Comparison of Short and Long Fusion

Koichiro Ono, Kazuo Ohmori, and Takeshi Hori

Center for Spinal Surgery, Nippon Koukan Hospital, Kawasaki 210-0852, Japan

Correspondence should be addressed to Koichiro Ono; koichirono@gmail.com

Guest Editor: Yasushi Oshima

Despite the accumulated knowledge of spinal alignment and clinical outcomes the full corrective surgery cannot be applied to all the deformity patients as it requires considerable surgical burden to the patients. The aim of this study was to investigate the clinical and radiological outcomes of the patients who have received short and long fusion for ASD. A total of 21 patients who received surgical reconstructive spinal fusion procedures and were followed up for at least one year were retrospectively reviewed. Sixteen cases have received spinal corrective surgery that upper instrumented vertebrate (UIV) was thoracic level (group T), or 5 cases were with UIV in lumbar level (group L). Group L had shorter operation time, smaller intraoperative estimated blood loss, and shorter postoperative hospitalization days. Group T tends to improve more in the magnitude of VAS of lumbar pain compared to group L. Improvement of spinal alignment revealed the advantage of long fusion compared to short fusion, in Cobb angle, sagittal vertical axis (SVA), lumbar lordosis (LL), PI-LL C7 plum line (C7PL), and center sacral vertebral line (CSVL). Pelvic tilt (PT) did not differ between the groups. Disc lordosis was the most acquired in XLIF compared to TLIF and PLF and maintained one year. There were 9 adverse events, 3 cases of pulmonary embolism (PE), one case of delirium, and 6 cases of proximal junctional kyphosis. Current study elucidated that long fusion, UIV, is thoracic and can achieve better spinal alignment compared to short fusion, UIV, in lumbar. XLIF demonstrated strong ability to reconstruct the deformity on intervertebral space that is better to apply as much intervertebral space as possible. For the ASD patients with complications, short fusion can be one of the options.

1. Introduction

In world's fastest aging society, one of the issues for quality of daily livings (QOL) of aging population in Japan is adult spinal deformity (ASD). ASD are associated with broad range of clinical and radiological findings such as progressive spinal deformity, chronic back pain, and neurological symptoms. Pathology of ASD includes primary degenerative scoliosis ("de novo" form), progressive idiopathic scoliosis in adult life, and scoliosis secondary to vertebral fracture and/or asymmetric arthritic disease [1]. Among these, the number of degenerative and secondary scolioses is increasing in Japanese aging society. Advanced ASD presents loss of function, refractory to nonoperative treatment, and therefore requires the surgical intervention.

Surgical intervention for ASD with posterior-only procedure consists of pedicle screws, osteotomies, and transforaminal interbody fusion [2]. For advanced ASD, posterior-only procedure usually requires high volume osteotomies that carry increased technical demands, longer operation time, and greater blood loss and associated morbidity. Anterior procedure predominantly utilized the disc space to reconstruct spinal alignment that also have large surgical burden as posterior osteotomies [3].

In recent years, minimally invasive surgery (MIS) for spinal fusion has become increasingly popular. The extreme lateral interbody fusion (XLIF) [4] uses the dedicated retractor installed from lateral, abdominal, retroperitoneal, transpsoas approach to lateral portion of the intervertebral disc. XLIF demonstrates strong ability to reconstruct the deformity on intervertebral space [5].

In addition to XLIF, the sacral alar iliac (SAI) screw extends from the second sacral segment to the anterior inferior iliac spine and enabled powerful compression and distraction maneuvers against greater sciatic notch [6].

Lastly, rod rotation [7] and cantilever bending technique [8] enabled correction of scoliosis and enhanced lumbar lordosis.

This recent advance in techniques, instruments, and retractors provides the means to achieve a radiographic correction for ASD to improve clinical outcomes [9]. Despite the accumulated knowledge of spinal alignment and clinical outcomes [9, 10] the full corrective surgery cannot be applied to all the deformity patients as they require considerable surgical burden to the patients. The aim of this study was to investigate the clinical and radiological outcomes of the patients who have received short and long fusion for ASD with a minimum of one year of follow-up.

2. Material and Methods

2.1. Study Design and Patient Population. A total of 21 patients who received surgical reconstructive spinal fusion procedures for their adult spinal deformity at Nippon Koukan Hospital and were followed up for at least one year, from 2014 to 2017, were retrospectively reviewed. Inclusion criteria were symptomatic degenerative adult scoliosis that has failed conservative treatment of patients with Cobb angle of at least 10°, whereas Parkinson disease and deformity due to the vertebral fracture were excluded. The follow-up period was minimum 14.3 months to maximum 57.4 months and average follow-up was 38 months. The mean age was 75.1 years old (65-88 years old), 4 males and 17 females. Of the 21 patients, 16 cases have received spinal corrective surgery that upper instrumented vertebrate (UIV) [10] was thoracic level (group T), or 5 cases were with UIV in lumbar level (group L) (Table 1). Four cases in group T underwent the same day procedure, whereas 12 cases received staged combined anterior and posterior procedures (Table 1). Staged procedures were performed on 7- to 9-day interval; XLIF was performed for the first stage and posterior surgery for the second stage. Clinical and radiographical outcomes were compared between the groups. Also, disc lordosis (Figure 1(b)) was compared among XLIF, transforaminal lumbar interbody fusion (TLIF), or posterior lumbar fusion (PLF). Lastly, introduction of Bendini (Nuvasive, San Diego, CA, USA) was discussed.

2.2. Surgical Procedure. In all of staged procedures (12 cases), in the initial surgery, multilevel (2 to 4) XLIF was performed [4]. During XLIF, the retractor attached with the light source was docked on the lateral aspect of intervertebral disc *via* retroperitoneal, transpsoas approach. After the discectomy and trial placement, a lordotic interbody cage (Nuvasive, San Diego, CA, USA) was filled with ReFit (HOYA Technosurgical Corporation, Tokyo, Japan) and autologous bone was harvested from ilium.

For posterior surgery, patients were positioned to prone on the frame and their spine was approached in a standard open fashion. Transforaminal lumbar interbody fusion (TLIF) was performed on intervertebral disc, L1/2 to L5/S1 level, where XLIFs were not performed. After the complete exposure of posterior elements, pedicle screws were placed into all targeted segments. Interspinous ligament resection and facet osteotomies or Ponte osteotomy was performed from L1/2 to L5/S1 among instrumented levels as necessary. Rod rotation [7] and cantilever bending technique [8] were performed to correct scoliosis and enhance lumbar lordosis whenever possible. A curved temporary rod was applied to the convex side of the deformity from T12 to L5 and rod rotation maneuver was performed. A final rod was designed by Bendini spinal rod bending system (Nuvasive, after Mar. 2017) and applied to the concave side with sequential compression and rotation and cantilever technique [8]. Finally, the temporary rod was change to the final rod.

2.3. Clinical Assessment. Clinical outcomes were assessed preoperatively and one year and final follow-up using the Japanese Orthopedic Association (JOA) score and the Oswestry Disability Index (ODI). The visual analog scale (VAS) was used for back and leg pain. The medical record was searched for operative data and complications.

2.4. Radiological Evaluation. Standing neural anterior-posterior and lateral thoracolumbar films were obtained before surgery, one month and a year after the surgery for assessment. Coronal alignment parameters included Cobb angle and coronal imbalance by plum line deviation (Figure 1(a)). Cobb angle was determined from degree of most superior and most inferior vertebral body (VB) of the scoliotic curve. Coronal imbalance was measured as the distance between a C7 plumb line to the center sacral vertebral line (C7PL-CSVL). Sagittal alignment parameters included lumbar lordosis (LL) from L1 to S1, pelvic incidence (PI), sagittal vertical axis (SVA), and pelvic tilt (PT) (Figure 1(b)). SVA was measured by the horizontal offset from the center of C7 to posterosuperior corner of S1 (Figure 1(b)). Disc lordosis (DL) was determined from degree of inferior line of superior VB and superior line of inferior VB (Figure 1(b)). In addition to comparison study of groups T and L, DL change was compared among XLIF, TLIF, or PLF.

Proximal junctional kyphosis (PJK) was defined as proximal junctional angle and caudal endplate to UIV to the cephalad endplate of 2 proximal vertebrae increases more than 10 degrees. [11].

2.5. Data Analysis. For numerical variables, means and standard deviations were calculated, and comparisons were made using a 2-tailed Student's t-test. Categorical variables were compared using χ^2 test.

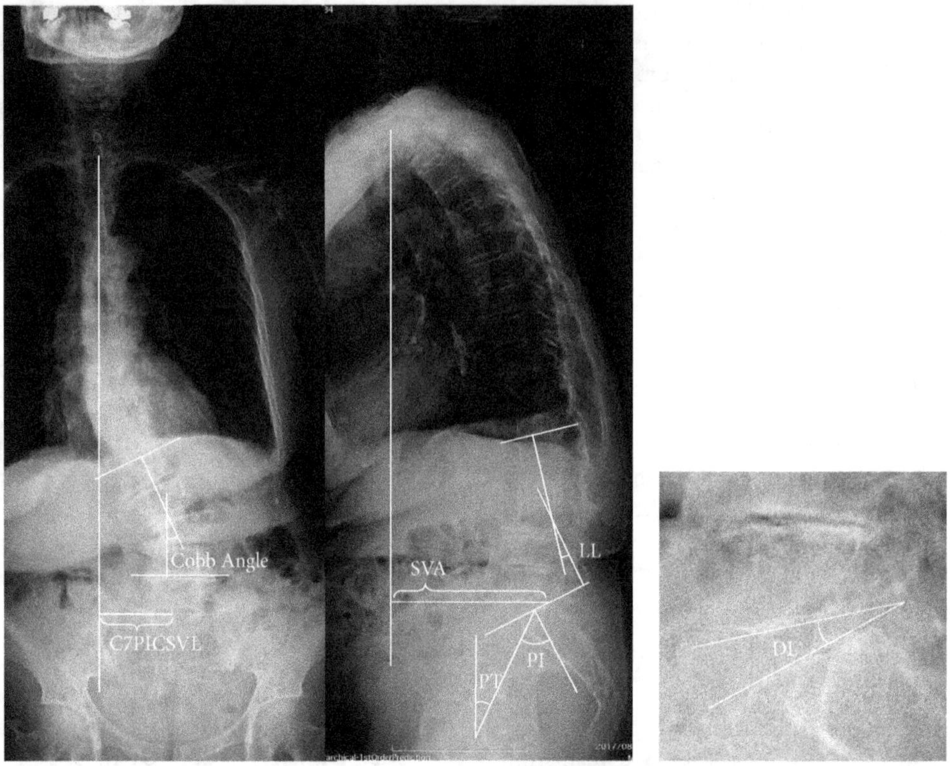

(a) (b)

FIGURE 1: (a) Measurements of sagittal spinal alignment. C7PL-CSVL, C7 plum line to center sacral vertebral line; Cobb angle; SVA, sagittal vertical axis; PT, pelvic tilt; PI, pelvic incidence; LL, lumbar lordosis. (b) DL, disc lordosis.

3. Results

3.1. Clinical and Operative Data. Sixteen patients in group T had a mean age of 76 years (67-88), while 5 cases in group L had 72.2 years (65-77) with no significance (Table 2). Body Mass Index (BMI) (group T versus L = 22.3 versus 23, p = 0.74) and sex (male/female = 2/14 versus 2/3, 0.17) were also similar between groups (Table 2). The mean operation time was significantly shorter in group L (404 versus 285 min., p < 0.01); as a consequence an intraoperative estimated blood loss was smaller in group L (870 versus 137 ml, p < 0.01), and postoperative hospitalization days were shorter in group L (43.9 versus 26.8 days, p = 0.03) (Table 2). There were 9 adverse events recorded. There were three cases of pulmonary embolism (PE) in group T (cases 10, 11, and 14; Table 1). Three cases were all staged cases. One case had episode of delirium in group T (case 17). PJK were developed in four cases of group T (cases 6, 7, 13, and 17; Table 1) and one case of group L (case 2). PJK developed 277.6 days (14-532), on average, after the surgery. PJK occurred 2 weeks after the surgery in the delirium case (case 17). Four of five PJK cases required the additional surgery to extend their instrumentation superiorly. Comparison of improvement ratio in clinical outcomes revealed no significant differences between groups T and L, at one year after the surgery, in JOA score, VAS of leg pain, and ODI (p = 0.49, p = 0.69, and p = 0.7, respectively). However, group T tends to improve more in the magnitude of VAS of lumbar pain compared to group L (p = 0.067). JOA score improved from 16.9 points and 15.8 points (groups T and L), preoperatively on average to 25.3 and 25.2 at 1 year follow-up (p = 0.96) and 25.1 and 25.2 at final (p = 0.96) (Figure 2(a)). VAS of lumbar pain decreased from 64.8 mm and 43 mm preoperatively on average to 13.4 and 13.3 at 1 year follow-up (p = 0.99) and 16 and 4.8 at final (p = 0.13) (Figure 2(b)). VAS of leg pain improved from 44.3 and 44.3 preoperatively on average to 37.5 and 13.3 at 1 year follow-up (p = 0.23) and 8 and 12.3 at final (p = 0.77) (Figure 2(c)). ODI improved from 41.8 and 32 preoperatively on average to 22.8 and 16.8 at 1 year follow-up (p = 0.7) and 25.1 and 25.2 at final (p = 0.41) (Figure 2(d)).

3.2. Radiological Data. Improvement of spinal alignment revealed the advantage of long fusion compared to short fusion (Figure 3). On average, Cobb angle improved from 26.3° and 24.2° (group T and L) to 8.2° and 14° at one month after the surgery and 8.1 and 17.4 at one year (Figure 3(a)) (p < 0.01 and p< 0.01, respectively). C7PL-CSVL did not differ between the groups during the course (Figure 3(b)). Global sagittal balance investigated by the SVA changed from 92.6 mm and 93.2 mm to 40.9 mm and 94.4 mm at one month and 55.6 mm and 107 mm at one year (Figure 3(c)) (p < 0.01 and p< 0.01, respectively). SVA improved more in group T, Δ-53.5 mm, compared to group L, and Δ1.2 mm, at one month (p < 0.01). LL changed from 9.9° and 16.2° to 33.3°

TABLE 1: Case summaries.

Group	Case No.	age	sex	stage	XLIF levels	UIS	instrumented levels	PJK
Group L	1	77	F	1	0	L	L2-SAI	
	2	65	M	1	0	L	L2-SAI	+
	3	67	M	1	2	L	L2-5	
	4	77	F	1	3	L	L2-5	
	5	75	F	1	2	L	L3-5	
Group T	6	78	M	1	0	T	T8-SAI	+
	7	72	F	1	0	T	T10-SAI	+
	8	81	M	1	0	T	T10-SAI	
	9	76	F	1	0	T	T10-SAI	
	10	76	F	2	2	T	T7-SAI	
	11	74	F	2	2	T	T8-SAI	
	12	73	F	2	3	T	T9-SAI	
	13	75	F	2	3	T	T10-SAI	+
	14	67	F	2	2	T	T9-SAI	
	15	74	F	2	3	T	T10-SAI	
	16	72	F	2	4	T	T9-SAI	
	17	69	F	2	2	T	T10-SAI	+
	18	79	F	2	3	T	T10-SAI	
	19	88	F	2	3	T	T10-SAI	
	20	76	F	2	3	T	T10-SAI	
	21	86	F	2	3	T	T10-SAI	

TABLE 2: Clinical and operative variables. BMI = Body Mass Index.

Variable	Group T	Group L	p Value
No. of cases	16	5	
age	76 (67-88)	72.2 (65-77)	0.24
BMI	22.3	23	0.74
Sex (M/F)	2/14	2/3	0.17
Operation time	404**	285	<0.01*
Intra-operative estimated blood loss	870	137	<0.01*
Post-operative hospitalization days	43.9	26.8	0.03*

* Statistically significant.
** In staged cases, time of second surgery was adopted.

and 19.4° at one month and 19.5° and 14.2° at one year. LL improved more in group T, Δ23.3°, compared to group L, and Δ3.2°, at one month (Figure 3(d)) ($p < 0.01$). Similarly, PI-LL changed from 42.6 and 33.2 to 20.7 and 30 at one month, 22 and 35.2 at one year, improved more in group T, Δ-23.5, compared to group L, Δ-3.2°, at one month (Figure 3(e)) ($p < 0.01$). PT did not differ between the groups during the course (Figure 3(f)). Disc lordosis was the most acquired in XLIF compared to TLIF and PLF ($p < 0.01$) and maintained till one year (Figure 4) ($p < 0.01$).

Four cases in group T and one case in group L developed PJK after the surgery. In group T, patients were divided into PJK and non-PJK group and were compared. Four cases of PJK had larger SVA (82.5 versus 50.2 mm, $p = 0.11$), whereas other parameters did not reach significance. One case in group L had the largest SVA.

4. Case

Eighty-six-year-old female (case no. 21) received staged spinal corrective surgery on her ASD (Figures 5(a) and 5(b)). XLIF was performed on L2/3,3/4,4/5 with 2 hours 29 min., estimated bleeding of 30 ml. Eight days later, open posterior surgery was conducted from T10 to S2 level with 7 hours and 27 min., estimated bleeding of 1100ml. Postoperative hospitalization days were 64 days. Clinical outcomes improved in

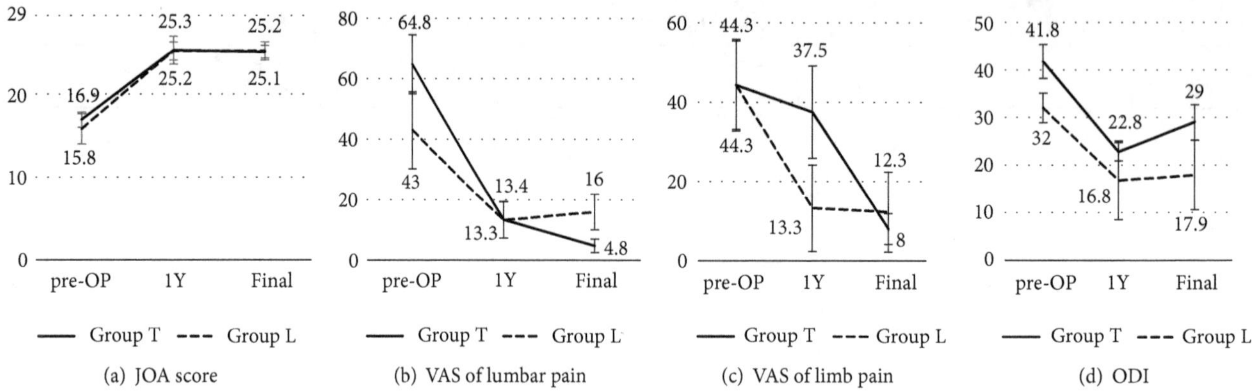

FIGURE 2: Mean values of clinical outcomes at preoperative, 1 year after the surgery and final follow-up of (a) JOA score, (b) VAS of lumbar pain, (c) VAS of limb pain, and (d) ODI. JOA, Japanese Orthopedic Association; VAS, Visual Analog Scale; ODI, Oswestry Disability Index.

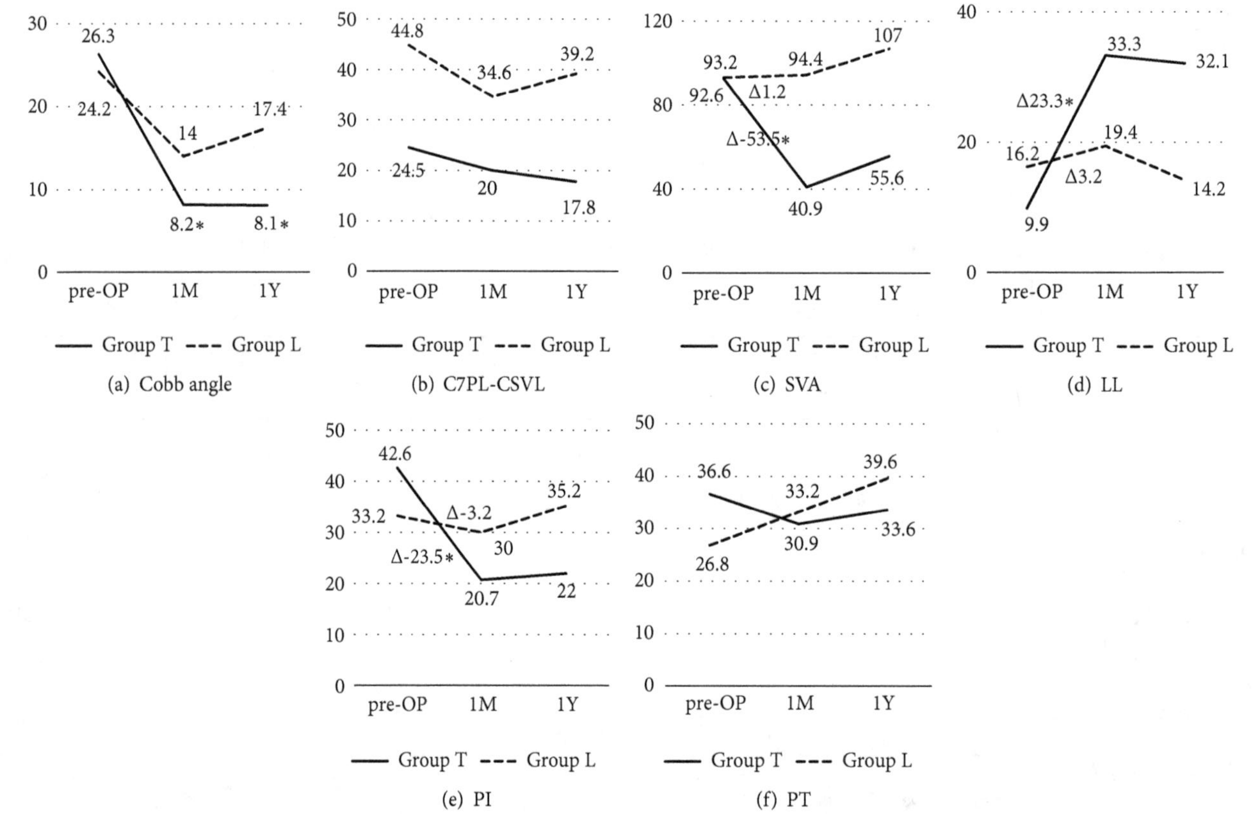

FIGURE 3: Mean values of radiological measurements at preoperative, 1 month after the surgery and 1 year of (a) Cobb angle, (b) C7PL-CSVL= C7 plum line, central sacral vertical line, (c) SVA = Sagittal vertical axis, (d) LL = lumbar lordosis, and (e) PI = Pelvic incidence. (f) PT = pelvic tilt. ∗ Difference is significant compared to group L.

magnitude of JOA score, VAS of lumbar pain and leg pain, ODI from 23, 64.8, 44.3, and 41.8, preoperatively to 23, 46, and 37, and no data at one month after the surgery, 25, 12, 20, and 17.8 at one year, respectively (Table 3(a)). C7PL-CSVL improved from 62 mm to 3 mm at one month after the surgery and 2 mm at one year. SVA decreased from 119 mm to 12 mm at one month after the surgery and 11 mm at one year (Table 3(b)). Cobb angle improved from 29° to 4° at one month after the surgery and 8° at one year. LL increased from 4° to 42° at one month and 45° at one year. In consequence, PI-LL improved from 50 to 12 at one month and 9 at one year. PT did not change during the course, from 24° to 21° at one month after the surgery and 27° at one year (Table 3(b)).

5. Discussion

ASD are associated with broad range of clinical and radiological findings such as progressive spinal deformity, chronic

TABLE 3: Clinical scores and alignment parameters of case no. 21.

(a)

Clinical scores	pre-OP	1 M	1 Y
JOA score	19	23	25
VAS of lumbar pain	69	46	12
VAS of leg pain	51	37	20
ODI	33.3	-	17.8

(b)

Alignment parameters	pre-OP	1 M	1 Y
C7PL-CSVL	62	3	2
SVA	119	12	11
Cobb angle	29	4	8
LL	4	42	45
PT	24	21	27
PI-LL	50	12	9

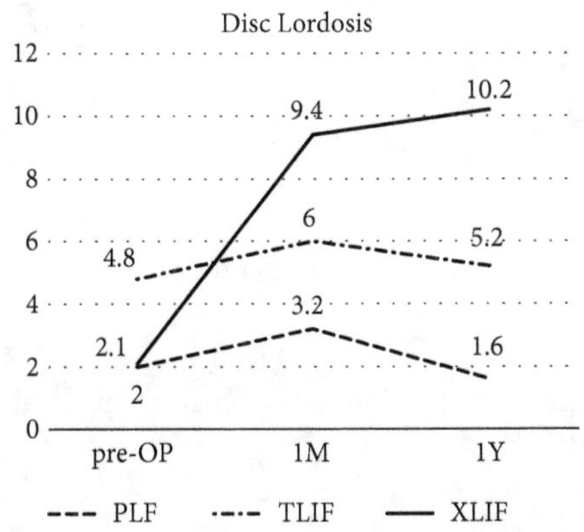

FIGURE 4: Disc lordosis before operation, 1 month after the surgery, and 1 year.

back pain, and neurological symptoms. Previous studies have shown the spinal sagittal alignment and global balance is essential for patients QOL [9, 10, 12, 13]. To achieve proper spinopelvic alignment in the ASD patients, some of operative interventions require more surgical burden for the patient and more technical and physical demand on the spine surgeons. For advanced ASD, posterior-only procedure usually requires high volume osteotomies. Instead of osteotomies, anterior procedure predominantly utilized the disc space to reconstruct spinal alignment that also has large surgical burden [3]. Recently introduced XLIF [4] can be alternative to the anterior procedure. Combined with XLIF and posterior correction and instrumentation, favorable clinical outcomes have been reported [12, 14, 15]. XLIF use the dedicated retractor which requires smaller incision than open anterior procedure and approach from lateral, abdominal, retroperitoneal, transpsoas approach to lateral portion of the intervertebral disc. Surgical field is bright with light source so that retroperitoneal organs and psoas are visible and surgeon can carefully approach the lateral aspect of the disc without bleeding or damaging vital organs. In this manner, XLIF extremely reduced surgical burden compared to the conventional anterior procedure. In addition to reduction of surgical burden, XLIF demonstrates strong ability to reconstruct the deformity on intervertebral space [5]. It restores disc height and indirectly decompression spinal canal. Previous studies have reported XLIF is effective for coronal correction and only mild effect on improvement of sagittal alignment [16, 17]. Therefore, we perform conventional open surgery for posterior procedure to acquire adequate sagittal alignment. Sagittal correction is enhanced using facet osteotomies, rod rotation [7], and cantilever bending technique [8]. Open conventional procedure requires a decent amount of surgical burden that the long fusion needs to consider for their application on the ASD patients with complications. According to our comparison study, group T had longer operation time, intraoperative estimated blood loss, and longer postoperative hospital stay (Table 2). As expected, this result indicated that surgical burden was higher in group T.

It is known that sagittal balance is the most important and reliable radiographic predictor for clinical outcomes [13]. Schwab established the threshold value for the proper spinopelvic alignment in ASD patients, SVA less than 5 cm, PT less than 25°, and PI-LL under 10 [13]. In the current study, improvement of spinal alignments was better in group T compared to group L (Table 3). In group L, the SVA has not changed between before and after; rather it worsened little whereas LL increased after surgery. This might be because the thoracic kyphosis exceeded improved LL. These results indicate that the long fusion is required to achieve adequate sagittal alignment. However, most of the spinal parameters in group T did not satisfy the threshold value of sagittal balance. Correction of coronal deformity is also important in ASD patients. Cobb angle improved in both groups, where group T achieved better correction at one month and one year follow-up. Current study showed correction of Cobb angle was identical to previous report [18]. C7PL-CSVL, however, did not improve to targeted threshold [19]. These insufficient corrections may be because the age of patient of this study was high and bone quality could not tolerate the correction. The other factor for the substandard of the threshold can be the technical issues. For the earlier patients, the rod rotation [7] and cantilever bending technique [8] were not applied, where correction may be inadequate. After these techniques are introduced in combination with Ponte osteotomy and XLIF, postoperative spinal alignment improved compared to previous cases (Figure 5). In addition, disc lordosis was most acquired in the XLIF than TLIF or PLF that XLIFs are performed on many disc spaces as possible (Figure 4). In three cases in group T, Bendini spinal rod bending system was applied for rod bending. This system will save surgeon from the stress of rod bending. Time for rod bending, alignment assessment, and complication such as rod failure needs to be investigated in future.

JOA and some of patients-based outcomes are not significantly different as the spinal parameters. In this study, JOA score is collected by the operators that may cause the bias. Importantly, VAS of lumbar pain improved better in group T compared to group L at the final follow-up, which was parallel to improvement of spinal alignment (Figure 2(b)).

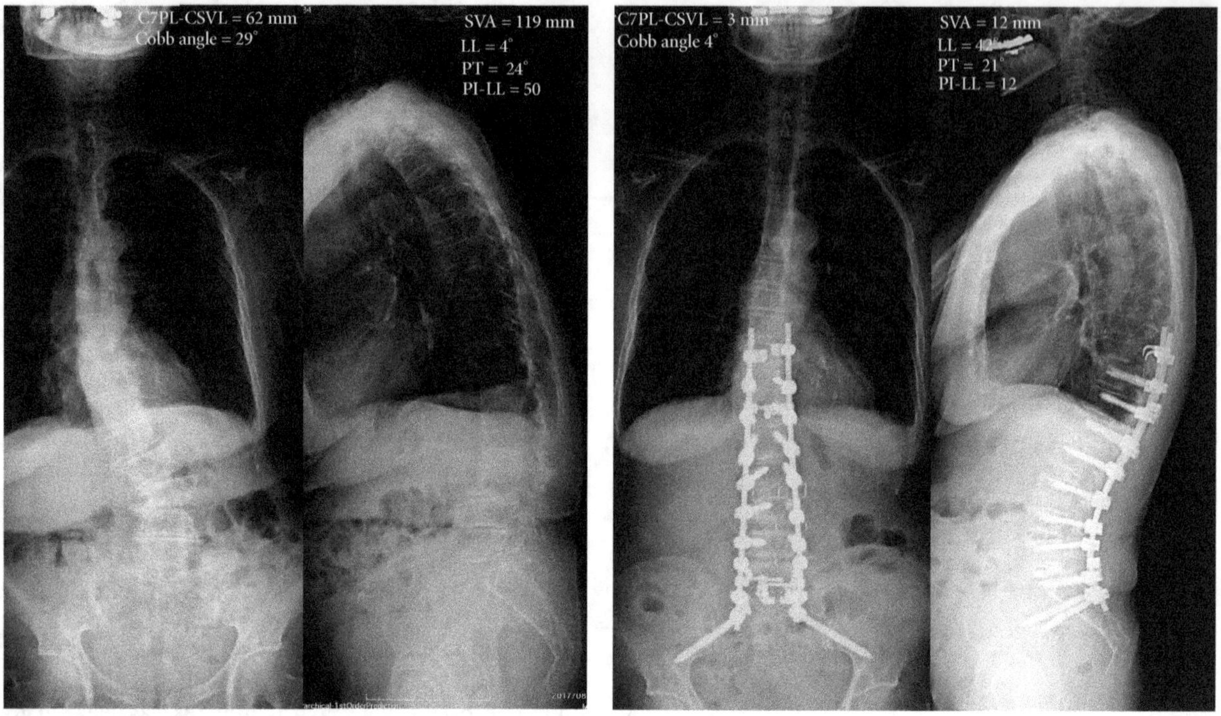

(a) (b)

FIGURE 5: Before and after images of total spine of the case. The after images were 1 month after the surgery.

The complication rate was 38%, and there were no mortalities related to the procedure. Seven out of 16 cases developed complications in group T and 1 case out of 5 in group L. Although it was not significantly high, group T seems to have more complications compared to group L. Three cases developed PE in our series (14.3%). The ratio was higher than previous report [18, 20]. After compression stockings and intermittent pneumatic compression device were adopted for precaution during the surgery, no symptomatic PE case was observed. The ratio of PJK was lower in current series (28.3%) [11, 21, 22]. It is known that LL change more than 30° is the risk for PJK [22]. Therefore, lower PJK ratio can be our moderate correction of LL. However, large SVA was found as a risk factor for PJK. These results indicated optimal spinal alignment is required for favorable postoperative clinical outcomes. Further clinical study is required to understand optimal spinal alignment. Additionally, wearing hard corset for more than a year after the surgery might help to avoid PJK.

5.1. Study Limitation. This was the retrospective study and the limitation in this study is selection bias and incomplete data. And the number of cases was small to describe conclusion. In future, prospective study with large number of the patients will provide sufficient data to assess defined study.

5.2. Conclusion. Current study elucidated that to acquire harmonious spinal alignment and favorable clinical outcomes, long fusion is better than short fusion. XLIF demonstrated strong ability to reconstruct the deformity on intervertebral space that is better to apply as much as possible. For the ASD patients with complications, short fusion can be one of the options [10].

Acknowledgments

Current study was performed with the funding support of Nippon Koukan Hospital.

References

[1] M. Aebi, "The adult scoliosis," *European Spine Journal*, vol. 14, no. 10, pp. 925–948, 2005.

[2] I. G. Dorward and L. G. Lenke, "Osteotomies in the posterior-only treatment of complex adult spinal deformity: a comparative review," *Neurosurgical Focus*, vol. 28, no. 3, pp. 1–10, 2010.

[3] I. G. Dorward, L. G. Lenke, K. H. Bridwell et al., "Transforaminal versus anterior lumbar interbody fusion in long deformity constructs: a matched cohort analysis," *The Spine Journal*, vol. 38, no. 12, pp. E755–E762, 2013.

[4] B. M. Ozgur, H. E. Aryan, L. Pimenta, and W. R. Taylor, "Extreme lateral interbody fusion (XLIF): a novel surgical technique for anterior lumbar interbody fusion," *The Spine Journal*, vol. 6, no. 4, pp. 435–443, 2006.

[5] A. M. Caputo, K. W. Michael, T. M. Chapman Jr. et al., "Clinical outcomes of extreme lateral interbody fusion in the treatment of adult degenerative scoliosis," *The Scientific World Journal*, vol. 2012, Article ID 680643, 5 pages, 2012.

[6] A. Jain, J. T. Brooks, K. M. Kebaish, and P. D. Sponseller, "Sacral alar iliac fixation for spine deformity," *JBJS Essential Surgical Techniques*, vol. 6, no. 1, article no e10, 2016.

[7] A. Matsumura, T. Namikawa, M. Kato et al., "Posterior corrective surgery with a multilevel transforaminal lumbar interbody fusion and a rod rotation maneuver for patients with degenerative lumbar kyphoscoliosis," *Journal of Neurosurgery: Spine*, vol. 26, no. 2, pp. 150–157, 2017.

[8] K.-W. Chang, "Cantilever bending technique for treatment of large and rigid scoliosis," *The Spine Journal*, vol. 28, no. 21, pp. 2452–2458, 2003.

[9] F. J. Schwab, V. A. Smith, M. Biserni, L. Gamez, J.-P. C. Farcy, and M. Pagala, "Adult scoliosis: a quantitative radiographic and clinical analysis," *The Spine Journal*, vol. 27, no. 4, pp. 387–392, 2002.

[10] B. Blondel, A. M. Wickman, A. Apazidis, V. C. Lafage, F. J. Schwab, and J. A. Bendo, "Selection of fusion levels in adults with spinal deformity: an update," *The Spine Journal*, vol. 13, no. 4, pp. 464–474, 2013.

[11] T. Ohba, S. Ebata, H. Oba, K. Koyama, and H. Haro, "Correlation between postoperative distribution of lordosis and reciprocal progression of thoracic kyphosis and occurrence of proximal junctional kyphosis following surgery for adult spinal deformity," *Clinical Spine Surgery*, vol. 31, no. 9, pp. E466–E472, 2018.

[12] H. Taneichi, "Update on pathology and surgical treatment for adult spinal deformity," *Journal of Orthopaedic Science*, vol. 21, no. 2, pp. 116–123, 2016.

[13] F. Schwab, A. Patel, B. Ungar, J.-P. Farcy, and V. Lafage, "Adult spinal deformity-postoperative standing imbalance: how much can you tolerate? an overview of key parameters in assessing alignment and planning corrective surgery," *The Spine Journal*, vol. 35, no. 25, pp. 2224–2231, 2010.

[14] N. Anand, E. M. Baron, G. Thaiyananthan, K. Khalsa, and T. B. Goldstein, "Minimally invasive multilevel percutaneous correction and fusion for adult lumbar degenerative scoliosis: a technique and feasibility study," *Journal of Spinal Disorders & Techniques*, vol. 21, no. 7, pp. 459–467, 2008.

[15] M. Y. Wang and P. V. Mummaneni, "Minimally invasive surgery for thoracolumbar spinal deformity: initial clinical experience with clinical and radiographic outcomes," *Neurosurgical Focus*, vol. 28, no. 3, article E9, 2010.

[16] F. L. Acosta Jr., J. Liu, N. Slimack, D. Moller, R. Fessler, and T. Koski, "Changes in coronal and sagittal plane alignment following minimally invasive direct lateral interbody fusion for the treatment of degenerative lumbar disease in adults: a radiographic study," *Journal of Neurosurgery: Spine*, vol. 15, no. 1, pp. 92–96, 2011.

[17] G. Costanzo, C. Zoccali, P. Maykowski, C. M. Walter, J. Skoch, and A. A. Baaj, "The role of minimally invasive lateral lumbar interbody fusion in sagittal balance correction and spinal deformity," *European Spine Journal*, vol. 23, supplement 6, pp. S699–S704, 2014.

[18] S. J. Lewis, S. G. Keshen, S. Kato, T. E. Dear, and A. M. Gazendam, "Risk factors for postoperative coronal balance in adult spinal deformity surgery," *Global Spine Journal*, vol. 8, no. 7, pp. 690–697, 2018.

[19] H. Koller, C. Pfanz, O. Meier et al., "Factors influencing radiographic and clinical outcomes in adult scoliosis surgery: a study of 448 European patients," *European Spine Journal*, vol. 25, no. 2, pp. 532–548, 2016.

[20] H. J. Kim, S. Iyer, B. G. Diebo et al., "Clinically significant thromboembolic disease in adult spinal deformity surgery: incidence and risk factors in 737 patients," *Global Spine Journal*, vol. 8, no. 3, pp. 224–230, 2018.

[21] Y. Ha, K. Maruo, L. Racine et al., "Proximal junctional kyphosis and clinical outcomes in adult spinal deformity surgery with fusion from the thoracic spine to the sacrum: a comparison of proximal and distal upper instrumented vertebrae," *Journal of Neurosurgery: Spine*, vol. 19, no. 3, pp. 360–369, 2013.

[22] T. Yasuda, T. Hasegawa, Y. Yamato et al., "Proximal junctional kyphosis in adult spinal deformity with long spinal fusion from T9/T10 to the ilium," *Journal of Spine Surgery*, vol. 3, no. 2, pp. 204–211, 2017.

20

Sacral Anatomical Orientation in the Lebanese Population

Joseph Maalouly,[1] Fouad Jabbour,[1] Elias Saidy,[1] Georgio Lati,[1] Gerard El-Hajj,[2] Dany Aouad,[1] Rami Ayoubi,[1] and Alexandre Nehme[1]

[1]*Department of Orthopedic Surgery and Traumatology, Saint George Hospital University Medical Center, Balamand University, P.O. Box 166378, Achrafieh, Beirut 1100 2807, Lebanon*
[2]*Department of Radiology, Saint George Hospital University Medical Center, Balamand University, P.O. Box 166378, Achrafieh, Beirut 1100 2807, Lebanon*

Correspondence should be addressed to Joseph Maalouly; josephmaalouly2@gmail.com

Academic Editor: Benjamin Blondel

Introduction. PI is currently used as the gold standard measurement in spinopelvic anatomy. There is a need for a reliable method to calculate sacral anatomic orientation (SAO) independent of posture and to establish its association with PI, which was previously established in a single study (Peleg et al., 2007). Therefore, the aim of our study is the application and verification of this association on a Lebanese sample. *Methods.* Methods for measuring SAO and PI on living individuals are described. The study was carried out on 200 adult individuals using CT 3D images (volume-rendering method). Reliability (intratester and intertester) was evaluated using the intraclass correlation test. A regression analysis was carried out to evaluate the association between the two measurements. *Results.* There were 103 females (51%) and 97 males (49%) with a mean age of 58.68 ± 19.6 years (min = 20; max = 93). The mean SAO and PI in our population were found to be 52.65° (SD = 8.16°) and 59.08° (SD = 12.53°), respectively. SAO and PI measurements were highly correlated (Pearson correlation test; $r = -0.296$, $P < 0.0001$ for our general population). PI can be predicted via SAO, i.e., SAO = $(-0.193 \times \text{PI}) + 64.057$. *Conclusions.* SAO may be an important tool, alongside PI, in defining the sagittal shape of the spine and useful for understanding its association with spinal diseases as they are not affected by postural changes.

1. Introduction

A previous study by Peleg et al. [1] has already established an association between SAO and PI. But, in order to correctly assess SAO or PI on individuals of different ancestry or from different populations, it is fundamental that the method be tested on the specific population one is working on. Therefore, the aim of the present study is the application and verification of the already described method of measuring SAO and its association with PI on a Lebanese population sample.

Pelvic orientation (PO) is considered a key factor in spinal shape and has been shown to significantly influence spino-pelvic balance in normal and pathologic conditions. This finding has important clinical and anthropologic implications and has fostered a renewed interest in the radiologic evaluation of PO. Usual parameters of its evaluation are sacral slope (SS), pelvic tilt (PT), and pelvic incidence (PI) [2, 3].

SS is defined as the angle created between a line running parallel to the superior surface of the first sacral vertebra and a horizontal line. PT is defined as the angle between the vertical line and the line joining the middle of the sacral endplate and the axis of the femoral heads. PI is defined as the angle between the line perpendicular to the sacral endplate at its midpoint and the line connecting this point to the joined axis of the femoral heads [4]: PI = SS + PT.

PI is the gold standard measurement, and it has been proven many times to correlate with spinal parameters like lumbar lordosis and thoracic kyphosis.

Increased PI and decreased pelvic lordosis were found in low-grade isthmic spondylolisthesis [4, 5]. In the past decade, extensive research was conducted on this subject, and PI and pelvic lordosis were found correlated with the severity of spondylolisthesis [6]. Recently, Mays [7] based on observation and measurements taken on the skeletal material concluded that high PI may have heightened the risk of developing pars interarticularis defects.

The advantage of PI over SS and PT is that its angular values are unaffected by posture. Its disadvantage is that individuals with similar SS may manifest different values of PI due to a different location of the sacrum within the pelvis and/or dissimilarity in the anteroposterior size of the superior surface of the first sacral vertebra. Moreover, as angles in both methods are measured from standing lateral radiographs, the angle obtained may be affected by the superimpositioning of anatomic structures, magnification of structures further from the film. Recently, CT scan with 3D reconstruction has become more widely available and is helpful in determining spinal pathology.

Those disadvantages and the clinical significance of those angles were behind the search for a new method to calculate sacral anatomic orientation (SAO) independent of posture and to establish the association between PI and SAO.

2. Materials and Methods

The study sample consisted of 200 randomly selected pelvic CTscans performed in the radiology department of Saint George Hospital, Beirut, Lebanon, between January 2006 and December 2007. All selected individuals were adults (>20 years) from Lebanese origin (verified by phone). Information on age and sex was recorded for every individual when the CT scan was done. Informed written consent was obtained from all patients. There were 103 females (51%) and 97 males (49%) with a mean age of 58.68 (SD = 19.6) years (min = 20; max = 93).

After acquisition of the data on a General Electric CT scan machine, with a thickness of cut of 1 to 3 mm, each set of data was copied on a CD for each individual and subsequently imported on a Sony Vaio laptop computer. Each examination was then opened using the Amira 4.1 volume rendering software. Every stack of images was imported through Amira and opened first as three orthogonal slices in the 3 spatial planes. This allows using the cropping module which narrows the region of interest to the pelvis excluding thus the lumbar spine and any additional artifact. An isosurface was then generated using the Amira 3D rendering module which allows obtaining a volumetric representation of the pelvis. 2D and 3D measurements of distances and angles were then carried on the buildup. All measurements were verified by three observers.

2.1. Measurement of SAO Angle. SAO is the angle created between the intersection of a line running parallel to the superior surface of the sacrum and a line running between the anterior superior iliac spine (ASIS) and the anterior-superior edge of the symphysis pubis (Figure 1, angle α). It was measured using Amira 4.1 using the following steps. Using the module isolines, a sagittal plane was created at the middle of the sacrum and perpendicular to the sacral plate. The pelvis was rotated until we obtained complete superimpositionning of both hemipelvises verified with the perfect alignment of both iliac crests and both anterior inferior iliac spines. The hemipelvis at the front was then cropped at the mid-sagittal isoline plane. This allowed exposure of the sacral plate and the drawing of a line running parallel to the superior surface of the sacrum, as well as another line running between the anterior superior iliac spine (ASIS) and the anterior-superior edge of the symphysis pubis. The 2D angle formed between those 2 lines was measured and recorded for each individual.

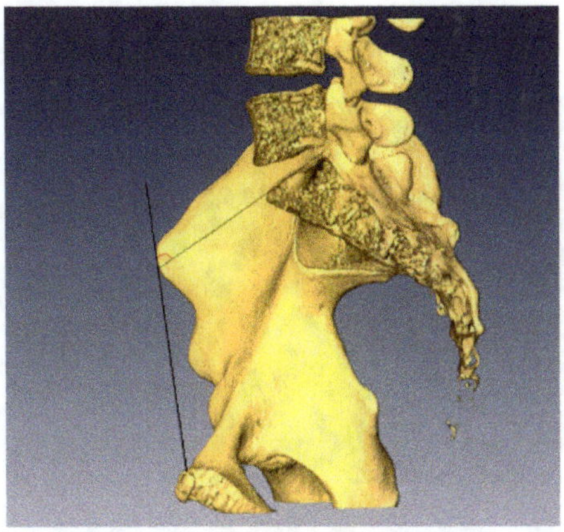

Figure 1: Sacral anatomic orientation.

2.2. Measurement of PI Angle. PI is defined as the angle between the line perpendicular to the sacral plate at its midpoint and the line connecting this point to the middle of the axis connecting the centers of both femoral heads (Figure 2). To be able to obtain exactly the line connecting the centers of both femoral heads, we used the intersection of two orthogonal planes (coronal and horizontal) cutting simultaneously both femoral heads into identical halves. The pelvis was then rotated until we obtained complete superimpositionning of both hemi pelvises, which allowed the projection of the line connecting the centers of both femoral heads as a single point. A line was then drawn on the sagittal plane to connect this point to the center of the sacral plate and also the perpendicular to the sacral plate at its midpoint. The 2D angle formed between those 2 lines was measured and recorded for each individual.

2.3. Statistical Analysis. In order to determine the association between SAO and PI, Pearson correlation analysis was done and then a linear regression analysis was carried out. The measurements were taken by one observer (AN – $n = 200$). The intraclass correlation coefficient was used to determine the intratester reliability of the measurements. An independent t-test was done between the spondylolisthesis group (grades 1 and 2) and the control group.

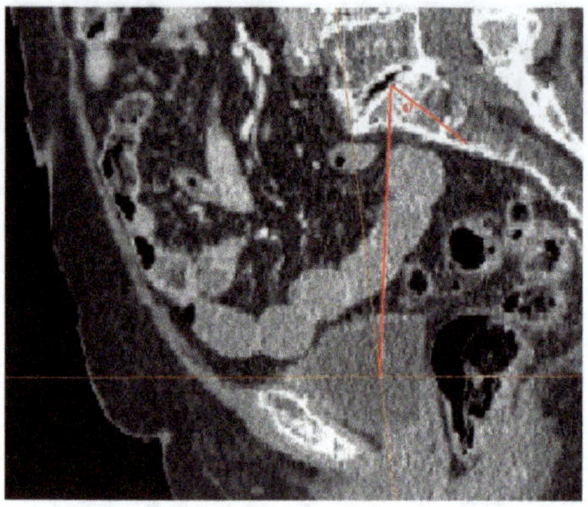

Figure 2: Pelvic incidence.

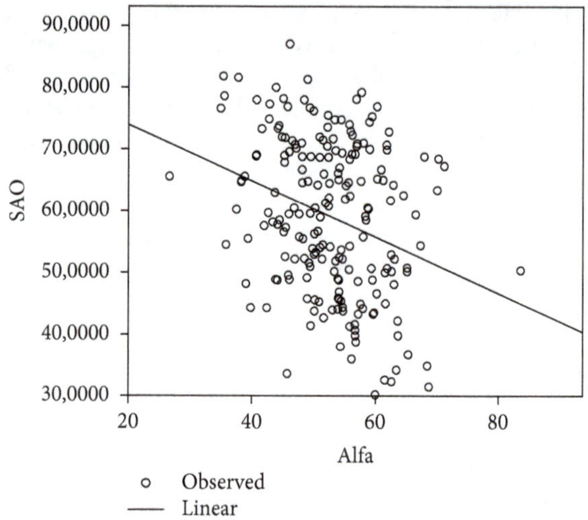

Figure 3: Association between PI (alfa) and SAO.

3. Results

3.1. SAO and PI Reliability

SAO. Reliability was high. Intraclass correlation coefficient for intratester reliability was 0.967 ($P < 0.001$). Intertester reliability was 0.89 ($P < 0.001$).

PI. Reliability was similarly high. Intraclass correlation coefficient for intratester reliability was 0.971 ($P < 0.001$). Intertester reliability was 0.82 ($P < 0.001$).

3.2. Assosciation between SAO and PI. SAO and PI were correlated (Figure 3) negatively with a pearson correlation coefficient $r = -0.296$ ($P < 0.0001$). PI and SAO can be deduced from each other according to the following formulas: $\text{SAO} = (-0.193 \times \text{PI}) + 64.057$; $\text{PI} = (-0.455 \times \text{SAO}) + 83.05$.

3.3. Comparison of SAO and PI Values between Spondylolisthesis Population and Control Group. The mean value of SAO is significantly lower in the spondylolisthesis group while the mean of PI is higher in the spondylolisthesis group (Table 1). The Student *t*-test, after assuming equal variances according to Levene's test, shows significant difference between the two groups for SAO (Table 2).

4. Discussion

The present study validates the described method for assessing SAO, based on the anatomic position of the human pelvis. SS and PT vary with posture and they are measured relative to a horizontal line and a vertical line, while SAO is measured relative to the ASIS-pubis line located in humans on the same coronal plane. Thus, it can be measured constantly despite postural change.

The finding that SAO is correlated with PI lends validity to the former as a measurement that takes into consideration not only the physiologic aspect of sacral orientation (measured relative to the axis of gravity), but also the anatomic ones. Today, PI is the main parameter measured for pelvic morphology and its association with spinopelvic alignment and spinal deformities [4]. Nonetheless, our findings show a negative correlation, an inverse linear curve, between SAO and PI in a significant part of the Lebanese adult population, and PI cannot be explained by SAO alone. To our knowledge, no such study was done using pelvis CT scans for comparison of SAO and PI and their correlation in a living Lebanese population.

Berthonnaud et al. [3], in a review of 160 asymptomatic adult volunteers, have shown that the pelvis and spine in the sagittal plane can be considered as a linear chain linking the head to the pelvis where the shape and orientation of each anatomical section is tightly connected and affects the neighboring section to preserve a stable posture with the least amount of energy expenditure. Changes in shape or orientation at one level will directly affect the adjacent segment. Knowledge of these normal relationships is of prime importance for the comprehension of the sagittal balance in normal and pathologic conditions of the spine and pelvis. The pelvic shape, which was quantified by the PI angle and now by the SAO angle, determines the position of the sacral end. The spine reacts to this position by changing the lumbar lordosis (LL) accordingly; the amount of lordosis increases as the SS increases to maintain the balance of the trunk in the upright position.

Thus, the decision as to which angle is more appropriate depends largely on the question asked. For example, issues relating to spinal malalignment could benefit from both parameters.

We speculate that in the etiology of spondylolysis and spondylolisthesis, pelvic incidence is a significant variable. By definition, a vertically oriented sacral endplate is associated with a high grade of pelvic incidence [8]. The vertical sacral endplate increases the shear forces acting across L5-S1 disc, which will cause increased traction on the L5 pars interarticularis. This, in turn, may break the pars under these conditions due to the traction effect. Therefore, slipping of the vertebra anteriorly will ensue. It has been demonstrated that increased slip angle, female sex, a vertical orientation of the L5-S1 intervertebral disc, and early age at the onset of symptoms are associated with progression of spondylolisthesis [9–11]. In our study, SAO decreases in the spondylisthesis group as opposed to the PI which increases

Table 1: Group statistics of SAO and PI between control and spondylolisthesis groups.

Group statistics	Spondylolisthesis	N	Mean	Std. deviation	Std. error mean
SAO	Yes	20	44.8944	8.71987	2.17997
	No	180	53.3404	7.72541	.57582
PI	Yes	20	62.9688	11.60263	2.90066
	No	180	58.7667	12.42240	.92591

Table 2: Student t-test and Levene's test for SAO and PI between control and spondylolisthesis groups.

	Levene's test for equality of variances						
	F	Sig.	T	df	Sig. (2-tailed)	Mean difference	Std. error difference
SAO							
Equal variances assumed	0.516	0.473	−4.147	198	0.000	−8.446	2.03660
Equal variances not assumed			−3.746	17.159	0.002	−8.4465	2.25473
PI							
Equal variances assumed	0.125	0.724	1.303	198	0.194	4.202	3.22466
Equal variances not assumed			1.380	18.197	0.184	4.202	3.04485

(Table 1). This further demonstrates the inverse relationship between the two parameters. In addition, a significant difference of SAO values between both groups was noticed by using the Student t-test (Table 2).

In contrast, there are less shear forces acting on the pars when the L5-S1 junction is oriented more horizontally, such as when the sacral slope is less than approximately 40° and lower pelvic incidence [8].

Although modifications in human posture do not affect the angular values of PI and SAO, the most significant distinction between the two measurements is that PI portrays pelvic morphology rather than pelvic orientation, while SAO defines both. Furthermore, SAO angle has an inverse linear relationship with PI [12].

Peleg et al.'s hypothesis is that the curves of the spine must adjust to the orientation of the sacrum's body [13]. In reality, this means that a horizontal sacrum results in an almost vertical orientation of the superior disk surface of S1. To cope with such an orientation of the disk surface; if a vertical spine is to be maintained, the lumbar lordosis must increase. Therefore, the more horizontally oriented the sacrum, the deeper the lordosis [13]. This, in turn, results in an increase in the lever arm of the lumbar extensors.

Several articles reported in the literature support the above hypothesis. For instance, it has been shown that the final segmental spinal alignment starts with increased lumbar lordosis in adolescence especially during growth spurt ages 13 to 15 accompanied by a more horizontally oriented sacrum [14]. Roussouly and Pinheiro-Franco [15] demonstrated that spinal curve shapes in adults are associated with PI grade. For example, an increase in lordosis is associated with a high PI.

The importance of these findings lies in emphasizing the role of sacral orientation in establishing normal spinal configuration. Once epiphyseal rings ossification is complete for the vertebral bodies (at 14–16 years of age), no more changes can occur [16]. Adolescent growth spurt studies show that anterior vertebral development exceeds posterior vertebral growth, leading to reduced thoracic kyphosis and increased lumbar lordosis [14, 17, 18].

As we now know, the benefit of using PI and SAO is that their values are unaffected by posture. The main drawback from using PI is that certain individuals with similar SS values may have different values of PI due to a variable location of the sacrum within the pelvis with the possible addition of dissimilarity in the anteroposterior size of the superior surface of the first sacral vertebra. Furthermore, as angles in both methods are usually measured from standing lateral radiographs, the angle obtained can be affected by the overlap of anatomic structures, magnification of structures further from the film. In our series, the measurements of PI and SAO were made on CT scan with 3D reconstruction which benefits from the precision associated with the imaging modality chosen [19–21].

5. Conclusion

To sum up, we think that there is a connection between spinal alignment and sacral orientation as demonstrated by the inverse linear curve, similar to Peleg et al. This demonstrates that SAO changes with PI and it can be used across different populations. According to our data and the literature review, it is the orientation of the sacrum that helps dictate the shape of the spine. Therefore, a combination of both PI and SAO, as both parameters are not affected by postural changes, help in gaining a thorough understanding of the spino-pelvic pathologies, including spondylolisthesis. Further studies are warranted for proving the correlation between SAO, lumbar lordosis, and thoracic kyphosis, which has been proven for PI.

Abbreviations

PO: Pelvic orientation

SAO: Sacral anatomical orientation
PI: Pelvic incidence
PT: Pelvic tilt
SS: Sacral slope
CT: Computed tomography
ASIS: Anterior superior iliac spine
LL: Lumbar lordosis.

Additional Points

Limitaions. This is a retrospective study, using only pelvis CT scan of 200 patients for assessment of spinopelvic parameters.

Authors' Contributions

Dr. Alexandre Nehme conceptualized this research project.

Acknowledgments

Data were imported to the software used in this article with the help of Saint George Hospital University Medical center, Beirut.

References

[1] S. Peleg, G. Dar, N. Steinberg, N. Peled, I. Hershkovitz, and Y. Masharawi, "Sacral orientation revisited," *Spine*, vol. 32, no. 15, pp. E397–E404, 2007.

[2] G. Vaz, P. Roussouly, E. Berthonnaud, and J. Dimnet, "Sagittal morphology and equilibrium of pelvis and spine," *European Spine Journal*, vol. 11, no. 1, pp. 80–87, 2002.

[3] E. Berthonnaud, J. S. Dimnet, P. Roussouly, and H. Labelle, "Analysis of the sagittal balance of the spine and pelvis using shape and orientation parameters," *Journal of Spinal Disorders & Techniques*, vol. 18, no. 1, pp. 40–47, 2005.

[4] J. Legaye, G. Duval-Beaupère, C. Marty, and J. Hecquet, "Pelvic incidence: a fundamental pelvic parameter for three-dimensional regulation of spinal sagittal curves," *European Spine Journal*, vol. 7, no. 2, pp. 99–103, 1998.

[5] C. Marty, B. Boisaubert, H. Descamps et al., "The sagittal anatomy of the sacrum among young adults, infants, and spondylolisthesis patients," *European Spine Journal*, vol. 11, no. 2, pp. 119–125, 2002.

[6] C. Boulay, C. Tardieu, J. Hecquet et al., "Sagittal alignment of spine and pelvis regulated by pelvic incidence: standard values and prediction of lordosis," *European Spine Journal*, vol. 15, no. 4, pp. 415–422, 2006.

[7] S. Mays, "Spondylolysis, spondylolisthesis, and lumbo-sacral morphology in a medieval English skeletal population," *American Journal of Physical Anthropology*, vol. 131, no. 3, pp. 352–362, 2006.

[8] P. Roussouly, S. Gollogly, E. Berthonnaud, H. Labelle, and M. Weidenbaum, "Sagittal alignment of the spine and pelvis in the presence of L5-S1 isthmic lysis and low-grade spondylolisthesis," *Spine*, vol. 31, no. 21, pp. 2484–2490, 2006.

[9] L. J. Grobler, P. A. Robertson, J. E. Novotny, and M. H. Pope, "Etiology of spondylolisthesis," *Spine*, vol. 18, no. 1, pp. 80–91, 1993.

[10] R. N. Hensinger, "Spondylolysis and spondylolisthesis in children and adolescents," *The Journal of Bone & Joint Surgery*, vol. 71, no. 7, pp. 1098–1107, 1989.

[11] T. Ikata, R. Miyake, S. Katoh, T. Morita, and M. Murase, "Pathogenesis of sports-related spondylolisthesis in adolescents," *The American Journal of Sports Medicine*, vol. 24, no. 1, pp. 94–98, 1996.

[12] S. Peleg, G. Dar, B. Medlej et al., "Orientation of the human sacrum: anthropological perspectives and methodological approaches," *American Journal of Physical Anthropology*, vol. 133, no. 3, pp. 967–977, 2007.

[13] S. Peleg, G. Dar, N. Steinberg, Y. Masharawi, and I. Hershkovitz, "Sacral orientation and Scheuermann's kyphosis," *SpringerPlus*, vol. 5, pp. 1–9, 2016.

[14] A. Cil, M. Yazici, A. Uzumcugil et al., "The evolution of sagittal segmental alignment of the spine during childhood," *Spine*, vol. 30, pp. 93–100, 2004.

[15] P. Roussouly and J. L. Pinheiro-Franco, "Biomechanical analysis of the spinopelvic organization and adaptation in pathology," *European Spine Journal*, vol. 20, no. 5, pp. 609–618, 2011.

[16] E. M. Bick and J. W. Copel, "The ring apophysis of the human vertebra," *The Journal of Bone & Joint Surgery*, vol. 33, no. 3, pp. 783–787, 1951.

[17] J.-M. Mac-Thiong, H. Labelle, E. Berthonnaud, R. R. Betz, and P. Roussouly, "Sagittal spinopelvic balance in normal children and adolescents," *European Spine Journal*, vol. 16, no. 2, pp. 227–234, 2007.

[18] S. Pasha, A. P. Sangole, C.-E. Aubin, S. Parent, J.-M. Mac-Thiong, and H. Labelle, "Characterizing pelvis dynamics in adolescent with idiopathic scoliosis," *Spine*, vol. 35, no. 17, pp. E820–E826, 2010.

[19] R. C. Brink, L. Vavruch, T. P. C. Schlösser et al., "Three-dimensional pelvic incidence is much higher in (thoraco) lumbar scoliosis than in controls," *European Spine Journal*, vol. 28, no. 3, pp. 544–550, 2019.

[20] H.-F. Chen, J. Mi, H.-H. Zhang, and C.-Q. Zhao, "Pelvic incidence measurement using a computed tomography data-based three-dimensional pelvic model," *Journal of Orthopaedic Surgery and Research*, vol. 14, no. 1, p. 13, 2019.

[21] C.-H. Jeon, K.-S. Kwack, S. Park, H.-D. Lee, and N.-S. Chung, "Combination of whole-spine lateral radiograph and lateral scanogram in the assessment of global sagittal balance," *The Spine Journal*, vol. 18, no. 2, pp. 255–260, 2018.

21

Prospective, Multicenter Evaluation of a Polyherbal Supplement alongside Standard-of-Care Treatment for Mild Knee Osteoarthritis

Zbigniew Żęgota[1] **Joanna Goździk**[2] **and Joanna Głogowska-Szeląg**[2,3]

[1]*Zbigniew Żęgota Specjalistyczny Ośrodek Leczniczo-Badawczy, Ostróda, Poland*
[2]*Silmedic Ltd., Katowice, Poland*
[3]*Department of Pathophysiology and Endocrinology, Medical University of Silesia, Zabrze, Poland*

Correspondence should be addressed to Joanna Głogowska-Szeląg; a.ruksztо@iestat.pl

Academic Editor: Paulo Adriano Schwingel

Background. This study aimed to provide clinical information on general and joint performance from individuals taking Tregocel® (containing curcuminoid and extracts of the herbs *Harpagophytum procumbens*, *Boswellia serrata*, *Apium graveolens*, and *Zingiber officinale*) alongside a standard therapy of symptomatic mild knee osteoarthritis (OA). *Methods.* This was a multicenter, open-label, prospective, single-arm study, in which Tregocel® was supplemented for 36 weeks. Participants with symptomatic mild knee OA requiring pharmacologic treatment for pain were enrolled. Physical performance (6-minute walk test, WOMAC-pain and functional domain, and heel-thigh distance flexion test), general performance (WOMAC questionnaire), and VAS (Visual Analogue Scale) assessment of knee pain, as well as anti-inflammatory and analgesic medication consumption, were assessed. *Results.* Between January and April 2019, 107 participants were enrolled and analysed in per protocol population. Mean age was 59.7 (SD 10.8) years, and there were 68.2% women. Mean observation time was 291.1 (SD 7.7) days. Mean increase in 6MWT result observed at the end of the study was 26.0 (SD 30.4) m ($p < 0.001$). Median VAS score decreased from 60.0 (IQR 50–72) mm at the beginning of the study to 21.0 (IQR 14–30) mm after 36 weeks of product administration ($p < 0.001$). Regular knee OA medications were taken in 99.1% of subjects at baseline decreasing to 55.1% at the end of the Tregocel® supplementation. *Conclusions.* During Tregocel® supplementation, participants observed improved functional capacity confirmed in the distance in 6MWT and in the heel-thigh distance flexion test, decreased level of pain, and improved WOMAC scores for all domains.

1. Introduction

Osteoarthritis (OA) is the predominant form of arthritis and often hands, knees, feet, and hips are involved. Pain is the main symptom that leads people to present to healthcare providers with a subsequent diagnosis of OA. Data modelling from the 2017 Global Burden of Disease study estimated that there were about 303.1 million (95% CI 273.3 to 338.6 million) prevalent cases of hip and knee OA, with a 9.3% increase from 1990 to 2017 [1].

The lifetime risk of developing knee OA is estimated at about 46% [2], with an incidence that increases with age and affects more women than men. Symptomatic knee OA rates increase rapidly around 50 years of age and then level off after the age of 70 [3].

The rapid increase in OA prevalence results in a growing impact and major challenges for healthcare systems. This is very true when we realize that OA is frequently associated with disturbed sleep, depression, increased sedentary behaviour, less physical activity, obesity, and polypharmacy, leading to decreased quality of life and overall physical and mental performance. Currently, treatment of OA varies widely from lifestyle changes (e.g., weight reduction with exercise and diet), physical aids (e.g., canes or braces), physical therapies, and medications including acetaminophen, nonsteroidal anti-inflammatory drugs (NSAIDs), corticosteroids, and/or complementary and alternative medicines (CAMs) [4–7].

A proprietary form of CAM developed in Australia, called Tregocel®, is a herbal composite supplement that may provide supportive benefits to standard therapy for OA. It contains a patented curcuminoid preparation and extracts of the herbs *Harpagophytum procumbens*, *Boswellia serrata*, *Apium graveolens*, and *Zingiber officinale*. Curcumin is an active phenolic compound found in turmeric (*Curcuma longa*). In Tregocel® curcumin is incorporated into a phospholipid complex (also trademarked as Meriva®), which was shown to be 29-fold more absorbed than the natural, unformulated curcuminoids [8]. It also contains an extract of *Harpagophytum procumbens*, with a few active ingredients including harpagoside as the primary one. Tregocel® also contains an extract of *Boswellia serrata*, in which boswellic acids are primary active constituents. *Apium graveolens* (celery) seeds are another component, which contain volatile oils such limonene and selinene, flavonoid compounds, and celeroside glucosides and phthalide glycosides, as well as aromatic and lignin glucosides. Finally, Tregocel® contains an extract of *Zingiber officinale* (ginger) with main phytochemicals such as phenols (gingerol, shogaols, and paradols), diarylheptanoids, gingerdiols, and sesquiterpenes [9].

Natural therapies involving supplementation with curcuminoids, boswellic acids, ginger, harpagosides, and luteolin (a type of flavonoid compound of celery) have been demonstrated to support pain relief and physical performance in OA. However, until now, these substances have not been evaluated clinically in a single dosage form or in the specific combination used in Tregocel® [10].

This study aimed to provide clinical information on general and joint performance from individuals taking Tregocel® as a dietary supplement in addition to standard therapies for symptomatic mild knee OA.

2. Materials and Methods

2.1. Study Design and Study Population. This was a multicenter, open-label, prospective, single-arm study which included a 1-week screening/run-in period, followed by 36 weeks of diet supplementation and a 4-week follow-up period after the last dose of supplementation. Five clinic visits were performed: baseline (visit 1), after 12 weeks (visit 5), after 24 weeks (visit 9), after 36 weeks (visit 13), and visit 14–4 weeks after the end of supplementation (additionally there were 9 remote visits). The study population consisted of participants with symptomatic mild knee OA requiring pharmacologic treatment for pain and meeting the following requirements at baseline: (1) presence of pain in the target knee at least half of the days in the past month (target knee was defined as the one with worse pain; if both knees presented the same level of pain, then the right knee was defined as the target knee); (2) maximal pain score ≥ 30 on a 100 mm VAS (Visual Analogue Scale) at screening and confirmed at baseline, and (3) use of pain killers as required (PRN) within the preceding month on at least 10 days (including at least 2 days in run-in period). After enrolment, both PRN treatment and regular OA treatment were able to be adjusted by an investigator to suit participant needs. Detailed inclusion and exclusion criteria are presented in Supplementary Table 1. During the study, patients were allowed to take acetaminophen (paracetamol) or NSAIDs. The following substances were prohibited: systemic steroids, intra-articular injections, glucosamine, chondroitin sulfate, diacerein, avocado/soya extracts, or other forms of herbal, vitamin, mineral, amino acid or related supplements.

2.2. Study Product. Subjects enrolled into the study received Tregocel® supplementation in an open-label fashion. After enrolment at the baseline visit, 2 tablets of Tregocel® were taken once daily with or after meals, for a duration of 36 weeks. The daily dose was equivalent to 1 g of curcuminoid-phospholipid complex, which is the primary active ingredient. Each Tregocel® film coated tablet contains curcuma phospholipid (500 mg; equiv. curcumin 90 mg), *Boswellia serrata* (Indian frankincense) gum oleoresin extract (500 mg; equiv. boswellic acids–81.25 g), *Harpagophytum procumbens* (devil's claw) tuber (500 mg), *Apium graveolens* (celery) seed (500 mg), and *Zingiber officinale* (ginger) rhizome (165 mg).

2.3. Study Objectives. The primary study objective was to assess physical performance with 6-minute walk test (6MWT) in participants with symptomatic mild knee OA taking standard therapy with Tregocel® supplementation. The secondary objectives were to assess perception of pain, general performance, the need for standard pharmacological treatment, and the safety profile of Tregocel®.

2.4. Study Assessments and Procedures. Subjects with OA involving other joints were allowed, and providing pain in the target knee was the most predominant OA symptom, with no expected impact of pain in other OA locations on the primary outcome measure. Data from the subject medical history, including ongoing treatment and/or therapies and medications, were gathered. Osteoarthritis severity was assessed based on Kellgren–Lawrence classification (grades 0–4). Pain perception was assessed using a VAS scale, where 0 represented "no pain," and 100 represented "extreme pain." Subjects rated the perception of maximal pain during the last 24 hours on a daily basis and at clinic visits. For physical performance, 6-minute walk test (6MWT) and heel-thigh distance flexion test were performed during clinic visits, based on recording of the distance covered (in meters) during 6 minutes of walking in a straight line. In heel-thigh distance flexion tests, the investigator evaluated the angle and distance between heel and thigh at maximum knee flexion, in both supine and prone positions. For assessment of physical and general performance, the Western Ontario and McMaster Universities Osteoarthritis Index (WOMAC) questionnaire was also used. WOMAC is a widely used, proprietary health status questionnaire used to evaluate the condition of patients with OA of the knee and hip, including pain (5 items), stiffness (2 items), and physical functioning (17 items). The translated and validated Polish version of the WOMAC (VAS-based) was used in this study, with permission from Prof Nicholas Bellamy, University of Queensland, Herston, Australia (copyright holder, http://www.womac.org).

Vital signs were measured after 5 minutes of rest and included temperature, systolic and diastolic blood pressure, and heart rate. Additionally, standard clinical laboratory tests were performed as follows: haematology (red blood cell count [RBC], white blood cell count [WBC], haemoglobin, haematocrit, and platelets count), chemistry (aspartate aminotransferase [AST], alanine aminotransferase [ALT], total bilirubin, phosphates, creatinine, sodium, and potassium), C-reactive protein as an inflammation parameter, and urinalysis.

2.5. Statistics. A sample size of 150 was calculated as sufficient to determine a statistically significant mean difference of approximately 30% of standard deviation, assuming use of paired Student's t-test, at a significance level $\alpha = 0.05$ and power of 90%. Continuous data are presented as mean and standard deviation (SD) for normally distributed variables and median with 1st and 3rd quartiles in case of nonnormally distributed variables. Categorical data are presented as numbers and percentages. Distribution of categorical variables was compared between time points using McNemar's test. The distribution of continuous variables was first evaluated with the Shapiro-Wilk test, then the normally distributed variables were compared between two time points using the paired Student's t-test; otherwise, the Wilcoxon test for paired data was used. To assess time effect on efficacy measure values in repeated measures design in case of analysing more than two time points, Skillings-Mack test was applied. The significance level was set at $\alpha = 0.05$. Two-sided tests were used. Statistical analyses were performed with the statistical package R, version 3.4.1 (R Foundation for Statistical Computing, Vienna, Austria).

2.6. Ethical Consideration. The study conformed to the STROBE statement for reporting of observational studies. Local Ethics Committee in Wroclaw (Poland) approved the study (No 08/03/2018). The study was conducted in accordance with the Declaration of Helsinki. It was registered at ClinicalTrials.gov (NCT03636035).

3. Results

3.1. Study Population. Between January and April 2019, a total number of 151 participants were screened across 8 different investigation sites across Poland. Of those screened, 137 were enrolled, with 107 participants completing the 36-week Tregocel® intervention. This group was subsequently analysed as the per protocol population. The study flowchart is presented in Figure 1. Mean observation time was 291.1 ± 7.7 days. The mean age was 59.7 ± 10.8 years, and there were 68.2% ($n = 73$) of women in the study population, with right knee in 62.6% ($n = 67$) identified as the target knee. The median duration of OA was 1.8 [1.2, 4.6] years (min 0.4, max 17.7 years). The distribution of knee OA severity as per Kellgren–Lawrence classification was found to be as follows: class 0–4.7%, class 1–50.5%, and class 2–44.9%. Detailed dataset characteristics are presented in Table 1. Of the compliant individuals (98.1% of the per protocol group), compliance was equal to or greater than 94.5%.

3.2. Physical and Global Performance. The primary endpoint was to assess physical performance with 6MWT in subjects with symptomatic mild knee OA taking standard therapy with Tregocel® supplementation. At baseline, the mean 6MWT result was 382.8 ± 88.1 m, and at the end of the study was 408.8 ± 96.3 m. The difference of 26.0 ± 30.4 m was statistically significant ($p < 0.001$, Student's t-test) (Figure 2).

Regarding heel-thigh distance flexion test, distances (supine and prone) were significantly improved from visit V5 comparing to baseline V1, with further differences observed also at visits V9 and V13 ($p < 0.001$, Skillings-Mack test) (Figure 3). Supine and distance angle values did not significantly change in time.

WOMAC scores assessed before the 6MWT in all domains (pain, stiffness, physical function, and total) had improved progressively throughout the study. The scores on the subsequent visits statistically significantly decreased in time ($p < 0.001$ for all WOMAC scores, Skillings-Mack test). The level of decrease was the greatest on V5 (about 50% in all domains) and continued to improve in subsequent visits (Figure 4).

3.3. Pain Assessment and Concomitant Medications. With the duration of the study, subjective pain levels significantly decreased from baseline [60.0 (IQR 50.0–72.0) at V1] to 37.0 (IQR 24.5–51.5) at V5, 27.0 (IQR 19.0–39.0) at V9 and 21.0 (IQR 14.0–30.0) at V13 ($p < 0.001$, Skillings-Mack test). The overall decrease was statistically significant and the value at the end of the study stood at approximately 30% of baseline pain scores (Figure 5).

As a consequence, the decrease in the administration of regular knee OA medications was also observed. At baseline, 99.1% of patients regularly took anti-inflammatory/analgesic drugs, whereas this progressively declined after 12 weeks (V5, 76.6%), 24 weeks (V9, 69.2%), and 36 weeks (V13, 55.1%).

3.4. Safety Conclusions. All patients who received at least one dose of Tregocel® were included in the safety analysis; therefore, the safety population counted 137 participants.

A total number of 32 AEs (adverse events) were reported in 25 (23.4%) subjects, including one (0.7%) SAE (serious adverse event). The SAE was associated with a right knee injury, and not related to the study product. In 25% of AEs, concomitant therapy was initiated; in 15.6%, supplement suspension/discontinuation was ordered; in 21.9%, other actions were taken; and in 37.5%, no actions were required to be taken. No vital signs or lab test abnormalities were found except for mild and transient increase in AST/ALT. A listing of all AEs is provided in Table 2.

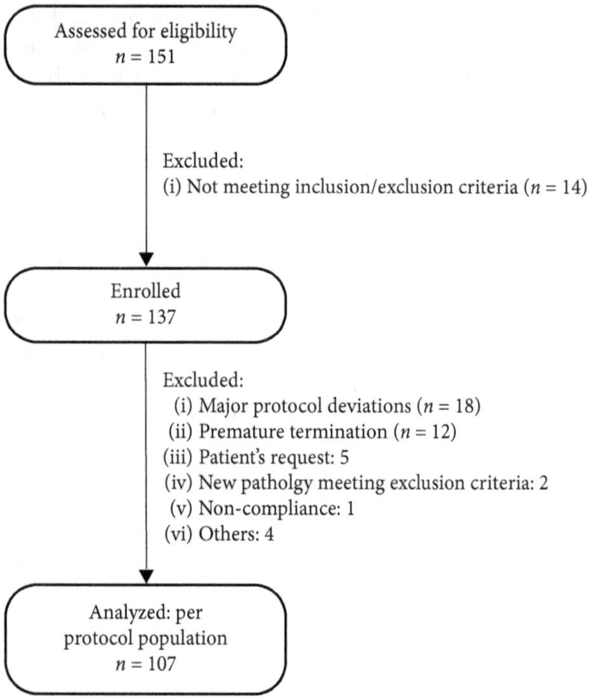

Figure 1: Study flowchart.

Table 1: Baseline characteristics.

Parameter	Value
Demographics	
Mean age, mean (SD)	59.7 ± 10.8
Female, n (%)	73 (68.2)
Race – Caucasians, n (%)	107 (100)
Vital signs	
Weight (kg), mean (SD)	74.97 ± 11.97
Height (m), mean (SD)	1.66 ± 0.1
BMI (kg/m^2), mean (SD)	27.12 ± 3.51
Sitting pulse (beats/min), mean (SD)	70.6 ± 6.8
Systolic blood pressure (mm Hg), mean (SD)	129 ± 9
Diastolic blood pressure (mm Hg), mean (SD)	78.7 ± 7.5
Knee osteoarthritis	
Duration (years), median (IQR)	1.81 (1.16, 4.58)
Mean observation time (days), mean (SD)	291.1 ± 7.7
Target knee	
Right, n (%)	67 (62.6)
Left, n (%)	40 (37.4)
Kellgren–Lawrence classification: n (%)	
0	5 (4.7)
1	54 (50.5)
2	48 (44.9)
3	0
4	0
Treatment: n (%)	
Anti-inflammatory/analgesic drugs	106 (99.1)
Physiotherapy	27 (25.2)
Orthopaedic supply	1 (0.7)

4. Discussion

This was the first study to evaluate the safety and efficacy of the polyherbal product, Tregocel®, given as a dietary supplement in parallel with standard medications for mild knee osteoarthritis. Subjects in the per protocol group displayed improved functional capacity, confirmed in the distance in 6MWT and in the heel-thigh distance flexion test, decreased level of pain (VAS scale), and improvements in all WOMAC domains. These differences were observed as early as after 12 weeks of supplementation and improved even further with maximal effect at 36 weeks. Moreover, Tregocel® supplementation was characterized by a favourable safety profile.

With population aging, the problem of osteoarthritis will continue to grow, with the knee being one of the most common joints prone to injury. And this might predispose to osteoarthritis even more. Suter et al. [11] projected the cumulative incidence of symptomatic knee OA requiring total knee repair in the following scenarios: no prevalent or incident injury; isolated anterior acute ligament tear, surgically treated; isolated anterior acute ligament tear, nonoperatively treated; or a prevalent history or surgically treated anterior acute ligament and meniscal tear. The authors observed that the estimated lifetime risk of symptomatic knee OA was 34% for patients with an anterior acute ligament injury and meniscal tear, compared to 14% for the no-injury cohort. Anterior acute ligament injury without meniscal tear was associated with a lifetime risk of knee OA between 16% and 17%. Moreover, subjects in the anterior acute ligament injury and meniscal tear cohort developed OA approximately 1.5 years earlier (55.7 vs. 57.1) than patients without knee injuries. These results prompted us to investigate dietary supplements aimed to preserve knee joint health and function.

The results of this study with Tregocel® (improvement in walking distance, pain reduction, and improved general performance) were consistent with the observations of previous clinical studies involving the curcuminoids-phytosome complex used in the formulation [8, 12]. Curcuminoids are of special interest mostly due to unique properties of curcumin, which has been shown to downregulate the expression of matrix metalloproteinase-3 in OA. They also display antioxidant activity, which is associated with amelioration of joint tissue damage. As a result, curcumin has the potential to restrain inflammation and tissue damage in OA [13, 14].

Recently, Shep et al. [15] compared curcumin with diclofenac in patients with knee OA. One hundred and thirty-nine patients with knee OA were randomized to receive a curcumin 500-mg capsule three times daily or a diclofenac 50-mg tablet two times daily for one month. At days 14 and 28, patients receiving curcumin showed comparable betterment in pain severity and in Knee Injury and Osteoarthritis Outcome Score (KOOS) values, when compared with diclofenac. However, at day 7, patients in the curcumin group experienced a significantly larger increase in the number of episodes of flatulence compared with diclofenac ($p < 0.01$). At the end of the study, a weight-lowering effect ($p < 0.01$) and antiulcer effect ($p < 0.01$) of curcumin were registered. In the curcumin group, no patients required H_2 blockers, and 19 patients in the diclofenac group (0% vs. 28%, respectively; $p < 0.01$). Moreover, adverse effects overall were significantly less frequent in the

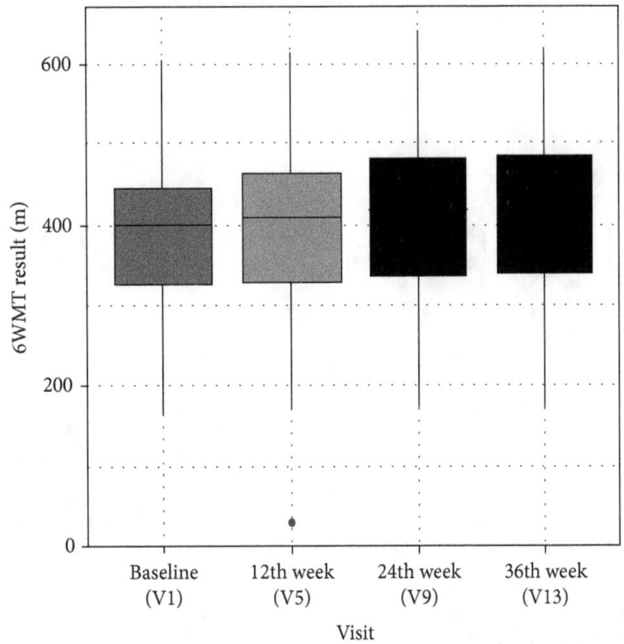

FIGURE 2: Results of 6-minute walk test (6MWT) at visit 1, visit 5 (after 12 weeks), visit 9 (after 24 weeks), and visit 13 (after 36 weeks).

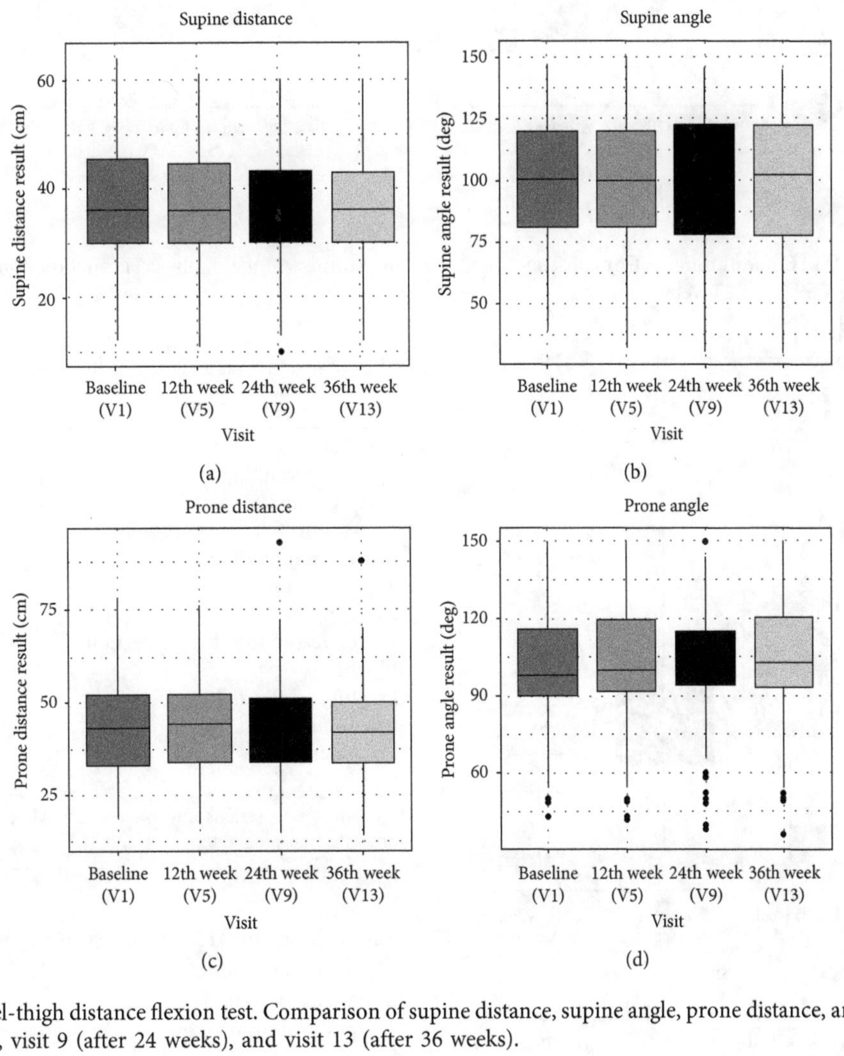

FIGURE 3: Results of heel-thigh distance flexion test. Comparison of supine distance, supine angle, prone distance, and prone angle at visit 1, visit 5 (after 12 weeks), visit 9 (after 24 weeks), and visit 13 (after 36 weeks).

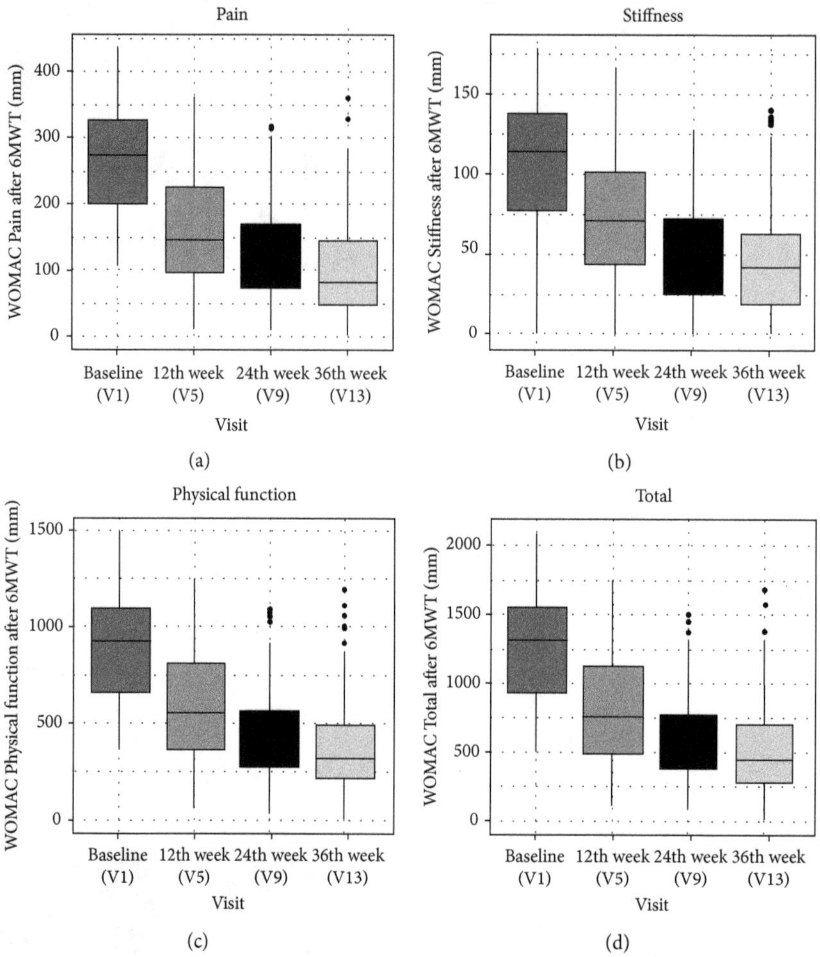

FIGURE 4: Results of WOMAC questionnaire. Comparison of pain domain, stiffness domain, physical function domain, and total at visit 1, visit 5 (after 12 weeks), visit 9 (after 24 weeks), and visit 13 (after 36 weeks). Results are presented as median with interquartile range (IQR).

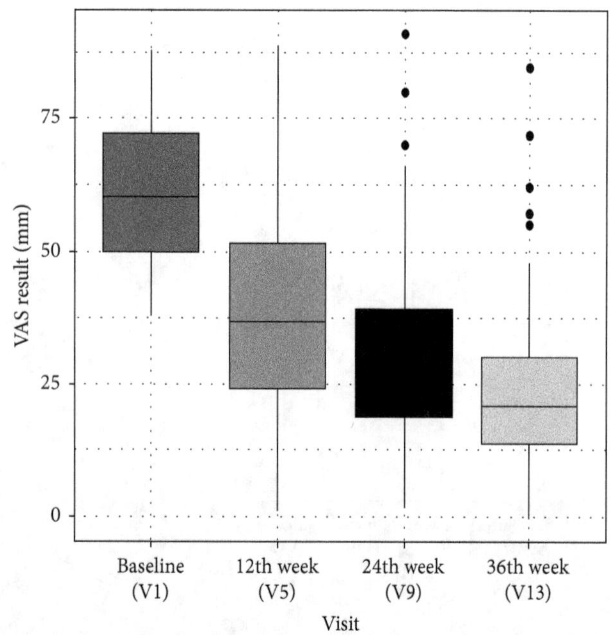

FIGURE 5: Pain assessment in VAS scale at visit 1, visit 5 (after 12 weeks), visit 9 (after 24 weeks), and visit 13 (after 36 weeks). Results are presented as median with interquartile range (IQR).

TABLE 2: Adverse events in the safety population ($n = 137$).

Adverse event	N (%) $N = 32$
Anemia	6 (4.4)
Diarrhea/vomiting	4 (2.9)
AST/ALT increase	4 (2.9)
Increase in C-reactive protein	3 (2.2)
Muscle stiffness/numbness	3 (2.2)
Stomach pain	3 (2.2)
Knee injury	2* (1.6)
Upper respiratory tract infection	2 (1.6)
Bloating	1 (0.7)
Fracture of the right upper limb	1 (0.7)
Leg swelling	1 (0.7)
Leucopenia	1 (0.7)
Sciatica	1 (0.7)

*Including one serious adverse event. ALT: alanine transaminase; AST: aspartate transaminase;

curcumin group (13% vs. 38%; $p < 0.01$). Other studies also confirmed the beneficial use of curcuminoids in knee OA management [16, 17].

In a systematic review, Onakpoya et al. [18] investigated the efficacy of curcuminoids administered orally in OA. The authors included seven studies with a total number of 797 patients with primarily knee OA. Compared with placebo, the use of curcuminoids significantly decreased knee pain ($p = 0.001$) and improved quality of life ($p < 0.001$). Curcuminoid use was also associated with significant improvements in WOMAC total scores as well as with significant reductions in the use of rescue medication. No SAEs were reported.

Haroyan et al. [19] proved that curcuminoid complex extract from turmeric rhizome with turmeric volatile oil, combined with an extract of boswellic acids, performed better than placebo in physical performance tests and the WOMAC joint pain index, while when only the curcuminoid complex extract was used, it was more effective than placebo only in terms of physical performance tests. A further meta-analysis by Bannuru et al. [20] confirmed that curcuminoids and *Boswellia* formulations might pose a valuable additive to the knee OA treatment regimens. They effectively relieve pain symptoms and simultaneously reduce safety risks.

Recently, there was published an interesting study aimed to understand whether any pharmacokinetic interactions are among the major constituents of *Boswellia serrata* extract, curcumin, pine bark extract, and methylsulfonylmethane so as to provide information when considering the combination use of these supplements. The pharmacokinetics of each constituent was characterized, and there were no significant differences in the pharmacokinetic profiles of the constituents when administered as a combination, relative to the constituents when administered alone [21].

Safety analysis of Tregocel® supplementation was also favourable. There were 32 registered AEs (affected 23.4% of population) and they were reported, including one SAE (affected 0.7% of population). No deaths were reported. Only seven of the AEs were determined by the investigators to be related to the study product. Also, the increase in AST/ALT levels was transient and in the opinion of investigators was also not related to the study product.

Although this was the first clinical study to evaluate Tregocel® supplementation in OA, there are two main limitations. The first is the lack of a control group for comparison, and the second is the potential influence of concomitant drugs (e.g., NSAID) on the observed effects. While the use of standard medications had decreased during the course of the study, future randomized, placebo-controlled trials combined with regression analyses would be required to confirm the observed effects of Tregocel® on OA symptoms.

This was the first study with the use of dietary supplement Tregocel® in subjects with mild knee osteoarthritis. During Tregocel® supplementation (36 weeks), subjects observed improved functional capacity confirmed in the distance in 6MWT and in the heel-thigh distance flexion test, decreased level of pain (VAS scale), and improved general performance (WOMAC score). These differences were observed as early as after 12 weeks of supplementation and improved even further with maximal effect at 36 weeks. Tregocel® supplementation also characterized a favourable safety profile. The results are encouraging and warrant verification in a randomized placebo-controlled study.

Authors' Contributions

All authors contributed to the analysis plan and the interpretation of the results, and all reviewed the final submitted manuscript.

Acknowledgments

The authors thank Jacek Bil, MD, PhD, for providing medical writing support in accordance with Good Publication Practice (GPP3) guidelines (http://www.ismpp.org/gpp3). This study was funded by Max Biocare, South Yarra, Australia, and Max Biocare Pty. Ltd., Melbourne, Australia.

References

[1] S. Safiri, A. A. Kolahi, E. Smith et al., "Global, regional and national burden of osteoarthritis 1990-2017: a systematic analysis of the Global Burden of Disease Study 2017," *Annals of the Rheumatic Diseases*, vol. 79, no. 6, pp. 819–828, 2020.

[2] E. Losina, A. M. Weinstein, W. M. Reichmann et al., "Lifetime risk and age at diagnosis of symptomatic knee osteoarthritis in the US," *Arthritis Care & Research*, vol. 65, no. 5, pp. 703–711, 2013.

[3] Y. Zhang and J. M. Jordan, "Epidemiology of osteoarthritis," *Clinics in Geriatric Medicine*, vol. 26, no. 3, pp. 355–369, 2010.

[4] J. Sokolove and C. M. Lepus, "Role of inflammation in the pathogenesis of osteoarthritis: latest findings and interpretations," *Therapeutic Advances in Musculoskeletal Disease*, vol. 5, no. 2, pp. 77–94, 2013.

[5] M. S. M. Persson, J. Stocks, G. Varadi et al., "Predicting response to topical non-steroidal anti-inflammatory drugs in osteoarthritis: an individual patient data meta-analysis of randomized controlled trials," *Rheumatology*, vol. 59, no. 9, pp. 2207–2216, 2020.

[6] N. Kakatum, P. Pinsornsak, P. Kanokkangsadal, B. Ooraikul, and A. Itharat, "Efficacy and safety of sahastara remedy extract capsule in primary knee osteoarthritis: a randomized double-blinded active-controlled trial," *Evidence-Based Complementary and Alternative Medicine*, vol. 2021, Article ID 6635148, 10 pages, 2021.

[7] H. R. Farpour, F. Estakhri, M. Zakeri, and R. Parvin, "Efficacy of piroxicam mesotherapy in treatment of knee osteoarthritis: a randomized clinical trial," *Evidence-Based Complementary and Alternative Medicine*, vol. 2020, Article ID 6940741, 8 pages, 2020.

[8] G. Belcaro, M. R. Cesarone, M. Dugall et al., "Product-evaluation registry of Meriva(R), a curcumin-phosphatidylcholine complex, for the complementary management of osteoarthritis," *Panminerva Medica*, vol. 52, no. 2 Suppl 1, pp. 55–62, 2010.

[9] A. Al-Nahain, R. Jahan, and M. Rahmatullah, "Zingiber officinale: A potential plant against rheumatoid Arthritis," *Arthritis*, vol. 2014, Article ID 159089, 8 pages, 2014.

[10] K. V. Peddada, K. V. Peddada, S. K. Shukla, A. Mishra, and V. Verma, "Role of curcumin in common musculoskeletal disorders: a review of current laboratory, translational, and clinical data," *Orthopaedic Surgery*, vol. 7, no. 3, pp. 222–231, 2015.

[11] L. G. Suter, S. R. Smith, J. N. Katz et al., "Projecting lifetime risk of symptomatic knee osteoarthritis and total knee replacement in individuals sustaining a complete anterior cruciate ligament tear in early adulthood," *Arthritis Care & Research*, vol. 69, no. 2, pp. 201–208, 2017.

[12] G. Belcaro, M. R. Cesarone, M. Dugall et al., "Efficacy and safety of Meriva(R), a curcumin-phosphatidylcholine complex, during extended administration in osteoarthritis patients," *Alternative Medicine Review*, vol. 15, no. 4, pp. 337–344, 2010.

[13] J.-J. Zeng, H.-D. Wang, Z.-W. Shen, X.-D. Yao, C.-J. Wu, and T. Pan, "Curcumin inhibits proliferation of synovial cells by downregulating expression of matrix metalloproteinase-3 in osteoarthritis," *Orthopaedic Surgery*, vol. 11, no. 1, pp. 117–125, 2019.

[14] R. S. Ahmad, M. B. Hussain, M. T. Sultan et al., "Biochemistry, safety, pharmacological activities, and clinical applications of turmeric: a mechanistic review," *Evidence-Based Complementary and Alternative Medicine*, vol. 2020, Article ID 7656919, 14 pages, 2020.

[15] D. Shep, C. Khanwelkar, P. Gade, and S. Karad, "Safety and efficacy of curcumin versus diclofenac in knee osteoarthritis: a randomized open-label parallel-arm study," *Trials*, vol. 20, no. 1, p. 214, 2019.

[16] K. Hashemzadeh, N. Davoudian, M. R. Jaafari, and Z. Mirfeizi, "The effect of nanocurcumin in improvement of knee osteoarthritis: a randomized clinical trial," *Current Rheumatology Reviews*, vol. 16, no. 2, pp. 158–164, 2020.

[17] Y. Panahi, A.-R. Rahimnia, M. Sharafi, G. Alishiri, A. Saburi, and A. Sahebkar, "Curcuminoid treatment for knee osteoarthritis: a randomized double-blind placebo-controlled trial," *Phytotherapy Research*, vol. 28, no. 11, pp. 1625–1631, 2014.

[18] I. J. Onakpoya, E. A. Spencer, R. Perera, and C. J. Heneghan, "Effectiveness of curcuminoids in the treatment of knee osteoarthritis: a systematic review and meta-analysis of randomized clinical trials," *International Journal of Rheumatic Diseases*, vol. 20, no. 4, pp. 420–433, 2017.

[19] A. Haroyan, V. Mukuchyan, N. Mkrtchyan et al., "Efficacy and safety of curcumin and its combination with boswellic acid in osteoarthritis: a comparative, randomized, double-blind, placebo-controlled study," *BMC Complementary and Alternative Medicine*, vol. 18, no. 1, p. 7, 2018.

[20] R. R. Bannuru, M. C. Osani, F. Al-Eid, and C. Wang, "Efficacy of curcumin and Boswellia for knee osteoarthritis: systematic review and meta-analysis," *Seminars in Arthritis and Rheumatism*, vol. 48, no. 3, pp. 416–429, 2018.

[21] X. Liu, D. J. Hunter, J. Eyles et al., "Pharmacokinetic assessment of constituents of Boswellia serrata, pine bark extracts, curcumin in combination including methylsulfonylmethane in healthy volunteers," *The Journal of Pharmacy and Pharmacology*, vol. 72, no. 1, pp. 121–131, 2020.

22

Swiss Orthopaedics Minimal Dataset: First Pilot Report of Reliability and Validity

Thorsten Jentzsch,[1] **Claudio Dora**,[2] **Urs Müller**,[3] **and Mazda Farshad**[1]

[1]*Department of Orthopedics, Balgrist University Hospital, University of Zurich, Zurich, Switzerland*
[2]*Swiss Orthopaedics, Bourg-en-Lavaux, Switzerland*
[3]*Onaxis Ltd, Bern, Switzerland*

Correspondence should be addressed to Thorsten Jentzsch; thorsten.jentzsch@gmail.com

Academic Editor: Andreas K. Demetriades

Background. The Swiss Orthopaedics Minimal Dataset (SOMD) was launched seven years ago. It is a standardized, generic, and patient-reported outcome questionnaire, comprising ten items (location of disease, pain within the past four weeks, limitations at work/leisure/sleep/autonomy, subjective value of a body part, employment status, work disability (sick leave/pension), and household support). We conducted this study about the SOMD to report its reliability, validity, and clinical applicability. *Methods.* A retrospective observational cohort study was conducted. The test-retest study population ($n = 60$; lost to follow-up: $n = 7$ (12%)) was drawn from three retirement homes (in 2013), while the test study population ($n = 14{,}180$; excluded (e.g., duplicates): $n = 1{,}990$ (14%)) consisted of patients from a university hospital (in 2014–2017). In the test-retest study population, the same questionnaire was completed twice (at days 0 and 7). In the test study population, only the first questionnaire was included (to avoid duplicates). In a subgroup of the test study population ($n = 302$), only those patients who completed the SOMD and Western Ontario and McMaster Universities Osteoarthritis Index (WOMAC) of the hip within 14 days were considered (to minimize recall bias). Reliability (test-retest and internal consistency), criterion validity for the item of pain, and return rates were analyzed. *Results.* The test-retest study population ($n = 53$) showed very high test-retest reliability for all tested items of the SOMD (intraclass correlation coefficient = 0.96–1.00 (95% confidence interval 0.93–1.00), $p < 0.001$). The test study population ($n = 12{,}190$) revealed good internal consistency reliability for all ten items (Cronbach's alpha = 0.80). The return rates of the SOMD were improvable (43% in 2016 and 31% in 2017). The subgroup of the test study population ($n = 302$) displayed a borderline acceptable criterion validity (correlation of the item of pain between SOMD and WOMAC hip: rho = 0.62, $p < 0.001$). *Conclusion.* This is the first report about the validation of the SOMD. A relatively high reliability (test-retest and internal consistency), borderline acceptable (criterion) validity for the item of pain, and improvable clinical implementation were observed. This analysis serves as the basis for a structured modification of the SOMD to improve its value.

1. Introduction

Health-related quality of life (HRQoL) describes the perceived well-being of individuals [1]. This can change over time (e.g., after treatment of disease). Accurate measurements (e.g., questionnaires) to detect this change are important not only for internal and external quality control but also for the evaluation of treatment success and costs. There are many questionnaires to choose from, but the gold standard remains elusive.

The Swiss Orthopaedics Minimal Dataset (SOMD) was introduced seven years ago, in 2013, as a measuring tool for HRQoL in order to assess the indications and results of all orthopaedic surgeries. It is a standardized, generic, and patient-reported outcome questionnaire. It consists of ten items: location of disease (only at one body part), pain within the past four weeks (score of 0–100), limitations at work/leisure/sleep/autonomy (0–100 each), subjective value of a body part (0–100), employment status (training, employed, and retired), work disability ((A) sick leave and (B) pension)

(0–100), and household support (0, <1, 1–2, 3–5, and >5 hours per day and a care assistant). The interpretation is based on a rating scale for each item without a single index value. It is free-of-charge, available in four languages (German, English, French, and Italian), accessible in electronic- and paper-based forms, and can be completed within five minutes. In our institution, it is used at first consultation and intermediate and final follow-ups.

The psychometric properties (i.e., reliability, validity, and sensitivity) of the SOMD have not been adequately provided yet. So far, only content validity (i.e., expert opinion) has been established. The reliability, criterion validity, and clinical implementation (i.e., return rate) remain unknown. Reliability is defined as the consistency of an item. It can be assessed with a test-retest method providing an intraclass correlation coefficient (ICC) and internal consistency across different items within a test providing Cronbach's alpha (α). Criterion validity describes the correlation between an item of a new questionnaire with the same item of an established questionnaire providing Spearman's rho. A well-established, reliable, and valid questionnaire for comparison with the SOMD is the Western Ontario and McMaster Universities Osteoarthritis Index (WOMAC), which was first described by Bellamy in a Master's thesis in 1982 [2–7]. It is one of the most commonly used questionnaires for the hip, available in around 100 languages, and consists of 24 questions about pain, stiffness, and daily activities. The item of pain refers to the last two days and different situations (walking, stairs, bed, sitting, and standing), which is particularly detail-oriented. Scoring is performed on a five-point (or level) Likert scale from none, over, and moderate to extreme.

We conducted the first study about the validation of the SOMD. The study hypothesis was that the SOMD is highly reliable, valid, and clinically applicable.

2. Methods

A retrospective observational cohort study was conducted. The cantonal ethics committee issued a waiver to allow this study with anonymous data without the need for informed consent (BASEC Request-Nr. 2018-00276).

The test-retest study population ($n = 60$) was drawn from retirement homes in 2013. The loss to follow-up was acceptable ($n = 7$ (12%)). The retirement homes offered assisted but autonomous living. After thorough instruction of individuals, the German version of the SOMD was completed twice, initially at day 0 and again at day 7. Two items, employment status and work disability (sick leave/pension), were not evaluated in this elderly study population.

The test study population ($n = 14{,}180$) consisted of all patients that filled out the questionnaire from a university hospital from April 2014 until December 2017. Only the first SOMD was considered. Duplicates and test questionnaires were excluded ($n = 1{,}990$ (14%)). Furthermore, a subgroup of the test study population was chosen, in which the WOMAC of the hip had also been completed within 14 days (to minimize recall bias) ($n = 302$).

Data were given as medians (interquartile range (IQR)). For the test-retest study population, the test-retest reliability (ICC (95% confidence interval (CI))) was calculated. For the test study population, the internal consistency (Cronbach's α of all ten items and item-rest correlations for each item), criterion validity (Spearman's correlation (rho) of the item of pain in the SOMD and WOMAC of the hip), and return rates were calculated. A scatterplot is provided for illustration. The significance level was set at $p < 0.05$. For a test-retest reliability test, it was previously suggested that a sample size of ≥46 individuals would be needed to measure an ICC of 0.9 with a power of 0.8 at a significance level of 5% [8]. For internal consistency, it was also suggested that a sample size of ≥300 individuals would be sufficient [9]. Both of our study populations surpassed these numbers. Stata (IC13.1; StataCorp, College Station, Texas, United States of America) was used for analysis.

3. Results

In the test-retest study population ($n = 53$), the median age was 75 (IQR 69–79) years. There were more females than males (females: $n = 34$ (57%) vs males: $n = 26$ (43%)). The scores for each item were moderate (e.g., pain: median = 50 (IQR 30–90)).

The test-retest reliability for all tested separate items of the SOMD was very high (e.g., pain: ICC = 1.00 (95% CI 1.00–1.00), $p < 0.001$) (Table 1). The best reliabilities were found for the items of pain, limitation at leisure and autonomy, subjective value of a body part, and household support (ICC = 1.00, each with CIs between 0.97 and 1.00).

In the test study population ($n = 12{,}190$), the median age was 49 years (IQR 35–61). There were less females than males (females: $n = 5{,}872$ (48%) and males: $n = 6{,}318$ (52%)). The scores for each item were moderate (e.g., pain: median = 50 (IQR 30–70)) (Table 2). The right side was most commonly affected (right: $n = 6{,}186$ (51%); left: $n = 4{,}615$ (38%); axial: $n = 1{,}376$ (11%); not applicable: $n = 13$ (0%)). The shoulder, knee, and foot were most commonly impaired (shoulder: $n = 2{,}390$ (20%); knee: $n = 2{,}348$ (20%); foot: $n = 1{,}969$ (17%); pelvis: $n = 1{,}393$ (11%); axial: $n = 1{,}376$ (11%); hand: $n = 664$ (5%); ankle: $n = 411$ (3%); hip: $n = 339$ (3%); elbow: $n = 253$ (2%); thigh: $n = 228$ (2%); calf: $n = 204$ (2%); wrist: $n = 359$ (3%); upper arm: $n = 156$ (1%); lower arm: $n = 87$ (0%); not applicable: 13 (0%)).

The internal consistency for all ten items was very high (Cronbach's $\alpha = 0.80$). The item-rest correlations were the lowest for employment status (0.18), work disability (sick leave (0.40), pension (0.24)), and household support (0.36). After the removal of these items from the calculation of the internal consistency, Cronbach's α increased to 0.85. The return rates of the SOMD were improvable (43% in 2016 and 31% in 2017).

TABLE 1: Descriptive data and test-retest reliability for the test-retest sample ($n = 60$).

Item	Test ($n = 60$) Median (IQR)	Retest ($n = 53$) Median (IQR)	ICC (95% CI)	P value*
Pain	50 (30–90)	60 (40–90)	1.00 (1.00–1.00)	<0.001
Work limitation	80 (25–100)	80 (40–100)	0.99 (0.99–1.00)	<0.001
Leisure limitation	50 (15–100)	60 (20–100)	1.00 (1.00–1.00)	<0.001
Sleep limitation	90 (25–100)	90 (40–100)	0.96 (0.93–0.98)	<0.001
Independence limitation	90 (25–100)	90 (50–100)	1.00 (0.97–0.99)	<0.001
Subjective body part value	70 (50–90)	70 (50–90)	1.00 (1.00–1.00)	<0.001

*F-test. IQR: interquartile range; ICC: intraclass correlation coefficient; %: percent; CI: confidence interval. Note: interpretation of intraclass correlation coefficient (ICC): 0.00–0.19 = very weak; 0.20–0.39 = weak; 0.40–0.59 = moderate; 0.60–0.79 = high; 0.80–1.00 = very high.

TABLE 2: Descriptive data for the test sample ($n = 12{,}190$).

Item	Median (IQR)
Pain	50 (30–70)
Work limitation	50 (20–70)
Leisure limitation	70 (50–90)
Sleep limitation	30 (10–60)
Independence limitation	20 (0–50)
Subjective body part value	50 (30–70)
Sick leave	10 (10–10)

IQR: interquartile range.

In the subgroup of the test study population ($n = 302$), the criterion validity for pain was borderline acceptable (correlation of the item of pain between the SOMD and WOMAC of the hip: rho = 0.62) (Figure 1).

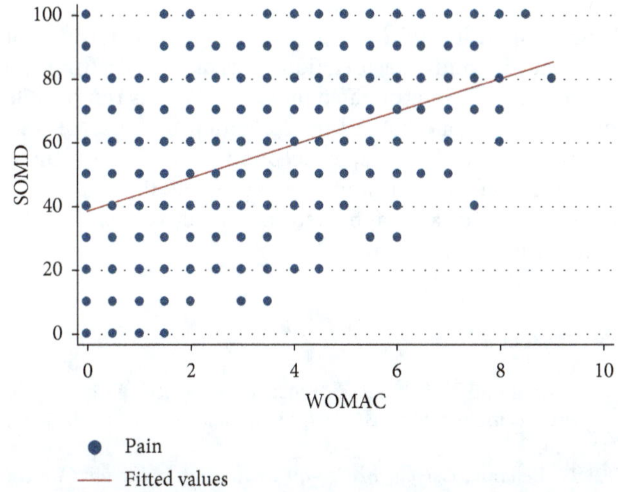

FIGURE 1: Item-rest correlations of all ten items of the test study population ($n = 302$).

4. Discussion

This is the first study reporting on the validation of the SOMD. Our findings show that the SOMD is highly reliable (i.e., very high test-retest reliability and internal consistency) but has borderline acceptable validity (i.e., correlation of the item of pain in the SOMD and WOMAC of the hip) and improvable clinical implementation (return rates).

Overall, the SOMD appears as a valid measurement tool for the quantification of a joint-specific HRQoL. However, several modifications are necessary for revised future versions. In general, improvement of reliability can be achieved with item homogeneity (i.e., identical minimum and maximum of different items) and item selectivity (i.e., substantial differences in minimum and maximum of a single item). For improved internal and external quality control of surgical indications and outcomes, economic analyses, and research, a highly validated questionnaire, such as the EuroQol 5-Items (EQ-5D) [10], should be integrated into the SOMD to allow calculation of a single index value and quality-adjusted life years (QALYs). The EQ-5D is a standardized, generic, self-reported, fast, generalized, and validated questionnaire. It is available in 120 languages, highly reliable and valid, and commonly used to measure HRQoL. The first version with three levels was designed in 1990 and its current form with five levels (no, slight, moderate, severe, and extreme) has been used since 2009. It allows the calculation of 3,125 (5^5) different HRQoL states. Using crosswalk links, a single index value and QALYs (0 = dead to 1 = perfect health) can be calculated [11]. Using population value sets, this permits utility analyses. Furthermore, questions from the validated Core Outcome Measures Index (COMI) questionnaire [12] could be added to quantify the joint-specific HRQoL and level of pain. Additionally, survey reports can vary according to the educational level [13], which should be quantified by an additional question. We have proposed a revised version of the SOMD, which was drafted by a subcommittee of the Swiss Orthopaedics Panel of Quality and Methodology together with the general manager of the Swiss Implant Register (SIRIS) [14] and has been approved by Swiss Orthopaedics board of directors [15].

5. Conclusion

In conclusion, this is the first report about the validation of the SOMD. A relatively high reliability (test-retest and internal consistency), borderline acceptable (criterion) validity for the item of pain and improvable clinical implementation was observed. The analysis serves as the basis for a structured modification of an improved version of the SOMD.

Disclosure

The subcommittee of the Swiss Orthopaedics Panel of Quality and Methodology of Swiss Orthopaedics consisted of the authors MF and CD, as well as Anne Lübbeke, MD, M.Sc., DSc, and Anne Mannion, MD, PhD. The general manager of the Swiss Implant Register (SIRIS) is Andreas Mischler. The abstract was presented as an oral presentation at the Annual Conference of the Swiss Orthopaedics, Montreux, Switzerland, June 06–08, 2018.

Authors' Contributions

TJ was responsible for conception and design, acquisition of data, analysis and interpretation of data, and drafting the manuscript. CD interpretated the data. UM was responsible for acquisition of data and interpretation of data. MF was responsible for the idea, conception and design, ethics, interpretation of data, and supervision of the study. All authors revised and approved the final version of the manuscript.

References

[1] I. Daig and A. Lehmann, "Procedures to measure quality of life," *Zeitschrift für Medizinische Psychologie*, vol. 16, pp. 5–23, 2007.

[2] N. Bellamy, *Osteoarthritis—an Evaluative Index for Clinical Trials*, McMaster University, Hamilton, Canada, 1982.

[3] N. Bellamy, W. W. Buchanan, C. H. Goldsmith, J. Campbell, and L. W. Stitt, "Validation study of WOMAC: a health status instrument for measuring clinically important patient relevant outcomes to antirheumatic drug therapy in patients with osteoarthritis of the hip or knee," *The Journal of Rheumatology*, vol. 15, no. 12, pp. 1833–1840, 1988.

[4] F. Wolfe and S. X. Kong, "Rasch analysis of the Western Ontario MacMaster questionnaire (WOMAC) in 2205 patients with osteoarthritis, rheumatoid arthritis, and fibromyalgia," *Annals of the Rheumatic Diseases*, vol. 58, no. 9, pp. 563–568, 1999.

[5] F. Angst, T. Ewert, S. Lehmann, A. Aeschlimann, and G. Stucki, "The factor subdimensions of the Western Ontario and McMaster Universities Osteoarthritis Index (WOMAC) help to specify hip and knee osteoarthritis. a prospective evaluation and validation study," *The Journal of Rheumatology*, vol. 32, no. 7, pp. 1324–1330, 2005.

[6] F. Angst, A. Aeschlimann, and G. Stucki, "Smallest detectable and minimal clinically important differences of rehabilitation intervention with their implications for required sample sizes using WOMAC and SF-36 quality of life measurement instruments in patients with osteoarthritis of the lower extremities," *Arthritis & Rheumatism*, vol. 45, no. 4, pp. 384–391, 2001 Aug.

[7] N. J. Collins, D. Misra, D. T. Felson, K. M. Crossley, and E. M. Roos, "Measures of knee function: international knee documentation committee (IKDC) subjective knee evaluation form, knee injury and osteoarthritis outcome score (KOOS), knee injury and osteoarthritis outcome score physical function short form (KOOS-PS), knee outcome survey activities of daily living scale (KOS-ADL), lysholm knee scoring scale, Oxford knee score (OKS), western Ontario and McMaster Universities osteoarthritis index (WOMAC), activity rating scale (ARS), and tegner activity score (TAS)," *Arthritis Care & Research*, vol. 63, no. S11, pp. S208–S228, 2011.

[8] T. Ngo, M. Stupar, P. Côté, E. Boyle, and H. Shearer, "A study of the test-retest reliability of the self-perceived general recovery and self-perceived change in neck pain questions in patients with recent whiplash-associated disorders," *European Spine Journal*, vol. 19, no. 6, pp. 957–962, 2010.

[9] J. C. Nunnally and I. H. Bernstein, *Psychometric Theory*, McGraw-Hill, New York, NY, USA, 3rd edition, 1994.

[10] The EuroQol Group, "EuroQol-a new facility for the measurement of health-related quality of life," *Health Policy*, vol. 16, no. 3, pp. 199–208, 1990.

[11] R. Rabin and F. d. Charro, "EQ-SD: a measure of health status from the EuroQol Group," *Annals of Medicine*, vol. 33, no. 5, pp. 337–343, 2001.

[12] A. F. Mannion, F. Porchet, F. S. Kleinstück et al., "The quality of spine surgery from the patient's perspective. Part 1: the Core Outcome Measures Index in clinical practice," *European Spine Journal*, vol. 18, no. S3, pp. 367–373, 2009.

[13] M. E. Greene, O. Rolfson, S. Nemes, M. Gordon, H. Malchau, and G. Garellick, "Education attainment is associated with patient-reported outcomes: findings from the Swedish Hip Arthroplasty Register," *Clinical Orthopaedics and Related Research*, vol. 472, no. 6, pp. 1868–1876, 2014.

[14] Swiss National Joint Registry, "SIRIS report 2012-2016: annual report of the swiss national joint registry, hip and knee," Technical Report, pp. 23–38, University of Bern, Bern, Switzerland, 2016.

[15] Foundation for quality assurance in implant surgery—SIRIS, 2020, https://www.siris-implant.ch/en/Downloads?category=32.

23

Comparison of Effectiveness between Cobalt Chromium Rods versus Titanium Rods for Treatment of Patients with Spinal Deformity

Frank D. Shega,[1,2] HongQi Zhang,[1] Daudi R. Manini,[1,3] MingXing Tang,[1] and ShaoHua Liu[1]

[1]*Department of Spine Surgery, Xiangya Hospital of Central South University, Changsha City 410008, Hunan Province, China*
[2]*Department of Orthopedic Surgery, Mount Meru Regional Referral Hospital, P.O Box 3092, Arusha City, Tanzania*
[3]*Department of Orthopedic Surgery, Mwananyamala Regional Referral Hospital, P.O Box 61665, Dar-es-salaam City, Tanzania*

Correspondence should be addressed to ShaoHua Liu; liushaohua509@163.com

Academic Editor: Benjamin Blondel

Background. Biomechanical properties of rods determine their ability to correct spinal deformity and prevention of postoperative sagittal and coronal changes. The selection of a proper rod material is crucial due to their specific mechanical properties that influence the surgical outcome. The purpose of this study is to compare the effectiveness of cobalt chromium rods versus titanium rods for the treatment of spinal deformity by a systematic review and meta-analysis. *Methods.* PubMed, EMBASE, and the Cochrane library were searched for observational and biomechanical studies comparing cobalt chromium and titanium rods in terms of correction rate, thoracic kyphosis, lumbar lordosis, incidence of rod fracture, fatigue life of contoured rod, bending stiffness of rods, and occurrence of proximal junctional kyphosis. The demographic data and mean values of outcomes of interest were extracted from each group and compared by their mean difference as an overall outcome measure. The Review Manager software (RevMan 5.3) was utilized at a 95% significance level. *Results.* Eleven eligible studies with 641 participants for 7 observational studies and 35 samples for 4 biomechanical studies were identified. There were no significant differences between cobalt chromium and titanium rods in the correction rate of spinal deformity. Postoperative thoracic kyphosis was well restored in the cobalt chromium group with statistical significance (p value = 0.009). The incidence of rod fracture was high in titanium rods compared to cobalt chromium rods with significant difference (p value = 0.0001). Proximal junctional kyphosis occurs more in the cobalt chromium group with a significant difference (p value = 0.0009). No statistical significance between two materials in terms of lumbar lordosis, fatigue of life, and bending stiffness of rods. *Conclusion.* The cobalt chromium rod is better than titanium rod for effective correction of spinal deformity and postoperative stability of the spine. However, the use of cobalt chromium rods is associated with increased risk of proximal junctional kyphosis.

1. Introduction

Spinal deformity, one of the commonest orthopedic disorders, is a malformation or malalignment of the vertebral column. It presents as unnatural curvature, as in scoliosis, kyphosis, lordosis, or combined deformities [1]. Apart from idiopathic and congenital etiologies, spinal deformity also occurs due to multiple fractures or ankylosing spondylitis. Its prevalence is reported to increase with age and estimated to be 30%–68% in the elderly population [2]. Pain and disabilities caused by spinal deformities lead to poor health-related quality of life [3].

Management of spinal deformity is based on extensive assessment of the spine with thorough physical examinations, plain radiography, computed tomography scan (CT scan), and magnetic resonance imaging (MRI) to come up with the best treatment plan and determination of prognosis [4]. Posterior spinal instrumentation and fusion using pedicle screws and rigid rods have been a recommended surgical treatment for the correction of spinal deformities in the coronal, sagittal, and axial planes [5–10]. The ultimate aim of corrective surgery in spinal deformities is to prevent progression and to stabilize the spine. The factors influencing postoperative correction outcome include the magnitude of the curve, flexibility of a curve, type of surgical technique, points of fixation, selection of instrumented levels, type of implants used, and postoperative care.

The size of the posterior implant typically determines its biomechanical profile in terms of diameter and material properties. Currently, different types of rods such as stainless-steel rods, titanium alloys rods, and cobalt chromium rods are widely used for the treatment of diverse spine deformities for stability and correction of the spinal deformity. The selection of a proper rod material is critical as each of them possesses different mechanical properties, which are determined by their chemical composition. Cobalt chromium (CoCr) and titanium alloy TA6V (Ti) are mostly used rods as they exhibit favorable biomechanical properties such as resistance to corrosion and compatibility with magnetic resonance imaging (MRI) [11]. However, the titanium has greater elasticity, whereas cobalt chromium has greater stiffness [12]. Contouring of rods plays a significant role in overall postoperative correction outcomes as it can diminish their fatigue strength and increases the risk of rod fracture after implantation [13–15].

Despite the availability of many studies on the surgical outcome of spinal deformities, very few of them focused on the postoperative effectiveness of surgical rods. This study compared cobalt chromium rods with titanium rods, in terms of deformity correction rate, change in thoracic kyphosis angle, change in lumbar lordosis angle, incidence of rod fracture, fatigue life of contoured rod, bending stiffness of rods, and occurrence of proximal junctional kyphosis (PJK), by systematic review and meta-analysis of the available published literature.

2. Methods

2.1. Eligibility Criteria. Studies comparing the effectiveness of cobalt chromium rods and titanium rods for correction of spinal deformity regardless of age, gender, or follow-up time were eligible for inclusion. Only observational and experimental studies comparing the two groups and has the outcome of interest (correction rate, thoracic kyphosis, lumbar lordosis, incidence of rod fracture, fatigue life of contoured rod, bending stiffness of rods, or occurrence of proximal junctional kyphosis) were eligible for inclusion. Only English and full-text published literature were eligible for inclusion. Studies across the world that abide by the inclusion criteria mentioned above were included.

2.2. Information Sources. Three online databases, namely, PubMed, EMBASE, and the Cochrane library, were searched to come up with the list of eligible included studies. No date range customization of searches was set. Corresponding authors of articles searched could be contacted to provide further information or settle unclear explanations. Secondary referencing of eligible studies was done to extend the scope of the searches. The online databases were accessed via the Central South University library's website: http://lib.csu.edu.cn/. The last date of the search was 30th January 2020.

2.3. Study Search. To generate a set of citations that are relevant to our study's search question, an advanced search tool was used in all of the three databases previously mentioned. Free text words, as well as MeSH terms, were used to search. Using PubMed, advanced search was customized to "human species" and "full text" as (((("cobalt"[MeSH Terms] OR "cobalt"[All Fields]) AND ("chromium"[MeSH Terms] OR "chromium"[All Fields]) AND rods[All Fields]) AND (("titanium"[MeSH Terms] OR "titanium"[All Fields]) AND rods[All Fields])) AND ("scoliosis"[MeSH Terms] OR "scoliosis"[All Fields])) OR ("kyphosis"[MeSH Terms] OR "kyphosis"[All Fields]). The advance search in EMBASE was done by using a combination of keywords (cobalt AND chromium AND titanium AND rods AND scoliosis OR kyphosis) and filtered with "human" and "article or review." Two authors independently performed the searches: FS and DM. Any differences of thought were settled through discussion with the third and fourth authors: ZQ and TX. Results were exported to computer software known as *Mendeley Desktop*, which was used to manage and keep track of references throughout this study.

2.4. Study Selection Process. All studies resulting from online database search independently conducted by two authors were initially screened by their titles and abstracts to assess their relevance to our study question, and grossly irrelevant articles were discarded. This was level-one screening and was done by the same two authors, FS and DM. Compiled search results of level-one screening were then searched for their full-text articles from which eligibility for inclusion was sought. This was level-two screening, and any differences of thoughts in the search process were settled by ZQ and TX. The study search, screening, and selection process are summarized in Figure 1.

2.5. Data Extraction. Data from included articles were independently extracted by two authors, namely, FS and DM. Disagreements were solved through discussion with ZQ, TX, and LH. Data derived from each of the included studies were study title, author name, and year of publication; study design; comparison group (cobalt chromium rods versus titanium rods); study participants' demographics including mean ages and sex; participants' number; surgical technique; mean and standard deviation of the follow-up time and clinical outcomes (correction rate, thoracic kyphosis, lumbar lordosis, rod fracture, rod fatigue life, and proximal junctional kyphosis (PJK))

2.6. Quality Assessment. The quality assessment of the 11 eligible studies with their design, content, and ease of use in the interpretation of results was done by using the Newcastle-Ottawa scale (NOS). The assessment was done independently by two authors, FS and DM. The disagreement

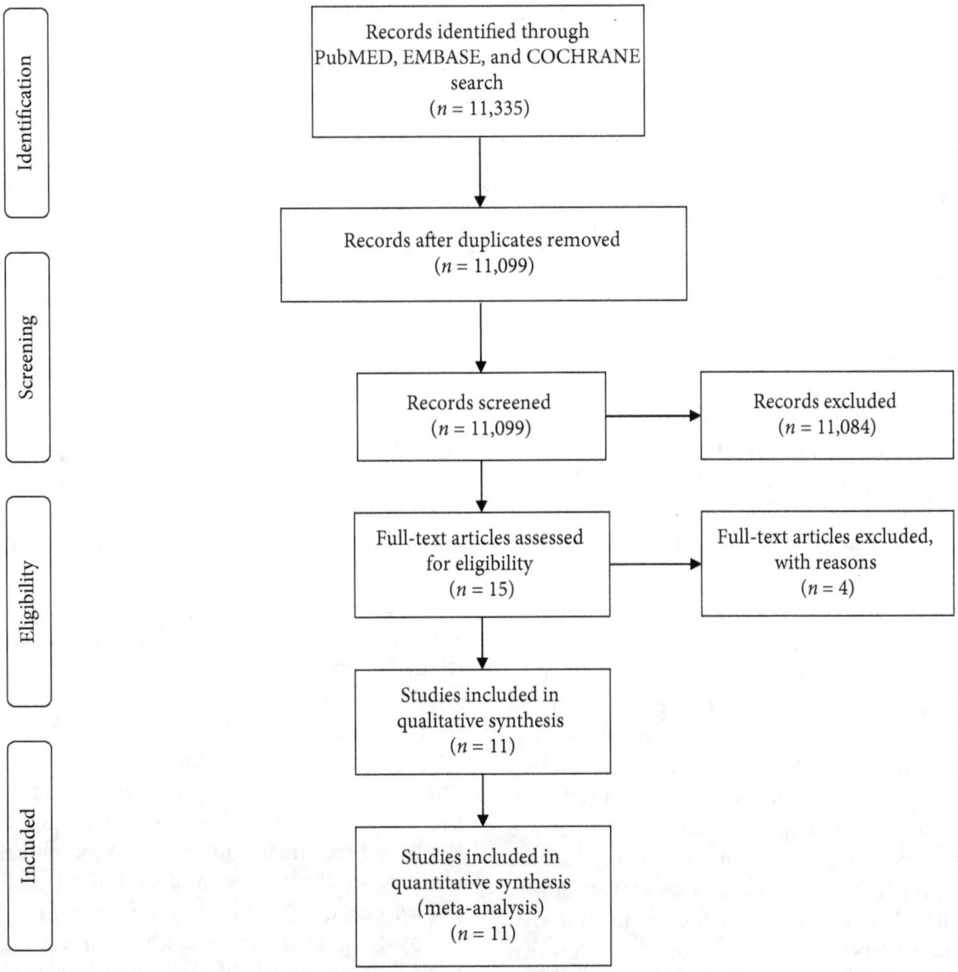

FIGURE 1: Study selection process according to PRISMA guidelines.

was solved through discussion with third, fourth, and fifth authors, ZQ, TX, and LH. All included studies scored more than 7 stars on the Newcastle-Ottawa scale (NOS). The score indicated that the quality of all included studies was good as defined by a scale "good quality: 3 or 4 stars in selection domain, 1 or 2 stars in comparability domain, and 2 or 3 stars in outcome/exposure domain". The results for the NOS score for each study are summarized in Table 1.

2.7. Statistical Analysis. Data were analyzed separately according to individual components and then it gave rise to five separate analyses: comparison of cobalt chromium and titanium rods in sagittal correction (correction rate, thoracic kyphosis, and lumbar lordosis), rod fracture, rod fatigue life, bending stiffness, and proximal junctional kyphosis (PJK). The mean difference was used to measure and compare the overall effect modified by the two-rod constructs. Forest-plots diagrammatically illustrated the overall effect. The Review Manager software (RevMan 5.3, the Cochrane Collaboration, Oxford, UK) was used to perform statistical analysis and generation of forest plots. Continuous variables were reported as mean difference (MD), standard deviation (SD) and 95% confidence interval (95% CI), while dichotomous data were presented as odds ratio (OR) and 95% confidence interval (95% CI). The software was customized to a random or fixed effect model depending on the heterogeneity (I^2) of the studies when analyzing the outcomes. The fixed effect model was used when heterogeneity was less than 50%, and the random effect model was used when heterogeneity was more than 50%. Collected data were entered into the computer and rechecked by two authors, FS and DM. Some articles gave raw data; to get the data we need, we computed the mean and standard deviation by using Statistical Package for the Social Sciences (SPSS) version 25.

2.8. Assumptions and Simplifications. All participants, despite the study country's economic status and technological differences, were considered to have received standard surgical care.

3. Results

3.1. Study Selection. A total of fifteen full-text studies were identified through database searching for eligibility assessment. Four of these were excluded due to various reasons; Etemadifar et al. [26] compared our outcome of interest but it was randomized clinical trial rather than observational or biomechanical study; Smith et al. [27] assessed the risk factors for rod fracture and not rod fracture as an outcome;

TABLE 1: Newcastle-Ottawa scale for quality assessment of the eligible studies.

Study name	Selection	Comparability	Outcome	Total score
Sabah et al. 2018 [12]	4	2	3	9
Angelliaume et al. 2016 [16]	4	2	3	9
Han et al. 2017 [17]	4	2	3	9
Han et al. 2017 [18]	4	2	3	9
Shinohara et al. 2016 [19]	4	1	3	8
Sia et al. 2019 [20]	4	1	3	8
Nguyen et al. 2011 [21]	3	2	2	7
Demura et al. 2014 [22]	3	2	2	7
Noshchenko et al. 2011 [23]	4	1	2	7
Shah et al. 2018 [24]	3	2	2	7
Smith et al. 2012 [25]	4	2	2	8

Slivka et al. [28] did not compare the outcome of our interest; Serhan et al. [29] was excluded because it did not assess the outcome of our interest. A total of eleven studies met the criteria for inclusion and included in our study.

3.2. Study Characteristics. The summary of the study characteristics of our eleven studies that were eligible for inclusion in our study is given in Table 2. The total number of participants with respect to the study type was 641 for observational studies and 35 for biomechanical studies. Regarding participants demographics, while observational studies recorded age and follow-up time and recruited both genders equally, biomechanical studies did not because are not applicable but were included because our study focuses only on the effectiveness of surgical rods to correct spinal deformity regardless of age, gender, or follow-up time. All observational studies reported a participant's age central tendencies by mean. While other studies used a larger sample size, others used smaller sample sizes.

Five were cohort observational studies; one was a case-control observational study; one was case series observational study, and four were biomechanical studies. Studies were conducted in different countries across continents that increase the external validity of the study. Four studies were done in USA [21, 23–25], two studies in France [12, 16], two studies in South Korea [17, 18], two studies in Japan [19, 22], and one study in Malaysia [20].

Even though the search was not set to any specified range of dates, all included studies were published after the year 2010. These studies reported the different outcomes of interest concerning our study questions. Four studies compared correction rate [12, 16, 19, 20]; five studies compared rod fracture [17–19, 24, 25]; three studies compared thoracic kyphosis [12, 16, 20], proximal junctional kyphosis [12, 17, 18], and fatigue life [21–23] each; two studies compared lumbar lordosis [12, 16] and bending stiffness [22, 23] each. Studies comparing similar outcomes were analyzed together in the same forest plot.

3.3. Sources of Bias. Eligible studies were assessed for risk of bias in two levels, at study level and the review level. The bias assessment at the study level shows that studies used different sample sizes. Some included studies used a large sample size, while others had a small sample size. Even though none of them reported to have calculated the required sample size before their conduction, the smaller the sample size, the less representative of the general population.

All studies compared cobalt chromium rods versus titanium rods with respect to our question of interest. Confounding factors might have been introduced to our research as factors such as gender, mean age, BMI, rod diameter, implant density, follow-up time, location of rod fracture, required bending angle, influence of rod contouring on rod strength, and stiffness were reported to some studies while other studies did not. All studies utilized posterior spinal fusion but with different constructs and maneuvers; some studies (observational studies) used patients. In contrast, others (biomechanical studies) used lumbar vertebrectomy models, but all of these studies reported our question of interest even though they use different designs. Different studies had different rod bending technique and used different type of rod bender as well as introduced different bending angles. These unusual conditions across every included study were thought to increase heterogeneity hence influence our results.

While at the review level, the risk of biases was identified as some studies had our data of interest to be extracted; other studies need calculation to obtain the required data for analysis. The overall mean age of participants in two groups could not be calculated as median was used rather than mean in some studies [20] and not reported in some studies [21–24]. Also, the overall follow-up time could not be calculated as data were not reported in some studies [20–24]. To reduce biases, the authors firstly evaluated all eligible studies by conducting database search and data extraction from different sources. Assessment for methodological biases was done before the data extraction from eligible full-text articles. To minimize reporting biases, the PRISMA (Preferred Reporting Items for Systematic Reviews and Meta-Analyses) tool was used in the study write-up.

3.3.1. Correction Rate. Figure 2 elucidates four [12, 16, 19, 20] of the eleven included studies that compared correction rate outcomes in percentage between cobalt chromium rods versus titanium rods. The overall mean difference between the two implants was −0.24, 95% CI (−3.32, 2.84) favouring cobalt chromium rods, but the difference did not reach statistical significance with p value = 0.88 (i.e. p value >0.05).

TABLE 2: Characteristics of included studies.

Study name, year	Study type	Comparison group	Number of participants	Mean age (years)	Sex F/M	Follow-up time (months)	Surgical technique	Country of study	Outcome
Sabah et al. 2018 [12]	Retrospective cohort study	CoCr Ti	30 33	15 ± 2 15 ± 2	27/3 27/6	45 ± 24 41 ± 9	PSF (PS + ST2R)	France	CR, TK, LL, and PJK
Angelliaume et al. 2016 [16]	Retrospective cohort study	Ti CoCr	35 35	16.6 ± 4 15.7 ± 2	28/7 31/4	53 ± 5 49 ± 6	PSF (HC + PTT)	France	CR, TK and LL
Han et al. 2017 [17]	Retrospective case-control study	CoCr Ti	20 34	67.7 (55–74) 64.8 (50–77)	19/1 33/1	13.7 (12–23) 56.4 (14–168	PSF (PS + Rods)	South Korea	PJK and RF
Han et al. 2017b [18]	Retrospective cohort study	CoCr Ti	50 50	69 (22–89) 67 (30–79)	36/14 31/19	25 (25–51) 28.5 (24–110)	PSF (PS + Rods)	South Korea	RF and PJK
Shinohara et al. 2016 [19]	Retrospective cohort study	Ti CoCr	4 9	6.7 (5–9) 13.8	12/1	68.5 (59–72) 26.1 (20–39)	PSF (DGRT)	Japan	CR, RF
Sia et al. 2019 [20]	Prospective case series	Ti CoCr	10 11	16 17	NR	NR	PSF (PS + Rods)	Malaysia	CR and TK
Nguyen et al. 2011 [21]	Biomechanical study	Ti CoCr	6 9	NA	NA	NA	LBVM	USA	FL
Demura et al. 2014 [22]	Biomechanical study	CoCr Ti	1 3	NA	NA	NA	TPBT	Japan	BS and FL
Igarashi et al. 2011 [23]	Biomechanical study	CoCr	5 Ti	NA 5	NA	NA	TPBT	USA	BS and FL
Burger et al. 2018 [24]	Biomechanical study	CoCr Ti	3 3	NA	NA	NA	PSOM	USA	RF
Smith et al. 2012 [25]	Retrospective review	CoCr Ti	110 210	NR	NR	NR	PSO	USA	RF

CoCr = cobalt chromium, Ti = titanium, PSF = posterior spinal fusion, PS = pedicle screw, ST2R = simultaneous translation on two rods maneuver, HC = hybrid constructs, PTT = posteromedial translation technique, CR = correction rate, TK = thoracic kyphosis, LL = lumbar lordosis, PJK = proximal junctional kyphosis, DGRT = dual growing rod technique, RF = rod fracture, FL = fatigue life, LVM = lumbar vertebrectomy models, BS = bending stiffness, TPBT = three-point bending test, PSO = pedicle subtraction osteotomy, PSOM = pedicle subtraction osteotomy models, NA = not applicable, NR = not recorded.

Study or subgroup	Cobalt chromium rods Mean	SD	Total	Titanium rods Mean	SD	Total	Weight	Mean difference IV, fixed, 95% CI
Angelliaume 2016	65.45	20	35	67.24	27.3	35	7.6%	−1.79 [−13.00, 9.42]
Sabah 2018	76	9	30	75	7	33	59.1%	1.00 [−3.01, 5.01]
Shinohara 2016	51	6.2	9	52.5	5.2	4	22.4%	−1.50 [−8.01, 5.01]
Sia 2019	66.7	10.7	11	70	11	10	11.0%	−3.30 [−12.60, 6.00]
Total (95% CI)			*85*			*82*	*100.0%*	*−0.24 [−3.32, 2.84]*

Heterogeneity: $chi^2 = 1.00$, $df = 3$ ($P = 0.80$); $I^2 = 0\%$

Test for overall effect: $Z = 0.15$ ($P = 0.88$)

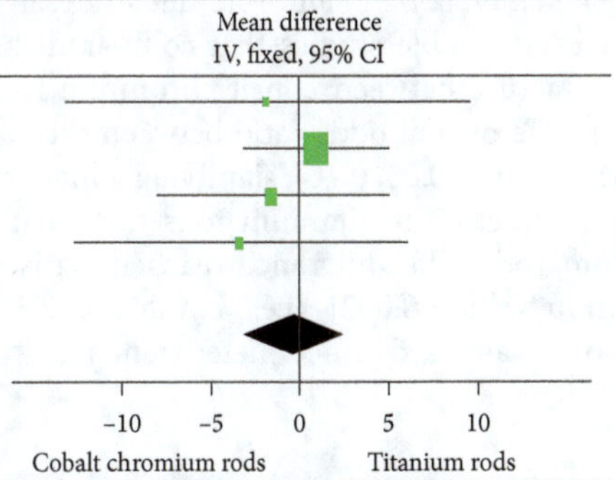

FIGURE 2: Forest plot for correction rate in percentage between cobalt chromium rods and titanium rods.

A fixed-effect model was used since heterogeneity, I^2, was 0% (i.e. $I^2 < 50\%$).

3.3.2. *Thoracic Kyphosis.* Figure 3(a) elucidates two [12, 16] of eleven eligible studies that compared changes in thoracic kyphotic angles in degrees between cobalt chromium rods versus titanium rods. The overall mean difference between the two implants was 3.99, 95% CI (1.00, 6.98), signifying better restoration of thoracic kyphotic angle in cobalt chromium rods. The difference reached statistical significance with p value = 0.009 (i.e., p value <0.05). A fixed-effect

Study or subgroup	Cobalt chromium rods Mean	SD	Total	Titanium rods Mean	SD	Total	Weight	Mean difference IV, fixed, 95% CI
Angelliaume 2016	40	10	35	34	8	35	49.8%	6.00 [1.76, 10.24]
Sabah 2018	32	9	30	30	8	33	50.2%	2.00 [−2.22, 6.22]
Total (95% CI)			*65*			*68*	*100.0%*	*3.99 [1.00, 6.98]*

Heterogeneity: chi^2 = 1.72, df = 1 (P = 0.19); I^2 = 42%

Test for overall effect: Z = 2.61 (P = 0.009)

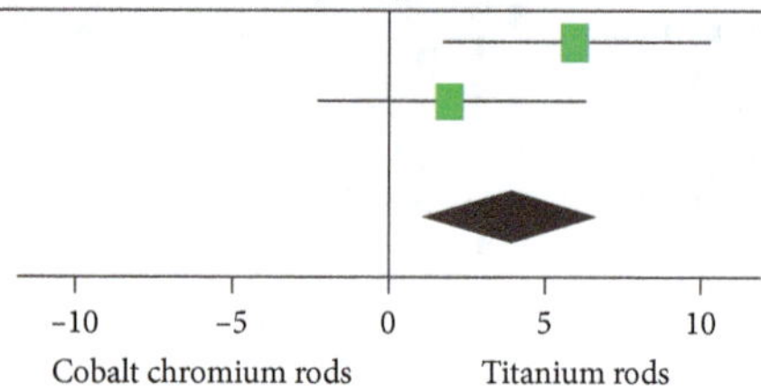

(a)

Study or subgroup	Cobalt chromium rods Mean	SD	Total	Titanium rods Mean	SD	Total	Weight	Mean difference IV, fixed, 95% CI
Angelliaume 2016	53	10	35	53	17	35	39.5%	0.00 [−6.53, 6.53]
Sabah 2018	63	8	30	64	13	33	60.5%	−1.00 [−6.28, 4.28]
Total (95% CI)			*65*			*68*	*100.0%*	*−0.61 [−4.71, 3.50]*

Heterogeneity: chi^2 = 0.05, df = 1 (P = 0.82); I^2 = 0%

Test for overall effect: Z = 0.29 (P = 0.77)

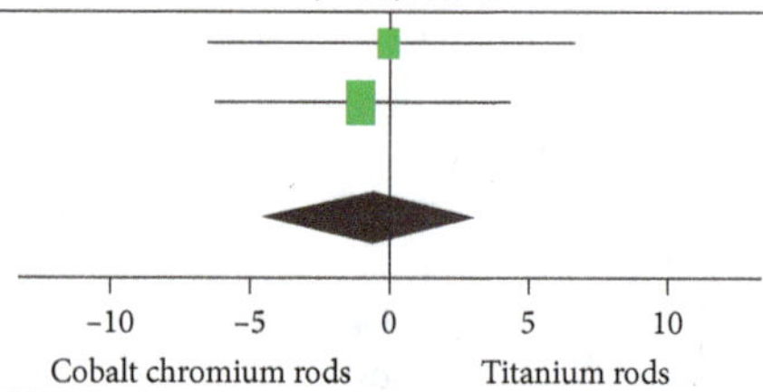

(b)

FIGURE 3: Forest plot between CoCr and Ti rods. (a) Illustrating two of eleven studies comparing thoracic kyphosis outcome results. (b) Illustrating two of eleven studies comparing lumbar lordosis outcome results.

model was used since heterogeneity, I^2, was 42% (i.e. $I^2 < 50\%$).

3.3.3. Lumbar Lordosis. Figure 3(b) illustrates two [12, 16] of eleven eligible studies that compared lumbar lordosis outcomes in degrees between cobalt chromium rods versus titanium rods. The overall mean difference between the two implants was −0.61, 95% CI (−4.71, 3.50) without reaching statistical significance as p value = 0.77 (i.e., p value >0.05). A fixed-effect model was used since heterogeneity, I^2, was 0% (i.e. $I^2 < 50\%$).

3.3.4. Rod Fracture. Figure 4(a) illustrates five [17–19, 24, 25] of eleven eligible studies that compared the occurrence of rod fracture between cobalt chromium rods and titanium rods. The overall odds ratio between the two implants was 0.15, 95% CI (0.06, 0.40), signifying a higher occurrence rate of rod fracture in titanium rods than that of cobalt chromium rods. The difference reached statistical significance with p value = 0.0001 (i.e., p value <0.05). A fixed-effect model was used since heterogeneity, I^2, was 0% (i.e., $I^2 < 50\%$).

3.3.5. Proximal Junctional Kyphosis. Figure 4(b) illustrates three [12, 17, 18] of eleven eligible studies that compared the rate of occurrence of proximal junctional kyphosis between cobalt chromium rods versus titanium rods. The odds ratio between the two implants was 3.16, 95% CI (1.61, 6.20), signifying a higher occurrence rate in cobalt chromium rods. The difference reached statistical significance with p value = 0.0009 (i.e., p value <0.05). A fixed-effect model was used since heterogeneity, I^2, was 13% (i.e., $I^2 < 50\%$).

3.3.6. Fatigue of Life. Figure 5(a) elucidates three [21–23] of eleven eligible studies that compared fatigue of life in terms of a number of loading cycles between cobalt chromium rods versus titanium rods. The overall mean difference between the two implants was 1250.36, 95% CI (−672.18, 3172.89) favouring titanium rods, but the difference did not reach statistical significance as p value = 0.20 (p value >0.05). A random effect model was used since heterogeneity was high, $I^2 = 99\%$ (i.e., $I^2 > 50\%$).

3.3.7. Bending Stiffness. Figure 5(b) elucidates two [22, 23] of eleven eligible studies that compared bending stiffness outcomes in terms of newtons per millimetre between cobalt chromium rods versus titanium rods. The overall mean difference between the two implants was 664.79, 95% CI (−468.65, 1798.23) without reaching statistical significance as p value = 0.25 (i.e., p value >0.05). A random effect model was used since heterogeneity was very high, I^2, was 100% (i.e. $I^2 > 50\%$).

3.4. Sensitivity Analysis. Excluding one study as it was a randomized clinical trial conducted in Iran [26] has an impact on the statistical significance of thoracic kyphosis outcome results; however, the outcome results for deformity correction rate and lumbar lordosis did not change the statistical significance. When included, the new results were as follows: the overall mean difference of deformity correction rate was 1.57 (−3.32, 6.47), p value = 0.53, and $I^2 = 64\%$; the overall mean difference of thoracic kyphosis was 1.77 (−-3.09, 6.62), p value = 0.48, and $I^2 = 84\%$; the overall mean difference of lumbar lordosis was −0.85 (−3.30, 1.61), p value = 0.50, and $I^2 = 0\%$.

Study or subgroup	Cobalt chromium rods Events	Cobalt chromium rods Total	Titanium rods Events	Titanium rods Total	Weight	Odds ratio M-H, fixed, 95% CI
Han 2017a	0	20	11	34	25.8%	0.05 [0.00, 0.90]
Han 2017b	0	50	8	50	25.8%	0.05 [0.00, 0.88]
Shah 2018	2	3	3	3	4.0%	0.24 [0.01, 8.62]
Shinohara 2016	1	9	2	4	7.5%	0.13 [0.01, 2.18]
Smith 2012	3	110	18	210	36.9%	0.30 [0.09, 1.04]
Total (95% CI)		*192*		*301*	*100.0%*	*0.15 [0.06, 0.40]*
Total events	6		42			

Heterogeneity: $chi^2 = 2.34$, $df = 4$ ($P = 0.67$); $I^2 = 0\%$

Test for overall effect: $Z = 3.88$ ($P = 0.0001$)

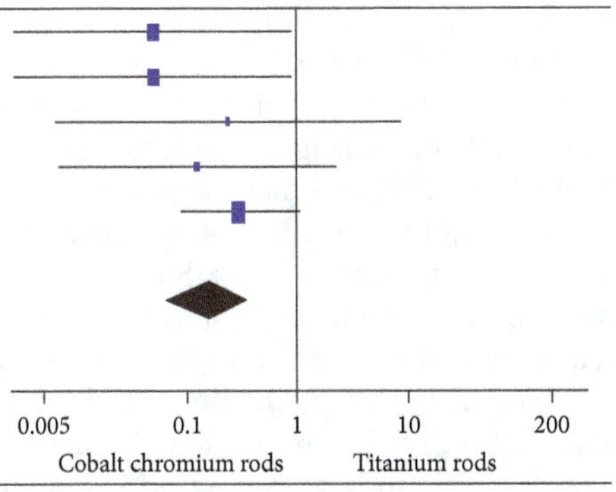

(a)

Study or subgroup	Cobalt chromium rods Events	Cobalt chromium rods Total	Titanium rods Events	Titanium rods Total	Weight	Odds ratio M-H, fixed, 95% CI
Han 2017a	12	20	9	34	27.9%	4.17 [1.29, 13.49]
Han 2017b	22	50	9	50	52.8%	3.58 [1.44, 8.91]
Shah 2018	1	30	2	33	19.3%	0.53 [0.05, 6.21]
Total (95% CI)		*100*		*117*	*100.0%*	*3.16 [1.61, 6.20]*
Total events	35		20			

Heterogeneity: $chi^2 = 2.30$, $df = 2$ ($P = 0.32$); $I^2 = 13\%$

Test for overall effect: $Z = 3.34$ ($P = 0.0009$)

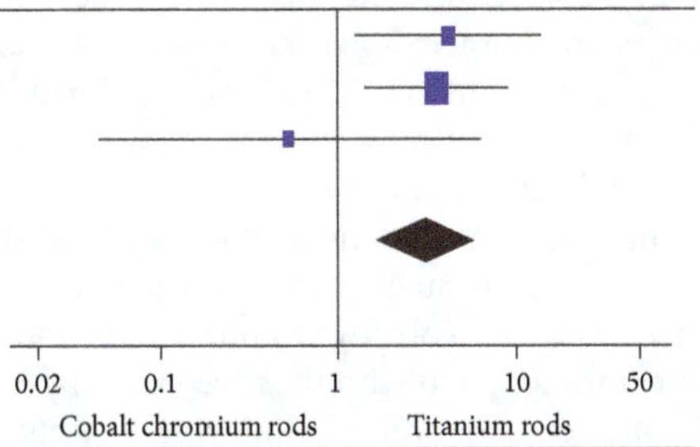

(b)

FIGURE 4: Forest plot between CoCr and Ti rods. (a) Illustrating five of eleven studies comparing rod fracture outcome results. (b) Illustrating three of eleven studies comparing proximal junctional kyphosis outcome results.

Study or subgroup	Cobalt chromium rods Mean	Cobalt chromium rods SD	Cobalt chromium rods Total	Titanium rods Mean	Titanium rods SD	Titanium rods Total	Weight	Mean difference IV, fixed, 95% CI
Demura 2014	476	65.7	1	509.7	245	3	46.7%	-33.70 [-339.38, 271.98]
Nguyen 2011	16,822	2,563.39	9	11,478.67	8,841.89	6	6.1%	5343.33 [-1927.04, 12613.70]
Noshchenko 2011	6,591	125.3	5	4,598	23.6	5	47.2%	1993.00 [1881.24, 2104.76]
Total (95% CI)			*15*			*14*	*100.0%*	*1250.36 [-672.18, 3172.89]*

Heterogeneity: $tau^2 = 2035432.72$; $chi^2 = 149.89$, $df = 2$ ($P < 0.0001$); $I^2 = 99\%$

Test for overall effect: $Z = 1.27$ ($P = 0.20$)

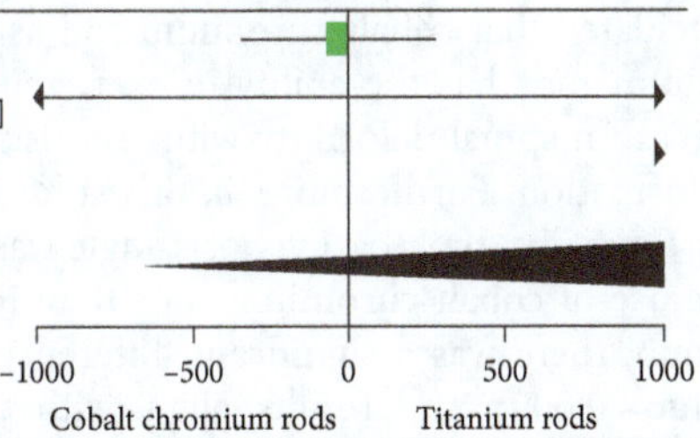

(a)

Study or subgroup	Cobalt chromium rods Mean	Cobalt chromium rods SD	Cobalt chromium rods Total	Titanium rods Mean	Titanium rods SD	Titanium rods Total	Weight	Mean difference IV, random, 95% CI
Demura 2014	208.7	18.8	1	120.1	15	3	50.2%	88.60 [48.03, 129.17]
Noshchenko 2011	3,816.6	162.7	5	2,571.4	10.7	5	49.8%	1245.20 [1102.28, 1388.12]
Total (95% CI)			*6*			*14*	*100.0%*	*664.79 [-468.65, 1798.23]*

Heterogeneity: $tau^2 = 665988.98$; $chi^2 = 232.83$, $df = 1$ ($P < 0.0001$); $I^2 = 100\%$

Test for overall effect: $Z = 1.15$ ($P = 0.25$)

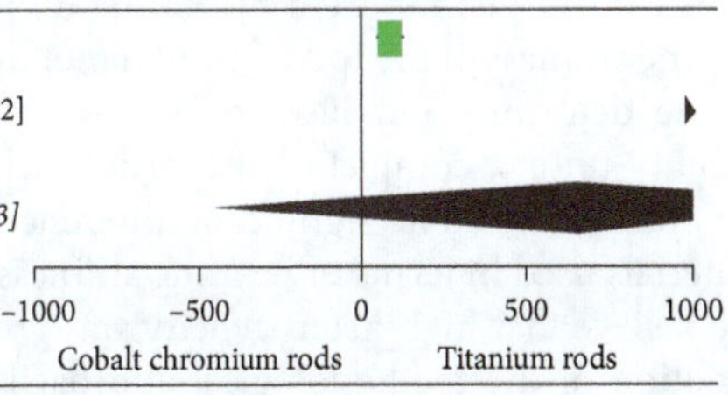

(b)

FIGURE 5: Forest plot between CoCr and Ti rods. (a) Illustrating two of eleven studies comparing fatigue of life outcome results. (b) Illustrating two of eleven studies comparing bending stiffness outcome results.

4. Discussion

The effectiveness of spinal rods after posterior instrumentation is influenced by several factors, including the body weight (BMI), rod diameter, fusion levels (implant density), rod contouring, required bending angle, and type of bender used. Biomechanical properties of rods determine their ability to correct spinal deformity and to prevent postoperative sagittal changes. Stainless steel with various diameters was previously commonly used but recently replaced by titanium rods and cobalt chromium rods [16]. The cobalt chromium gained popularity for correction of spinal deformity due to its higher mechanical strength hence less likely to have correction loss after surgery [26]. This study aimed to compare the effectiveness of cobalt chromium rods with titanium rods, in terms of their deformity correction rate; the occurrence of rod fracture; changes in thoracic kyphosis; changes in lumbar lordosis; and fatigue life of contoured rods and bending stiffness of rods, by systematic review and meta-analysis of available published literature.

The results of our meta-analysis revealed no significant difference in the main curve correction rate of spinal deformity between cobalt chromium rods and titanium rods. These findings align with those reported by Etemadifar et al. [26]; in their randomized clinical trial study on 59 patients, the authors concluded that cobalt chromium rods and titanium rods provide a similar significant primary curve correction rate, but the success rate of cobalt chromium rods was superior on spinal deformity correction. Results are also consistent with those reported by Watanabe et al. [30] and Thompson et al. [31] whereby no significant difference was observed in the correction rate between two groups implanted with titanium rods or cobalt chromium rods. Serhan et al. [29], in their biomechanical study of 80 rods, elucidated that cobalt chromium rod as compared with titanium rods has the ability to exert remarkable corrective forces on spinal deformity with less risk of developing rod deformation. Furthermore, in this study, we found that the postoperative thoracic kyphosis angle was well restored with the use of cobalt chromium rods than in the titanium rod group; there was a significant difference between them (p value = 0.009); the results align with those reported by Etemadifar et al. [26]. On the other hand, the findings of our study showed that there is no statistical significance in changes of lumbar lordosis with a p value of 0.77, which align with results reported by Han et al. [17].

The stiffness of the rod is essential not only for correction of the deformity but also for the maintenance of spine stability until a complete bone fusion achieved. However, our study revealed no significant difference between the two materials used in terms of bending stiffness (p value = 0.25). We believe that high heterogeneity was probably due to the variation of the methodological approach during the conduction of the respective study. Our results for bending stiffness contradicts with those reported by Noshchenko et al. [23] and Demura et al. [22] that cobalt chromium rods demonstrated higher bending stiffness than titanium rods, and there was a significant difference between them. Slivka et al. [28] elucidated that the rebending of the rods has to be avoided as it is a potential increased risk of implant failure.

In our study, we also found that the incidence of rod fracture is lower in cobalt chromium than that in titanium with a significant difference (p value = 0.0001), which aligns with those reported by Smith et al. [27], Han et al. [17], Shah et al. [24], Han et al. [18], and Shinohara et al. [19]. The follow-up duration for the occurrence of rod fracture is among important factors to be considered as revealed by Han et al. [17], whereby it was longer in the titanium group (56.4 ± 39.8 months) than that in the cobalt chromium group (14.0 ± 3.3 months). This means that the longer the follow-up time in the titanium group would likely show a higher incidence of rod fracture than the cobalt chromium group.

Moreover, from our study, the proximal junctional kyphosis occurs more in the cobalt chromium group with a significant difference (p value = 0.0009). These findings concur with the previous literature by Han et al. [17] and Han et al. [18] who reported a higher incidence of PJK in the cobalt chromium group than in the titanium group. The authors also showed a significant difference between the two groups in terms of the meantime of PJK occurrence after the operation. They reported a mean time of 3.6 months (range, 2–7 months, median: 3 months) in the cobalt chromium group and 26.3 months (range, 2–84 months, median: 24 months) in the titanium group; therefore, the follow-up duration has to be considered for the postoperative occurrence of PJK. Regarding fatigue of life, our study found that there is no statistical significance on the fatigue of life between contoured cobalt chromium rods and titanium rods (p value = 0.20). This result contradicts with those of Nguyen et al. [21] who concluded that the fatigue life of contoured CoCr rods is greater than that of Ti rods. The results of our meta-analysis suggest that the fatigue of life of an implant may vary due to material type used and loading condition.

Our study has some limitations, including the analysis of different studies with different designs and sample sizes; also, none of these eleven studies reported to have calculated the required sample size before their conduction. There was variability among studies concerning surgical technique as well as variability in terms of follow-up duration among included studies. The excluded randomized trial study had an impact on the statistical significance of thoracic kyphosis outcome results when included in our study but did not change the statistical significance of deformity correction rate and lumbar lordosis. Despite the presence of proximal junctional kyphosis in cobalt chromium rods, the authors of this study call upon a larger series and extensive research on the occurrence of PJK on CoCr rods to further assess its impact as a mechanical risk factor.

5. Conclusion

In conclusion, the cobalt chromium rod is better than a titanium rod to enhance correction of the spinal deformity as its uses increase the effectiveness and stability of the postoperative spine in a coronal and sagittal plane. However, the use of cobalt chromium rods is associated with increased risk of proximal junctional kyphosis.

References

[1] M.-S. Moon, B.-J. Lee, and S.-S. Kim, "Spinal deformity," *Indian Journal of Orthopaedics*, vol. 44, no. 2, pp. 123–126, 2010.

[2] C. Smith, N. Lamba, Z. Ou et al., "The prevalence of complications associated with lumbar and thoracic spinal deformity surgery in the elderly population: a meta-analysis," *Journal of Spine Surgery*, vol. 5, no. 2, pp. 223–235, 2019.

[3] S. Bess, O. Boachie-Adjei, D. Burton et al., "Pain and disability determine treatment modality for older patients with adult scoliosis, while deformity guides treatment for younger patients," *Spine*, vol. 34, no. 20, pp. 2186–2190, 2007.

[4] A. I. Tsirikos, A. Saifuddin, and M. H. Noordeen, "Spinal deformity in neurofibromatosis type-1: diagnosis and treatment," *European Spine Journal*, vol. 14, no. 5, pp. 427–439, 2005.

[5] R. A. Lehman, L. G. Lenke, K. A. Keeler et al., "Operative treatment of adolescent idiopathic scoliosis with posterior pedicle screw-only constructs," *Spine*, vol. 33, no. 14, pp. 1598–1604, 2008.

[6] Y.-J. Kim, L. Lenke, K. Bridwell, and B. Sides, "P77. Comparative analysis of pedicle screw versus hybrid instrumentation in posterior spinal fusion of adolescent idiopathic scoliosis: a match cohort analysis," *The Spine Journal*, vol. 4, no. 5, p. S85, 2004.

[7] Y. J. Kim, L. G. Lenke, J. Kim et al., "Comparative analysis of pedicle screw versus hybrid instrumentation in posterior spinal fusion of adolescent idiopathic scoliosis," *Spine*, vol. 31, no. 3, pp. 291–298, 2006.

[8] H. Halm, T. Niemeyer, T. Link, and U. Liljenqvist, "Segmental pedicle screw instrumentation in idiopathic thoracolumbar and lumbar scoliosis," *European Spine Journal*, vol. 9, no. 3, pp. 191–197, 2000.

[9] J. E. Lowenstein, H. Matsumoto, M. G. Vitale et al., "Coronal and sagittal plane correction in adolescent idiopathic scoliosis," *Spine*, vol. 32, no. 4, pp. 448–452, 2007.

[10] U. R. Liljenqvist, H. F. H. Halm, and T. M. Link, "Pedicle screw instrumentation of the thoracic spine in idiopathic scoliosis," *Spine*, vol. 22, no. 19, pp. 2239–2245, 1997.

[11] M. Lamerain, M. Bachy, M. Delpont, R. Kabbaj, P. Mary, and R. Vialle, "CoCr rods provide better frontal correction of adolescent idiopathic scoliosis treated by all-pedicle screw fixation," *European Spine Journal*, vol. 23, no. 6, pp. 1190–1196, 2014.

[12] Y. Sabah, J.-L. Clément, F. Solla, O. Rosello, and V. Rampal, "Cobalt-chrome and titanium alloy rods provide similar coronal and sagittal correction in adolescent idiopathic scoliosis," *Orthopaedics & Traumatology: Surgery & Research*, vol. 104, no. 7, pp. 1073–1077, 2018.

[13] X. Wang, L. Boyer, F. Le Naveaux, R. M. Schwend, and C.-E. Aubin, "How does differential rod contouring contribute to 3-dimensional correction and affect the bone-screw forces in adolescent idiopathic scoliosis instrumentation?" *Clinical Biomechanics*, vol. 39, pp. 115–121, 2016.

[14] C. Lindsey, V. Deviren, Z. Xu, R.-F. Yeh, and C. M. Puttlitz, "The effects of rod contouring on spinal construct fatigue strength," *Spine*, vol. 31, no. 15, pp. 1680–1687, 2006.

[15] K. R. Cidambi, D. A. Glaser, T. P. Bastrom, T. N. Nunn, T. Ono, and P. O. Newton, "Postoperative changes in spinal rod contour in adolescent idiopathic scoliosis," *Spine*, vol. 37, no. 18, pp. 1566–1572, 2012.

[16] A. Angelliaume, E. Ferrero, K. Mazda et al., "Titanium vs cobalt chromium: what is the best rod material to enhance adolescent idiopathic scoliosis correction with sublaminar bands?" *European Spine Journal*, vol. 26, no. 6, pp. 1732–1738, 2017.

[17] S. Han, S.-J. Hyun, K.-J. Kim, T.-A. Jahng, S. Lee, and S.-C. Rhim, "Rod stiffness as a risk factor of proximal junctional kyphosis after adult spinal deformity surgery: comparative study between cobalt chrome multiple-rod constructs and titanium alloy two-rod constructs," *The Spine Journal*, vol. 17, no. 7, pp. 962–968, 2017.

[18] S. Han, S.-J. Hyun, K.-J. Kim, T.-A. Jahng, and H.-J. Kim, "Comparative study between cobalt chrome and titanium alloy rods for multilevel spinal fusion: proximal junctional kyphosis more frequently occurred in patients having cobalt chrome rods," *World Neurosurgery*, vol. 103, pp. 404–409, 2017.

[19] K. Shinohara, T. Takigawa, M. Tanaka et al., "Implant Failure of Titanium Versus Cobalt-Chromium Growing Rods in Early-onset Scoliosis," *Spine*, vol. 41, no. 6, pp. 502–507, 2016.

[20] U. Sia, B. B. Tan, B. Tan, Y. Teo, and C. C. Wong, "Post-implantation deformation of titanium rod and cobalt chrome rod in adolescent idiopathic scoliosis," *Malaysian Orthopaedic Journal*, vol. 13, no. 1, pp. 14–19, 2019.

[21] T.-Q. Nguyen, J. M. Buckley, C. Ames, and V. Deviren, "The fatigue life of contoured cobalt chrome posterior spinal fusion rods," *Proceedings of the Institution of Mechanical Engineers, Part H: Journal of Engineering in Medicine*, vol. 225, no. 2, pp. 194–198, 2011.

[22] S. Demura, H. Murakami, H. Hayashi et al., "Influence of Rod Contouring on Rod Strength and Stiffness in Spine Surgery," *Orthopedics*, vol. 38, no. 6, pp. e520–e523, 2015.

[23] A. Noshchenko, Y. Xianfeng, G. A. Armour et al., "Evaluation of spinal instrumentation rod bending characteristics for in-situ contouring," *Journal of Biomedical Materials Research Part B: Applied Biomaterials*, vol. 98B, no. 1, pp. 192–200, 2011.

[24] K. N. Shah, G. Walker, S. C. Koruprolu, and A. H. Daniels, "Biomechanical comparison between titanium and cobalt chromium rods used in a pedicle subtraction osteotomy model," *Orthopedic Reviews*, vol. 10, pp. 32–35, 2018.

[25] J. S. Smith, C. I. Shaffrey, C. P. Ames et al., "Assessment of Symptomatic Rod Fracture After Posterior Instrumented Fusion for Adult Spinal Deformity," *Neurosurgery*, vol. 71, no. 4, pp. 862–868, 2012.

[26] M. R. Etemadifar, A. Andalib, A. Rahimian, and S. M. H. T. Nodushan, "Cobalt chromium-Titanium rods versus Titanium-Titanium rods for treatment of adolescent idiopathic scoliosis; which type of rod has better postoperative outcomes?" *Revista da Associação Médica Brasileira*, vol. 64, no. 12, pp. 1085–1090, 2018.

[27] J. S. Smith, E. Shaffrey, E. Klineberg et al., "Prospective multicenter assessment of risk factors for rod fracture following surgery for adult spinal deformity," *Journal of Neurosurgery: Spine*, vol. 21, no. 6, pp. 994–1003, 2014.

[28] M. A. Slivka, Y. K. Fan, and J. C. Eck, "The effect of contouring on fatigue strength of spinal rods: is it okay to re-bend and which materials are best?" *Spine Deformity*, vol. 1, no. 6, pp. 395–400, 2013.

[29] H. Serhan, D. Mhatre, P. Newton, P. Giorgio, and P. Sturm, "Would CoCr rods provide better correctional forces than stainless steel or titanium for rigid scoliosis curves?" *Journal of Spinal Disorders and Techniques*, vol. 26, pp. 70–74, 2013.

[30] K. Watanabe, K. Uno, T. Suzuki et al., "Risk factors for complications associated with growing-rod surgery for early-onset scoliosis," *Spine*, vol. 38, pp. 464–468, 2013.

[31] G. H. Thompson, B. A. Akbarnia, and R. M. Campbell, "Growing rod techniques in early-onset scoliosis," *Journal of Pediatric Orthopaedics*, vol. 27, no. 3, pp. 354–361, 2007.

Comparison of the Separate and Combined Effects of Physiotherapy Treatment and Corticosteroid Injection on the Range of Motion and Pain in Nontraumatic Rotator Cuff Tear

Shaahin Hajivandi[1] **Atousa Dachek**[2] **Amirhossein Salimi**[3] **Hesan Jelodari Mamaghani**[4] **Seyed Peyman Mirghaderi**[4] **Javad Dehghani**[5] **Roham Borazjani**[6] **Amirmohammad Babaniamansour**[7] **Rojin Sarallah**[8] **Salar Javanshir**[8] **and Maryam Salimi**[5,9]

[1]*Department of Orthopedic Surgery, Dezful University of Medical Sciences, Dezful, Iran*
[2]*Student Research Committee, Dezful University of Medical Sciences, Dezful, Iran*
[3]*Student Research Committee, Shahid Sadoughi University of Medical Sciences, Yazd, Iran*
[4]*Students' Scientific Research Center (SSRC), Tehran University of Medical Sciences, Tehran, Iran*
[5]*Bone and Joint Diseases Research Center, Department of Orthopedic Surgery, Shiraz University of Medical Sciences, Shiraz, Iran*
[6]*Trauma Research Center, Shahid Rajaee (Emtiaz) Ttauma Hospital, Shiraz University of Medical Sciences, Shiraz, Iran*
[7]*Department of Orthotics and Prosthetics, School of Rehabilitation Sciences, Iran University of Medical Sciences, Tehran, Iran*
[8]*Islamic Azad University Medical Branch of Tehran, Tehran, Iran*
[9]*Student Research Committee, Shiraz University of Medical Sciences, Shiraz, Iran*

Correspondence should be addressed to Maryam Salimi; salimimaryam7496@gmail.com

Academic Editor: Benjamin Blondel

Background. Surgical treatment and conservative treatment is the options to improve pain, function, and range of motion following rotator cuff tear. In this study, we aimed to compare the effects of physiotherapy and corticosteroid injections on the function, pain, and range of motion in patients with full-thickness rotator cuff tearing separately and simultaneously. *Methods.* A total of 96 patients were randomly assigned to the study and divided into 3 groups of 32 patients. DASH questionnaire and VAS criterion were completed by all three groups, and the range of motions of all groups was measured by a goniometer. Then, the first group underwent 12 sessions of physiotherapy twice a week for 6 weeks; the second group received 80 mg of methylprednisolone and 1 ml of lidocaine 2% in two stages, 21 days apart; and the third group received 80 mg of methylprednisolone and 1 ml of lidocaine 2%, and after 2 days, 6 sessions of physiotherapy twice a week for 3 weeks were prescribed. In the end, the questionnaire was filled out by the patient, and the range of emotions was assessed with a goniometer. *Results.* More than 80% of patients in each group were female. There was no significant difference between the gender and age distribution of the groups. The mean age in physiotherapy, steroid, and physiotherapy + steroid groups was 51.78 ± 7.37, 52.37 ± 6.61, and 50.87 ± 5.65, respectively. The combination of physiotherapy + steroid intervention was more effective in reducing VAS and DASH scores than physiotherapy or steroid injection alone. Goniometric findings showed that treatments that included the steroid injection approach (steroid injection and steroid + physiotherapy) had a more dramatic effect on improving the patients' range of motion than physiotherapy alone. *Conclusions.* Among the conservative approaches of treating full-thickness rotator cuff tear, a combination of steroid injection and physiotherapy is more effective significantly in comparison with either treatment alone. This trial is registered with IRCT20200102045987N1.

1. Introduction

The shoulder is one of the largest joints and the most mobile and unstable joint in the body due to the shallow depth of the glenoid cavity. Therefore, the tendons and muscles around the joint including the rotator cuffs (e.g., supraspinatus, infraspinatus, teres minor, and subscapularis) play an important role in joint stability as well as joint movements [1]. Furthermore, shoulder pain with muscle-associated origin is one of the most common complaints of patients who visit orthopedists (30% to 70%), among which rotator cuff ruptures are considered as the most prevalent ones (23% to 49%) [2].

Pain, weakness, and limited range of motion are the most common symptoms of complete rotator cuff rupture, which can impair the function and quality of life [3]. Likewise, magnetic resonance imaging (MRI) was recognized as a gold standard diagnostic test regarding rotator cuff tearing [4].

The prevalence and size of the ruptures increase with age, and the clinical success of the tendon repair decreases within the ruptures [5]. In this regard, treatment is performed in conservative or surgical management including open surgery and arthroscopy. Based on the patient's condition and the rapture size as well as available equipment and facilities, the type of treatment is selected; in fact, not all patients with rotator cuff ruptures need surgery. Moreover, the treatment choice for rotator cuff tearing was varied in the studies with different lengths of the follow-up period and complications [6].

Although many studies have reported the results of complete rotator cuff rupture surgery, there are few studies on the effectiveness of conservative treatment. Likewise, conservative and physiotherapy treatments are diverse and choosing the best and most appropriate treatment for these patients requires further research.

Therefore, due to the high prevalence and functional disability caused by rotator cuff tearing, disagreement about the appropriate treatment method and the limited evidence regarding the role of physiotherapy and exercise programs in reducing pain and disability of these patients, and lack of sufficient objective evidence of complete recovery of patients following surgery, a randomized clinical trial was needed to reduce the complications, pain, and costs of surgical treatment and determine the effects of physiotherapy and corticosteroid injections (CSI) in these patients.

Numerous studies have been performed in recent years on the effects of physiotherapy and CSI in patients with other pathologies of the rotator cuff muscles such as impingement syndrome and frozen shoulder, which are pathologically different from the complete tendon rupture. In the present study, the separate and combined effect of physiotherapy and CSI on motor function and pain in patients with complete rupture of the rotator cuff was investigated.

2. Materials and Methods

In the present randomized clinical trial study, 96 patients (15 males and 81 females) with a mean age of 51 years who had complete rotator cuff rupture in the period of February 2017 to November 2016 were identified and enrolled in the study.

According to the specific purpose of comparing the performance in the three groups under study, the opinion of the relevant experts and previous studies [7] and considering $p1 = 0.63$ (percentage of the effect of physiotherapy and CSI on motor function in patients with rotator cuff rupture) and $p2 = 0.3$ (percentage of the effect of physiotherapy on motor function of patients with rupture of the rotator cuff), the sample size was calculated using the following formula in the three intervention groups.

$$n = \frac{\left(z_{1-(a/2)} + z_{1-\beta}\right)^2 \left[p^1\left(1 - p^1\right) + p^{2\left(1-p^2\right)}\right]}{\left(p^1 - p^2\right)^2},$$

$$n = \frac{(1/96 + 0.85)2\ [0/63\,(1 - 0.3) + 0.3\,(1 - 0.7\,)]}{(0/63 - 0/3)2} = 32. \tag{1}$$

Therefore, the first group (physiotherapy and CSI) of 32 people, the second group (physiotherapy) of 32, and the third group (CSI) of 32 were calculated.

Inclusion criteria were patients with an age range of 30 to 70 years who were diagnosed with complete rotator cuff degenerative rupture with MRI and clinical examination and were consciously and cooperatively willing to participate in the study. Exclusion criteria were any concomitant shoulder disease such as infection, fracture, and tumor as well as trauma during treatment and therapeutic intervention by other people. Patients were referred to the orthopedic clinic and assessed after signing the informed consent. The variables studied were pain and active range of motion of patients. The severity of pain was evaluated based on the visual pain scale (VAS), and the active range of motion was assessed by goniometer and disabilities of the arm, shoulder, and hand (DASH) questionnaire.

The DASH questionnaire has 30 questions, of which 23 are about functional limitations in work, play, and interaction and examine the inadequacy of the upper extremity in performing functional activities, and 7 questions are about the severity of symptoms such as pain and weakness in impairing a person's functional ability. Likewise, the questionnaire is scored using a Likert scale with a range of 1 to 5 for each question. Score 1 indicates the absence of difficulty or limitation in the activities in question, and score 5 indicates the high intensity of the constraint. According to the instructions to convert the scores resulting from the questionnaire to standard scores in the range of 0 to 100 with the standard deviation of 50 ± 10, the raw scores obtained from each questionnaire are included in the following formula:

$$\left(\frac{\text{total answers to questions}}{\text{number of answered questions}} - 1\right) \times 25. \qquad (2)$$

Therefore, the overall score of this questionnaire is between zero and 100, and the higher scores indicate a higher level of disability. [8] Furthermore, it has shown that the DASH questionnaire is well able to distinguish between different levels of functional disability [9]; consequently, it is inferred that scores close to 100 in the DASH questionnaire represent higher levels of functional disability and inadequacy in comparison with the scores close to zero, which are considered as functional adequacy, and in the same way, scores close to 50 are in the intermediate range of this spectrum.

In addition to the 30 questions in this questionnaire, there are two series of questions with four items that are optional to answer and are called sports/arts DASH and work DASH and are scored similarly above. This part is not used in the present study. Mousavi et al. [10] prepared a Persian version of this tool and standardized the process in 271 Iranian patients with musculoskeletal disorders of the upper extremities such as painful arch syndrome, carpal tunnel syndrome, joint capsule adhesions, ulnar nerve entrapments, tendonitis, and bursitis. Cronbach's alpha was 0.96, and the intraclass correlation coefficient was 0.82. The present study uses the validated Persian version of this questionnaire.

Visual pain scale (VAS) is the pain ruler that contains a horizontal line that is scaled from zero to 10; zero indicates absolutely no pain, and 10 signs the unbearable and worst pain [11].

After the initial evaluation, the patients were randomly divided into 3 groups of 32 patients with block static method, so that based on 9-person blocks (AABBCC), all its subitems were calculated and randomly assigned to each intervention group.

The first group underwent 12 sessions of physiotherapy in the form of massage, rotator cuff and scapular muscle stretching exercises, strengthening exercises and modalities including laser, transcutaneous electrical nerve stimulation (TENS), and ultrasound (US) twice a week for 6 weeks with a duration of 45 minutes per session including 30 minutes of electrotherapy and 15 minutes of manual therapy training. Normal tense current with a frequency of 120 Hertz, a pulse width of 120 microseconds in 15 minutes and current with a frequency of 50 Hertz, a pulse width of 350 microseconds, an 8 second contraction time, and a 2 second rest time for 10 minutes were used. Ultrasound with 1 to 2 watts per frequency of 3 MHz continuously and intensity of 5 cm square in 5 minutes was performed by a specialized rehabilitation physiotherapist. The first stage included the first 4 sessions to achieve shoulder movements, especially internal and external rotation equal to the opposite side and arm abduction less than 90°; with Cadman pendulum exercises and passive range of motion exercises, bending the shoulder, straightening the shoulder, and internal and external rotation were started. Capsule stretching exercises for the anterior, posterior, and inferior capsules were taught to patients using the contralateral arm and gradually moved toward active range-of-motion exercises such as wall walking. All inactive exercises at this stage were performed up to the maximum range of motion that did not aggravate the patient's pain, with the aim of controlling pain and creating shoulder movements below 90° and elbow movements.

The second phase consisted of 4 second sessions performed with the aim of improving the strength, power, and endurance of the shoulder set. Pain control methods such as the first step were also performed in this step. The goal of the shoulder movements at this stage was to equalize the active range of motion of the affected shoulder joint with the opposite shoulder in all movement plates. For this purpose, exercises included passive range of motion, capsular stretching, and auxiliary-active movement exercises; then, the range-of-motion exercises were performed. To gain muscle strength, we performed the exercises twice a week, with 8 to 12 repetitions for three periods. Exercises included strengthening the remaining rotator cuff muscles, starting closed-chain isometric reinforcement (internal and external rotation and abduction), and progressing to open-chain strengthening.

The third step was performed in the third 4 sessions with the aim of improving neuromuscular control and shoulder depth sense, preparing for a gradual return to functional activities. At the end of the sessions, motor function and pain according to DASH and VAS questionnaires and measurements with a goniometer (flexion, extension, abduction, and external and internal rotation) were evaluated.

The second group was injected with 8 mg of methylprednisolone and 1 ml of 2% lidocaine with a posterior approach in the subacromial region in two stages 21 days apart. Two weeks after the second injection, the patient completed a questionnaire, and functional assessments were examined with a goniometer.

The third group was injected with 8 mg of methylprednisolone and 1 ml of lidocaine 2% and, two days later, underwent 6 sessions of physiotherapy by a rehabilitation specialist twice a week for 3 weeks. The duration of each session was 45 minutes, including 30 minutes of electrotherapy and 15 minutes of manual therapy training; after 6 sessions of physiotherapy at the end of the third week, the injection was performed, and the other 6 sessions of physiotherapy twice a week for 2 weeks were performed with a duration of 45 minutes per session. (The steps of physiotherapy were the same as the first group.)

All groups were instructed not to use NSAIDs or herbal and home remedies either orally or systemically or topically during the study. At the end of the sessions, function and pain were assessed according to the DASH and VAS questionnaires and goniometer measurement. At the end of the study, the data before and after the intervention of all three groups were compared.

Ethical considerations were applied in accordance with the approval of the ethics committee of Dezful University of Medical Sciences with the code number IR.DUMS.-REC.1398.045. All the patients who agreed to participate in the trial provided written informed consent. Likewise, the patients' personal information was also preserved. The study protocol, including the statistical analysis plan, is available at fa.irct.ir with the code number IRCT20200102045987N1. Quality control of verification and screening of adherence to protocols were performed on a regular basis by the trial coordinators. This research has been approved by the IRB of the authors' affiliated institutions. One-way analysis of variance within the subjects and Friedman test were used to investigate the relationship between separate and combined physiotherapy treatment and CSI and the studied variables. Statistical analysis was performed using SPSS software version 23. Alpha less than 0.05 was considered significant.

3. Results

In this study, 32 patients in each treatment group were present. More than 80% of the patients in each group were female. The chi-square test shows that there is no significant difference between the gender distribution of groups ($p = 0.789$). The gender frequency distribution of patients in different groups was summarized in Table 1. The mean age in the physiotherapy, steroid, and physiotherapy + steroid groups was 51.75 ± 7.37, 52.37 ± 6.61, 50.87 ± 5.65 years, respectively. ANOVA test showed that there was no significant difference in the age of the three groups ($p = 0.658$).

Paired samples *T*-test shows that in all three groups, the DASH and VAS scores have decreased significantly after the intervention. In other words, all three interventions have been effective in reducing the DASH and VAS scores. Also, the ANOVA test showed that there was no difference in DASH and VAS scores between patients before the intervention, but after the intervention, Bonferroni and Scheffe post hoc test showed that DASH and VAS scores were not different in the physiotherapy and steroid groups, but the DASH as well as VAS score in the physiotherapy + steroid group was significantly lower than the other two groups. In other words, the combined physiotherapy + steroid intervention was more effective in reducing the DASH and VAS scores ($p < 0.05$; Table 2).

Paired samples *T*-test shows that in all three groups, after the intervention, the flexion angle increased significantly. In other words, all three interventions were effective in increasing the flexion angle. The ANOVA test showed that there was no difference in the patients' flexion angle before the intervention, but this difference was significant after the intervention. Bonferroni and Scheffe post hoc tests showed that the flexion angle in the steroid group and physiotherapy + steroids were not different, but the angle of flexion in the physiotherapy group was significantly less than the other two groups. In other words, physiotherapy was less effective in increasing the angle of flexion than treatments containing steroids ($p < 0.05$; Table 2).

After intervention in the steroid and physiotherapy + - steroid groups, the extension angle increased significantly (p value = 0 and 0.029, respectively), but this increase was little. The ANOVA test also showed that there was no difference in the extension angle of patients before and after the intervention. Therefore, the interventions performed did not change the extension angle clinically and significantly (Table 2).

Table 1: Gender frequency distribution of patients in the three intervention groups.

Variable		Frequency n (%)	p value
Physiotherapy	Female	27 (84.4)	
	Male	5 (15.6)	
Corticosteroid injection	Female	28 (87.5)	
	Male	4 (12.55)	
Physiotherapy + corticosteroid injection	Female	26 (81.3)	0.789
	Male	6 (18.8)	
Total	Female	81 (84.4)	
	Male	15 (15.6)	

In all three groups, the abduction angle increased significantly after the intervention. In other words, all three interventions were effective in increasing the abduction angle. Also, the ANOVA test showed that there was no difference in the abduction angle of patients before the intervention, but after the intervention, this difference was significant. Bonferroni and Scheffe post hoc test showed that the abduction angle in the physiotherapy + steroid group was more than in the other two groups, and in the steroid group, it was more than the physiotherapy group. In other words, physiotherapy + steroid was the most effective treatment in increasing the abduction angle, and physiotherapy alone was less effective ($p < 0.05$; Table 2).

Paired samples *T*-test showed that in all three groups, after the intervention, the internal and external rotation angles increased significantly. In other words, all three interventions were effective in increasing the internal and external rotation angles. ANOVA test also showed that there was no difference in the patients' internal and external rotation angles before the intervention, but this difference was significant after the intervention. Bonferroni and Scheffe post hoc test showed that there was no significant difference in the internal and external rotation angles in the steroid group and physiotherapy + steroid, but this angle in the sole physiotherapy group was significantly less than the other two groups, which received containing steroid therapies ($p < 0.05$).

4. Discussion

Management of rotator cuff complete rapture is a dilemma due to the controversial opinion among various surgical and nonsurgical treatment modalities. Nowadays with respect to surgical complications (e.g., stiffness, infection, neurologic injury, bleeding, prolonged hospital stays, and so on), there is an increasing trend for shifting from operative techniques to more conservative, nonoperative, and less invasive methods [12]. Likewise, with respect to fewer side effects and cost as well as more accessibility of conservative treatment, it seems that it is more preferable the first-line treatment in comparison to surgery. Furthermore, Ryösä et al. concluded in a systematic review that the surgical approach did not perform significantly better in terms of pain and function than conservative treatment [13]. Moreover, there are several studies that also suggested conservative therapy as the first-line treatment of degenerative rotator cuff tears except in those with acute traumatic rapture [14–17]. On the other hand, the American Academy Orthopaedic Surgeons (AAOS)

TABLE 2: The effect of different management on pain-related scores and range of motions.

Variable	Physiotherapy			Corticosteroid injection			Physiotherapy + corticosteroid injection			p value	
	Before INT[a]	After INT	p value	Before INT	After INT	p value	Before INT	After INT	p value	Before INT	After INT
DASH[b]	57.21 ± 4.15	48.77 ± 4.0	0.000	57.29 ± 3.60	47.83 ± 3.52	0.000	56.77 ± 3.65	45.91 ± 4.12	0.000	0.797	0.013
VAS[c]	5.53 ± 0.62	4.00 ± 0.91	0.000	5.78 ± 0.70	4.18 ± 0.64	0.000	5.59 ± 0.66	3.56 ± 0.66	0.000	0.299	0.004
Flexion°	144.9 ± 9.7	164.9 ± 7.9	0.000	142.1 ± 10	169.6 ± 7.6	0.000	141.2 ± 9.2	170.6 ± 7	0.000	0.281	0.007
Extension°	61.9 ± 5.39	62.46 ± 7.79	0.406	59.4 ± 4.9	60.5 ± 4.43	0.000	60 ± 5.63	60.96 ± 5.63	0.029	0.140	0.290
Abduction°	119.1 ± 10.36	143.0 ± 8.97	0.000	116.34 ± 10.2	148.9 ± 8.8	0.000	118.7 ± 12.5	154.7 ± 9.8	0.000	0.555	0.000
Internal rotation°	36.6 ± 4.3	56.9 ± 3.2	0.000	33.81 ± 4.7	59.5 ± 3.2	0.000	35.4 ± 4.9	60.1 ± 4.12	0.000	0.060	0.001
External rotation°	50.4 ± 5.5	66.7 ± 4.2	0.000	48.6 ± 5.5	70.9 ± 4.3	0.000	49.0 ± 5.5	70.7 ± 3.8	0.000	0.236	0.000

[a]INT: intervention; [b]DASH: disabilities of the arm, shoulder, and hand; and [c]VAS: visual pain scale.

guidelines claimed that surgical repair is a superior valid option for patients with symptomatic full-thickness rotator cuff tears even though there is also a lack of supporting evidence for conservative treatment [18]. Moreover, the superiority of surgical over the conservative treatment is challenging to demonstrate, due to the heterogeneity of studies' findings. According to the recent meta-analysis, significant differences were reported in terms of the Constant–Murley score and VAS only at 1 year follow-up in favor of the surgical group compared with the conservative group [12]. On the other study, the short time follow-up of both the surgical and conservative groups was the same, while the long-term function of the surgical group was better. A hypothesis proposed to explain this phenomenon in the long term is based on the inherent disadvantages of conservative treatment [19]. On the basis of the points mentioned above, it would seem that there are also many controversies on the optimal management of rotator cuff tears.

There are also many controversies among the choice of the optimal and most effective nonoperative managements including ice, simple exercises, medications, and progress to more intensive physical therapy, hyaluronic acid injections, CSI, biological augmentation with platelet-derived products (PRP), marrow stimulation, and so on [20]. Therefore, we found it essential to compare the efficacy of some of the most common conservative therapies including physiotherapy and CSI separately and simultaneously.

In the present study, despite the significant decrease in VAS and DASH scores in all three groups, no significant differences were observed between the two physiotherapy treatment approaches and CSI in the VAS and DASH scores. Instead, people who received both treatments showed significantly lower VAS as well as DASH scores than the other two groups. Regarding this issue, there are some studies that reported similar aforementioned results and recommended the combination of CSI and physical therapy in comparison with physical therapy or CSI alone [21, 22]. Burger et al. and Mehtap et al. also did not find any significant difference in the efficacy between physiotherapy and CSI, but they did not evaluate the influence of the simultaneous therapies [23, 24]. Hay et al., on the other hand, reported a significant better long-term outcome in the physiotherapy group in comparison with CSI even though he did not apply the combined therapies [25]. On the contrary, Koester et al. did not suggest the CSI in rotator cuff tears [26]. Therefore, it can be said that the combination therapy of CSI and physiotherapy is superior to each management alone for decreasing the pain and disability in rotator cuff tearing. Further studies are required regarding the exact dose and duration of corticosteroid therapy and finding the optimal technique of physiotherapy.

As to the ROM evaluation, in the present study, it was observed that therapies containing the steroid injection approach (steroid injection and steroids + physiotherapy) had a more dramatic effect on improving the patients' ROM than physiotherapy alone. Similar results were reported by Boudreault et al., reporting that corticosteroid injection had a significant effect on the range of motion of the shoulder in abduction. Conversely, Burger et al. and Mehtap et al. did not report a significant difference between the two treatment approaches, which is inconsistent with the present study. This may be due to the fact that in the Burger et al.'s study, the subjects were the patients with rotator cuff syndrome, and in the Mehtap et al.'s study, the patients with shoulder pain were evaluated, but the present study was performed on patients with complete rotator cuff rupture. To sum up, everything that has been stated so far, the effect of combined treatment (corticosteroids + physiotherapy) can be far better than any of the treatments alone in the range of motion and performance of individuals.

Despite many positive considerations, this study had few limitations. No program was designed for long-term follow-up of patients. Furthermore, there was no control group to compare the effect of any interventions with no treatment. Likewise, although the patients were instructed not to use NSAIDs or herbal and home remedies either orally or systemically or topically during the study, we cannot be sure about it. Because we cannot follow the patients when they are out of the clinic.

5. Conclusions

Among the conservative approaches to complete rotator cuff rupture, a combination of steroid injection and physiotherapy can be more effective than either approach alone in both reducing pain and improving shoulder function and range of motions.

Consent

Written informed consent was obtained from all individual participants included in the study. The purpose of this research was completely explained to the patients, and they were assured that their information will be kept confidential by the researcher. Written informed consent was also obtained from the patients regarding the publication of this study.

Acknowledgments

The authors would like to thank Shiraz University of Medical Sciences, Shiraz, Iran, and also the Center for Development of Clinical Research of Nemazee Hospital and Dr. Nasrin Shokrpour for editorial assistance.

References

[1] A. Yamamoto, K. Takagishi, T. Osawa et al., "Prevalence and risk factors of a rotator cuff tear in the general population," *Journal of Shoulder and Elbow Surgery*, vol. 19, no. 1, pp. 116–120, 2010.

[2] H. Kijima, H. Minagawa, T. Nishi, K. Kikuchi, and Y. Shimada, "Long-term follow-up of cases of rotator cuff tear treated conservatively," *Journal of Shoulder and Elbow Surgery*, vol. 21, no. 4, pp. 491–494, 2012.

[3] K. J. Hippensteel, R. Brophy, M. V. Smith, and R. W. Wright, "A comprehensive review of physical examination tests of the cervical spine, scapula, and rotator cuff," *Journal of the American Academy of Orthopaedic Surgeons*, vol. 27, no. 11, pp. 385–394, 2019.

[4] M. J. Tuite, M. F. Sanford, D. S. Levey et al., Rotator Cuff Injury MRI, 2018.

[5] M. Karasuyama, M. Gotoh, K. Tahara et al., "Clinical results of conservative management in patients with full-thickness rotator cuff tear: a meta-analysis," *Clinics in Shoulder and Elbow*, vol. 23, no. 2, pp. 86–93, 2020.

[6] K. Vachhani, C. Whyne, D. Nam, J. Wong, J. Chou, and R. Paul, "Comparing surgical techniques for irreparable rotator CUFF tear management: a cadaveric biomechanical study," in *Orthopaedic Proceedings: 2020*, The British Editorial Society of Bone & Joint Surgery, London, UK, 2020.

[7] E. Maman, C. Harris, L. White, G. Tomlinson, M. Shashank, and E. Boynton, "Outcome of nonoperative treatment of symptomatic rotator cuff tears monitored by magnetic resonance imaging," *Journal of Bone and Joint Surgery American Volume*, vol. 91, no. 8, pp. 1898–1906, 2009.

[8] P. L. Hudak, P. C. Amadio, C. Bombardier et al., "Development of an upper extremity outcome measure: the DASH (disabilities of the arm, shoulder, and head)," *American Journal of Industrial Medicine*, vol. 29, no. 6, pp. 602–608, 1996.

[9] A. Jester, A. Harth, G. Wind, G. Germann, and M. Sauerbier, "Disabilities of the arm, shoulder and hand (DASH) questionnaire: determining functional activity profiles in patients with upper extremity disorders," *Journal of Hand Surgery*, vol. 30, no. 1, pp. 23–28, 2005.

[10] S. J. Mousavi, M. Parnianpour, M. Abedi et al., "Cultural adaptation and validation of the Persian version of the Disabilities of the Arm, Shoulder and Hand (DASH) outcome measure," *Clinical Rehabilitation*, vol. 22, no. 8, pp. 749–757, 2008.

[11] M. E. Wewers and N. K. Lowe, "A critical review of visual analogue scales in the measurement of clinical phenomena," *Research in Nursing & Health*, vol. 13, no. 4, pp. 227–236, 1990.

[12] U. G. Longo, L. R. Ambrogioni, V. Candela et al., "Conservative versus surgical management for patients with rotator cuff tears: a systematic review and META-analysis," *BMC Musculoskeletal Disorders*, vol. 22, no. 1, pp. 1–10, 2021.

[13] A. Ryösä, K. Laimi, V. Äärimaa, K. Lehtimäki, J. Kukkonen, and M. Saltychev, "Surgery or conservative treatment for rotator cuff tear: a meta-analysis," *Disability & Rehabilitation*, vol. 39, no. 14, pp. 1357–1363, 2017.

[14] N. D. Clement, Y. X. Nie, and J. M. McBirnie, "Management of degenerative rotator cuff tears: a review and treatment strategy," *Sports Medicine, Arthroscopy, Rehabilitation, Therapy & Technology: SMARTT*, vol. 4, no. 1, pp. 48–55, 2012.

[15] F. Franceschi, R. Papalia, A. Palumbo, A. Del Buono, N. Maffulli, and V. Denaro, "Operative management of partial-and full-thickness rotator cuff tears," in *Rotator Cuff Tear*, pp. 100–113, Karger Publishers, Basel, Switzerland, 2012.

[16] C. C. Schmidt, C. D. Jarrett, and B. T. Brown, "Management of rotator cuff tears," *The Journal of hand surgery*, vol. 40, no. 2, pp. 399–408, 2015.

[17] J. R. Bytomski and D. Black, "Conservative treatment of rotator cuff injuries," *Journal of Surgical Orthopaedic Advances*, vol. 15, no. 3, pp. 126–131, 2006.

[18] R. Z. Tashjian, "AAOS clinical practice guideline: optimizing the management of rotator cuff problems," *American Academy of Orthopaedic Surgeon*, vol. 19, no. 6, pp. 380–383, 2011.

[19] S. Moosmayer, G. Lund, U. S. Seljom et al., "Tendon repair compared with physiotherapy in the treatment of rotator cuff tears," *Journal of Bone and Joint Surgery*, vol. 96, no. 18, pp. 1504–1514, 2014.

[20] S. Weber and J. Chahal, "Management of rotator cuff injuries," *Journal of the American Academy of Orthopaedic Surgeons*, vol. 28, no. 5, pp. e193–e201, 2020.

[21] B. Gialanella and M. Bertolinelli, "Corticosteroids injection in rotator cuff tears in elderly patient: pain outcome prediction," *Geriatrics and Gerontology International*, vol. 13, no. 4, pp. 993–1001, 2013.

[22] V. B. Vad, R. F. Warren, D. W. Altchek, S. J. O'Brien, H. A. Rose, and T. L. Wickiewicz, "Negative prognostic factors in managing massive rotator cuff tears," *Clinical Journal of Sport Medicine*, vol. 12, no. 3, pp. 151–157, 2002.

[23] M. Burger, C. Africa, K. Droomer et al., "Effect of corticosteroid injections versus physiotherapy on pain, shoulder range of motion and shoulder function in patients with subacromial impingement syndrome: a systematic review and meta-analysis," *South African Journal of Physiotherapy*, vol. 72, no. 1, p. 318, 2016.

[24] A. C. Mehtap, "Comparison of the efficacy of physiotherapy and local corticosteroid injections on painful shoulder," *Journal of Arthritis*, vol. 5, no. 4, pp. 1–5, 2016.

[25] E. M. Hay, E. Thomas, S. Paterson, K. Dziedzic, and P. Croft, "A pragmatic randomised controlled trial of local corticosteroid injection and physiotherapy for the treatment of new episodes of unilateral shoulder pain in primary care," *Annals of the Rheumatic Diseases*, vol. 62, no. 5, pp. 394–399, 2003.

[26] M. C. Koester, W. R. Dunn, J. E. Kuhn, and K. P. Spindler, "The efficacy of subacromial corticosteroid injection in the treatment of rotator cuff disease: a systematic review," *Journal of the American Academy of Orthopaedic Surgeons*, vol. 15, no. 1, pp. 3–11, 2007.

25

Thromboembolism in Malignant Musculoskeletal Tumour

Achmad Fauzi Kamal,[1] Didi Saputra Ramang,[1] and Marcel Prasetyo[2]

[1]*Department of Orthopaedic and Traumatology, Faculty of Medicine Universitas Indonesia, Cipto Mangunkusumo General Hospital, Jakarta, Indonesia*
[2]*Department of Radiology, Faculty of Medicine Universitas Indonesia, Cipto Mangunkusumo General Hospital, Jakarta, Indonesia*

Correspondence should be addressed to Didi Saputra Ramang; dsramang@gmail.com

Academic Editor: Andreas K. Demetriades

Malignant musculoskeletal tumour may cause considerable burden to general health. The fast growth combined with the tumour characteristics and its invasion capability resulted in the poor prognosis of malignant musculoskeletal tumour. Malignant musculoskeletal tumour may cause significant disability by destroying normal tissue that plays important role in body kinematics. Thromboembolism, including deep vein thrombosis, pulmonary embolism, and other kinds of venous thromboembolism, is one of the most underestimated complications of musculoskeletal tumour. Normally, thrombosis ensues when pathologic factors overcame the body hemostatic regulatory capabilities, which will predispose the body to the formation of thrombus. Venous thromboembolism in musculoskeletal tumour may develop as a result of interaction between the tumour pathologic capabilities and its interaction with normal bodily functions. In this study, we reviewed the burden of musculoskeletal tumour and its complication on global health. Then, the review will focus on the pathologic and clinical aspect of thromboembolism in malignant musculoskeletal tumour, including pathophysiology, diagnosis, and treatment based on recent findings and literature.

1. Introduction

In recent years, malignant cancers are currently on the rise with an estimated incidence of 15.2 million of new cases of cancer with a death count of 8.8 million for year 2015. In terms of incidence, musculoskeletal tumours are relatively rare compared to other types of cancer in adults and are more often seen in pediatric and adolescents. Musculoskeletal tumour only makes up for around 0.2–0.5% of all tumour cases in adults, and the distribution varies greatly across the globe. Musculoskeletal tumour can be differentiated into benign and malignant tumours based on the tumour invasiveness, rate of growth, and many other different factors. Compared to its benign counterpart, malignant musculoskeletal tumour generally grows much more extensively in a faster rate. If not adequately treated as soon as possible, malignant musculoskeletal tumour mainly has fatal outcome. Osteosarcoma and Ewing sarcoma are two of the most encountered types of musculoskeletal tumour, and both types are malignant. The mainstay treatment for malignant musculoskeletal tumour is complete excision of the tumour followed by reconstruction of tumour-associated defects. Limb-salvaging treatment options are much more preferable than ablative treatments [1].

Some complications are associated with malignant musculoskeletal tumour, ranging from surgical site infection after tumour excision to loss of limb function and even mortality. One of the most concerning complication associated with malignant musculoskeletal tumour is thromboembolism, including pulmonary embolism and deep vein thrombosis. Thromboembolism is deeply correlated with both orthopedic surgery and orthopedic tumour. Literature studies reported the incidence of thromboembolism in orthopedic cases ranging from <1 to 22% [2]. Symptomatic thromboembolism is associated with poor prognosis, and Iwata et al. found the incidence rate of symptomatic thromboembolism to be 1.18% in patients with bone and soft tissue sarcomas [3]. Morbidity and mortality caused by thromboembolism urged the need for a rapid and accurate diagnostic method for diagnosing thromboembolism in malignant musculoskeletal cancer patients. At the same time, it also signals the importance of early treatment of thromboembolism in malignant musculoskeletal tumour in order to avoid unwanted disabilities.

2. Methods

Comprehensive literature search was done by searching PubMed, Scopus, EBSCOHost, ProQuest, ScienceDirect, SpringerLink, and Wiley on November 2020. The literature search included all articles regarding thromboembolism in malignant musculoskeletal tumour, including systematic reviews, clinical trials, cohorts, case controls, and case reports. Articles on different aspects of thromboembolism in malignant musculoskeletal tumour including pathophysiology, diagnosis, and treatment modalities are included in this study in order to provide comprehensive review about thromboembolism in malignant musculoskeletal tumours. Letters, editor opinion, and commentary studies are excluded. Analysis of the articles obtained from the search is done on December 2020. Findings are screened and extracted by a single reviewer. The result of the literature search is described and summarized in Table 1.

3. Literature Search Results

3.1. The Mechanism of Thromboembolic Formation. The exact mechanism triggering clotting in patients with thromboembolism is not fully understood. It is thought that arterial thrombus may be incited by disruption of endothelial integrity, while venous thromboembolism was found to be preceded by venous stasis. It is agreed that intact vasculature microstructure is vital in preventing thromboembolism, and disturbance of the vessel wall integrity may initiate pathophysiologic cascade that resulted in the formation of thrombus, which may get unattached to form emboli that travel and block vessels smaller in size compared to the emboli distant to the thrombus formation location. Hemostasis is the balancing process that maintains the blood flow system inside blood vessels. When pathologic factors exceeded the protective and regulatory features of hemostasis, blood coagulation will be initiated. Blood coagulation is a very complex process that happens as a result of interplay between many different intravascular elements, including shear stress on the inner lining of the vessel wall, blood coagulation factors, and other contributing agents, which ends in the generation of thrombus. Physiologically, thrombosis is actually an important protective sequence that protects the body from excessive blood loss [4, 5].

In general, thromboembolism may happen as a combination of dysfunctional vascular endothelium, activity of an intravascular tissue factor, the existence of anticoagulant endovascular proteins, and the inhibition of fibrinolysis. Normally, endothelium prevents the formation of thrombus by producing thromboregulator agents, including nitric oxide, prostacyclin, and ectonucleotidase CD39. Following endothelial disruption, exposure of collagen and intravascular tissue factor to blood will initiate the generation of thrombus by accumulation and activation of accumulated thrombocytes. Collagen and intravascular tissue participated in the thrombus regulatory equilibrium by acting as hemostatic barrier in order to maintain the integrity of the circulatory system. Intravascular tissue factor, a transmembrane glycoprotein, is expressed in vessel wall tissue and functions as a receptor and cofactor of factor VII that ultimately plays vital role in the activation of factor IX [6]. Intravascular tissue factor may also activate platelets in the absence of endothelium disruption by cleaving protease-activated receptor-4 on the surface of platelets, thereby causing platelets to release thromboxane A_2, adenosine diphosphate, and serotonin that will activate other platelets and enhance thrombus formation [7]. Anticoagulant endovascular proteins including thrombin-activatable fibrinolysis inhibitor (TAFI), antithrombin, protein S, and protein C are a group of proteins that hinder thrombosis by inactivating blood-clotting factors including factor VIIIa and factor Va. Endogenous fibrinolysis is another protective factor that broke down formed thrombus by the activation of plasminogen into plasmin. Plasmin degrades the fibrin clot into soluble products and plays a major role in fibrin removal [8, 9].

3.2. Thromboembolism in Musculoskeletal Tumours: Pathophysiology. The risk of venous thromboembolism in cancer patients is almost five-fold higher compared to general population [10]. In cancer patients, it is thought that increased risk of thrombosis is attributed to some factors coined as Virchow's triad, including stasis of the blood flow, endothelial dysfunction, and state of hypercoagulability. Malignant musculoskeletal tumour patients may have limited mobility resulting from the invasion and the growth of tumour tissue. The immobilization of musculoskeletal tumour patients may cause stasis in the blood flow, contributing to the formation of thrombus. Other factors that contribute to the immobility of musculoskeletal tumour patients include the disability of the patients in the advanced stage of the disease and the damage to the musculoskeletal tissue caused by surgery. Decreased blood flow participated in the formation of blood clot by causing improper clearance of blood-clotting factor while also increasing blood viscosity. The accumulation of blood clotting factors combined with the slow blood flow may overwhelm anticoagulant regulatory systems, resulting in the hypercoagulable state of musculoskeletal tumour patients and therefore predisposing musculoskeletal tumour patients to the formation of thromboemboli. The invasion of tumour into the vascular tissue or treatment interventions for the tumour such as vascular catheters and surgery might also disturb the endothelial integrity, favoring the formation of thromboemboli [4, 11].

Some literature studies found that the musculoskeletal tumour itself may contribute to the formation of thrombus. Tumour tissue can induce hypercoagulable state by increasing the activation of coagulative factors and inactivating the anticoagulant factors at the same time.

Table 1: List literatures reviewed.

Studies	Year	Type of study	Findings of the study
Pathophysiology			
Falanga et al.	2012	Literature review	Risk of VTE in cancer patients is significantly higher compared to normal population
Walder et al.	2012	Case report	Invasion of tumour into vascular tissue and invasive treatment such as catheters may affect incidence
Falanga et al.	2015	Literature review	Musculoskeletal tumour inhibit fibrinolysis and cytokine production while increasing platelet aggregation
Hisada et al.	2015	Literature review	Central venous line, transfusion, and chemotherapy increase the risk of thrombus formation in cancer patients
Yoshimura et al.	2018	Prospective cohort	High BMI increases the risk of thrombus formation
Groot et al.	2018	Retrospective cohort	Risk of VTE increases significantly in patents with long bone metastasis receiving surgical therapy
Tukaye et al.	2016	Literature review	Thrombosis may be the first finding of occult tumour
Dickmann et al.	2013	Prospective cohort	Increased cumulative probability of VTE in cancer patients with metastases
Diagnosis			
Mitsunaga et al.	2013	Case report	Contrast-enhanced MRI may be helpful in finding tumour thrombus
Navalkele et al.	2013	Case report	The utilization of ultrasound in diagnosis of thromboembolism in cancer patients
Kaiser et al.	2017	Retrospective cohort	Preoperative complete blood examination may help in screening patients with risk of postoperative VTE
Treatment			
Haase et al.	2020	Retrospective cohort	Tranexamic acid may decrease the risk of postoperative VTE with insignificant result
Mendez et al.	2017	Retrospective cohort	Aspirin decreases the risk of thromboembolism in several types of cancer when administered as thromboprophylaxis
Farge et al.	2016	Guideline	LMWH has been widely used to prevent postoperative thromboembolism in patients with a high risk of immobilization
Watson et al.	2015	Guideline	LMWH may be used as a preventive and treatment agent for VTE
Kearon et al.	2016	Guideline	LMWH may be used as a preventive and treatment agent for VTE
Farge et al.	2019	Literature review	The limitation of LMWH is that it is an expensive drug and is administered by injection, therefore lowering compliance

VTE: venous thromboembolism; LWMH: low molecular weight heparin.

Musculoskeletal tumour also hampers the fibrinolytic cascade by upregulating plasminogen activator inhibitor-1 (PAI-1), producing proinflammatory cytokines including IL-6 and TGF-β which were found to induce the hypercoagulable state by increasing the expression of intravascular tissue factor, and increases platelet aggregation on the vessel [12]. Modalities used in anticancer therapies such as central venous line, blood transfusion, chemotherapy, and surgical therapy which were also found to increase the risk of thrombus formation [13]. Yoshimura et al. found that the risk of venous thromboembolism postoperatively in patients receiving surgery for malignant bone and soft tissue tumours in the lower extremity is increased, with high body mass index (BMI) which was found to be a significant risk factor contributing to the formation of thrombus [14]. Groot et al. found that the risk of postoperative venous thromboembolism increased significantly in patients receiving surgery for the treatment of long bone metastases [15].

Thrombosis may be one of the first signs of undetected neoplasm. The likelihood of the existence of tumour in patients with bilateral deep vein thrombosis is almost five times higher than in general population. Patients with metastatic cancers were especially predisposed for venous thromboembolism even when compared to other cancer patients without metastases. The Vienna Cancer and Thrombosis Study found an increased cumulative probability of venous thromboembolism in metastasized cancer patients [16, 17].

3.3. Diagnosing Thromboembolism in Musculoskeletal Cancer Patients. Thrombus in cancer patients is mainly diagnosed by imaging modalities. Imaging modalities that can be used include CT, MRI, Doppler ultrasound, and positron emission tomography. Contrast-enhanced MRI may be used to find intraluminal soft tissue enhancement along the suspected vessel [18]. Ultrasound imaging may be used to diagnose the tumour initially and followed up using CT or PET [19]. Laboratory diagnostic for measuring coagulation markers such as D-dimer was found to be of no use in diagnosing thromboembolism in cancer patients. Yoshimura et al. found that only 1 case out of 8 VTE cases diagnosed using enhanced CT was found to have elevated level of D-dimer above 10 μg/mL [14]. However, Kaiser et al. found that high preoperative white blood cell count is a significant independent risk factor for venous thromboembolism in primary osteosarcoma patients. This signals the utility of routine preoperative blood examination in musculoskeletal tumour patients to help determine which patients may develop venous thromboembolism after surgical intervention [20].

3.4. Treatment of Thromboembolism in Musculoskeletal Tumour Patients. Vascular surgery is one of the main treatments for thromboembolism in musculoskeletal tumour patients. Venous thrombectomy is one of the most used procedures, where the intravascular thrombus is taken out from the blood vessel. However, recent advances in medical science noted the availability of pharmacological agent as treatment and prevention modality for thromboembolism in cancer. Haase et al. found that the usage of tranexamic acid in cancer patients undergoing endoprosthetic reconstruction decreased the number of patients with venous thromboembolism postoperatively. However, the result was statistically insignificant, and the main purpose of tranexamic acid is to decrease blood loss and not to decrease or change the risk of postoperative venous thromboembolism in musculoskeletal cancer patients [21]. Thromboprophylaxis is a new approach used to prevent the occurrence of postoperative venous thromboembolism, in which a pharmacologic agent is administrated in order to decrease the risk of thrombus formation. Mendez et al. found that aspirin decreases the risk of postoperative venous thromboembolism formation in patients diagnosed with malignant soft tissue carcinoma, metastatic carcinoma, lymphoma, or multiple myeloma when compared to another group that did not receive any thromboprophylaxis treatment [22]. The finding was found to be statistically significant. The study also identifies predicting factors that helps to determine which patients may benefit from thromboprophylaxis using aspirin, including patients with history of venous thromboembolism, history of diabetes melitus, operative blood loss around 250–1000 mL, and history of postoperative transfusion.

Another widely known agent that may be used as thromboprophylaxis is heparin, particularly low molecular weight heparins (LMWH). LMWH has been widely known as a pharmacological agent with beneficial role in preventing and treating thromboembolism. Medical guidelines have stated the utilization of LMWH injections to prevent postoperative thromboembolism in patients suffering from neoplasms with a risk of long-term immobilization [23]. Past clinical trials have found the efficacy of LMWH for cancer-associated thrombosis. LMWH is also recommended as a preventive and treatment agent for established venous thromboembolism and is used for at least 3 months [24, 25]. Even though LWMH may be considered as the best anticoagulant choice for patients with cancer, it also comes with downside. In some countries, LMWH is considered as an expensive drug, and the use of injection may lower compliance of some patients [26].

4. Conclusion

Malignant musculoskeletal tumour poses a threat to public health since it may cause significant morbidity and mortality. One of the most concerning complication associated with musculoskeletal tumour is the incidence of thromboembolism, which may happen as result of disturbance in the hemostatic equilibrium. Timely diagnosis using accurate diagnostic methods, while also considering significant predisposing factors together with right treatment, is beneficial in preventing disabilities caused by cancer-associated thromboembolism.

References

[1] M. Bergovec, O. Kubat, M. Smerdelj, S. Seiwerth, A. Bonevski, and D. Orlic, "Epidemiology of musculoskeletal tumors in a national referral orthopedic department. A study of 3482 cases," *Cancer Epidemiology*, vol. 39, no. 3, pp. 298–302, 2015.

[2] D. V. Congiusta, K. M. Amer, J. Thomson, J. Ippolito, K. S. Beebe, and J. Benevenia, "Risk factors of venous thromboembolism in patients with benign and malignant musculoskeletal tumors: a dual database analysis," *International Orthopaedics*, vol. 44, no. 10, pp. 2147–2153, 2020.

[3] S. Iwata, A. Kawai, T. Ueda, and T. Ishii, "Symptomatic venous thromboembolism in patients with malignant bone and soft tissue tumours: a prospective multicenter cohort study," *Annals of Surgical Oncology*, 2020.

[4] E. Vazquez-Garza, C. Jerjes-Sanchez, A. Navarrete, J. Joya-Harrison, and D. Rodriguez, "Venous thromboembolism: thrombosis, inflammation, and immunothrombosis for clinicians," *Journal of Thrombosis and Thrombolysis*, vol. 44, no. 3, pp. 377–385, 2017.

[5] C. A. Karcutskie, J. P. Meizoso, J. J. Ray et al., "Association of mechanism of injury with risk for venous thromboembolism after trauma," *JAMA Surgery*, vol. 152, no. 1, pp. 35–40, 2017.

[6] R. De Caterina, S. Husted, L. Wallentin et al., "General mechanisms of coagulation and targets of anticoagulants (section I): position paper of the ESC working group on thrombosis—task force on anticoagulants in heart disease," *Thrombosis and Haemostasis*, vol. 109, no. 4, pp. 569–579, 2013.

[7] P. A. Gurbel and U. S. Tantry, "Antiplatelet and anticoagulant agents in heart failure," *JACC: Heart Failure*, vol. 2, no. 1, pp. 1–14, 2014.

[8] K. Date, C. Ettelaie, and A. Maraveyas, "Tissue factor-bearing microparticles and inflammation: a potential mechanism for the development of venous thromboembolism in cancer," *Journal of Thrombosis and Haemostasis*, vol. 15, no. 12, pp. 2289–2299, 2017.

[9] B. R. Branchford and S. L. Carpenter, "The role of inflammation in venous thromboembolism," *Frontiers in Pediatrics*, vol. 6, p. 142, 2018.

[10] A. Falanga and L. Russo, "Epidemiology, risk and outcomes of venous thromboembolism in cancer," *Hamostaseologie*, vol. 32, no. 2, pp. 115–125, 2012.

[11] E. Walder and M. L. Usher, "Tumor thrombus arising from osteosarcoma," *Journal for Vascular Ultrasound*, vol. 41, no. 3, pp. 123–125, 2017.

[12] A. Falanga, M. Marchetti, and L. Russo, "The mechanisms of cancer-associated thrombosis," *Thrombosis Research*, vol. 135, pp. S8–S11, 2015.

[13] Y. Hisada, J. E. Geddings, C. Ay, and N. Mackman, "Venous thrombosis and cancer: from mouse models to clinical trials," *Journal of Thrombosis and Haemostasis*, vol. 13, no. 8, pp. 1372–1382, 2015.

[14] Y. Yoshimura, S. Ikegami, K. Aoki et al., "Incidence, diagnosis, and risk factors of venous thromboembolism after

surgery for malignant bone and soft tissue tumour of lower extremity," *International Journal of Physical Medicine & Rehabilitation*, vol. 6, no. 1, 2018.

[15] O. Q. Groot, P. T. Ogink, S. J. Janssen et al., "High risk of venous thromboembolism after surgery for long bone metastases: a retrospective study of 682 patients," *Clinical Orthopaedics & Related Research*, vol. 476, no. 10, pp. 2052–2061, 2018.

[16] D. N. Tukaye, H. Brink, and R. Baliga, "Venous thromboembolism in cancer patients: risk assessment, prevention and management," *Future Cardiology*, vol. 12, no. 2, pp. 221–235, 2016.

[17] B. Dickmann, J. Ahlbrecht, C. Ay et al., "Regional lymph node metastases are a strong risk factor for venous thromboembolism: results from the Vienna cancer and thrombosis study," *Haematologica*, vol. 98, no. 8, pp. 1309–1314, 2013.

[18] M. M. Mitsunaga, C. Bateni, and J. Bindra, "Venous tumor thrombus from a pelvic osteosarcoma," *Radiology Case Reports*, vol. 8, no. 3, p. 864, 2013.

[19] P. Navalkele, S. M. Jones, J. K. Jones et al., "Osteosarcoma tumour thrombus," *Texas Heart Institute Journal*, vol. 40, no. 1, pp. 75–78, 2013.

[20] C. L. Kaiser, M. K. Freehan, D. A. Driscoll, J. H. Schwab, K. D. A. Bernstein, and S. A. Lozano-Calderon, "Predictors of venous thromboembolism in patients with primary sarcoma of bone," *Surgical Oncology*, vol. 26, no. 4, pp. 506–510, 2017.

[21] D. R. Haase, K. J. Templeton, H. G. Rosenthal, and K. R. Sweeney, "Tranexamic acid in patients with cancer undergoing endoprosthetic reconstruction: a retrospective review," *Journal of the American Academy of Orthopaedic Surgeons*, vol. 28, no. 6, pp. 248–255, 2020.

[22] G. M. Mendez, Y. M. Patel, D. A. Ricketti, J. P. Gaughan, R. D. Lackman, and T. W. B. Kim, "Aspirin for prophylaxis against venous thromboembolism after orthopaedic oncologic surgery," *Journal of Bone and Joint Surgery*, vol. 99, no. 23, pp. 2004–2010, 2017.

[23] D. Farge, H. Bounameaux, B. Brenner et al., "International clinical practice guidelines including guidance for direct oral anticoagulants in the treatment and prophylaxis of venous thromboembolism in patients with cancer," *The Lancet Oncology*, vol. 17, no. 10, pp. e452–e466, 2016.

[24] H. G. Watson, D. M. Keeling, M. Laffan, R. C. Tait, M. Makris, and British Committee for Standards in Haematology, "Guideline on aspects of cancer-related venous thrombosis," *British Journal of Haematology*, vol. 170, no. 5, pp. 640–648, 2015.

[25] C. Kearon, E. A. Akl, J. Ornelas et al., "Antithrombotic therapy for VTE disease: CHEST guideline and expert panel report," *Chest*, vol. 149, no. 2, pp. 315–352, 2016.

[26] D. Farge and C. Frere, "Recent advances in the treatment and prevention of venous thromboembolism in cancer patients: role of the direct oral anticoagulants and their unique challenges," *F1000Research*, vol. 8, 2019.

26

Surgical Treatment of Severe Idiopathic Flexible Flatfoot by Evans–Mosca Technique in Adolescent Patients

Vincenzo De Luna, Fernando De Maio, Alessandro Caterini, Martina Marsiolo, Lidio Petrungaro, Ernesto Ippolito, and Pasquale Farsetti

Department of Clinical Sciences and Traslational Medicine, Division of Orthopaedic Surgery, University of "Tor Vergata", Rome, Italy

Correspondence should be addressed to Pasquale Farsetti; farsetti@uniroma2.it

Academic Editor: Allen L. Carl

Flexible idiopathic flatfoot is very common in growing age and rarely causes pain or disability. Surgery is indicated only in severe symptomatic cases that are resistant to conservative treatment, and numerous surgical procedures have been proposed. Lateral column calcaneal lengthening as described by Evans and modified by Mosca is a widely used surgical technique for the correction of severe symptomatic flexible flatfoot. In the present study, we report the long-term clinical and radiographic results in 14 adolescent patients (mean age: 12.8 years) affected by severe symptomatic flexible flatfoot, surgically treated by Evans–Mosca procedure, for a total of 26 treated feet (12 cases bilateral and 2 unilateral). In all cases, surgery was indicated for the presence of significant symptoms resistant to nonsurgical management. Clinical evaluation was made according to the American Orthopedic Foot and Ankle Society (AOFAS) Ankle-Hindfoot Scale, the Foot and Ankle Disability Index (FADI) Score, and Yoo et al.'s criteria. Radiographic evaluation was made using anteroposterior and lateral weight-bearing radiographs of the feet to evaluate Meary's angle and Costa–Bertani's angle and to evaluate possible osteoarthritic changes in the midtarsal joints. At follow-up (mean: 7 years and 7 months), we observed a satisfactory result in all patients. The mean average score of the AOFAS Ankle-Hindfoot Scale improved from 60.03 points to 95.26; the mean FADI score improved from 71.41 to 97.44; and according to Yoo et al.'s criteria, the average clinical outcome score was 10.96. At radiographic examination, nonunion of the calcaneal osteotomy was never observed. Meary's angle improved from an average preoperative value of 25° to 1.38° at follow-up; Costa–Bertani's angle improved from an average preoperative value of 154.2° to 130.9° at follow-up. In no case, significant radiographic signs of midtarsal joint arthritis were observed. According to our results, we believe that Evans–Mosca technique is a valid option of surgical treatment for severe idiopathic flexible flatfoot and allows a satisfactory correction of the deformity with a low rate of complications.

1. Introduction

Flexible flatfoot is a very common foot condition observed during skeletal growth, characterized by a depression of the medial arch with an associated hindfoot valgus and forefoot abduction [1–3]; also, a short Achilles tendon is often present [4]. Flexible flatfoot rarely causes pain or disability in growing age patients and generally does not require treatment because in the majority of cases, the medial arch spontaneously elevates during the first decade of life. Moreover, it is well known that many adults have a flexible flatfoot without any significant limitation in activities of daily living or sport activities [5]. Surgery is indicated only in severe symptomatic cases with diffuse activity-related pain and medial foot calluses, observed usually in adolescents, in which conservative treatment has failed [5, 6]. The correct indication, time, and methods of surgical treatment for the correction of severe symptomatic flatfoot are however still debated, and several surgical procedures have been proposed [7–11]. The most common operations performed are arthroereisis, lateral calcaneal lengthening osteotomy, and triple arthrodesis [8–11]. Soft tissue surgical procedures have also been reported, but when they are performed alone, they lead to unsatisfactory results [5]. Evans, more than forty years ago [10], introduced the lateral column lengthening for the treatment of severe symptomatic flatfoot and proposed a calcaneal lengthening osteotomy for its correction. More recently, Mosca elaborated a modification of this technique, proposing an opening wedge osteotomy with a trapezoidal, tricortical iliac crest wedge [11].

The aim of the present study was to report the long-term results obtained in a series of 14 adolescents affected by severe symptomatic flexible flatfoot, surgically treated by Evans–Mosca technique associated to a soft tissue procedure of the medial side of the foot and, in almost 50% of cases, percutaneous lengthening of the Achilles tendon.

2. Materials and Methods

We reviewed 14 patients affected by severe idiopathic symptomatic flexible flatfoot, surgically treated by lateral column lengthening according to Evans–Mosca procedure associated to the tibialis posterior tendon and talonavicular joint capsule strain and, in some cases, percutaneous lengthening of the Achilles tendon. Eight patients were male, and 6 were female. The mean age of the patients at surgery was 12.8 years (range: from 11 to 14.6 years); 12 cases were operated bilaterally, for a total of 26 feet. In all our patients treated bilaterally, we performed the two procedures at different times, with a distance between the two operations that ranged from 8 months to one year.

Regarding the clinical evaluation before surgery, all patients had a medial longitudinal arch abnormally depressed or absent with a normal subtalar joint mobility. In 12 feet, a short Achilles tendon was also present with an associated limitation of the ankle dorsiflexion. Preoperatively, standard weight-bearing radiographs of the foot in anteroposterior and lateral projections confirmed the presence of a flexible flatfoot in all cases. Conservative treatment aims to improve or solve foot pain without changing the foot shape. In our series, it was based on strengthening exercises, custom orthosis, or corrective shoes, but failed in all patients (Figure 1). The surgical technique was performed under general anesthesia with a thigh tourniquet. The incision was made with an oblique direction over the sinus tarsi towards the inferior border of the calcaneus. The calcaneus was exposed, and the osteotomy was performed approximately 1.5 cm proximally from the calcaneocuboid joint, between the anterior and middle facets of the subtalar joint. The osteotomy should be oriented from posterolateral to anteromedial to avoid damage of the middle facet. After the distraction osteotomy was performed with a spreader, a tricortical iliac crest autologous bone graft, taken from the same side of the operated side, was inserted into the space to obtain a lengthening of the lateral column through the anterior part of the calcaneus. The osteotomy was stabilized with one or two Kirschner or Steinmann wires, according to the age of the patients and the size of the foot. A second incision was made along the medial border of the foot. The tibialis posterior was strained through a tendon release, and the talonavicular joint capsule, including the spring ligament, was incised and plicated plantarmedially. In 12 feet, in which a short Achilles tendon was present, percutaneous lengthening was also performed. After surgery, a nonweight bearing below the knee cast was applied for 6–8 weeks. Weight bearing was permitted only after radiographic healing of the osteotomy was observed.

All patients were evaluated clinically, analyzing the preoperative function of the foot in comparison to the follow-up examination, using the American Orthopedic Foot and Ankle Society (AOFAS) Ankle-Hindfoot Scale [12], the Foot and Ankle Disability Index (FADI) Score [13], and, only at follow-up, Yoo et al. criteria [14]. From a radiographic point of view, all patients were evaluated by an anteroposterior and lateral weight-bearing examination of both feet, taken before surgery and at follow-up, to measure both Meary's and Costa–Bertani's angles.

Moreover, at follow-up radiographic examination, we looked for possible subluxation or osteoarthritic changes of the calcaneocuboid or talonavicular joints as well as the remodeling of the tricortical bone graft into the calcaneal osteotomy (Figure 2).

Statistical analysis was performed using paired Student's t-test, which was considered significant when p value measured <0.05.

3. Results

All patients were reviewed after a mean follow-up of 7 years and 7 months (from 6 y and 5 m to 12 y).

According to the AOFAS system [12], the average preoperative score was 69.03 points (from 59 to 78 points), while the average score at follow-up improved to 95.26 (from 88 to 100). According to the FADI method [13], the average preoperative score was 71.41 (from 59.5 to 75.3), while the average score at follow-up was 97.44 (from 88.5 to 100). The difference between the preoperative and final score evaluated at follow-up was statistically significant for both clinical rating scales adopted ($p < 0.01$). According to Yoo et al.'s criteria [14], the average clinical outcome score at follow-up was 10.96 (from 8 to 12); since a score equal to or greater than 8 corresponds to a satisfactory clinical result, we obtained a satisfactory clinical result in all patients. We found no difference in terms of clinical results and satisfaction between patients treated on one foot or both feet (Table 1).

At radiographic examination, nonunion of the calcaneal osteotomy was never observed, and the tricortical bone graft was always remodeled. Meary's angle improved from an average preoperative value of 25° (from 22° to 32°) to an average value of 1.4° (from 0° to 4°) at follow-up. Costa–Bertani's angle improved from an average preoperative value of 154.2° (from 150° to 160°) to an average value of 130.9° (from 124° to 138°) at follow-up. Also, for both radiographic parameters, the difference between preoperative and final angle values was statistically significant ($p < 0.01$). Calcaneocuboid joint subluxation was observed in only 3

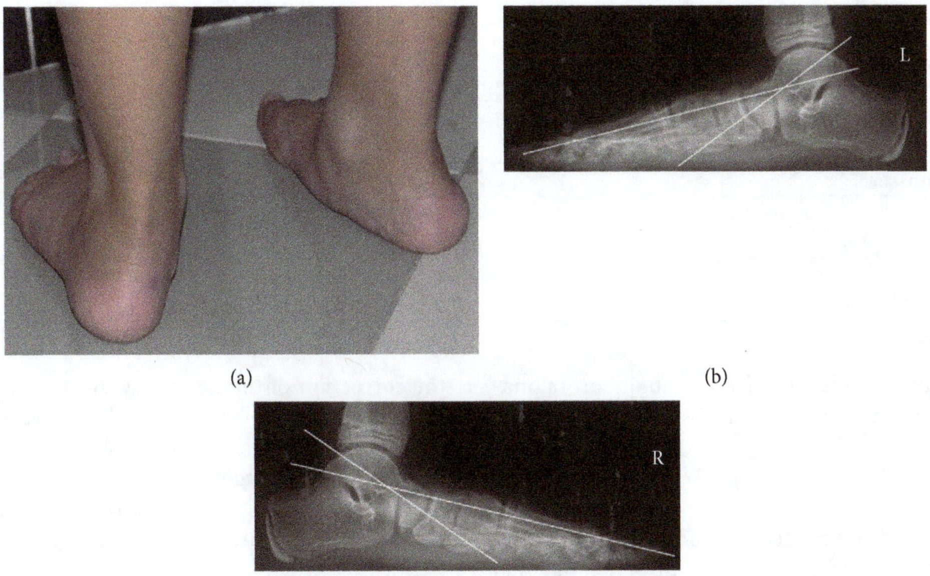

(a) (b) (c)

Figure 1: Clinical aspect of an 11-year-old boy with bilateral painful idiopathic flexible flatfoot (a). At radiographic examination, Meary's angle measured 26° of the left foot (b) and 23° of the right foot (c). The patient was treated conservatively by an insert sole, but this treatment failed, and a surgical procedure was proposed.

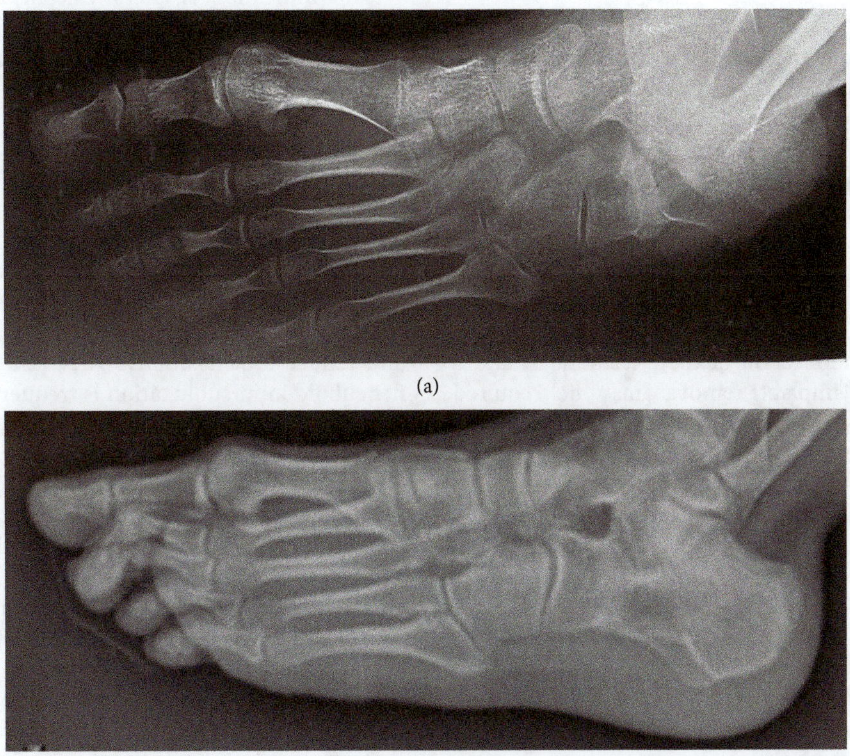

(a) (b)

Figure 2: Same patient of Figure 1, three years later. The patient was surgically treated by Evans–Mosca procedure bilaterally with an interval of six months. The radiographic examination of the left foot, performed in oblique view 3 months after surgery, showed good lengthening of the calcaneus with the presence of the tricortical bone graft (a). At an intermediate follow-up, 7 years later, the graft was perfectly remodeled in the calcaneal bone with the maintenance of calcaneal lengthening and without any sign of osteoarthritis of the calcaneocudoid joint (b).

Table 1: Preoperative and final (at follow-up) clinical and radiographic results in 26 flatfeet surgically treated by Evans–Mosca technique.

AOFAS (preop) AOFAS (follow up)	69.03 (59–79) 95.26 (88–100)	*p* value <0.01
FADI (preop) FADI (follow up)	71.41 (59.5–75.3) 97.44 (88.5–100)	*p* value <0.01
Yoo et al. (follow up)	10.96 (8–12)	—
Meary's angle (preop) Meary's angle (follow up)	25° (22°–32°) 1.4° (0°–4°)	*p* value <0.01
Costa-Bertani angle (preop) Costa-Bertani angle (follow up)	154.2° (150°–160°) 130.9° (124°–138°)	*p* value <0.01

feet (11.5%), while significant calcaneocuboid or talonavicular joint osteoarthritis was never observed (Figure 3).

4. Discussion

Flexible idiopathic flatfoot is very common in children and rarely causes pain or disability. On the contrary, congenital flatfoot caused by tarsal coalition, Marfan syndrome, or other congenital disorders, is usually painful, but uncommon in comparison to other congenital, pediatric, orthopedic diseases [15–18]. However, in some cases, especially in adolescents, flexible flatfoot may cause pain and disability, and surgery may be indicated when conservative treatment fails [19].

In severe idiopathic symptomatic adolescent flatfoot, surgical indication and the type of surgical treatment to perform are still controversial. Arthroereisis of the subtalar joint for the correction of severe flexible flatfoot in growing children is a widely used technique [20, 21]. This surgical procedure restricts excessive subtalar joint eversion by placing a synthetic implant. Different devices have been proposed over time including bioabsorbable implants. Good results have been reported in the literature for the correction of flexible flatfoot in growing children with arthroereisis of the subtalar joint [9, 20, 22], but pain at the level of the sinus tarsi is a possible complication of these techniques, and a second surgery for implant removal may be required [5, 23, 24]. For this reason, we preferred Evans–Mosca surgical procedures instead of arthroereisis in our series of adolescent patients.

Evans [10] believed that the lateral column in flatfeet was shorter than the medial column and first proposed a calcaneal lengthening osteotomy for the correction of valgus deformity, without an opening wedge osteotomy. This concept was elaborated by Mosca [5, 11] that published a modified technique utilizing a trapezoidal, tricortical iliac crest wedge to perform both an opening wedge and a distracting osteotomy and reported correction of all components of the deformity.

The calcaneal lengthening osteotomy for the surgical treatment of severe symptomatic idiopathic flexible flatfoot was later used by other authors with satisfactory results. Dogan et al. [25], in a series of 13 patients (25 feet) treated for flexible pes planovalgus by calcaneal lengthening osteotomy, reported that foot pain was eliminated in all patients but one. They concluded that the advantages of this procedure are the preservation of subtalar joint motion and the correction of the deformity in multiple plans. Moraleda et al. [26] also reported good clinical and radiographic results in a series of 21 children (33 feet) with symptomatic flexible flatfoot surgical treatment with a calcaneal lengthening osteotomy. More recently, Kumar and Sonanis [27] reported a systematic review on lateral column lengthening performed in adolescent pes planovalgus deformity. These authors identified seven studies with 103 patients involving 156 feet and concluded that lateral column lengthening leads to good clinical and radiological outcome with high patient satisfaction and acceptable complication rate. They also concluded that the literature is mostly retrospective, and there is need for other studies.

The indication of lateral calcaneal lengthening osteotomy for idiopathic flatfoot in children has been extended to other forms of flatfoot with a low incidence of complications [26]. Marengo et al. [28] reported the clinical and radiological outcome of calcaneal lengthening osteotomy for flatfoot deformity of various etiologies in 27 skeletally immature patients (38 feet). Clinical outcome was satisfactory in 89% of cases, and all radiographic parameters improved significantly. They concluded that calcaneal lengthening osteotomy is not contraindicated in symptomatic flatfoot of different etiologies, except neuromuscular disease-related flatfoot that can affect bone quality and reduce foot flexibility. They also reported that calcaneocuboid joint subluxation is frequently observed but has little functional impact as it tends to remodel over time. Similar to other CT studies that analyzed the results of treatment of the congenital clubfoot [29], Canavese et al. [30] published a study on postoperative CT-scan 3D reconstruction of the calcaneus following lateral calcaneal lengthening osteotomy performed in 14 children (20 feet) affected by symptomatic flatfoot with different etiologies. This study showed that subtalar anatomy presented significant anatomical variations among these examined patients; however, clinical evaluation at follow-up showed satisfactory outcome in 80% of cases. Calcaneal lengthening for flatfoot deformity in patients with cerebral palsy has also been reported with good results [31]. Andreacchio et al. [32] concluded that calcaneal lengthening is a successful treatment for flexible planovalgus foot deformity in ambulatory children with spastic CP. Regarding other etiologies, Mosca and Bevan [33] reported good results for correcting deformity and relieving pain in rigid flatfeet of 8 patients (13 feet), affected by talocalcaneal tarsal coalition, treated by calcaneal lengthening osteotomy with

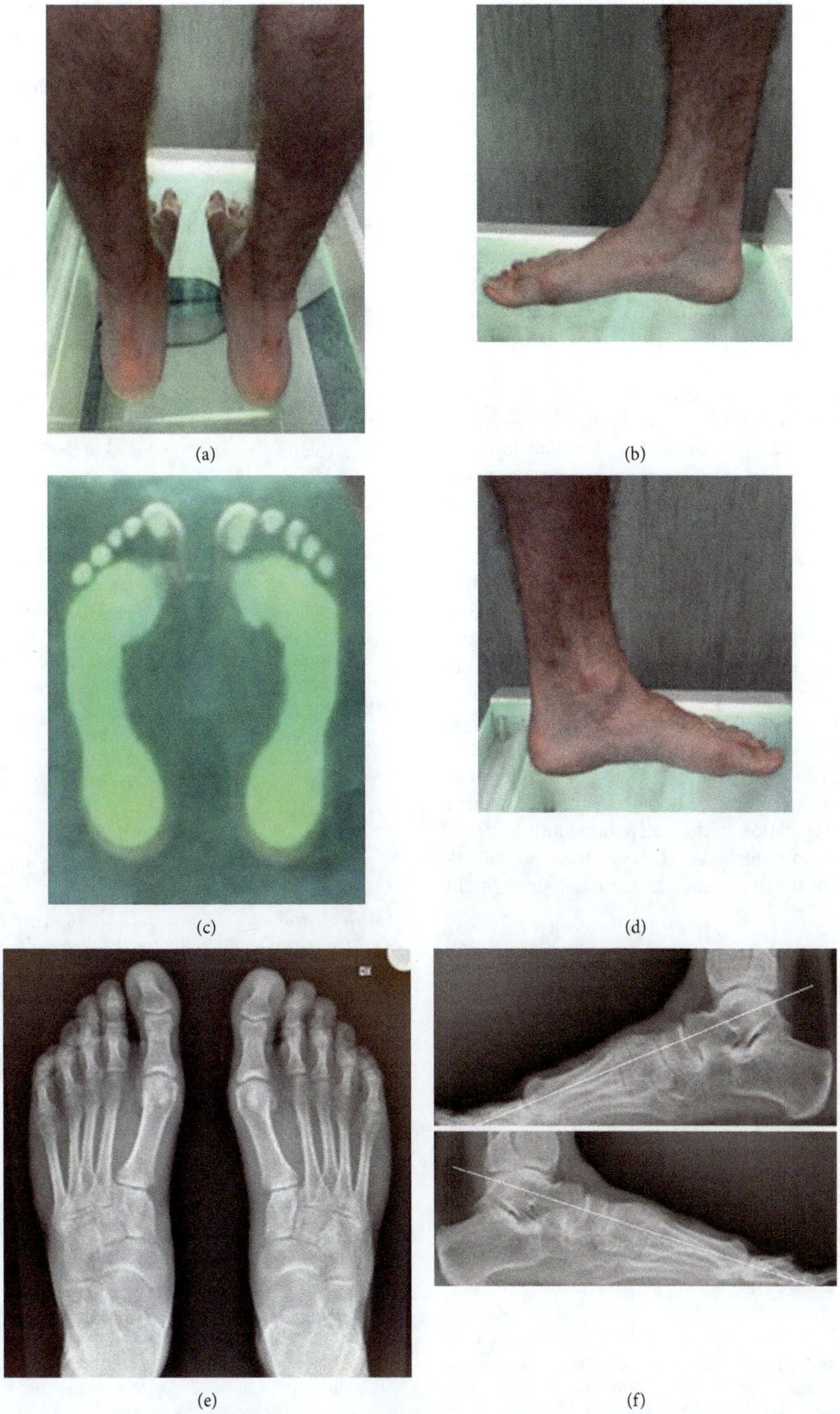

FIGURE 3: Same patient of Figure 1, at the final follow-up, 11 years after surgery. The patient was pain free. Clinical and podoscopic aspects of both feet showed an excellent result ((a)–(d)). At radiographic examination, Meary's angle was normal bilaterally (0°), in the absence of midtarsal joint osteoarthritis ((e) and (f)).

gastrocnemius or Achilles tendon lengthening. Guha and Perera [34] reported that calcaneal lengthening osteotomy may be performed even in the correction of adult flexible flatfoot, but they concluded that an essential prerequisite for using this technique is the absence of arthritis of the subtalar joint.

Our long-term results in a group of adolescents surgically treated for severe symptomatic idiopathic flexible flatfoot by the Evans–Mosca technique, in association with a strain of the tibialis posterior tendon and joint capsule, confirmed the good results reported by the aforementioned studies. All our patients were satisfied with the final result and referred a significant improvement of the preoperative symptoms.

In our patients, we paid particular attention to performing the calcaneal osteotomy into the interval between the anterior and middle facets of the subtalar joint as suggested by Ragab et al. [35], and at follow-up, we never observed significant radiographic changes of the midtarsal joint as reported by some studies [36, 37]. We always used a tricortical iliac crest autologous bone graft inserted into the osteotomy, as described by Mosca [11], to obtain lengthening of the lateral column of the calcaneus and never observed complications in terms of nonunion or loss of correction. Also, we never observed any patient morbidity from graft harvesting at the level of the iliac crest; however, some authors reported satisfactory results using autogenous bone graft from a different donor site or allogenic bone graft [38–40]. We had no personal experiences with titanium wedge insertion. We prefer to use bone autograft to obtain a better and faster integration in the native bone and to better maintain the correction obtained. However, to avoid the risk of pain at the level of the donor site, the use of allograft might be considered.

5. Conclusion

According to our long-term results, we believe that Evans–Mosca surgical procedure is an effective solution for the treatment of idiopathic symptomatic flexible flatfoot resistant to conservative treatment and allows the maintenance of the surgical correction without the development of osteoarthritic changes.

References

[1] L. T. Staheli, D. E. Chew, and M. Corbett, "The longitudinal arch. a survey of eight hundred and eighty-two feet in normal children and adults," *The Journal of Bone and Joint Surgery. American Volume*, vol. 69, no. 3, pp. 426–428, 1987.

[2] R. Vanderwilde, L. T. Staheli, D. E. Chew, and V. Malagon, "Measurements on radiographs of the foot in normal infants and children," *The Journal of Bone & Joint Surgery*, vol. 70, no. 3, pp. 407–415, 1988.

[3] E. J. Harris, "The natural history and pathophysiology of flexible flatfoot," *Clinics in Podiatric Medicine and Surgery*, vol. 27, no. 1, pp. 1–23, 2010.

[4] R. I. Harris and T. Beath, "Hypermobile flat-foot with short tendo achillis," *The Journal of Bone & Joint Surgery*, vol. 30, no. 1, pp. 116–150, 1948.

[5] V. S. Mosca, "Flexible flatfoot in children and adolescents," *Journal of Children's Orthopaedics*, vol. 4, no. 2, pp. 107–121, 2010.

[6] N. M. Blitz, R. J. Stabile, R. J. Giorgini, and L. A. DiDomenico, "Flexible pediatric and adolescent pes planovalgus: conservative and surgical treatment options," *Clinics in Podiatric Medicine and Surgery*, vol. 27, no. 1, pp. 59–77, 2010.

[7] B. S. Jones, "Flatfoot. a preliminary report of an operation for severe cases," *Journal of Bone and Joint Surgery British Volume*, vol. 57, no. 3, pp. 279–282, 1975.

[8] P. Angus and H. Cowell, "Triple arthrodesis. a critical long-term review," *The Journal of Bone and Joint Surgery. British Volume*, vol. 68-B, no. 2, pp. 260–265, 1986.

[9] S. Giannini, F. Ceccarelli, M. G. Benedetti, F. Catani, and C. Faldini, "Surgical treatment of flexible flatfoot in children," *The Journal of Bone and Joint Surgery-American Volume*, vol. 83, no. suppl. 2, pp. 73–79, 2001.

[10] D. Evans, "Calcaneo-valgus deformity," *The Journal of Bone and Joint Surgery. British Volume*, vol. 57-B, no. 3, pp. 270–278, 1975.

[11] V. S. Mosca, "Calcaneal lengthening for valgus deformity of the hindfoot. results in children who had severe, symptomatic flatfoot and skewfoot," *The Journal of Bone & Joint Surgery*, vol. 77, no. 4, pp. 500–512, 1995.

[12] H. B. Kitaoka, I. J. Alexander, R. S. Adelaar et al., "Clinical rating systems for the ankle-hindfoot, midfoot, hallux, and lesser toes," *Foot & Ankle International*, vol. 15, no. 7, pp. 349–353, 1994.

[13] R. L. Martin, R. G. Burdett, and J. J. Irrgang, "Development of the foot and ankle disability index (FADI)," *Journal of Orthopaedic & Sports Physical Therapy*, vol. 29, pp. A32–A33, 1999.

[14] W. J. Yoo, C. Y. Chung, I. H. Choi, T.-J. Cho, and D. H. Kim, "Calcaneal lengthening for the planovalgus foot deformity in children with cerebral palsy," *Journal of Pediatric Orthopaedics*, vol. 25, no. 6, pp. 781–785, 2005.

[15] S. J. Kumar, J. T. Guille, M. S. Lee, and J. C. Couto, "Osseous and non-osseous coalition of the middle facet of the talocalcaneal joint," *The Journal of Bone & Joint Surgery*, vol. 74, no. 4, pp. 529–535, 1992.

[16] F. De Maio, A. Fichera, V. De Luna, F. Mancini, and R. Caterini, "Orthopaedic aspects of marfan syndrome: the experience of a referral center for diagnosis of rare diseases," *Advances in Orthopedics*, vol. 2016, Article ID 8275391, , 2016.

[17] P. Farsetti, M. Dragoni, and E. Ippolito, "Tibiofibular torsion in congenital clubfoot," *Journal of Pediatric Orthopaedics B*, vol. 21, no. 1, pp. 47–51, 2012.

[18] P. Farsetti, R. Caterini, V. Potenza, and E. Ippolito, "Developmental dislocation of the hip successfully treated by preoperative traction and medial open reduction: a 22-year mean followup," *Clinical Orthopaedics and Related Research*, vol. 473, no. 8, pp. 2658–2669, 2015.

[19] J. V. Basmajian and G. Stecko, "The role of muscles in arch support of the foot," *The Journal of Bone & Joint Surgery*, vol. 45, no. 6, pp. 1184–1190, 1963.

[20] V. Pavone, A. Vescio, C. A. Di Silvestri, A. Andreacchio, G. Sessa, and G. Testa, "Outcomes of the calcaneo-stop procedure for the treatment of juvenile flatfoot in young athletes," *Journal of Children's Orthopaedics*, vol. 12, no. 6, pp. 582–589, 2018.

[21] C. Indino, J. H. Villafañe, R. D'Ambrosi et al., "Effectiveness of subtalar arthroereisis with endorthesis for pediatric flexible flat foot: a retrospective cross-sectional study with final follow up at skeletal maturity," *Foot and Ankle Surgery*, vol. 26, no. 1, pp. 98–104, 2020.

[22] D. Y. Chong, B. A. Macwilliams, T. A. Hennessey, N. Teske, and P. M. Stevens, "Prospective comparison of subtalar arthroereisis with lateral column lengthening for painful flatfeet," *Journal of Pediatric Orthopaedics B*, vol. 24, no. 4, pp. 345–353, 2015.

[23] C. Faldini, A. Mazzotti, A. Panciera, F. Perna, N. Stefanini, and S. Giannini, "Bioabsorbable implants for subtalar arthroereisis in pediatric flatfoot," *Musculoskeletal Surgery*, vol. 102, no. 1, pp. 11–19, 2018.

[24] A. Bernasconi, F. Lintz, and F. Sadile, "The role of arthroereisis of the subtalar joint for flatfoot in children and adults," *EFORT Open Reviews*, vol. 2, no. 11, pp. 438–446, 2017.

[25] A. Dogan, G. Zorer, E. I. Mumcuoglu, and E. Y. Akman, "A comparison of two different techniques in the surgical treatment of flexible pes planovalgus: calcaneal lengthening and extra-articular subtalar arthrodesis," *Journal of Pediatric Orthopaedics B*, vol. 18, no. 4, pp. 167–175, 2009.

[26] L. Moraleda, M. Salcedo, T. P. Bastrom, D. R. Wenger, J. Albiñana, and S. J. Mubarak, "Comparison of the calcaneo-cuboid-cuneiform osteotomies and the calcaneal lengthening osteotomy in the surgical treatment of symptomatic flexible flatfoot," *Journal of Pediatric Orthopaedics*, vol. 32, no. 8, pp. 821–829, 2012.

[27] S. Kumar and S. V. Sonanis, "Lateral column lengthening for adolescent idiopathic pes planovalgus deformity-systematic review," *Journal of Orthopaedics*, vol. 14, no. 4, pp. 571–576, 2017.

[28] L. Marengo, F. Canavese, M. Mansour, A. Dimeglio, and F. Bonnel, "Clinical and radiological outcome of calcaneal lengthening osteotomy for flatfoot deformity in skeletally immature patients," *European Journal of Orthopaedic Surgery & Traumatology*, vol. 27, no. 7, pp. 989–996, 2017.

[29] P. Farsetti, F. De Maio, L. Russolillo, and E. Ippolito, "CT study on the effect of different treatment protocols for clubfoot pathology," *Clinical Orthopaedics and Related Research*, vol. 467, no. 5, pp. 1243–1249, 2009.

[30] F. Canavese, A. Dimeglio, and F. Bonnel, "Postoperative CT-scan 3D reconstruction of the calcaneus following lateral calcaneal lengthening osteotomy for flatfoot deformity in children. is the surgical procedure potentially associated with subtalar joint damage?" *Foot and Ankle Surgery*, vol. 24, no. 5, pp. 453–459, 2018.

[31] A. M. Aboelenein, M. L. Fahmy, H. M. Elbarbary, A. Z. Mohamed, and S. Galal, "Calcaneal lengthening for the pes planovalgus foot deformity in children with cerebral palsy," *Journal of Clinical Orthopaedics and Trauma*, vol. 11, no. 2, pp. 245–250, 2020.

[32] A. Andreacchio, C. A. Orellana, F. Miller, and T. R. Bowen, "Lateral column lengthening as treatment for planovalgus foot deformity in ambulatory children with spastic cerebral palsy," *Journal of Pediatric Orthopaedics*, vol. 20, no. 4, pp. 501–505, 2000.

[33] V. S. Mosca and W. P. Bevan, "Talocalcaneal tarsal coalitions and the calcaneal lengthening osteotomy: the role of deformity correction," *The Journal of Bone and Joint Surgery-American Volume*, vol. 94, no. 17, pp. 1584–1594, 2012.

[34] A. R. Guha and A. M. Perera, "Calcaneal osteotomy in the treatment of adult acquired flatfoot deformity," *Foot and Ankle Clinics*, vol. 17, no. 2, pp. 247–258, 2012.

[35] A. A. Ragab, S. L. Stewart, and D. R. Cooperman, "Implications of subtalar joint anatomic variation in calcaneal lengthening osteotomy," *Journal of Pediatric Orthopaedics*, vol. 23, no. 1, pp. 79–83, 2003.

[36] P. S. Cooper, M. D. Nowak, and J. Shaer, "Calcaneocuboid joint pressures with lateral column lengthening (Evans) procedure," *Foot & Ankle International*, vol. 18, no. 4, pp. 199–205, 1997.

[37] K. H. Sung, S.-S. Kwon, C. Y. Chung, K. M. Lee, and M. S. Park, "Radiographic changes of the mid-tarsal joint after calcaneal lengthening for planovalgus foot deformity," *Foot and Ankle Surgery*, vol. 26, no. 1, pp. 110–115, 2020.

[38] D. Templin, K. Jones, and D. S. Weiner, "The incorporation of allogeneic and autogenous bone graft in healing of lateral column lengthening of the calcaneus," *The Journal of Foot and Ankle Surgery*, vol. 47, no. 4, pp. 283–287, 2008.

[39] J. Rhodes, A. Mansour, A. Frickman et al., "Comparison of allograft and bovine xenograft in calcaneal lengthening osteotomy for flatfoot deformity in cerebral palsy," *Journal of Pediatric Orthopaedics*, vol. 37, no. 3, pp. e202–e208, 2017.

[40] K. M. S. Mohamed, C. Fenelon, J. G. Galbraith, and L. G. D'Souza, "Obtaining local bone graft for evans calcaneal osteotomy in pes planovalgus deformity correction," *Foot and Ankle Surgery*, vol. 23, no. 3, pp. 208–210, 2017.

27

Musculoskeletal Corticosteroid Injection during COVID-19 Pandemic in Sabah: Is It Safe?

Mohamad Azwan Aziz,[1] Redzal Abu Hanifah,[2] and Azmi Mohamed Mohd Nahar[1]

[1] *Sports Medicine Department, University Malaya Medical Centre, Kuala Lumpur, Malaysia*
[2] *Sports Medicine Unit, Queen Elizabeth Hospital, Kota Kinabalu, Sabah, Malaysia*

Correspondence should be addressed to Mohamad Azwan Aziz; kassemkoya69@gmail.com

Academic Editor: Paulo Adriano Schwingel

Musculoskeletal corticosteroid injection is commonly used as an adjunct to help patients in pain management. In this current COVID-19 pandemic, many clinicians would differ from this treatment as steroid is considered an immunosuppressive drug and could risk the patient of developing severe adverse effects if contracting COVID-19. This is a retrospective study based in Sabah, Malaysia, examining the prevalence of COVID-19 infection following musculoskeletal corticosteroid injection from 1 December 2019 until 30 June 2020 in the sports medicine clinic and the orthopedic clinic. Patients who received musculoskeletal corticosteroid injection were called by telephone and asked about visits to the emergency department or government health clinic for influenza-like illness symptoms or severe acute respiratory infection that would require screening of COVID-19. Thirty-five patients who responded to the call were included, with mean ages of 47.9 years ± 15.1. 52% were male respondents, while 48% were female. 25% of them were diabetics, and 2.9% of them had a history of lymphoproliferative disorders. The mean pain score before injection was 6.74 ± 1.03 and after injection pain was 2.27 ± 1.63. In this study, there were 11.4% ($n = 4$) with minor complications of steroid injection, that is, skin discoloration. Nonetheless, there were no severe complications due to corticosteroids reported. There were no reported cases of COVID-19 among the respondents following corticosteroid injection. Musculoskeletal pain would affect a person's well-being and activities; thus, its management requires that careful consideration with risk-benefit analysis be made before administering musculoskeletal corticosteroid injection during COVID-19 pandemic.

1. Introduction

Musculoskeletal corticosteroid injection is a common procedure seen in a sports medicine clinic. The injection is used as an adjunct to treat various musculoskeletal diseases such as arthritic joint pain, bursitis, tendinopathy, and synovial inflammation. Robust studies have shown that corticosteroid injection helps patients control debilitating arthritic joint pain, improve the quality of daily living activities, improve range of motion, and an early return to work and, in certain patients, it helps delay or prevent surgical intervention [1]. Musculoskeletal corticosteroid injection is a safe procedure with a small risk of complications [1].

With the current public health emergency of COVID-19 outbreak, a careful decision of performing corticosteroid injection should be considered. Corticosteroid has an immunosuppressive effect. Numerous studies have reported that epidural steroid injection causes hypothalamic-pituitary axis (HPA) suppression from 4 to 12 weeks, and a single dose of intra-articular steroid injection could cause HPA suppression for up to 4 weeks [2–6]. Thus, in the early pandemic era, many professional national bodies have recommended against the usage of corticosteroid injection during this pandemic, as the fear of an asymptomatic patient infected with SARS-CoV-2 could put them at increased risk of an adverse outcome from the virus if they had received the injection [7]. The rising concern for use of injectable corticosteroids in musculoskeletal care comes from established guidelines from World Health Organization for systemic steroid use in patients under treatment for active COVID-

19. According to the recommendation by the interim guidelines of the World Health Organization during early pandemic, use of systemic corticosteroids is not recommended for treating severe COVID-19 infection as no good evidence shows the benefits of steroid usage and there was persuasive evidence of adverse short- and long-term harm [8]. In a retrospective study by Sytsma et al., they have shown an increased risk of contracting influenza infection during the influenza season in patients given a corticosteroid injection [9]. However, this study was unable to demonstrate the timeline between time of receiving corticosteroid injection, time of influenza vaccine delivered, and time of contracting influenza infection. In early global COVID-19 pandemic, the British Society for Rheumatology and the British Society of Skeletal Radiologists published a recommendation against musculoskeletal steroid injection except for severe debilitating pain despite optimum conservative therapy [10, 11].

We are concerned with the clear wholesale withdrawal of musculoskeletal steroid injection as a beneficial treatment option for patients who have severe and painful musculoskeletal conditions during the COVID-19 pandemic. As patients suffer and surgical management options seem months away, surgical alternatives are unlikely to be available, and it is good practice to consider conservative management with injection before committing to surgery. The latest guidelines by the National Health Service (England) on 16 June 2020, were for musculoskeletal steroid injections to be considered for severe symptoms after failed physical rehabilitation and splinting [12]. Currently, the evidence of increased risk of systemic infection including COVID-19 following intra-articular and periarticular corticosteroid injection is limited. A recent study by Chang et al. reported no significant elevation in the risk of developing COVID-19 infection following steroid injection compared to the general population [13]. McKean et al. also demonstrate a low incidence of COVID-19 following corticosteroid injection with no major adverse outcomes [14]. We hypothesize that there will be a very low risk of developing COVID-19 infection following musculoskeletal steroid injection. The study aims to determine the prevalence of COVID-19 infection following musculoskeletal steroid injection during the pandemic in Sabah, Malaysia.

2. Methods and Materials

2.1. Study Design. This study was conducted retrospectively from 1 December 2019 until 30 June 2020 during the COVID-19 pandemic in the state of Sabah, Malaysia. The date was chosen with respect to the first reported case of COVID-19 by the World Health Organization on 31 December 2019. Numerous studies conclude that a single dose of intra-articular steroid injection can cause HPA suppression of up to 4 weeks [2–6]. Thus, this study begins at 1 December 2019. All medical case notes were retrieved. Patients included in the study were those that had sought treatment in the sports medicine clinic and the orthopedic clinic in Queen Elizabeth Hospital and Queen Elizabeth 2 Hospital, Sabah, with presentation of inflammatory arthritis, non-inflammatory arthritis, bursitis, tenosynovitis, epicondylitis, and carpal tunnel syndrome, and were treated with corticosteroid injection with further follow-up given for 2 weeks. Demographic data including name, identification number, age, ethnicity, medical comorbidity, and diagnosis for clinical visitation were included in this study. The date of injection was recorded. Patients were excluded from this study if they had intramuscular steroid injections due to nonmusculoskeletal issues, intra-articular or soft tissue injections without using steroids, or incomplete data in their case notes. For injection over the finger, a dose of 20 mg triamcinolone was used per body part, while, in other parts of the body, a dose of 40 mg triamcinolone was used per body part. Once the patients were identified and included in this study, the investigator would call the patients, and the purpose of the study was explained. When consent was given by the patients, they were asked about any visit to the emergency department, government clinic, or private hospital for COVID-19 screening with symptoms of Influenza-Like Illness (ILI) or Severe Acute Respiratory Infection (SARI).

This study was conducted in compliance with ethical principles outlined in the Declaration of Helsinki and Malaysian Good Clinical Practice Guideline with approval from the Medical Research Ethics Committee.

2.2. Statistical Analysis. Descriptive analysis was done for this research. The participant's baseline characteristics, types of musculoskeletal corticosteroid injection, complication, and improvement were recorded in this study.

3. Results

Out of 52 intra-articular/periarticular injection procedures, 11 procedures did not use corticosteroids as an agent and 6 patients had incomplete or missing data. Table 1 shows the demographic characteristics of 35 patients enrolled in this study, with ages ranging from 27 to 85 years and a mean age of 47.9 ± 15.1 years. 52% were male and 48% were female. 25% are diagnosed with diabetes mellitus and 2.9% had a history of lymphoproliferative disorders. 17% of the patients were above 65 years of age.

All 35 patients required musculoskeletal corticosteroid injection as an adjunct for pain management. In Table 2, the most common sites of injections were knee ($n = 15$, 42.9%) and shoulder ($n = 7$, 20%). The most common indication for the injection was for knee osteoarthritis (Table 3). All patients received triamcinolone as steroid injection with 2% lignocaine as local anaesthetic. 34.3% of the patients had a corticosteroid injection with additional prolotherapy of Dextrose 50%. Three patients received 20 mg triamcinolone over fingers, 2 patients received 80 mg triamcinolone in bilateral knees in the same day, and the rest received 40 mg triamcinolone.

In this study, only 11.4% had minor complications of steroid injection as in Table 4. All were skin discoloration. Nonetheless, there were no serious or severe complications due to corticosteroids. There were no complications

Table 1: Demographic data of patients who received musculoskeletal steroid injections.

Characteristic	Range (years)	Mean (years)	SD
Age	27–85	47.9	15.1
		n	%
Race	Malay	5	14.3
	Chinese	14	40
	Bumiputera, Sabah	16	45.7
Comorbid	No comorbids	23	65.7
	Diabetes mellitus	9	25
	Hypertension	6	17
	Gout	1	2.9
	Lymphoproliferative disorder	1	2.9

Note. Age is described in mean ± SD. Other demographic data are described in numbers and percentage.

Table 2: Characteristics of musculoskeletal steroid injections.

Characteristics of steroid injection		n	%
Area of injection	Ankle	2	5.7
	Elbow	2	5.7
	Finger	3	8.6
	Knee	15	42.9
	Shoulder	7	20
	Spine	1	2.9
	Wrist	5	14.3
Number of joint injections per day per person	Single joint injection	33	94.3
	Multiple joint injections	2	5.7
Type of steroid	Triamcinolone	35	100
Type of anaesthesia	2% lignocaine	35	100
Additional prolotherapy	With prolotherapy	12	34.3
	Without prolotherapy	23	65.7

reported for local anaesthesia. The mean pain score before injection was 6.74 ± 1.03, and in the following injection the mean pain score was 2.27 ± 1.63 one week after the procedure (Table 5). None of the patients reported symptoms of ILI, SARI, or confirmed cases of COVID-19 following musculoskeletal corticosteroid injection.

Table 3: Indications for musculoskeletal steroid injections.

Diagnosis	n	%
Acromioclavicular osteoarthritis	1	2.9
Carpal tunnel syndrome	1	2.9
De Quervain tenosynovitis	4	11.4
Frozen shoulder	2	5.7
Hallux valgus	1	2.9
Knee osteoarthritis	14	40
Pes anserinus	1	2.9
Ankle impingement syndrome	1	2.9
S1 radiculopathy	1	2.9
Subacromial impingement	4	11.4
Supraspinatus tendinitis	1	2.9
Tennis elbow	2	5.7
Trigger finger	2	5.7

4. Discussion

There were major concerns in administering musculoskeletal steroid injections during COVID-19 pandemic. Many clinicians believe that administering musculoskeletal corticosteroids risks the patient to adverse outcomes of COVID-19 [7]. The key finding in our study showed that all patients who had musculoskeletal corticosteroid injection do not have symptoms of Influenza-Like Illness or Severe Acute Respiratory Syndrome, which would mandate for both nasopharyngeal and oropharyngeal swabs real-time polymerase chain reaction (rt-PCR) for SARS-CoV-2 in government health facilities. This could be partly due to the prevalence of COVID-19 in Sabah being relatively low (9.7 per 100 000 population), with an efficient public health system in promoting good preventive methods for spreading COVID-19 such as wearing masks in public, avoiding crowded places, social distancing, and frequent handwashing [15].

TABLE 4: Complications following musculoskeletal injections.

Complications	N	%
Patients presenting to hospital, diagnosed as COVID-19 after injection	0	0
Skin discoloration	4	11.4
No reported complications	31	88.6

TABLE 5: Outcome of musculoskeletal steroid injections in terms of pain score before and after procedures.

Pain score	Mean	SD
Preinjection pain score	6.74	1.03
Postinjection pain score	2.27	1.63

34.3% of patients in our study had at least one comorbidity and 83% were below 65 years of age. Systma et al. have examined the outcome of corticosteroid injection on risk of contracting influenza [9]. In Systma et al.'s study, a total of 15,068 joint injections have been analyzed [9]. There was an increased relative risk of 1.5 for vaccinated subjects developing influenza after an intra-articular corticosteroid using methylprednisolone (79%), betamethasone (11%), and triamcinolone (10%). The corticosteroid dose was 66 mg with a range of 40–120 mg [9]. In our study, there were zero rates of COVID-19 infection. Our study used triamcinolone (100%). According to Systma et al.'s study (2018), women below 65 years of age have a higher risk of contracting infection [9]. They examined the risk of contracting influenza infection after patients received influenza vaccine [9]. High influenza rate in the younger population (2.28% ($n = 46$ of 2015) versus 1.18% in elderly patient >65 years ($n = 33$ of 2789); $P < 0.001$) is possibly due to high dose vaccine received by the geriatric population [9]. This was the first study to identify the risk of contracting infection following corticosteroid injection during pandemic seasons. However, this study was unable to show the timeline between time of receiving the vaccine to the time that the patient received steroid injection, and the time when patients contracted the infection.

A recent study by Chang et al. also demonstrated no increased risk of COVID-19 infection following corticosteroid injection [13]. Out of 66 subjects who completed follow-up in 45 ± 22 (19–83) days after injection, 1 subject was positive for COVID-19 infection following injection. The rate of infection was 1.52% [13]. The subject had mild symptoms that did not require any hospitalization [13]. A larger study with 504 steroid injections had a 2.7% rate of infection, of which 1.1% were asymptomatic. There were no severe adverse outcomes to COVID-19 infection reported in the study [14]. Compared to our study, where we have zero infection rates, the rate of infection of COVID-19 is still low with no severe adverse outcomes following steroid injection.

A careful consideration with risk-benefit analysis should be applied before administering corticosteroid injection. In this study, there was improvement seen in pain score in all patients. The incidence of skin discoloration in this study was higher than that in Stephens et al.'s study (2001) of <1% [1]. This may be due to a small sample size in our study. There were 4 patients (11.4%) who had skin discoloration in this study, which resolved after a few months. Robust cases have reported incidence of hypopigmentation after triamcinolone injection, which is the type of steroid (100%) used in this study [16–18]. The mechanism of hypopigmentation is not well understood, but biopsy study showed that there is a decrease in melanocyte function rather than actual loss of melanocytes [16–18]. One of the possible reasons for high cases of hypopigmentation was the use of high dose of steroid (40 mg) in small soft tissue such as wrist and fingers. A careful explanation regarding the possible adverse effects of corticosteroid injection, including skin pigmentation, should be highlighted before the procedure.

Robust studies have shown the usage of corticosteroids in managements of COVID-19. A single-blind randomized controlled clinical trial on the usage of pulse methylprednisolone showed a significant survival improvement in severe COVID-19 infection [19]. RECOVERY trial also demonstrated a significant beneficial survival effect of systemic corticosteroids in severe and critically ill COVID-19 patients requiring respiratory support [20]. A prospective meta-analysis of seven randomized clinical trials by the WHO Rapid Evidence Appraisal for the COVID-19 Therapies Working Group also showed a mortality benefit when using corticosteroids compared to placebo [21]. This shows that corticosteroids are useful and have a significant benefit in management of COVID-19.

Although this is a retrospective descriptive study, it is important to conduct further research of the risk of contracting respiratory infection with corticosteroid injection during influenza outbreaks and the COVID-19 pandemic. A further risk analysis study is required to strengthen the knowledge for improvement in delivering pain management in patients who are in need. The major limitation of our study is that the true number of COVID-19 infections remains unknown in this patient cohort, as all subjects did not undergo a screening test during this period as there were no symptoms. There is high possibility of the presence of asymptomatic COVID-19 patients in this population study. This is because the Ministry of Health in Malaysia is focusing on a targeted screening approach of COVID-19 rather than mass testing. One of the other possible reasons why this study has no COVID-19 infection following corticosteroid injection is the small sample group and low prevalence of COVID-19 in Malaysia. The situation of COVID-19 in Malaysia as of 11 July 2020 was 8704 positive cases, 26.7 per 100 000 population [15]. In Sabah, there were 379 positive cases, 9.7 per 100 000 population [15]. Our aim in the future is to examine a larger population in Malaysia on the complex interaction between the host immune response, steroid injection, and risk of COVID-19 infection. Other limitations that we identify during this study are that, due to a small sample size, we were unable to risk stratifying patients who are at higher risk of contracting COVID-19 infection. Sytsma et al. identified that female patients below 65 years of age have a higher risk of contracting influenza infection [9]. Future direction of research should focus on bigger populations to examine the risk of contracting COVID-19 following musculoskeletal steroid injections. Artificial intelligence technology has created its way in the research field to examine big databases. For example, Zhang et al. discussed the use of artificial intelligence technology in improving the patient care with acute lung injury and acute respiratory distress syndrome [22]. Similar things could be applied during COVID-19 pandemic era to examine a bigger dataset.

5. Conclusion

In this study, there was no COVID-19 infection following intra-articular and soft tissue corticosteroid injection. There was no reported case of major complications following corticosteroid injection. 11.4% of patients reported skin discoloration at the site of injection. Thus, we suggest a careful consideration of risk-benefit analysis before administering musculoskeletal corticosteroids injection to patients who would gain the benefit of corticosteroid's effect on pain and inflammation. However, due to the small sample size, we could not conclude that musculoskeletal steroid injection brings no risk of contracting COVID-19 infection.

Acknowledgments

The authors would like to thank the Director General of Health Malaysia for his permission to publish this article.

References

[1] M. B. Stephens, A. I. Beutler, and F. G. O'Connor, "Musculoskeletal injections: a review of the evidence," *American Family Physician*, vol. 78, no. 8, pp. 971–976, 2008.

[2] J. L. Friedly, B. A. Comstock, P. J. Heagerty et al., "Systemic effects of epidural steroid injections for spinal stenosis," *Pain* vol. 159, no. 5, pp. 876–883, 2018.

[3] A. Iranmanesh, D. Gullapalli, R. Singh, and J. D. Veldhuis, "Hypothalamo-pituitary-adrenal axis after a single epidural triamcinolone injection," *Endocrine*, vol. 57, no. 2, pp. 308–313, 2017.

[4] A. J. Abdul, B. Ghai, D. Bansal, N. Sachdeva, A. Bhansali, and S. S. Dhatt, "Hypothalamic pituitary adrenocortical axis suppression following a single epidural injection of methylprednisolone acetate," *Pain Physician*, vol. 20, pp. E991–E1001, 2017.

[5] T. Weitof and L. Ronnblom, "Glucocorticoid resorption and influence on the hypothalamic-pituitary-adrenal axis after intra-articular treatment of the knee in resting and mobile patients," *Annals of the Rheumatic Diseases*, vol. 65, pp. 955–957, 2016.

[6] G. S. Habib, "Systemic effects of intra-articular corticosteroids," *Clinical Rheumatology*, vol. 28, pp. 749–756, 2009.

[7] https://www.england.nhs.uk/coronavirus/wpcontent/uploads/sites/52/2020/03/CO0043_Specialty-guide-and-coronavirus_-MSK-corcosteroid_-v1-25.2020.

[8] World Health Organization, *Clinical Management of Severe Acute Respiratory Infection (SARI) when Novel Coronavirus Infection Is Suspected*, WHO, Geneva, Switzerland, 2020.

[9] T. T. Sytsma, L. K. Greenlund, and L. S. Greenlund, "Joint corticosteroid injection associated with increased influenza risk," *Mayo Clinic Proceedings: Innovations, Quality & Outcomes*, vol. 2, no. 2, pp. 194–198, 2018.

[10] D. Fascia, D. Dalili, W. Rennie, E. Rowbotham, A. Carne, and P. Robinson, "Recommendations of the British Society of Skeletal Radiologists: the safety of corticosteroid injections during the COVID-19 global pandemic," 2020, https://www.bssr.org.uk/static/uploads/forum/Musculoskeletal_Radiology_during_the_COVID-19_ Global_Pandemic.pdf.

[11] British Society for Rheumatology, "Clinical guide for the management of patients with musculoskeletal and rheumatic conditions on corticosteroids during the coronavirus pandemic," 2020, https://www.bssr.org.uk/static/uploads/forum/13._CO0043_Specialty-guide-and- coronavirus_-MSK-corcosteroid_-v1.pdf.pdf.

[12] "Management of patients with musculoskeletal and rheumatic conditions who: are on corticosteroids; require initiation of oral/IV corticosteroids; require a corticosteroid injection," 2020.

[13] C. Y. Chang, A. Prabhakar, S. J. Staffa et al., "Symptomatic COVID-19 infections in outpatient image-guided corticosteroid injection patients during the lockdown phase," *Skeletal Radiology*, vol. 1, p. 7, 2020.

[14] D. McKean, S. L. Chung, R. Fairhead et al., "Corticosteroid injections during the COVID-19 pandemic," *Bone & Joint Open*, vol. 1, no. 9, pp. 605–611, 2020.

[15] https://www.who.int/malaysia/internal-publications-detail/covid-19-in-malaysia-situation-report-08. 2020.

[16] P. Venkatesan and W. L. Fangman, "Linear hypopigmentation and cutaneous atrophy following intra-articular steroid injections for de Quervain's tendonitis," *Journal of Drugs in Dermatology: JDD*, vol. 8, no. 5, pp. 492-493, 2009.

[17] A. V. Evans and D. H. McGibbon, "Symmetrical hypopigmentation following triamcinolone injection for de Quervain's tenosynovitis," *Clinical and Experimental Dermatology*, vol. 27, no. 3, pp. 247–251, 2002.

[18] K. Okere and M. C. Jones, "A case of skin hypopigmentation secondary to a corticosteroid injection," *Southern Medical Journal*, vol. 99, no. 12, pp. 1393-1394, 2006.

[19] M. Edalatifard, M. Akhtari, M. Salehi et al., "Intravenous methylprednisolone pulse as a treatment for hospitalised severe COVID-19 patients: results from a randomised controlled clinical trial," *European Respiratory Journal*, vol. 56, no. 6, Article ID 2002808, 2020.

[20] T. R. C. Group and The RECOVERY Collaborative Group, "Dexamethasone in hospitalized patients with Covid-19 - preliminary report," *The New England Journal of Medicine*, vol. 36, 2020.

[21] WHO Rapid Evidence Appraisal for COVID-19 Therapies (REACT) Working Group, J. A. C. Sterne, and S. Murthy, "Association between administration of systemic corticosteroids and mortality among critically ill patients with COVID-

19: a meta-analysis," *JAMA*, vol. 324, pp. 1330–1341, 2020.
[22] Z. Zhang, E. P. Navarese, B. Zheng et al., "Analytics with artificial intelligence to advance the treatment of acute respiratory distress syndrome," *Journal of Evidence-Based Medicine*, vol. 13, no. 4, pp. 301–312, 2020.

28

Nerve Conduction Studies in Patients with Lumbosacral Radiculopathy Caused by Lumbar Intervertebral Disc Herniation

Safa Yousif,[1] Ammar Ahmed,[1] Ahmed Abdelhai,[2] and Afraa Musa[1]

[1]*Department of Physiology, Faculty of Medicine, University of Khartoum, Khartoum, Sudan*
[2]*Department of Orthopaedics Surgery and Traumatology, Faculty of Medicine, University of Khartoum, Khartoum, Sudan*

Correspondence should be addressed to Safa Yousif; safaayousif27@yahoo.com

Academic Editor: Andreas K. Demetriades

Background. Nerve conduction studies (NCS) are electrodiagnostic tests used to evaluate peripheral nerves functions and aid in the assessment of patients with neuromuscular complaints. There is contrasting evidence concerning the use of NCS in the assessment of patients with lumbosacral radiculopathy. *Objectives.* This study was conducted to evaluate nerve conduction studies abnormalities in patients with lumbosacral radiculopathy and to find out their relation to abnormal physical examination findings. *Materials and Methods.* Twenty-seven patients with lumbosacral radiculopathy caused by L4/5 or L5/S1 intervertebral disc prolapse confirmed by magnetic resonance imaging (MRI) were recruited in the study. Twenty-five healthy subjects matched in age and sex served as control. Motor nerve conduction study bilaterally for both common peroneal and tibial nerves, F-wave for both nerves, and H-reflex had been conducted. *Results.* No significant difference was found in the motor nerve conduction study parameters (latency, amplitude, and conduction velocity) between the patients group and the control group. There was significant prolongation in H-reflex latency of both symptomatic and asymptomatic side in the patients group compared to the control group ($P < 0.05$). Also, F-wave latencies (F minimum, F maximum, and F mean) of the tibial nerve were significantly prolonged ($P < 0.05$) compared to control. *Conclusion.* Prolonged H-reflex latency was the commonest encountered abnormality in our study followed by F-wave latencies of the tibial nerve.

1. Introduction

Back pain in the third and fourth decade of life is frequently caused by lumbar disc herniation. Most people relate their back and leg pain to a traumatic incident as the pain is usually brought on by repetitive twisting, bending, or heavy lifting [1]. 95% of the lumbar disc herniation involves L4/5 and L5/S1 level, the latter being the commonest [2].

Radiculopathy due to lumbar disc herniation is defined by North American Spine Society as localized displacement of disc material beyond the normal margins of the intervertebral disc space resulting in pain, weakness, or numbness in a myotomal or dermatomal distribution [3].

Lumbar disc herniation is suspected from the history and clinical examination. Plain radiographs can be used to exclude infection, tumors, or other anomalies but are limited in diagnosing lumbar disc herniation or other intraspinal lesions. Magnetic resonance imaging (MRI) is the most useful tool for identifying structural abnormalities in the intervertebral disc area [1]. Nerve conduction studies (NCS) are electrodiagnostic tests (EDX) that assess peripheral nerve functions and can be used to evaluate patients with neuromuscular complaints.

Radiculopathy is a pathological process that affects the nerves at the root level. Patients usually present with sensory symptoms but motor symptoms also can exist either mixed with sensory symptoms or alone. Because the nerve affected is proximal to the dorsal root ganglia, sensory nerve conduction study is usually normal. For assessing patients with lumbosacral radiculopathy, motor studies of the common peroneal nerve and posterior tibial nerve can be performed. Late responses (F-wave and H-reflex) provide information about the proximal nerve segment (nerve root) [4].

Studies evaluating the use of nerve conduction studies in the diagnosis and assessment of patients with lumbosacral radiculopathy vary widely [5–15]. Nerve conduction studies have the advantage of being a noninvasive, objective, and reproducible tool to assess the physiologic integrity of the nerve root. NCS are not widely used in assessing patients with lumbosacral radiculopathy. NCS might provide a useful aid in patients' management with regard to options of treatment, postoperative evaluation of recovery, and detection of recurrence. There is a need for more studies to be conducted to correlate the findings of the NCS in patients with lumbosacral radiculopathy with the clinical manifestations of the disease, provided that there is a limited number of published researches addressing this issue.

The objective of our study was to evaluate nerve conduction studies (NCS) abnormalities in patients with lumbosacral radiculopathy and to find out their relation to abnormal physical examination findings.

2. Materials and Methods

2.1. Study Design and Sample. This study was a cross-sectional analytic study conducted in the duration from July to November 2016. The sample size was calculated using G-power software. The sampling technique was convenient sampling.

2.2. Participants. Two groups of subjects were studied: patients and control. Twenty-seven patients were selected; their age ranged between 23 and 60 years (18 males and 9 females). Patients were selected from Ibrahim Malik Teaching Hospital referred clinic and Ribat University Hospital referred clinic. Also, patients were recruited from specialized clinic in the Royal Scan diagnostic center, Mr. Ahmed Abdelhai specialized clinic.

2.3. Patients Group

2.3.1. Inclusion Criteria. Patients with L4/5 and/or L5/S1 intervertebral disc prolapse confirmed by MRI examination in addition to one or more of the following were included in the study: symptoms appropriate with the MRI level of the disc prolapse, motor weakness, sensory impairment, absent ankle jerk, and/or positive straight leg raising test.

2.3.2. Exclusion Criteria. Patients with history suggestive of polyneuropathy (e.g., diabetes), radiculopathy due to other pathology (e.g., tumor, instability), and/or previous spinal surgery were excluded from the study.

2.3.3. Control Group. Twenty-five healthy subjects were selected for the control group. Control group participants were selected from volunteers who work or study in Faculty of Medicine of Khartoum University. The age range of the control group was between 24 and 60 years (15 males and 10 females). The control group was matched in age and gender with the patients group.

Inclusion criteria included subjects with no history of radiculopathy or neuromuscular problems or any risk factors for having impaired nerve function (alcohol abuse, diabetes, renal problem, neurotoxic drugs, and hypothyroidism), and normal neurological examination.

The study was approved by the ethics research committee of the Faculty of Medicine, Khartoum University. Informed written consent was taken from all participants, and their confidentiality was highly conserved.

2.4. Data Collection

2.4.1. Clinical Assessment. Clinical assessment was performed by the principal investigator and took place in Physiology Department, Faculty of Medicine, Khartoum University. History taking included duration of symptoms and the limb involved, in addition to the history of weakness or sphincteric disturbance, and the distribution of sensory symptoms. Pain and/or numbness radiating to the lateral malleolus, lateral foot, heel, or plantar surface of the foot was considered to arise from S1 nerve root involvement. If pain or numbness described by the patient radiated to the anterolateral leg, dorsum of the foot, or the great toe, symptoms were attributed to L5 nerve root involvement. Physical examination included the examination of gait, the motor examination of the lower limb (tone, power, ankle reflex), touch and pinprick sensation, and straight leg raising test.

2.4.2. MRI. Patients' lumbosacral MRI was reported by consultant radiologists blinded to the physical examination findings and the reports were used by the principal investigator to address inclusion criteria.

2.4.3. NCS. NCS were performed using the Digital Medelec Synergy machine software version (10.1) and performed by the principal investigator in Physiology Department, Faculty of Medicine, Khartoum University. Both limbs were studied and NCS reviewed by neurophysiologists blinded to the physical examination findings. Tests performed included motor nerve conduction study of the tibial and common peroneal nerves, F-wave latencies of both nerves, and H-reflex latency of the tibial nerve. Also, the sural nerve sensory nerve conduction study was performed to exclude patient with polyneuropathy.

The following is a description of the conducted NCS tests and the machine setting for each test illustrated in Table 1.

2.4.4. Tibial Nerve Compound Motor Action Potential (CMAP). A recording electrode was placed over the abductor halluces muscle. Two stimulation sites were used, distal and proximal. The distal stimulation site was placed 10 cm proximal to the recording electrode, posterior to the medial malleolus. An electrode placed in the middle of the popliteal crease, served as the proximal stimulation site. Distal latency, amplitude, and conduction velocity were the parameters studied.

TABLE 1: Machine setting for nerve conduction studies [16].

Setting	Sweep velocity (msec/division)	Sensitivity (μv/division)	Filters high/low (kHz/Hz)	Stimulator duration/rate (msec/Hz)
Motor NCS	2	5000	10/2	0.2/1
Sensory NCS	1	10	2/20	0.1/2
H-reflex	10	500	10/20	1/0.5
F-wave	10	500	10/20	0.2/1

2.4.5. Peroneal Nerve CMAP. A recording electrode was placed over the extensor digitorum brevis. Two stimulation sites were used, distal and proximal. The distal stimulation site was in the dorsal lower leg between the tendons of tibialis anterior and extensor hallucis longus 9 cm proximal to the recording electrode. The proximal stimulation site was about 3–4 cm distal to the proximal tip of the fibular head. Parameters studied were distal latency, amplitude, and conduction velocity.

2.4.6. F-Wave. F-wave of the common peroneal and tibial nerves was studied. Electrodes placement was similar to the CMAP recording. The distal stimulation site was used and ten subsequent stimuli were delivered. The latencies recorded and studied were the F-minimum, F-maximum, and F-mean.

2.4.7. H-Reflex. The posterior tibial nerve was stimulated in the center of the popliteal crease and recorded over the soleus muscle. The parameter studied was the shortest latency obtained.

2.4.8. Sural Nerve Sensory Nerve Action Potential (SNAP). The recording electrode was placed behind the lateral malleolus, and the stimulating electrode placed in the midcalf 14 cm proximal to the recording electrode. Parameters recorded were the latency, amplitude, and conduction velocity. Sural nerve SNAP was studied to exclude participants with polyneuropathy.

2.4.9. Data Analysis. Software Statistical Package for the Social Sciences (IBM SPSS) version 20 was used for data analysis. Mean and standard deviation were calculated to describe continuous variables and frequencies were calculated to describe categorical variables. Data obtained from both groups were compared using the independent *t*-test. Parameters of the symptomatic and asymptomatic side were compared using the paired *t*-test. Association between clinical findings and NCS studies abnormalities was carried out by Chi-Square/Fisher's Exact test. *P* value less than 0.05 was considered significant.

3. Results

The total number of patients included in the study was 27, the mean age was 41.6 ± 11.7 years (mean ± standard deviation), and 66.67% were male. The number of healthy subjects was 25, the mean age was 37.24 ± 10.4 years, and 60 % were male.

The mean duration of symptoms was 20.7 ± 26.9 months, and 55.6% had symptoms for more than 6 months. The left limb was involved in 62.96% of patients, right limb was involved in 29.63%, and only 7.4% of patients showed bilateral limb involvement. L5 dermatomal distribution of paresthesia was described in 37.04% of patients, S1 dermatome was involved in 59.26%, and 3.7% showed involvement of both dermatomes.

Regarding physical examination, an antalgic gait was detected in 8 patients and listing in 5 patients (29.6% and 18.5%, respectively). Ankle jerk was absent in 8 patients (29.6%), and impaired touch sensation was detected in 15 patients (55.6%). A positive straight leg raising (SLR) test was the most common encountered abnormality (16 patients, 59.3%).

Cut-off values obtained from the control group motor nerve conduction studies were used as a reference value to classify patients' values into normal or abnormal (Table 2). CMAP amplitude of the common peroneal nerve was reduced in 9.3% of the 54 recorded nerves, while velocity was reduced in 3.7% of nerves. There was no statistically significant difference between the patients group and the control group in the parameters of common peroneal nerve ($P > 0.05$). Tibial nerve CMAP amplitude was reduced in 3.7% of the 53 recorded nerves, and velocity decreased in 11.1%. Also, no statistically significant difference between the patients group and the control group was obtained ($P > 0.05$).

F-wave minimum, maximum, and mean latencies of the common peroneal nerve were measured in 40 nerves and F-wave was absent in 14 nerves. No statistically significant difference was found between the patients group and the control group ($P > 0.05$). No statistically significant difference was found between symptomatic and asymptomatic side in the patients group. Also, no statistically significant difference was found between symptomatic side in the patients group and the control group, or between the asymptomatic side in the patients group and the control group.

F-wave latencies of the tibial nerve were obtained in 54 nerves, and there was a statistically significant difference between the patients group and the control group in minimum, maximum, and mean latencies. The maximum latency was the most significant ($P < 0.05$) (Table 3). Tibial nerve F-wave latencies of symptomatic and asymptomatic sides, when compared to the control group, revealed a significant difference in the maximum latency (Table 4). No statistically significant difference was found between symptomatic and asymptomatic side.

Table 2: CMAP parameters (patients group and control group).

Variable	Group	N	Mean	SD	5th percentile	95th percentile
Common peroneal nerve distal latency (ms)	Control	49	4.37	0.87	—	6
	Patient	54	4.43	1.04	—	—
Common peroneal nerve amplitude (mv)	Control	49	4.34	1.69	1.6	—
	Patient	54	3.77	1.69	—	—
Common peroneal nerve CV (m/s)	Control	49	49.57	6.25	40.6	—
	Patient	54	47.38	4.16	—	—
Tibial nerve distal latency (ms)	Control	50	3.71	0.71	—	4.7
	Patient	53	3.99	0.80	—	—
Tibial nerve amplitude (mv)	Control	50	11.15	4.3	3.99	—
	Patient	53	9.2	3.38	—	—
Tibial nerve CV (m/s)	Control	50	45.13	5.02	38	—
	Patient	53	44.2	5.32	—	—

Table 3: F-wave latencies of the tibial nerve (patients group vs control group).

Variable	Group	N	Mean	Sd	P value
Tibial nerve F-wave minimum latency (ms)	Control	50	43.42	8.88	0.019
	Patient	54	47.42	8.86	
Tibial nerve F-wave maximum latency (ms)	Control	50	52.69	6.32	0.005
	Patient	54	56.21	6.22	
Tibial nerve F-wave mean latency (ms)	Control	50	48.71	6.27	0.014
	Patient	54	51.73	6.68	

Table 4: Tibial nerve F-max (control vs symptomatic side and control vs asymptomatic side).

Variable	Population	N	Mean	Std. deviation	P value
Tibial nerve F-max latency (ms)	Control	50	52.69	6.31	—
	Patient symptomatic side	27	56.14	6.95	0.03
	Patient asymptomatic side	27	56.42	5.71	0.012

H-reflex latencies obtained were compared with values adjusted for age and height [17]. Recorded H-reflex latencies were prolonged in 53.7% of the 54 studied tibial nerves. 40.7% of the symptomatic sides showed prolonged H-reflex latency. 29.6% of the asymptomatic sides showed prolonged H-reflex latency. There was a high statistically significant difference between patients and control in H-reflex latency (P value = 0.001) (Table 5). Both symptomatic and asymptomatic sides showed a statistically significant difference when compared to the control (P value = 0.005 for both) (Table 6). Interside differences of more than 1.5 ms were obtained in 83.3% of patients with abnormal H-reflex latency, but no statistically significant difference was found between symptomatic and asymptomatic sides.

Of the 27 of the studied patients, 21 (77,8%) showed abnormal physical examination; 14 of them (66.7%) showed abnormal nerve conduction studies findings. Of the 6 patients with a normal physical examination, 4 (66.7%) showed abnormal NCS. Both subjects with chronic symptoms (duration more than 6 months) and those being symptomatic for less than 6 months revealed the same percentage of having abnormal NCS (66.7% for both groups). 50% of patients with S1 distribution of symptoms had prolonged H-reflex latency compared to 30% of patients with L5 dermatomal distribution.

Ankle jerk was absent in 8 patients and prolonged H-reflex latency was found in 62.5% of them. The percentage of patients with hypoesthesia who had abnormal nerve conduction studies findings was 60%. The percentage of patients with positive SLR tests who had abnormal nerve conduction studies findings was 68.8%.

No statistically significant association was found between abnormal physical examination findings (abnormal gait, absent ankle jerk, hypoesthesia, or positive SLR) and the abnormal nerve conduction studies parameters (reduced amplitude or CV of CMAP, prolonged F-wave latency, or prolonged H-reflex latency) (Table 7). When the association was tested between individual physical examination and nerve conduction studies, it revealed no statistically significant association. Neither absent ankle jerk nor positive straight leg raise test showed statistically significant association with prolonged H-reflex latency (Table 8 and Table 9, respectively).

4. Discussion

Nerve conduction studies are considered part of the clinical evaluation of patients with neuromuscular complaints. We conducted our study to define abnormalities in CMAP and late responses (F-wave and H-reflex) latencies in patients with clinical radiculopathy due to L4/L5 or L5/S1 disc

Table 5: H-reflex latency (patients group vs control group).

Variable	Group	N	Mean	Std. deviation	*P* value
Tibial nerve H-reflex latency (ms)	Control	50	31.09	3.25	**0.001**
	Patient	54	33.42	3.56	

Table 6: H-reflex latency (control vs symptomatic side and control vs asymptomatic side).

Variable	Population	N	Mean	Std. deviation	*P* value
Tibial nerve H-reflex latency (ms)	Control	50	31.09	3.25	—
	Patient symptomatic side	27	33.47	3.81	0.005
	Patient asymptomatic side	27	33.37	3.34	0.005

Table 7: Association between abnormal clinical examination and abnormal NCS.

NCS / Clinical examination	Normal	Abnormal	*P* value
Normal	2	4	1.000
Abnormal	7	14	

Table 8: Association between abnormal ankle jerk and abnormal H-reflex.

H-reflex / Ankle jerk	Normal	Abnormal	*P* value
Normal	12	7	0.398
Abnormal	3	5	

Table 9: Association between abnormal SLR and abnormal H-reflex.

H-reflex / SLR	Normal	Abnormal	*P* value
Normal	5	6	0.452
Abnormal	10	16	

herniation and, in addition, to find the association between clinical manifestations and the abnormal nerve conduction study findings.

Our study showed no significant difference in the CMAP parameters of both common peroneal and tibial nerves between patients and the control group. This finding goes with the findings of many previous studies [5, 8, 18] and contradicts other studies [6, 12]. In a study conducted by Matsui et al. [6], patients with different grades of motor weakness are included; their results showed a decrease in CMAP amplitude and prolonged latency that correlate with the degree of motor weakness [6], while in our study none of the patients suffered from any degree of motor weakness; this might explain the lack of the significant difference between the control and the patient group. Nafissi et al. reported significant abnormality in CMAP amplitude of peroneal nerve in patients with pretibial muscle weakness [12].

In the current study, F-wave of both common peroneal and tibial nerves was obtained, and minimum, maximum, and mean latencies were evaluated. There was a statistically significant difference between patients and normal subjects in the tibial F-wave minimum, maximum, and mean latencies, which coincide with previous studies [5, 11]. The maximum latency was the most significant of the three. When compared with control, both symptomatic and asymptomatic sides showed a statistically significant difference in the maximum latency. A study conducted by Toyokura and Murakami in 1996 reported high sensitivity (70%) of F-minimum, F-maximum, F-difference, and F-duration on the affected side [5]. Toyokura et al. carried out another study in 2002; they studied F-minimum and F-duration of tibial nerve in mild S1 radiculopathy. They concluded that F-minimum and F-duration corrected by the subject's height (F-min/H) were both significantly longer on the affected side than on the unaffected side and longer than the normal group. However, the incidence of abnormality was very low for both parameters [8].

Our study showed no statistically significant difference between controls and patients in peroneal F-wave latencies, contrary to a study carried out by Weber, who concluded from his study that tibial nerve F-wave is not sensitive and more cases of S1 radiculopathy can be detected by F-wave of the common peroneal nerve [18]. Their findings might be explained by the fact that most of their patients had L5 radiculopathy or combined L5 and S1 radiculopathy, while our study included more cases with S1 radiculopathy than L5 radiculopathy (59.26% and 37.04%, respectively).

Significant prolongation of H-reflex latency was obtained in this study and the percentage of tibial nerves that showed prolonged H-reflex was more on the symptomatic side; this was consistent with previous studies [7, 9, 10, 19]. Both symptomatic and asymptomatic sides revealed significant prolongation in latency when compared to the control group. This could be explained by the fact that disc prolapse tends to affect both nerve roots though one side remains subclinical. In contrast to the results of Haroun et al. and Alrowayeh et al., who studied H-reflex in S1 radiculopathy, our study result failed to show a statistically significant difference between symptomatic and asymptomatic sides [7, 10].

From patients with abnormal ankle jerk, 62.5% showed H-reflex latency prolongation in our study. This was lower than what was obtained by Haroun et al. in their study. They reported that all their patients with abnormal ankle jerk showed prolonged H-reflex latency [7]. Our study failed to show a statistically significant association between duration of symptoms and abnormal NCS in contrast to a previous study that reported a significant relationship between the duration of clinical symptoms and the electrophysiological findings [12].

Our current study showed no statistically significant association between physical examination and nerve conduction studies. Therefore, the physical examination is not an adequate predictor of abnormal nerve conduction studies in subjects with symptoms suggesting radiculopathy. This coincides with the conclusion of many previous studies [12–15]. Lauder et al. concluded that having at least one abnormal physical examination finding makes the probability of having an abnormal electrodiagnostic study more likely. However, having normal physical examination does not rule out the probability of finding abnormal EDX. They concluded also that history and clinical examination are not a perfect tool in diagnosing radiculopathy or predicting electrodiagnostic study but remain an essential part of clinical evaluation of patients to aid in formulating a differential diagnosis and guiding the electrodiagnostic study [14]. Inal et al. also emphasized that neurological examination and the electrodiagnostic test must be used and interpreted jointly [15]. Finally, NCS can be used to aid in the diagnosis when clinical findings do not coincide with MRI findings (e.g., non-compressive radiculopathy) [20], or when it is difficult to obtain MRI (e.g., a patient who has MRI-incompatible spinal cord stimulator).

5. Conclusion

We concluded from our findings that NCS is a valuable tool in evaluating subjects with lumbosacral radiculopathy, H-reflex latency prolongation being the commonest encountered abnormality in our study. Also, we concluded that normal physical examination was frequently encountered with abnormal NCS as well as abnormal physical examination detected in patients with normal NCS findings. Therefore, both of them should be evaluated simultaneously in patients with history suggesting radiculopathy.

References

[1] S. T. Canale, J. H. Beaty, *Campbell's Operative Orthopaedics*, Elsevier, Amsterdam, Netherlands, 12th edition, 2013.

[2] D. Moore, "Lumbar disc herniation," 2015, http://www.orthobullets.com/spine/2035/lumbar-disc-herniation.

[3] D. S. Kreiner, S. W. Hwang, J. E. Easa et al., "An evidence-based clinical guideline for the diagnosis and treatment of lumbar disc herniation with radiculopathy," *The Spine Journal*, vol. 14, no. 1, pp. 180–191, 2014.

[4] R. I. Chichkova and L. Katzin, "EMG and nerve conduction studies in clinical practice," 2010, http://practicalneurology.com/2010/02/emg-and-nerve-conduction-studies-in-clinical-practice.

[5] M. Toyokura and K. Murakami, "F-wave study in patients with lumbosacral radiculopathies," *Electromyography and Clinical Neurophysiology*, vol. 37, no. 1, pp. 19–26, 1996.

[6] H. Matsui, M. Kanamori, Y. Kawaguchi, H. Kitagawa,H. Nakamura, and H. Tsuji, "Clinical and electrophysiologiccharacteristics of compressed lumbar nerve roots," Spine, vol. 22, no. 18, pp. 2100–2105, 1997.

[7] N. S. Haroun, N. M. Sherief, M. M. Abdul-Hakiem, A. M. Al-Ganzoury, A. M. K. Al-Gogary, and M. R. S. Al-Helowe, "H-reflex in the diagnosis of lumbosacral radiculopathy," *Egyptian Rheumatology and Rehabilitation*, vol. 26, no. 4, pp. 763–769, 1999.

[8] M. Toyokura and T. Furukawa, "F wave duration in mild S1 radiculopathy: comparison between the affected and unaffected sides," *Clinical Neurophysiology*, vol. 113, no. 8, pp. 1231–1235, 2002.

[9] S. C. Cho, M. A. Ferrante, K. H. Levin, R. L. Harmon, and Y. T. So, "Utility of electrodiagnostic testing in evaluating patients with lumbosacral radiculopathy: an evidence-based review," *Muscle & Nerve*, vol. 42, no. 2, pp. 276–282, 2010.

[10] H. N. Alrowayeh and M. A. Sabbahi, "H-reflex amplitude asymmetry is an earlier sign of nerve root involvement than latency in patients with S1 radiculopathy," *BMC Research Notes*, vol. 4, no. 1, p. 102, 2011.

[11] M. Gencer, K. Uluc, Y. Cetinkaya et al., "Clinical utility of F wave parameters in unilateral S1 radiculopathy," *Neurosciences (Riyadh, Saudi Arabia)*, vol. 16, no. 3, pp. 237–241, 2011.

[12] S. Nafissi, S. Niknam, and S. S. Hosseini, "Electrophysiological evaluation in lumbosacral radiculopathy," *Iranian Journal of Neurology*, vol. 11, no. 3, pp. 83–86, 2012.

[13] T. D. Lauder, T. R. Dillingham, M. Andary et al., "Effect of history and exam in predicting electrodiagnostic outcome among patients with suspected lumbosacral radiculopathy," *American Journal of Physical Medicine & Rehabilitation*, vol. 79, no. 1, pp. 60–68, 2000.

[14] T. D. Lauder, "Physical examination signs, clinical symptoms, and their relationship to electrodiagnostic findings and the presence of radiculopathy," *Physical Medicine and Rehabilitation Clinics of North America*, vol. 13, no. 3, pp. 451–467, 2002.

[15] E. E. İnal, F. Eser, L. A. Aktekin, E. Öksüz, and H. Bodur, "Comparison of clinical and electrophysiological findings in patients with suspected radiculopathies," *Journal of Back and Musculoskeletal Rehabilitation*, vol. 26, no. 2, pp. 169–173, 2013.

[16] S. Yousif, A. Musa, A. Ahmed, and A. Abdelhai, "Correlation between findings in physical examination, magnetic resonance imaging, and nerve conduction studies in lumbosacral radiculopathy caused by lumbar intervertebral disc herniation," *Advances in Orthopedics*, vol. 2020, Article ID 9719813, 6 pages, 2020.

[17] R. Buschbach and N. Prahlow, *Manual of Nerve Conduction Studies*, Demos Medical Publishing, New York, NY, United States, 2nd edition, 2006.

[18] F. Weber, "The diagnostic sensitivity of different F wave parameters," *Journal of Neurology, Neurosurgery & Psychiatry*, vol. 65, no. 4, pp. 535–540, 1998.

[19] M. Wojtysiak, J. Huber, A. Wiertel-Krawczuk, A. Szymankiewicz-Szukała, J. Moskal, and J. Janicki, "Pre-and postoperative evaluation of patients with lumbosacral disc herniation by neurophysiological and clinical assessment," *Spine*, vol. 39, no. 21, pp. 1792–1800, 2014.

[20] M. J. Albeck, G. Taher, M. Lauritzen, and W. Trojaborg, "Diagnostic value of electrophysiological tests in patients with sciatica," *Acta Neurologica Scandinavica*, vol. 101, no. 4, pp. 249–254, 2000.

Evaluating Clinical Outcomes for Determining the Optimal Delay to Skin Incision under WALANT: A Prospective Series of 34 Patients from a Low-Resource Tertiary Setting

Alvin Hernandez, Mamer Rosario, Romina Mendoza-Torres, Carl Ryan Marino Taguba, Abigail Garcia, and Geoffrey Battad

Department of Orthopaedics, East Avenue Medical Center, East Avenue, Diliman, Quezon City 1101, Metro Manila, Philippines

Correspondence should be addressed to Mamer Rosario; msrosario@up.edu.ph

Academic Editor: Allen L. Carl

Background. Additional studies on clinical outcomes to determine the optimal time delay from injection of local anesthesia to skin incision for WALANT surgeries are needed. The authors aimed to propose the optimal time delay from local injection to skin incision for WALANT surgeries of the hand and wrist by analyzing intraoperative blood loss, postoperative pain scores, and complication rates. *Methods.* Thirty-four patients were consecutively recruited and allocated by either 7-min or 30-min delay for skin incision from local injection of epinephrine with lidocaine. Intraoperative bleeding and postoperative pain scores were analyzed between both groups by Mann–Whitney *U*-test, while complication rates were compared using Fisher's exact test. *Results.* The present study did not find significant differences in mean intraoperative blood loss (8 ± 5.8 mL vs. 5 ± 2.2 mL, $p = 0.074$), complication rates (18% vs. 0%, $p = 0.227$), and mean pain scores (1.2 ± 0.5 vs. 1.4 ± 0.5, $p = 0.307$) between the 7-min and 30-min groups. *Conclusion.* The authors conclude that a waiting time of 7 min from the injection of local anesthesia is sufficient to achieve comparable clinical outcomes for minor hand and wrist surgeries under WALANT.

1. Introduction

Hand surgeries traditionally rely on tourniquet to minimize intraoperative bleeding. However, upper arm tourniquet may cause pain and discomfort among wide-awake patients without general anesthesia or brachial plexus block [1, 2]. Minor procedures of the hand and wrist can be performed with local anesthesia without sedation on an outpatient basis. Use of upper arm tourniquet, however, can limit the duration of procedure due to excessive pain caused on some patients [2–4]. The wide-awake local anesthesia no tourniquet (WALANT) technique [5], in which lidocaine and epinephrine are injected for local anesthesia and vasoconstriction, respectively, has been increasingly used for hand surgeries [1, 6, 7]. The WALANT technique enables the surgery to be performed with the patient fully awake and without upper arm tourniquet, which allows intraoperative assessment of function during the procedure [1, 5].

Bleeding can be minimized with the WALANT technique by waiting for the optimal epinephrine effect after local anesthetic injection. Although vasoconstriction by epinephrine is traditionally believed to be optimal at approximately 7 to 10 minutes (min) from the time of injection [8], McKee et al. [8], in a prospective randomized trial, obtained the lowest cutaneous hemoglobin levels at roughly 26 min following injection of epinephrine. In their follow-up prospective comparative series [9] on carpal tunnel surgeries performed by WALANT, waiting roughly 30 min after injection of epinephrine resulted near three-fold reduction in mean quantity of intraoperative bleeding.

However, to the best of our knowledge, no additional studies on clinical outcomes to determine the optimal time delay to skin incision for WALANT surgeries of the hand or wrist have been published. In this regard, our study aimed to propose the optimal time delay from the injection to skin incision for most WALANT surgeries of the hand or wrist by analyzing not only intraoperative blood loss but also postoperative pain scores and complication rates, in a larger single-institutional cohort of patients.

2. Patients and Methods

In this prospective comparative study, healthy patients undergoing minor hand or wrist surgeries by WALANT on an outpatient basis at the East Avenue Medical Center, a public tertiary hospital in the Philippines, waited either 7 min or 30 min from the time of injection to the time of skin incision. Institutional review board approval was obtained. Patients undergoing repeat surgery, on anticoagulation medications, and with bleeding disorders were excluded. Thirty-four patients were consecutively recruited from January 1 to December 31, 2019, with our sample size based on the calculation performed by McKee et al. [8] for their study. The patients were not formally randomized but allocated prior to arriving at the operating room, based on surgeon scheduling factors. For 17 patients, we waited exactly 7 min following injection of local anesthesia before cutting, with each interval timed using a stopwatch, and then recorded. While for the other 17 patients, we waited exactly 30 min prior to skin incision.

For local anesthesia, we used up to 10 mL [10] of 1% lidocaine with 1 : 100,000 concentration of epinephrine (OCTOCAINE®; Novocol Pharma, Inc., Cambridge, Canada) introduced in a subcutaneous plane along the length of the planned incision. The same injector (AH) provided the anesthesia for all patients. All procedures were performed without the aid of surgical loupes. Intraoperative blood loss was estimated for each procedure using the method developed by Algadiem et al. [11]. Pain was assessed using the Verbal Rating Scale (VRS) [12], recorded from each patient at 1 hour after the procedure. Perioperative complications were documented and recorded. Median follow-up after surgery is 14 days (range 14 to 28 days).

Both the mean intraoperative blood loss in mL and mean VRS scores for both groups were analyzed using the Mann–Whitney *U*-test, while complication rates were compared using Fisher's Exact test. All statistical analyses were performed using SPSS version 21.0 (IBM Corp., Armonk, NY), with a p value of less than 0.05 considered statistically significant.

3. Results

We categorized patient-, disease-, and treatment-related variables according to the time delay from the injection of local anesthesia to skin incision (Table 1). The 7-min group and the 30-min group had a mean age of 48 years (range, 31 to 75 years) and 53 years (range, 39 to 75 years), respectively, and a male-to-female ratio of 1 : 1.12 for both groups. The mean time intervals of surgery from skin incision to closure, for the 7-min and 30-min groups, are 7.5 min (range, 6 to 12 min) and 6.8 min (range, 5 to 11 min), respectively, while the mean length of skin incision is 1.7 cm for both groups. Mean VRS scores at 1 hour postsurgery for the 7-min and 30-min groups are 0.6 (range, 0 to 1) and 0.5 (range, 0 to 1), respectively, while mean intraoperative bleeding for the 7-min and 30-min groups are 8 mL (range, 3 to 27 mL) and 5 mL (range, 3 to 12 mL), respectively. Three complications, one intraoperatively and two postoperatively, were documented in the 7-min group, while there was none in the 30-min group. Specifically, iatrogenic digital vessel injury during surgery, wound dehiscence, and development of neuroma occurred in three cases of trigger finger release (Table 2).

Our study did not find statistically significant differences in mean intraoperative blood loss (8 ± 5.8 mL vs. 5 ± 2.2 mL, $p = 0.074$), complication rates (18% vs. 0%, $p = 0.227$), and mean VRS scores (1.2 ± 0.5 vs. 1.4 ± 0.5, $p = 0.307$) between the 7-min and the 30-min groups (Table 3).

4. Discussion

When performing WALANT surgeries, waiting for the optimal epinephrine effect after local anesthetic injection shall minimize bleeding. Despite data by some authors [6, 7] showing significant reduction in intraoperative blood loss by waiting approximately 30 min from the time of epinephrine injection before incising skin, literature on clinical outcomes determining the optimal time delay to skin incision is scarce. Our study sought to propose the optimal time delay from injection to skin incision for most WALANT surgeries of the hand or wrist by analyzing clinical outcomes, particularly pain scores and complication rates, in addition to intraoperative blood loss.

The study has several limitations. First, our use of McKee et al.'s method [9] for measuring blood loss, although reliable, must be less accurate than that performed by other authors [9].However, we estimated the total intraoperative blood loss for each procedure, from skin incision to closure, to have better measure of intraoperative bleeding. Second, we included all hand and wrist surgeries in the analysis, instead of controlling confounders by limiting to a single hand procedure, like carpal tunnel release [8, 9]. Nonetheless, we upheld homogeneity of both groups, having found no significant differences in mean incision length (1.7 ± 0.5 cm vs. 1.7 ± 0.4 cm, $p = 0.807$), mean interval duration from skin incision to closure (7.5 ± 1.7 min vs. 6.8 ± 1.3 min, $p = 0.242$), and mean preoperative VRS scores (1.2 ± 0.7 vs. 1.4 ± 0.7, $p = 0.320$) between the 7-min and 30-min groups (Table 4). Third, randomization and blinding were not done. Although we have contributed additional data from a larger prospective cohort, more randomized controlled trials to fill the present lack of studies are recommended. Fourth, we did not use lidocaine for control measurements of bleeding. It has been reported by some authors [13, 14] that lidocaine has an initial vasodilatory effect in the skin. However, recent studies [15, 16] have shown no changes in perfusion following lidocaine infiltration on porcine eyelid flaps and flanks. Fifth, our study is limited by the relatively short follow-up period. Given our setting, it must be financially taxing for patients to pursue

TABLE 1: Patient characteristics.

	Total, $N = 34$	
	7-min ($n = 17$)	30-min ($n = 17$)
Age (years)*	48 (31 to 75)	53 (39 to 75)
Gender**		
Men	8 (47)	8 (47)
Women	9 (53)	9 (53)
Procedure**		
Trigger finger release	13 (76)	12 (70)
Carpal tunnel release	3 (18)	3 (18)
Excision of mass	1 (6)	2 (12)
Interval from skin incision to closure (min)*	7.5 (6 to 12)	6.8 (5 to 11)
Length of incision (cm)*	1.7 (1.5 to 3)	1.7 (1.5 to 2.5)
Preoperative VRS score*	1.2 (0 to 2)	1.4 (0 to 2)
VRS score 1-hour postsurgery*	0.6 (0 to 1)	0.5 (0 to 1)
Intraoperative blood loss (ml)*	8 (3 to 27)	5 (3 to 12)
Perioperative complications**	3 (18)	0 (0)

* Presented as the mean with the range in parentheses. **Presented as the number with the percentage in parentheses.

TABLE 2: List of perioperative complications.

Case no.	Group	Age/sex	Operation	Complication	Management	Outcome
13	7-min	53/F	Trigger finger release	Wound dehiscence	Debridement and primary closure	Improved
17	7-min	51/M	Trigger finger release	Digital vessel injury	Direct pressure	Improved
20	7-min	54/F	Trigger finger release	Painful neuroma	Oral pregabalin	Improved

TABLE 3: Analyses of intraoperative bleeding, postoperative VRS scores, and complication rates.

	N	Mean/proportion	p value
Blood loss			0.074
7-min	17	8 mL	
30-min	17	5 mL	
Postoperative VRS scores			0.307
7-min	17	1.2	
30-min	17	1.4	
Complications			0.227
7-min	17	18%	
30-min	17	0%	

TABLE 4: Analyses of preoperative VRS scores, duration of procedure, and length of skin incision.

	N	Mean/proportion	p value
Preoperative VRS scores			0.320
7-min	17	1.2	
30-min	17	1.4	
Duration of procedure			0.242
7-min	17	7.5 min	
30-min	17	6.8 min	
Length of skin incision			0.807
7-min	17	1.7 cm	
30-min	17	1.7 cm	

regular follow-up after surgery. In our experience, patients most commonly seek follow-up only for either the removal of wound sutures or development of a complication. A patient's nonappearance during follow-up somehow reassures there must be no postoperative complications. Lastly, multi-institutional studies involving larger cohorts must be necessary, in order to address the relatively small number of patients included in our analysis.

Having found no significant increase in blood loss with the 7 min delay from injection of local anesthesia, our findings seem in contrast with the controversial results of McKee et al. [8, 9].Although the disparity between our results and those of McKee et al.'s [9] study may be due to differences in the method of blood collection (by micropipette versus surgical gauze [11]), number of cases (15 versus 34), and length of skin incision (2.5 to 3 cm versus 1.7 cm), our findings must reflect the better estimates of total intraoperative bleeding since we opted to collect blood throughout the whole duration of each procedure (versus the 1 min interval by McKee et al. [9]). Therefore, a waiting time of 7 min seems acceptable, and sufficient, to reduce intraoperative bleeding when performing minor hand and wrist surgeries under WALANT. The epinephrine concentration used (1 : 100,000), anatomical location (hand and wrist), and patient demographics (age and sex) were similar in both studies.

Our findings are, moreover, in agreement with those by preceding authors [14–19]. Larrabee et al. [17] injected epinephrine with either lidocaine or saline into the skin of piglet trunks and found maximal vasoconstriction, measured by laser Doppler flowmetry, to occur at about 5 to 7 min in most of the cases. Similarly, O'Malley et al. [18] recorded maximal vasoconstriction following epinephrine injection in the neck of patients undergoing head and neck surgery after 3 to 4 min, while Ghali et al. [14] found maximal decrease in blood flow following injection of epinephrine to happen after 8 min in the face and 10 min in the forearm. Additionally, Hult et al. [19] estimated intra-operative bleeding in the eyelids of 16 patients undergoing upper eyelid blepharoplasty and found significant decrease in bleeding at 7 min following epinephrine injection, with no further decrease at 15 and 30 min thereafter. In a recent study by Sheikh et al. [15] on porcine flank flaps injected with epinephrine and lidocaine, low level of perfusion, measured by laser speckle contrast imaging and laser Doppler flowmetry, was already observed after approximately 2 minutes following the injection. In a similar study by the same authors [16] on porcine eyelid flaps, time to maximum hypoperfusion was found even shorter, recorded by laser speckle contrast imaging at 1.25 min following the injection.

The present study is the first to evaluate complication rates and pain scores for determining the optimal time delay from local anesthesia to skin incision when performing the WALANT technique. Despite the three complications that occurred in patients from the 7-min group, we found no significant difference in complication rates between the two groups. The digital vessel injury was adequately controlled by coagulation with direct pressure, while the wound dehiscence was formally debrided and then closed by suture repair. The neuroma was conservatively treated with 150 mg of oral pregabalin (LYRICA®; Pfizer, Inc., New York City, USA) daily for a week, which completely resolved the pain thereafter. Huang et al. [1], in a retrospective analysis of 24 distal radius fractures treated by open reduction and plating under WALANT, documented no complications following a mean follow-up period of 15 months. In contrast to Huang et al.'s study, the complication rate (9%) we found in our series must be high. We additionally analyzed a total of 19 patients who underwent minor hand procedures in our institution, but under local anesthesia with tourniquet in the same study period, and documented two (11%) complications after a median follow-up of 14 days (range, 14 to 121 days). Upon comparison with our WALANT cohort, no statistically significant difference in complication rates (9% vs. 11%, $p = 1.0$) was found. Aside from having analyzed nonfracture WALANT cases, the development of complications in our series must be explicable in the setting of a public tertiary facility in a developing country [20, 21].In our retrospective cohort that underwent surgery under local anesthesia with tourniquet, superficial surgical site infection and finger stiffness developed in two cases of trigger finger release. The former was successfully treated with 2-week regimen of 500 mg oral cefuroxime (CEFUREX®; Cathay Drug Co. Inc., Makati City, PH) twice daily and the latter, with six weeks of physical therapy. It has been recognized that traditional clinical research using standard follow-up is extraordinarily difficult in the developing world, where resources are limited [22]. It is financially challenging for our patients to pursue regular follow-up after surgery, and similar to the experiences of Young et al. [23], patients most commonly seek follow-up for the removal of wound sutures or due to development of a complication and less for surveillance. Moreover, we performed all procedures without the aid of surgical loupes, which could have promoted optimal tissue handling and dissection, and thus prevented iatrogenic soft tissue injury and wound complications. Although the low postoperative pain scores we found, in addition to those found by Huang et al. in their study [1], they must lay support to the latter authors' findings of significantly lower mean postoperative pain score under WALANT, in their subsequent comparative study on 47 distal radius fractures treated by volar plating, under either WALANT or general anesthesia with arm tourniquet [7].

5. Conclusion

In conclusion, we showed that a waiting time of 7 min from the injection of local anesthesia is sufficient to achieve comparable clinical outcomes for minor hand and wrist surgeries under WALANT. However, findings of the present study must be considered preliminary, and randomized clinical trials for larger cohort analyses are deemed necessary.

References

[1] Y. C. Huang, C. J. Hsu, J. H. Renn et al., "WALANT for distal radius fracture: open reduction with plating fixation via wide-awake local anesthesia with no tourniquet," *Journal of Orthopaedic Surgery and Research*, vol. 13, no. 195, 2018.

[2] G. Prodhomme, D. Mouraux, P.-M. Dugailly, C. Chantelot, C. Fontaine, and F. Schuind, "Tolerance of upper extremity pneumatic tourniquets and their effect on grip strength," *Journal of Hand Surgery (European Volume)*, vol. 33, no. 3, pp. 266–271, 2008.

[3] S. A. Edwards, G. D. Harper, G. E. B. Giddins et al., "Efficacy of forearm versus upper arm tourniquet for local anaesthetic surgery of the hand," *Journal of Hand Surgery*, vol. 25, no. 6, pp. 573-574, 2000.

[4] N. G. Yousif, B. K. Grumert, R. A. Forte et al., "A comparison of upper arm and forearm tourniquet tolerance," *The Journal of Hand Surgery*, vol. 18B, pp. 639–641, 2000.

[5] D. Lalonde, "Wide awake local anaesthesia no tourniquet technique (WALANT)," *BMC Proceedings*, vol. 9, no. S3, p. A81, 2015.

[6] D. Lalonde and A. Martin, "Epinephrine in local anesthesia in finger and hand surgery: the case for wide-awake anesthesia," *Journal of the American Academy of Orthopaedic Surgeons*, vol. 21, no. 8, pp. 443–447, 2013.

[7] Y.-C. Huang, C.-Y. Chen, K.-C. Lin, S.-W. Yang, Y.-W. Tarng, and W.-N. Chang, "Comparison of wide-awake local anesthesia no tourniquet with general anesthesia with tourniquet for volar plating of distal radius fracture," *Orthopedics*, vol. 42, no. 1, pp. e93–e98, 2019.

[8] D. E. McKee, D. H. Lalonde, A. Thoma, D. L. Glennie, and J. E. Hayward, "Optimal time delay between epinephrine injection and incision to minimize bleeding," *Plastic and Reconstructive Surgery*, vol. 131, no. 4, pp. 811–814, 2013.

[9] D. E. McKee, D. H. Lalonde, A. Thoma, and L. Dickson, "Achieving the optimal epinephrine effect in wide awake hand surgery using local anesthesia without a tourniquet," *Hand*, vol. 10, no. 4, pp. 613–615, 2015.

[10] M. R. Leblanc, J. Lalonde, and D. H. Lalonde, "A detailed cost and efficiency analysis of performing carpal tunnel surgery in the main operating room versus the ambulatory setting in Canada," *Hand*, vol. 2, no. 4, pp. 173–178, 2007.
[11] E. A. Algadiem, A. A. Aleisa, H. I. Alsubaie et al., "Blood loss estimation using gauze visual analogue," *Trauma Monthly*, vol. 21, no. 2, Article ID e34131, 2016.
[12] M. Haefeli and A. Elfering, "Pain assessment," *European Spine Journal*, vol. 15, no. S1, pp. S17–S24, 2006.
[13] E. M. Gessler, A. K. E. Hart, T. M. Dunlevy, and J. H. Greinwald, "Optimal concentration of epinephrine for vasoconstriction in ear surgery," *The Laryngoscope*, vol. 111, no. 10, pp. 1687–1690, 2001.
[14] S. Ghali, K. R. Knox, J. Verbesey, U. Scarpidis, K. Izadi, and P. A. Ganchi, "Effects of lidocaine and epinephrine on cutaneous blood flow," *Journal of Plastic, Reconstructive & Aesthetic Surgery*, vol. 61, no. 10, pp. 1226–1231, 2008.
[15] R. Sheikh, K. Memarzadeh, C. Torbrand, J. Blohmé, and M. Malmsjö, "Hypoperfusion in response to epinephrine in local anaesthetics: investigation of dependence on epinephrine concentration, spread of hypoperfusion and time to maximal cutaneous vasoconstriction," *Journal of Plastic, Reconstructive & Aesthetic Surgery*, vol. 70, no. 3, pp. 322–329, 2017.
[16] R. Sheikh, U. Dahlstrand, K. Memarzadeh, J. Blohmé, N. Reistad, and M. Malmsjö, "Optimal epinephrine concentration and time delay to minimize perfusion in eyelid surgery," *Ophthalmic Plastic and Reconstructive Surgery*, vol. 34, no. 2, pp. 123–129, 2018.
[17] W. J. F. Larrabee, B. J. Lanier, and D. Miekle, "Effect of epinephrine on local cutaneous blood flow," *Head & Neck Surgery*, vol. 9, no. 5, pp. 287–289, 1987.
[18] T. P. O'Malley, G. N. Postma, M. Holtel et al., "Effect of local epinephrine on cutaneous bloodflow in the human neck," *Laryngoscope*, vol. 105, no. 2, pp. 140–143, 1995.
[19] J. Hult, R. Sheikh, C. D. Nguyen, K. Tenland, U. Dahlstrand, and M. Malmsjö, "A waiting time of 7 min is sufficient to reduce bleeding in oculoplastic surgery following the administration of epinephrine together with local anaesthesia," *Acta Ophthalmologica*, vol. 96, no. 5, pp. 499–502, 2017.
[20] R. A. Gosselin, D. A. Spiegel, R. Coughlin et al., "Injuries: the neglected burden in developing countries," *Bulletin of the World Health Organization*, vol. 87, no. 4, pp. 246-247, 2009.
[21] T. A. Reynolds, B. Stewart, I. Drewett et al., "The impact of trauma care systems in low-and middle-income countries," *Annual Review of Public Health*, vol. 38, no. 1, pp. 507–532, 2017.
[22] S. Carsen, S. S.-H. Park, D. A. Simon, and R. J. Feibel, "Treatment with the SIGN nail in closed diaphyseal femur fractures results in acceptable radiographic alignment," *Clinical Orthopaedics and Related Research*, vol. 473, no. 7, pp. 2394–2401, 2015.
[23] S. Young, L. N. Banza, G. Hallan et al., "Complications after intramedullary nailing of femoral fractures in a low-income country," *Acta Orthopaedica*, vol. 84, no. 5, pp. 460–467, 2013.

30

Effectiveness of Surgical Treatment in Carpal Tunnel Syndrome Mini-Incision Using MIS-CTS Kits

Wongthawat Liawrungrueang and Sunton Wongsiri

Department of Orthopaedic Surgery, Faculty of Medicine, Prince of Songkla University, Hat Yai, Thailand

Correspondence should be addressed to Wongthawat Liawrungrueang; mint11871@hotmail.com

Academic Editor: Allen L. Carl

Introduction. Carpal tunnel syndrome (CTS) is caused by the compression of the median nerves in the wrist. Patients have pain and numbness in the hands. According to the records of Songklanagarind Hospital from 2015 to 2018, of 800 patients, 196 or 24.5% were treated with surgery. The novel tool of minimally invasive surgery for carpal tunnel syndrome (MIS-CTS) was developed to improve effectiveness and safety. *Purpose*. This study was performed to the effectiveness of visualization during surgery and the complete release of the transverse carpal ligament (TCL) and also the safety of using the MIS-CTS kits. *Methods*. Twenty fresh cadaveric forearms had surgery. Surgical techniques were (1) incision 15–18 mm at palmar hand; (2) the scissors and the navigator were inserted to create working space underneath the palmar aponeurosis; (3) the visual enhancer was inserted. The visual enhancer improves the visual field by shielding the soft tissue around the operative field; (4) the TCL was cut at the distal TCL by surgery scalpel, and then a flexible freer was used to detach the fibrous tissue from the median nerve and the TCL; and (5) the TCL cutting blade was pushed straight to cut the TCL completely from distal to proximal. TCL length was observed until the complete release. The median nerve and the recurrent branch of the median nerve were observed. *Results*. All TCL were cut completely. All median nerves, recurrent branches of the median nerve, and superficial palmar arches could be observed during the operation, and none were injured. This technique showed effectiveness and safety for minimally invasive carpal tunnel surgery. *Conclusions*. The study found that the new device, MIS-CTS kits, along with this technique is effective for CTS release in terms of minimally invasive open carpal tunnel surgery.

1. Introduction

Carpal tunnel syndrome is common and has a high prevalence of 6–10% in the elderly population with an average age of 54 years. It is twice more common in women than in men [1–6]. The initial treatment of mild symptoms can be conservative. However, if symptoms are more frequent or persistent, including muscular weakness and decreased handgrip or drooping, surgical treatment may be required; 20% of people with the disease need surgery [7–11]. Standard open surgery is a basic procedure with a 3–5 cm long incision and produces successful outcomes of carpal tunnel release, but wound complications are more frequent than with minimally invasive carpal tunnel surgery. The most common wound complications are wound infection, inflammation, wound dehiscence, and painful scar [9, 12–15]. Minimally invasive carpal tunnel surgery techniques, such as endoscopic surgery, have less wound complications and patients can return to work faster than with the standard open technique; however, minimally invasive carpal tunnel surgery has other complications, including recurrent incidents and incomplete release [12, 16–19]. Minimally invasive carpal tunnel surgery was developed to improve visualization. It is a surgical tool that is important for complete release [20–23].

Nowadays, the medical costs are high, because of expensive surgical devices; the cost of endoscopic surgery carpal tunnel surgery is higher than that of standard open and other minimally invasive methods [24, 25]. The complexity of tools and the surgical technique of endoscopic surgery require a longer learning curve for surgeons [26–28]. In order to eliminate the difficulties of use and cost, the first generation (PSU-CTR®) and the second generation (named MiniSURE®) of MIS-CTS kits were developed to help patients gain minimally invasive surgery outcomes (Figure 1). Now, surgery is easier because surgeons have greater visibility [22, 23, 29]. In previous studies of both generations of MIS-CTS kits, we found better outcomes with small wounds, less pain, and early return to work [29]. Nonetheless, we have improved some features in the next generation of kits, thus increasing effectiveness and safety. The new features include improved hand griping, antislipping with expandable visual enhancer, and insertion length of marker of TCL cutting blade and flexible freer. The purposes of this research are to study the effectiveness of visualization during surgery and the complete release of TCL and also the safety of using the MIS-CTS kits.

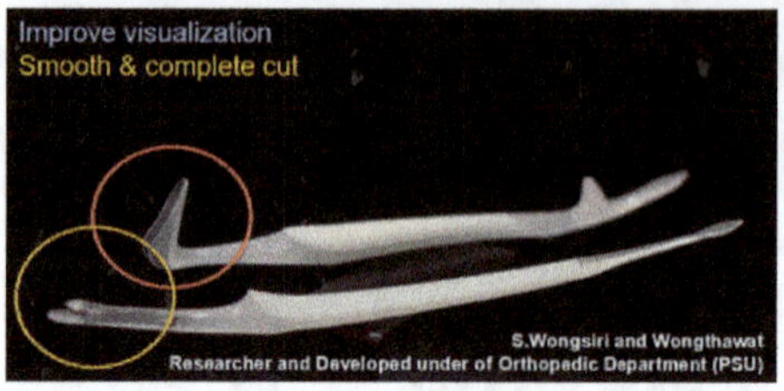

Figure 1: The minimally invasive surgery for carpal tunnel syndrome kits (MIS-CTS kits).

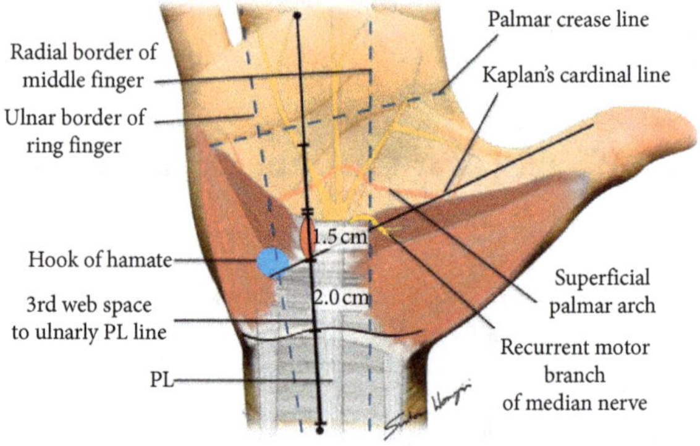

Figure 2: The landmark of anatomy of hand using Kaplan's cardinal line.

2. Methods

2.1. Study Subjects. This study was approved by the Institutional Review Board of Faculty of Medicine, Prince of Songkla University (IRB number EC 60-282-11-1). This study was performed on 20 forearms from 10 fresh cadavers obtained within 72 hours after death. The cadavers came from a donation center of faculty of science, Prince of Songkla University. The operation was performed by the same author. Procedures were performed in the supine position and described the landmark by Kaplan's cardinal line (Figure 2).

2.2. The Surgical Technique. The incision direction is the line between the middle finger and ring finger along the wrist crease. Incision of 15–18 mm, starts away from the wrist crease about 2 to 2.5 cm distally. (Figure 3)

The Palmaris longus tendon is retracted by Senn retractors, and then the TCL is observed at the base. Scissors are used to create working space underneath the PL tendon and palmar aponeurosis. Then, insert the navigator to increase the size of the space for visual enhancer insertion (Figure 4).

The visual enhancer is inserted in the space beneath the PL tendon and palmar aponeurosis. The transverse fiber of the TCL is observed from the bottom view. The visual enhancer improves the visual field by shielding the soft tissue around the operative field (Figure 5).

The TCL is cut by using a scalpel longitudinally at the top to create the long groove for the cutting guide and reducing the over prominence of TCL. The TCL is cut at the distal part for opening entry; then, a flexible freer is used to detach the fibrous tissue from the median nerve and the TCL (Figure 6).

The TCL cutting blade is pushed straight to cut the TCL from the distal to proximal along the groove until the antebrachial fascia that is 2 to 2.5 centimeters proximal to the wrist crease. (Figure 7). Finally, complete release can be directly checked by direct vision via the visual enhancer or through the use of a probe with the MIS-CTS kits, the TCL can be seen clearly through the small incision.

2.3. Statistical Analysis. The descriptive statistics was used in this study. Cadaveric data collected included sex, age, side of hand, transverse carpal ligament length, incision site for single portal, type of release (complete release/incomplete release), median nerve injury (yes/no), type of recurrent branch of median nerve, and recurrent branch of median nerve injury.

3. Results

This study was from 20 forearms from 10 fresh cadavers: age of 20 forearms ranged from 58–82 years (average 73.8 years); fresh cadavers were 4 male and 6 female; and forearms were 10 right and 10 left. The incision for Mini-CTS was 15–18 mm (average 16.2 mm). Transverse carpal ligaments were 26–36 mm (average 31 mm). All Mini-CTS of carpal tunnel release were complete with no median nerve injury and no recurrent branch of median nerve injury (Table 1). The recurrent branches of the median nerve, 13 were type A (65% in the extraligamentous type), 6 were type B (30% in the subligamentous branching type), and 1 were type C (5% in the transligamentous type) (Table 2). This technique was complete release TCL in all forearms.

4. Discussion

The new minimally invasive carpal tunnel release technique, the author's technique, using MIS-CTS kits, and enhanced visualization, offered a promising result in all 20 cadavers with complete release of TCL and no nerve or vascular injury. The modified minimally invasive technique using visual enhancer could improve the visualization for surgery. This technique can avoid incisions on the touching zone of

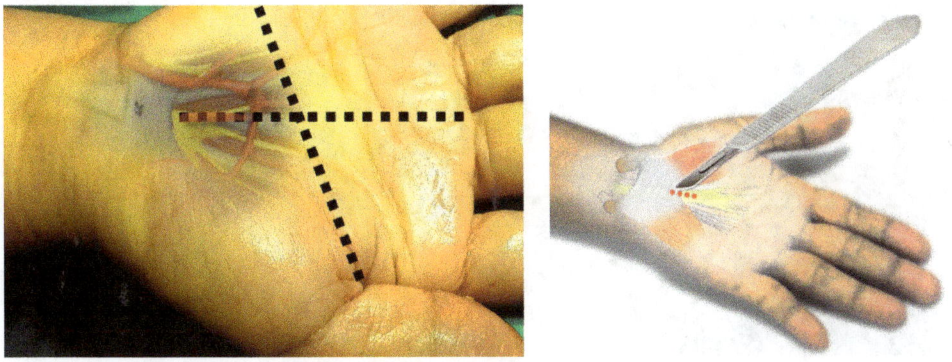

(a) (b)

FIGURE 3: The first step for the author's surgical technique using MIS-CTS kits.

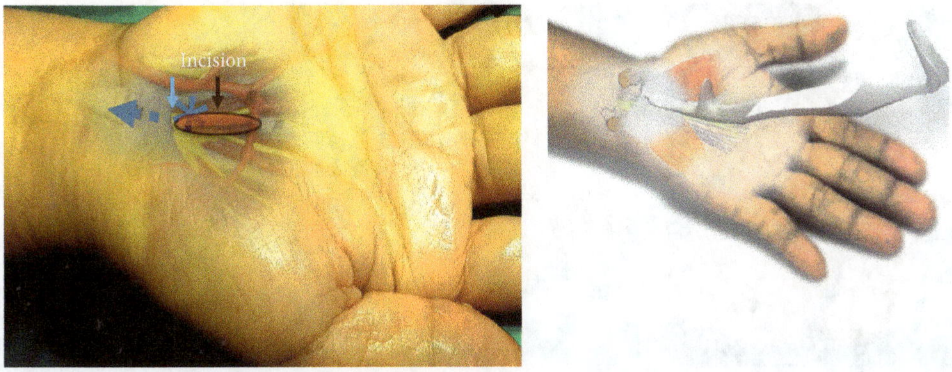

(a) (b)

FIGURE 4: The second step for the author's surgical technique using MIS-CTS kits.

the hand, 2–2.5 cm from the wrist crease, which is a sensitive area for touching and bending. The touching zones are composed of the palmar cutaneous branches of the median nerve, which lie superficial to the transverse carpal ligament [28, 30–33]. Palmar area operative scar may be related to the cause of chronic persistent pain, pillar pain, and slow return to work [14, 34–37]. Currently, the minimally invasive technique of carpal tunnel release is popular for patients due to its benefits and satisfaction.

In the previous study, the minimal invasive surgery of 1.5–1.8 cm skin incision was performed with the visual enhancer [22]. It showed significantly better maximal visual length compared with the Senn retractor (47.7 (8.1) mm vs. 39.2 (6.5) mm). For careful attention of safety, the author's approach by the distal approach can gain benefit to observe directly in the superficial palmar vascular arch and recurrence branch of the median nerve. Also, when the TCL cutting blade is pushed straight from the distal to the proximal end of TCL, it can cut the TCL all at once.

In contrast, the endoscopic technique needs to cut TCL many times because the scalpel is designed to cut by layers from the bottom to the top. Sometimes, surgeons may have difficultly determining the other fascia from TCL when looking from the bottom of the endoscope view [30, 38]. The brachial fascia look like TCL, and it also continues from TCL.

The author observed that the TCL cutting blade offered the promising result of complete detachment, and the smooth cutting edge did not fray any remnants. The author believes that the smooth cutting edge, without fraying remnants of TCL and both edges, can reduce the risk of recurrence. Usually, TCL requires many attempted cuts, such as using the scissors or the endoscope, which may risk fraying remnants with the rough edge of TCL. The author's technique using a scalpel is more effective. However, more research is required in order to determine the risks of recurrence, thus improving patient outcome. Because the lower tip is slim and short, pressure in the carpal tunnel is reduced. The concept of less pressure with a slim and short tip may be the right way to reduce nerve injury while inserting equipment; this aspect needs to be studied further. Most advice states not to insert an endoscope if there is severe compression or the tunnel is really tight. Because of a long incision of standard open CTS release, the complications and sequelae are mainly wound problems, scar pain, wound dehiscence, and slow return to work [9, 13, 31, 32]. The minimally invasive technique was introduced for improving wound complication.

Minimally endoscopic carpal tunnel release is used to minimize wound problems. The endoscopic technique can approach from either portal 2 or portal 1 and makes an impressive minimal skin incision of 1.5 cm [16, 18, 33, 39].

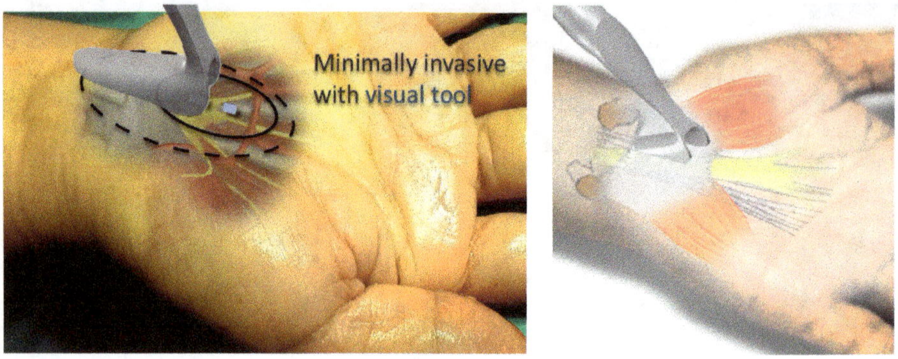

(a) (b)

FIGURE 5: The third step for the author's surgical technique using MIS-CTS kits.

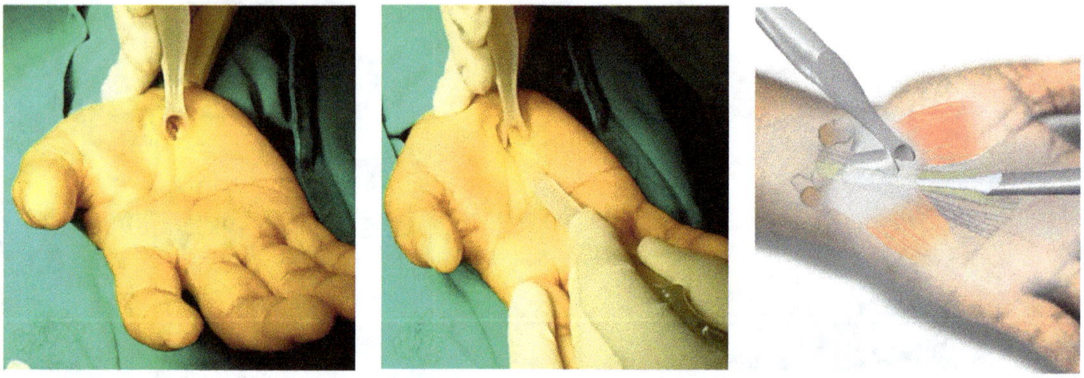

(a) (b) (c)

FIGURE 6: The fourth step for the author's surgical technique using MIS-CTS kits.

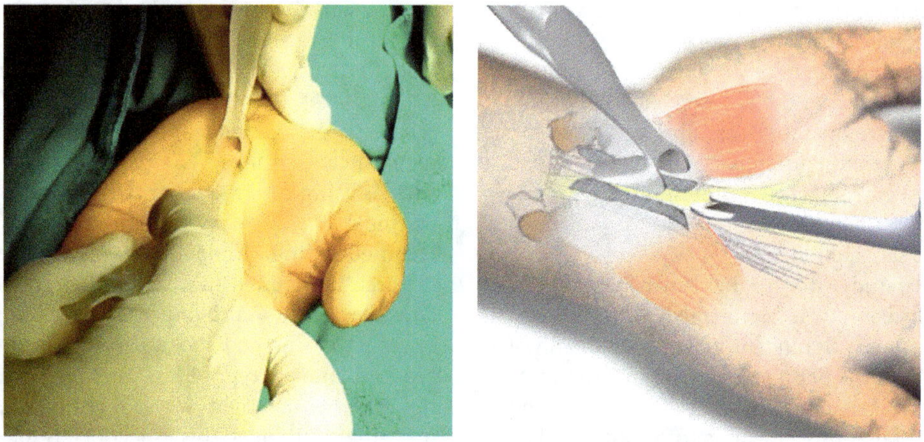

(a) (b)

FIGURE 7: The fifth step for the author's surgical technique using MIS-CTS kits.

The meta-analysis of randomized controlled trials in the endoscopic versus open carpal tunnel release for idiopathic carpal tunnel syndrome significantly reduced postoperative hand pain, it increased the possibility of reversible postoperative nerve injury in patients with idiopathic CTS but statistical difference in the overall complication rate, subjective satisfaction, the time to return to work, postoperative grip and pinch strength, and operative time. However, the endoscope is an imaging and IT technology tool that needs special training with a longer learning curve [40]. Many studies found that transient nerve problems may occur during operations, especially inserting dilators or metallic equipment in the pressured carpal tunnel. The endoscope is not a proper device to use in severe compression. Once the

TABLE 1: The results of carpal tunnel released by the MIS-CTS kits.

Sex	Cadaveric forearm (N)	Average age (years)	Average incision (mm)	Type of release (complete/ incomplete)	Average TCL length (mm)	Median nerve injury (%)	Recurrent branch of median nerve injury (%)
Male	Left (4) Right (4)	67	16	Complete (100%)	32.5	0	0
Female	Left (6) Right (6)	78	16.63	Complete (100%)	30	0	0
Total	20	73	16.2	Complete (100%)	31	0	0

TABLE 2: Type of recurrent branches of the median nerve.

Type	N (%)
Type A (extraligamentous type)	13 (65)
Type B (subligamentous branching type)	6 (30)
Type C (transligamentous type)	1 (5)

surgeon finds the obstacle during insertion of the tool, the surgeon must stop and convert to open carpal tunnel surgery because the median nerve may be damaged or torn.

The Indiana tome is a minimally invasive carpal tunnel surgery that uses local anesthesia and approaches the median nerve from the palm using a special scalpel to cut the TCL [41, 42]. The Indiana tome simplified carpal tunnel surgery. It transformed carpal tunnel surgery to a faster, same day procedure. It seems the Indiana tome and other carpal tunnel tools, such as the Safeguard and Knight light, offer promising results, including complete TCL dividing, short incision, short operative time, and early return to work. However, the literature review highlights some nerve problems that can occur while using this equipment, even though some new developments have reduced the size of equipment [41, 43, 44]. We have developed both a new equipment and a new technique to avoid using the cannula and dilator, which may increase pressure on the carpal tunnel. We believe that minimal insertion in high-pressured carpal tunnel will reduce the risk of transient neuropathy; however, further clinical studies are required. The AAOS published recommendations for CTS: visualization and completely dividing TCL are the major roles of CTS [45]. Authors also believe the same important points. Currently, we are developing a visualization tube for improving visualization and a specific TCL knife for complete release. It is possible to improve the technique and the tool. This technique and the tool can perform the minimally invasive technique [22, 23]. It offers a simplified technique with good outcomes of improved visualization and complete release. For the benefit of patients, it should reduce operative pain, touching scar pain, wound complication, and transient neuropathy and offer an early return to work. For the benefit of surgeons, the distal incision made using the special visual enhancer should improve visualization and improve safety while preventing injury of the median nerve, the ulnar-median nerve palmar communicating branch, and the superficial palmar arch. For the benefit of the healthcare system: it may reduce the currently critically high costs of surgery. In 2002, Martin reported that CTS cost 4 billion dollars annually. In 2003, the increasing cost of healthcare is 12%. The healthcare system could save from lower costs for equipment, minimal equipment usage, shortened operative service costs, no anesthetic team, one surgeon, and one nurse.

The author's technique and the novel tool can improve effectiveness from the original standard of open release of CTS with both practical benefits (simple to use, enhanced visualization, complete cut) and productivity benefits (MIS, save time, save cost, and quick return to work). In the current era of high-cost healthcare, the author hopes that author's method will provide affordability for more patients to receive quality service. If any surgical technique and equipment is developed with the same concept of value, the healthcare costs will be reduced for patients, including health insurance and government support. This is the only cadaveric study which proves the concept. However, the author believes that a clinical study is important for the next stage.

5. Conclusion

This study found that the author's device (MIS-CTS kits) with the author's technique was effective and safe for TCL completely release in terms of minimally invasive open carpal tunnel surgery.

Abbreviations

TCL: Transverse carpal ligament
CTS: Carpal tunnel syndrome
OCTR: Open carpal tunnel release
ECTR: Endoscopic carpal tunnel release
MIS-CTS kits: Minimally invasive surgery for carpal tunnel syndrome kits.

Authors' Contributions

Wongthawat Liawrungrueang carried out the experimental study, performed the statistical analysis, and drafted the manuscript. Wongthawat Liawrungrueang and Sunton

Wongsiri participated in surgery by the author's technique with MIS-CTS kits. All authors read and approved the final manuscript.

Acknowledgments

This research article was presented by W. Liawrungrueang at the Conference: JOA2019, the 92nd Annual Meeting of the Japanese Orthopaedic Association "The Power of Orthopeadics as the Power of Japan" JOA Congress 2019 Travel Award). The authors thank the Department of Orthopedic Surgery, Faculty of Medicine, Prince of Songkla University, for their support. This study was supported by the Faculty of Medicine, Prince of Songkla University research fund.

References

[1] I. Atroshi, C. Gummesson, R. Johnsson, and A. Sprinchorn, "Symptoms, disability, and quality of life in patients with carpal tunnel syndrome," *The Journal of Hand Surgery (American Volume)*, vol. 24, no. 2, pp. 398–404, 1999.

[2] A. Zyluk and P. Puchalski, "Natural history of carpal tunnel syndrome-a review," *Chirurgia Narzadów Ruchu i Ortopedia Polska*, vol. 75, no. 4, pp. 261–266, 2010.

[3] I. Atroshi, C. Gummesson, R. Johnsson, E. Ornstein, J. Ranstam, and I. Rosén, "Prevalence of carpal tunnel syndrome in a general population," *The Journal of the American Medical Association*, vol. 282, no. 2, pp. 153–158, 1999.

[4] L. E. Wessel, D. T. Fufa, M. I. Boyer, and R. P. Calfee, "Epidemiology of carpal tunnel syndrome in patients with single versus multiple trigger digits," *The Journal of Hand Surgery*, vol. 38, no. 1, pp. 49–55, 2013.

[5] L. Padua, D. Coraci, C. Erra et al., "Carpal tunnel syndrome: clinical features, diagnosis, and management," *The Lancet Neurology*, vol. 15, no. 12, pp. 1273–1284, 2016.

[6] M. Osterman, A. M. Ilyas, and J. L. Matzon, "Carpal tunnel syndrome in pregnancy," *Orthopedic Clinics of North America*, vol. 43, no. 4, pp. 515–520, 2012.

[7] G. A. Demopulos and J. R. Urbaniak, "Carpal tunnel release: comparing the options," *Journal of Musculoskeletal Medicine*, vol. 13, pp. 51–58, 1996.

[8] T. A. Tran and R. M. Szabo, "Surgical release of the carpal tunnel," in *Operative Dictations in Plastic and Reconstructive Surgery*, pp. 489–491, Springer, Berlin, Germany, 2017.

[9] A. W. Siegmeth and J. A. Hopkinson-Woolley, "Standard open decompression in carpal tunnel syndrome compared with a modified open technique preserving the superficial skin nerves: a prospective randomized study," *The Journal of Hand Surgery*, vol. 31, no. 9, pp. 1483–1489, 2006.

[10] J. H. J. English and D. P. Gwynne-Jones, "Incidence of carpal tunnel syndrome requiring surgical decompression: a 10.5-year review of 2,309 patients," *The Journal of Hand Surgery*, vol. 40, no. 12, pp. 2427–2434, 2015.

[11] M. Fajardo, S. H. Kim, and R. M. Szabo, "Incidence of carpal tunnel release: trends and implications within the United States ambulatory care setting," *The Journal of Hand Surgery*, vol. 37, no. 8, pp. 1599–1605, 2012.

[12] A. A. M. Gerritsen, B. M. J. Uitdehaag, D. Van Geldere, R. J. P. M. Scholten, H. C. W. De Vet, and L. M. Bouter, "Systematic review of randomized clinical trials of surgical treatment for carpal tunnel syndrome," *British Journal of Surgery*, vol. 88, no. 10, pp. 1285–1295, 2001.

[13] M. Tarallo, P. Fino, V. Sorvillo, P. Parisi, and N. Scuderi, "Comparative analysis between minimal access versus traditional accesses in carpal tunnel syndrome: a perspective randomised study," *Journal of Plastic, Reconstructive & Aesthetic Surgery*, vol. 67, no. 2, pp. 237–243, 2014.

[14] E. M. Mack, N. J. Callinan, M. Reams, D. C. Bohn, and T. L. Chmielewski, "Patient-reported outcomes after open carpal tunnel release using a standard protocol with 1 hand therapy visit," *Journal of Hand Therapy*, vol. 30, no. 1, pp. 58–64, 2017.

[15] S. Aroori and R. A. J. Spence, "Carpal tunnel syndrome," *The Ulster Medical Journal*, vol. 77, no. 1, pp. 6–17, 2008.

[16] I. Okutsu, S. Ninomiya, Y. Takatori, and Y. Ugawa, "Endoscopic management of carpal tunnel syndrome," *Arthroscopy: The Journal of Arthroscopic & Related Surgery*, vol. 5, no. 1, pp. 11–18, 1989.

[17] J. M. Agee, H. R. McCarroll, and E. R. North, "Endoscopic carpal tunnel release using the single proximal incision technique," *Hand Clinics*, vol. 10, no. 4, pp. 647–659, 1994.

[18] T. B. Hansen and H. G. Majeed, "Endoscopic carpal tunnel release," *Hand Clinics*, vol. 30, no. 1, pp. 47–53, 2014.

[19] J. C. Y. Chow and M. E. Hantes, "Endoscopic carpal tunnel release: thirteen years' experience with the chow technique," *The Journal of Hand Surgery*, vol. 27, no. 6, pp. 1011–1018, 2002.

[20] Y. Iwase, T. Ikai, A. Hara, K. Mori, and K. Kusonose, "Carpal tunnel release through a small incision using a special knife guide," *Techniques in Hand and Upper Extremity Surgery*, vol. 6, no. 4, pp. 193–195, 2002.

[21] M. K. Abouzahr, M. C. Patsis, and D. T. W. Chiu, "Carpal tunnel release using limited direct vision," *Plastic and Reconstructive Surgery*, vol. 95, no. 3, pp. 534–538, 1995.

[22] S. Wongsiri, P. Suwanno, B. Tangtrakulwanich, V. Yuenyongviwat, and E. Wongsiri, "A new tool for mini-open carpal tunnel release—the PSU retractor," *BMC Musculoskeletal Disorders*, vol. 9, no. 1, p. 126, 2008.

[23] S. Wongsiri, "The new wave of carpal tunnel syndrome (CTS) surgery," *The Bangkok Medical Journal*, vol. 6, no. 1, pp. 80–85, 2013.

[24] D. H. Palmer and L. P. Hanrahan, "Social and economic costs of carpal tunnel surgery," *Instructional Course Lectures*, vol. 44, no. 44, pp. 167–172, 1995.

[25] A. Thoma, V. H. Wong, S. Sprague, and E. Duku, "A cost-utility analysis of open and endoscopic carpal tunnel release," *Canadian Journal of Plastic Surgery*, vol. 14, no. 1, pp. 15–20, 2006.

[26] M. Chammas, "Carpal tunnel syndrome," *Chirurgie de la Main*, vol. 33, no. 2, pp. 75–94, 2014.

[27] J. D. Beck, J. H. Deegan, D. Rhoades, and J. C. Klena, "Results of endoscopic carpal tunnel release relative to surgeon experience with the agee technique," *The Journal of Hand Surgery*, vol. 36, no. 1, pp. 61–64, 2011.

[28] J. M. R. Serra, J. R. Benito, and J. Monner, "Carpal tunnel release with short incision," *Plastic and Reconstructive Surgery*, vol. 99, no. 1, pp. 129–135, 1997.

[29] S. Wongsiri, "Keyhole surgery of CTS using novel tool MiniSure," *BMC Proceedings*, vol. 9, no. S3, p. A79, 2015.

[30] S. Uchiyama, K. Nakamura, T. Itsubo et al., "Technical difficulties and their prediction in 2-portal endoscopic carpal tunnel release for idiopathic carpal tunnel syndrome," *Arthroscopy: The Journal of Arthroscopic & Related Surgery*, vol. 29, no. 5, pp. 860–869, 2013.

[31] P.-T. Kim, H.-J. Lee, T.-G. Kim, and I.-H. Jeon, "Current approaches for carpal tunnel syndrome," *Clinics in Orthopedic Surgery*, vol. 6, no. 3, pp. 253–257, 2014.

[32] S. Suppaphol, P. Worathanarat, V. Kawinwongkovit, and P. Pittayawutwinit, "The comparison between limited open carpal tunnel release using direct vision and tunneling technique and standard open carpal tunnel release : a randomized controlled trial study," *Journal of the Medical Association of Thailand*, vol. 95, pp. 532–536, 2012.

[33] M. A. Mirza, E. T. King, and S. Tanveer, "Palmar uniportal extrabursal endoscopic carpal tunnel release," *Arthroscopy: The Journal of Arthroscopic & Related Surgery*, vol. 11, no. 1, pp. 82–90, 1995.

[34] P. S.-H. Yung, L.-K. Hung, C. W.-C. Tong, and P.-C. Ho, "Carpal tunnel release with a limited palmar incision: clinical results and pillar pain at 18 months follow-up," *Hand Surgery*, vol. 10, no. 1, pp. 29–35, 2005.

[35] S. Avci and U. Sayli, "Carpal tunnel release using a short palmar incision and a new knife," *Journal of Hand Surgery*, vol. 25, no. 4, pp. 357–360, 2000.

[36] P. Cellocco, C. Rossi, S. El Boustany, G. L. Di Tanna, and G. Costanzo, "Minimally invasive carpal tunnel release," *Orthopedic Clinics of North America*, vol. 40, no. 4, pp. 441–448, 2009.

[37] K. S. Ludlow, J. L. Merla, J. A. Cox, and L. N. Hurst, "Pillar pain as a postoperative complication of carpal tunnel release," *Journal of Hand Therapy*, vol. 10, no. 4, pp. 277–282, 1997.

[38] T. Y. Law, S. Rosas, Z. S. Hubbard, L. O. Chieng, and H. W. Chim, "Trends in open and endoscopic carpal tunnel release utilization in the Medicare patient population," *Journal of Surgical Research*, vol. 214, pp. 9–13, 2017.

[39] L. S. Benson, A. A. Bare, D. J. Nagle, V. S. Harder, C. S. Williams, and J. L. Visotsky, "Complications of endoscopic and open carpal tunnel release," *Arthroscopy*, vol. 22, no. 9, pp. 924–924.e2, 2006.

[40] D. Zuo, Z. Zhou, H. Wang et al., "Endoscopic versus open carpal tunnel release for idiopathic carpal tunnel syndrome: a meta-analysis of randomized controlled trials," *Journal of Orthopaedic Surgery and Research*, vol. 10, no. 1, p. 12, 2015.

[41] W. P. A. Lee, B. M. Schipper, and R. J. Goitz, "13-Year experience of carpal tunnel release using the Indiana tome technique," *The Journal of Hand Surgery*, vol. 33, no. 7, pp. 1052–1056, 2008.

[42] C. B. Chapman, S. Ristic, and M. P. Rosenwasser, "Complete median nerve transection as a complication of carpal tunnel release with a carpal tunnel tome," *American Journal of Orthopedics*, vol. 30, no. 8, pp. 652-653, 2001.

[43] T. B. Hughes and M. Baratz, "Limited open carpal tunnel syndrome using the safeguard system," *Techniques in Orthopaedics*, vol. 21, no. 1, pp. 12–18, 2006.

[44] T. L. Atik, B. Smith, and M. E. Baratz, "Risk of neurovascular injury with limited-open carpal tunnel release: defining the "safe-zone"," *Journal of Hand Surgery*, vol. 26, no. 5, pp. 484–487, 2001.

[45] M. W. Keith, V. Masear, P. C. Amadio et al., "Treatment of carpal tunnel syndrome," *Journal of the American Academy of Orthopaedic Surgeons*, vol. 17, no. 6, pp. 397–405, 2008.

Sensory Disturbance of the Lower Extremity after Sural Artery Flap Elevation

Kaoru Tada, Seigo Suganuma, Mika Nakada, Masashi Matsuta, Atsuro Murai, and Hiroyuki Tsuchiya

Department of Orthopaedic Surgery, Graduate School of Medical Science, Kanazawa University, 13-1 Takaramachi, Kanazawa 920-8641, Japan

Correspondence should be addressed to Kaoru Tada; tdkr@med.kanazawa-u.ac.jp

Academic Editor: Paulo Adriano Schwingel

Purpose. Elevation of the sural artery flap with the sural nerve is associated with donor-site morbidities, such as postoperative sensory disturbance of the lower extremity. We evaluated the sensory disturbance of the lower extremity after elevation of the sural artery flap. *Methods.* This study included 7 patients who underwent surgery using the sural artery flap. The sensory disturbances immediately after surgery and at present were evaluated on a 10-point scale. The influences of surgery on activities of daily living and patient satisfaction were also evaluated. *Results.* The sensory disturbance was 4.48 immediately after surgery and 2.24 presently, and the difference between the timepoints was not statistically significant. The influence of surgery on activities of daily living was 2.30, and the patient satisfaction was 7.90. *Conclusion.* It may be necessary to consider the sural artery flap, which does not include the sural nerve, to avoid unnecessary complications. When it is unavoidable to use the sural artery flap, including the sural nerve, it is important to thoroughly inform patients beforehand about the postsurgery sensory disturbance in the lower extremities.

1. Introduction

The sural artery flap is generally elevated with the sural nerve and its accompanying artery, as well as the lesser saphenous vein and its accompanying artery. Since this flap is a pedicled flap that does not require vascular anastomosis and is easy to elevate, it is widely used to treat soft tissue defects in the lower limbs and feet; to date, there are numerous studies that report the use of the sural artery flap [1–7]. However, because the sural artery flap includes the sural nerve, sensory disturbance of the lower extremity (especially on the lateral part of the foot) often occurs postoperatively. Many studies on the sural artery flap focus on the survival rate of the flap, and there are only a few studies that have evaluated the extent and course of sensory disturbance of the lower extremity [8]. In recent reviews, sensory disturbance due to sacrifice of the sural nerve has not been considered as a major complication [3, 7].

In this case report, we investigated the sensory disturbance of the lower extremity in patients who were treated with the sural artery flap for soft tissue defects.

2. Methods

2.1. Patients. Between 2008 and 2018, 17 patients underwent reconstruction for soft tissue defects of the lower extremity in our hospital using the sural artery flap. 10 of 17 patients had a different address and could not be located. Of the remaining 7 patients (5 males and 2 females) who agreed to participate in the study were included and completed the questionnaire. In all patients, we elevated the sural artery flap, which included the sural nerve and its accompanying artery, as well as the small saphenous vein and its accompanying artery.

2.2. Evaluations. Evaluations were conducted using a questionnaire with a 10-point scale. Evaluation items included the sensory disturbance of the lower extremity (0 = no disturbance, 10 = extreme disturbance) immediately after surgery and at present, the current influence of surgery on activities of daily living (ADL) (0 = no trouble, 10 = troubling), and satisfaction with the reconstruction surgery (0 = unsatisfied, 10 = completely satisfied).

2.3. Statistical Analyses. Patient characteristics, including age and time since surgery, and questionnaire data, including the sensory disturbance and all other evaluations, were expressed as median (interquartile range (25th and 75th percentile)). The sensory disturbance between the two timepoints was compared using the Wilcoxon signed-rank test. $P < 0.05$ was considered statistically significant, and all P values were two-tailed. Statistical analyses were performed using SPSS software, version 22.0 (IBM Corp, NY, US).

2.4. Ethical Considerations. This retrospective research was approved by the institutional review board of our institution. All procedures were conducted in accordance with the ethical standards of the Committee on Human Experimentation in our institution and the Helsinki Declaration of 1975. Written informed consent was obtained from each patient prior to inclusion in the study.

3. Results

The median age at the time of surgery was 47.0 (21.5, 63.5) years, and the median time since surgery was 7.0 (5.5, 8.5) years. Soft tissue defects occurred due to a tumor in 4 cases and trauma in 3 cases. The site of the soft tissue defect was the knee joint in 1 patient, the lower leg in 2 patients, the medial condyle in 3 patients, and the heel in 1 patient. 5 flaps were distally based, while 2 were proximally based.

The sensory disturbance was 4.48 (2.85, 6.46) immediately after surgery and is 2.24 (1.33, 4.61) presently. Symptoms tended to improve, but the difference between the timepoints was not statistically significant ($P = 0.17$). The influence of surgery on ADL was 2.30 (1.03, 3.34), while the patient satisfaction with reconstruction surgery was 7.90 (6.01, 9.05). In one case where a proximally based flap was used, hyperesthesia at the tip of the flap and radiation pain to the lower extremity occurred, which was thought to be due to stump neuroma.

4. Discussion

As a result of this study, sensory disturbance after using a sural artery flap was proven to be mild but remained, and no significant improvement was observed even 7 years after the surgery. The sural artery flap does not necessarily need to include the sural nerve, so it may be necessary to consider the sural artery flap, which does not include the sural nerve, to avoid unnecessary complications.

Since the development of the sural artery flap, it remains debatable whether the sural nerve should be included in the flap. Donski et al. developed the prototype of the sural artery flap, defining it as a "distally based fasciocutaneous flap from the sural region," and reporting that the sural nerve should not be included in the flap, if possible [9]. In addition, Masquelet et al. defined the sural artery flap as a "skin island flap supplied by the vascular axis of the sensitive superficial nerves." They indicated that the flap includes the sural nerve and reported that one problem of the flap was that it sacrificed the sensory nerve [10]. Later, the results of an anatomical study by Aoki et al. suggested that the accompanying artery around the sural nerve seems to have the most significant impact on flap survival and that the sural nerve has fewer intrinsic vessels than its accompanying artery [11]. Their sural artery flap included the accompanying artery, which was detached from the sural nerve, and did not include the sural nerve itself. However, detachment of the sural nerve and its accompanying artery is complicated and time-consuming, especially in the proximal part of the lower leg where the nerve and artery run below the deep fascia [2, 12]. Therefore, many studies have selected the sural artery flap that includes the sural nerve [1, 2, 4–6]. Donor-site morbidities caused by sacrifice of the sural nerve have rarely been considered in previous studies. Cheema et al. reported that "the loss of sensation of the foot has not been a significant clinical problem in our patients" [1].

However, the sensory disturbance after using a sural artery flap was proven to be mild but remained in this study. Therefore, flap elevation without inclusion of the sural nerve should be carefully considered so that it does not affect flap survival. The methods of Donski and Fogdestam [9] and the method of Nakajima et al. [13], which involves the veno-accompanying artery fasciocutaneous flap and uses the accompanying artery of the lesser saphenous vein as a feeding vessel without including the sural nerve and its accompanying artery, are considered effective. Furthermore, the sural nerve splitting method recently reported by Kim et al. [8], which preserves the medial sural cutaneous nerve, is also a reasonable method. If including the sural nerve is unavoidable, the nerve should be sharply dissected (so that a stump neuroma will not form) and the nerve stump should be embedded in the adipose tissue.

Because the patients who were treated with the sural artery flap originally had tumors and trauma of the lower extremity, it is considered that the surgery was invasive. However, unlike pain, sensory disturbance is not a symptom caused by surgical invasion itself, so it is thought that the sacrifice of the sural nerve is the main cause of sensory disturbance.

We believe that the results were partially affected by insufficient communication about sensory disturbance prior to surgery. When using the sural nerve autograft for reconstruction of the peripheral nerve defect, doctors commonly inform patients of the expectations regarding recovery and sensory disturbance, which is due to the sacrifice of the healthy sural nerve [14]. On the other hand, when using the sural artery flap for soft tissue defects in the lower extremity, explanations about flap survival and functional prognosis of the lower extremity are prioritized, and information regarding sensory disturbance of the lower extremity after flap elevation may be insufficient. As a result, sensory disturbance is often considered as an unexpected complication by these patients leading to poor outcome. In particular, a recent systematic review indicated that preoperative patient education reduced postoperative patient complaints [15]. In order to reduce the complaints after elevation of the sural artery flap, the best thing is to not include the sural nerve in the flap. However, if including the sural nerve is unavoidable, it is important to share sufficient information beforehand regarding the postsurgery sensory disturbance in the lower extremities with the patients.

The limitations of this study include the small sample size and the presence of sampling and recall biases, especially for the sensory disturbance evaluated immediately after surgery. Therefore, caution is needed when interpreting our results. Also, because this study is designed as a questionnaire survey, it was not possible to evaluate the patients using the Semmes–Weinstein monofilament test or the two-point discrimination test. In future, we would like to compare these results with the results of the sural artery flap that does not include the sural nerve.

5. Conclusions

The sensory disturbance after using a sural artery flap was proven to be mild but remained, and no significant improvement was observed even 7 years after the surgery. It may be necessary to consider the sural artery flap, which does not include the sural nerve, to avoid unnecessary complications. When it is unavoidable to use the sural artery flap, including the sural nerve, it is important to thoroughly inform patients beforehand about the postsurgery sensory disturbance in the lower extremities.

References

[1] T. A. Cheema, E. S. Saleh, and A. F. De Carvalho, "The distally based sural artery flap for ankle and foot coverage," *The Journal of Foot and Ankle Surgery*, vol. 46, no. 1, pp. 40–47, 2007.

[2] S. J. Cheon, I. B. Kim, W. R. Park, and H. T. Kim, "The proximally-based sural artery flap for coverage of soft tissue defects around the knee and on the proximal third and middle third of the lower leg," *Acta Orthopaedica*, vol. 79, no. 3, pp. 370–375, 2008.

[3] C. De Blacam, S. Colakoglu, A. A. Ogunleye et al., "Risk factors associated with complications in lower-extremity reconstruction with the distally based sural flap: a systematic review and pooled analysis," *Journal of Plastic, Reconstructive & Aesthetic Surgery*, vol. 67, no. 5, pp. 607–616, 2014.

[4] S.-M. Chang, X. H. Li, and Y. D. Gu, "Distally based perforator sural flaps for foot and ankle reconstruction," *World Journal of Orthopedics*, vol. 6, no. 3, pp. 322–330, 2015.

[5] C. G. Finkemeier and R. Neiman, "Reverse sural artery pedicle flap," *Journal of Orthopaedic Trauma*, vol. 30, pp. S41–S42, 2016.

[6] H. J. Roberts and G. L. DeSilva, "Can sural fasciocutaneous flaps Be effective in patients older than 65?" *Clinical Orthopaedics & Related Research*, vol. 478, no. 4, pp. 734–738, 2020.

[7] D. A. Daar, S. A. Abdou, J. A. David, D. J. Kirby, S. C. Wilson, and P. B. Saadeh, "Revisiting the reverse sural artery flap in distal lower extremity reconstruction," *Annals of Plastic Surgery*, vol. 84, no. 4, pp. 463–470, 2020.

[8] H. Kim, J. Hu, H. Chang, and B. J. Kim, "Sural nerve splitting in reverse sural artery perforator flap: anatomical study in 40 cadaver legs," *Plastic and Reconstructive Surgery*, vol. 140, no. 5, pp. 1024–1032, 2017.

[9] P. K. Donski and I. Fogdestam, "Distally based fasciocutaneous flap from the sural region," *Scandinavian Journal of Plastic and Reconstructive Surgery*, vol. 17, no. 3, pp. 191–196, 1983.

[10] A. C. Masquelet, M. C. Romana, and G. Wolf, "Skin island flaps supplied by the vascular axis of the sensitive superficial nerves," *Plastic and Reconstructive Surgery*, vol. 89, no. 6, pp. 1115–1121, 1992.

[11] S. Aoki, K. Tanuma, I. Iwakiri et al., "Clinical and vascular anatomical study of distally based sural flap," *Annals of Plastic Surgery*, vol. 61, no. 1, pp. 73–78, 2008.

[12] M. M. Al-Qattan, "A modified technique for harvesting the reverse sural artery flap from the upper part of the leg: inclusion of a gastrocnemius muscle ???Cuff??? around the sural pedicle," *Annals of Plastic Surgery*, vol. 47, no. 3, pp. 269–278, 2001.

[13] H. Nakajima, N. Imanishi, S. Fukuzumi et al., "Accompanying arteries of the lesser saphenous vein and sural nerve: anatomic study and its clinical applications," *Plastic and Reconstructive Surgery*, vol. 103, no. 1, pp. 104–120, 1999.

[14] F. F. A. IJpma, J.-P. A. Nicolai, and M. F. Meek, "Sural nerve donor-site morbidity," *Annals of Plastic Surgery*, vol. 57, no. 4, pp. 391–395, 2006.

[15] C. Szeverenyi, Z. Kekecs, A. Johnson, G. Elkins, Z. Csernatony, and K. Varga, "The use of adjunct psychosocial interventions can decrease postoperative pain and improve the quality of clinical care in orthopedic surgery: a systematic review and meta-analysis of randomized controlled trials," *The Journal of Pain*, vol. 19, no. 11, pp. 1231–1252, 2018.

32

Posterior Occipitocervical Fusion for Unstable Upper Cervical Trauma in Old and Elderly Population, Although Decreases Upper Cervical Rotation, Does Not Significantly Increase Neck Disability Index

Panagiotis Korovessis, Vasileios Syrimpeis, Evangelia Mpountogianni, Ioannis Papaioannou, and Vasileios Tsekouras

Orthopaedics Department, General Hospital of Patras, Patras 26335, Greece

Correspondence should be addressed to Panagiotis Korovessis; korovess@otenet.gr

Academic Editor: Benjamin Blondel

Background. Despite the research progress in the thoraco-lumbo-pelvic balance, cervical spine balance has only recently gained increasing interest. To our knowledge, there is a lack of research regarding sagittal occipitocervical spine balance restoration following posterior occipitocervical fusion (POCF). *Purpose.* The primary outcome measure is the evaluation of sagittal cervical alignment roentgenographic parameters and the secondary is the functional outcome (NDI), following POCF for upper (C1 & C2) cervical trauma (UCT) in coexistence with upper cervical spine degeneration. *Patients and Methods.* Twenty old and elderly patients aged 62 ± 12 years with evident upper cervical degeneration, who received POCF for upper C1 & C2 unstable cervical spine injuries, were included. C2-C7 lordosis, C2-C7 SVA, spinocranial angle (SCA), T1-slope, neck tilt (NT), thorax inlet angle (TIA), cervical tilt (CT), cranial tilt (CrT), and C0-C1 angle were measured. The subfusion angle was used to study the behavior of the unfused cervical segments below fusion. The Neck Disability Index (NDI) was used for the functional outcome evaluation. 29 age-matched individuals were used as controls for radiographic analysis and self-reported functional status comparison. *Results.* The roentgenographic data were measured 3 and 39 ± 12 months postoperatively. Twelve patients showed no disability, and eight showed mild disability. Postoperatively, the patients stood with less C2-C7 lordosis, SCA, and CT ($P < 0.02$) but with higher NT ($P < 0.02$) in comparison to the controls. The patient's neck disability (NDI) was increasing as TIA increases ($P = 0.023$). Subfusion angle seems to adapt to C2-C7 lordosis ($P < 0.0033$) and C0-C2 angle ($P < 0.003$) without any changes till the last evaluation. *Conclusions.* POCF sufficiently restored occipitocervical sagittal balance along with functional outcome similar to controls in adult and elderly individuals with evident upper cervical degeneration. We do not recommend POCF for young active individuals without occipitocervical pathology, but in contrary, we recommend the removal of the spinocranial connection hardware after cervical fusion is completed.

1. Introduction

Posterior occipitocervical fusion (POCF) has been an effective surgical procedure for the treatment of occipitocervical and upper cervical instability (UCI) for a variety of pathologies (trauma, degeneration, etc.) [1–13]. POCF that is a demanding surgery, acts mechanically as a tension band required to promote immediately stability and subsequently permanent cervical fusion [14–16]. However, POCF restricts about 50% of the axial rotation and flexion-extension of the head and this is a significant disadvantage of this technique in young individuals without cervical degenerative disease [14–16]. POCF in inadequate sagittal position of the cervical spine, occipitocervical junction, and head may be associated with functional complications (loss/reduction of horizontal gaze, dysphagia, respiratory disturbance, and disability)

[12, 17–24]. In contrary, POCF in the elderly with often significant degeneration of the upper cervical spine and occipitocervical junction is often beneficial for reducing pain and technical issues such as loss of screw fixation due to osteoporosis, pseudarthrosis, and significant bleeding in C1-C2 fixation [12, 17–24].

There is evidence that several roentgenographic parameters such as C0-C2 angle, T1-slope, C2-C7 SVA, and spinocranial angle (SCA) should be reconstructed with surgery to achieve good functional outcome [18–21].

There is a lack of information regarding the restoration of the occipitocervical spine and the impact of postoperative sagittal occipitocervical alignment in neck disability following UCI and POCF in adult and elderly population.

The primary outcome measure is the roentgenographic sagittal occipitocervical alignment and the secondary outcome measure is the neck disability following POCF for acute upper cervical injury (UCI).

2. Materials and Methods

The authors' institution is the single Level 1 trauma center covering spine trauma in a region of over 1.2 million people. After institutional review board approval was obtained, the authors reviewed the institutional database and patients' files for POCF from 2012 to 2015. Twenty consecutive patients, 16 males and 4 females, suffering from acute UCI who had underwent early successful POCF by one experienced senior orthopedic spine surgeon in this period were recruited for evaluation. POCF surgery was defined as the operation with evident radiological completed fusion and without serious mechanical complications that required reoperation. The patients' age at the time of surgery was averaged, SD 61 ± 12 years, ranging from 43 to 78 years (Table 1).

The inclusion criteria were adult (>40 years) and elderly patients, acute trauma, and symptomatic degeneration of upper cervical or occipitocervical spine. The exclusion criteria were patients with C1-C2 fusion, congenital instability, or previous spinal surgeries. Preoperative imaging included (a) plain roentgenograms and (b) CT/MRI scans. An age-matched control group of 29 consecutive asymptomatic individuals was selected without history of spine injury or operation. The control group was subsequently selected to match in age to the patients' group. The average, SD age of the 29 controls was 63 ± 14 years with a range of 44–76 years. On admission, 2 patients (10%) had incomplete spinal cord injury (ASIA Grades C). The most common indication for POCF was C2 Levine IIa and/or traumatic spondylolisthesis that were diagnosed in 10/20 (50%) patients (Table 1). Only supine preoperative roentgenograms of the cervical spine were available, while standing AP and lateral roentgenograms were used for the final postoperative evaluation. Standing anteroposterior (AP) and lateral roentgenograms of the cervical spine were taken in the age-matched controls.

The cervical trauma AO-classification [25] was used, and the validated national version of the Neck Disability Index (NDI) questionnaire [26] was filled out for all the 20 survived patients at the final evaluation.

2.1. Roentgenographic Study. Sagittal occipitocervical balance was evaluated in the patients with successful POCF and compared to that of the age-matched controls (Figure 1) [27–31] in terms of the following: (1) C0-C2 lordosis (the angle created by McGregor's line and the inferior surface of the axis); (2) C2-C7 lordosis (the angle between the lower plate of C2 and the lower plate of C7 vertebra); (3) spinocranial angle (SCA) (the angle between the C7-slope and the straight line joining the middle of the C7 end plate and the middle of the sella turcica); (4) T1-slope (the angle between an horizontal line and the superior endplate of T1); (5) C2-C7 SVA (the distance from the vertical line from the center of the C2 body and the posterior-superior corner of C7); (6) neck tilt (NT) (the angle formed by the reference vertical line drawn in the upper end of the sternum and a line connecting the center of the T1 upper endplate and the upper end of the sternum); (7) thorax inlet angle (TIA) (the angle formed by a line perpendicular to the superior endplate of T1 and a line connecting the T1 upper endplate and the upper end of the sternum); (8) cervical tilt (CT) (the angle between two lines, both originating from the center of the T1 upper endplate; one is vertical to the T1 upper endplate, and the other passes through the tip of the dens); (9) cranial tilt (CrT) (the angle between two lines, both originating from the center of the T1 upper endplate, with one passing through the dens and the other being a vertical line).

The subfusion angle (SA) (the angle formed by a line perpendicular to the superior endplate of the lowermost instrumented cervical vertebra and a line connecting the C7 upper endplate) was measured in the 3-month follow-up and at the final observation, in order to evaluate the adaptation of the nonfused cervical segments to POCF (Figure 2).

Fifteen randomly selected digital lateral radiographs from patients and controls were blindly measured twice within a one-week interval by two independent orthopedic surgeons. The reproducibility and repeatability of all roentgenographic measurements were evaluated using the kappa values. P values were tested against the significance level of 0.05.

2.2. Statistical Data Analysis. Data were analyzed using SPSS, statistics version 24 (Inc., Chicago, IL, USA). Continuous data were reported as mean ± SD.

The skewness and kurtosis tests were used to test the data frequency.

Levene's test of variance homogeneity was used to assess the equality of variances for each variable calculated for the two groups. The paired t-test was used for the comparison of the same continuous variable change. The bivariate Pearson correlation coefficient (r) was used to correlate different continuous roentgenographic and categorical variables. The categorical variables (gender, age, and NDI score) were graded in two groups: gender (women: 0, men: 1); age groups in controls (≤66 years: 0, >66 years: 1) and age groups in patients (≤61 years: 0, >61 years: 1). The ages of 66 and 61 years old were chosen because they were the average age of controls and patients, respectively. No disability (NDI score:

TABLE 1: Demographic data of 20 patients that received occipitocervical fusion for upper cervical spine injuries.

ID	Gender	Age	Surgery diagnosis	Levels of fusion	Surgical complications	Follow-up in months
1	M	58	C2 D'Alonzotype 2	C0-C4	Superficial infection Surgical debridement	39
2	M	61	C2 Levine IIb C2 traumatic spondylolisthesis	C0-C4	No	31
3	F	75	C2 D'Alonzotype 2	C0-C4	No	52
4	M	49	C2 D'Alonzotype 3	C0-C3	No	25
5	M	51	C2 Levine IIa C2 traumatic spondylolisthesis	C0-C3	No	26
6	F	72	C2 D'Alonzotype 2	C0-C5	No	28
7	F	71	C1 IIIa/AO	C0-C3	No	24
8	M	75	C1 IIIa/AO	C0-C3	No	25
9	M	78	C2 Levine IIa C2 traumatic spondylolisthesis	C0-C4	No	29
10	M	56	C2 Levine II C2 traumatic spondylolisthesis C2 traumatic spondylolisthesis	C0-C4	No	41
11	M	68	C2 Levine II C2 traumatic spondylolisthesis	C0-C5	No	56
12	M	60	C1 IIIa/AO	C0-C3	Superficial infection Surgical debridement	27
13	M	44	C1 IIIb/AO	C0-C7	No	39
14	M	60	C2 Levine IIa C2 traumatic spondylolisthesis	C0-C3	No	47
15	M	38	C2 Levine IIa C2 traumatic spondylolisthesis	C0-C5	No	54
16	F	58	C2 Levine IIa C2 traumatic spondylolisthesis	C0-C4	No	52
17	M	60	C1 IIIa/AO	C0-C4	No	57
18	M	50	C2 Levine IIa C2 traumatic spondylolisthesis	C0-C4	No	49
19	M	75	C2 D'Alonzotype 3	C0-C4	No	53
20	M	69	C2 D'Alonzotype 3	C0-C6	Superficial infection	25

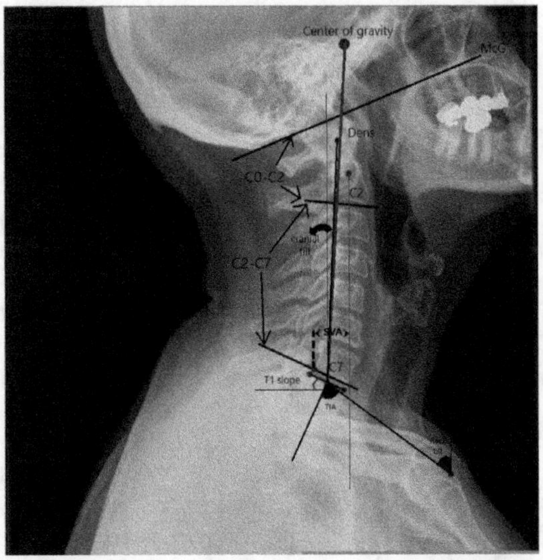

FIGURE 1: Lateral roentgenographic parameters used for sagittal cervical balance study.

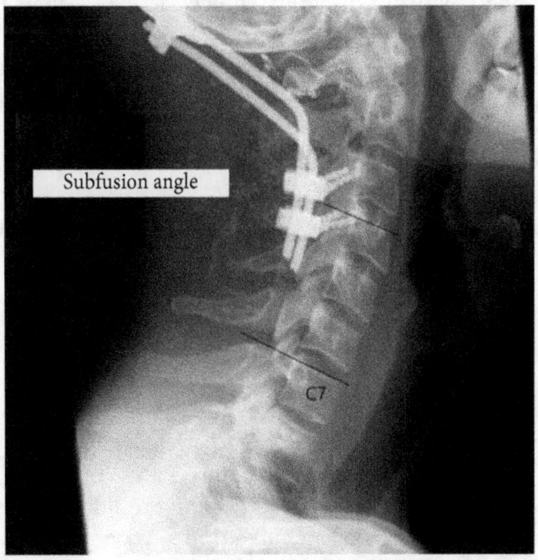

FIGURE 2: Lateral roentgenogram following POCF showing the subfusion angle measurement.

0–4) was graded (0) and mild disability (NDI > 4) was graded (1) at the final observation. The NDI scores in the patients at the final observation were tested for any significant correlation with each of the roentgenographic variables.

3. Results

There were no skewed data and no kurtosis issues while Levene's heterogeneity test showed homogeneity for all variables at baseline in both groups. The kappa values for both inter- and intraobserver agreements for the roentgenographic parameters measuring were 0.98–1.

The time elapsed between the trauma and the day of surgery ranged from 1 to 3 days (average: 1.4 days). The surgery duration averaged to 105 min (range: 90–120 min). The average hospital stay was 7 days (range: 3–21 days), although this was decreased to 3 days (range: 2–4 days) in cases of isolated UCI.

The follow-up observation averaged to 39 ± 12 (range: 25–57 months).

3.1. Functional Results. The average NDI score was 10% ± 8% (range: 2–24%). Twelve patients showed no disability (NDI: 0–8%), while 8 patients reported mild disability (10–28%).

3.2. Roentgenographic Results. There were no radiological changes in any sagittal roentgenographic parameter value between 3 months postoperatively and at the last observation (Figures 3(a)–3(c)).

Controls stood with increased C2-C7 lordosis, SCA, and CT (P = 0.019, <0.003, and <0.001, respectively) compared to their counterparts (patients), whereas patients showed higher NDI than controls postoperatively (P = 0.013).

Significant correlations were shown between anthropometric and roentgenographic parameters in both groups (Tables 2 and 3).

Female controls stood with more C2-C7 lordosis and SCA than their male counterparts (P = 0.008 and 0.017, respectively), while C2-C7 SVA was greater in men (P = 0.014). TIA was greater in controls aged ≥66 years (P = 0.041) than those aged <66 years.

Patients with no disability showed less TIA than those with mild disability (ANOVA, P = 0.023).

The subfusion angle (SA) that averaged 0.65 ± 13° three months postoperatively did not change at the last observation (2.6 ± 14°) (paired t-test, P = 0.76).

SCA is increasing with increasing C2-C7 lordosis (P = 0.0022 and 0.0001) and C0-C2 angle (P = 0.019 and 0.024). In contrary, SCA is decreasing with increasing T1-slope (P = 0.038) and CT (P = 0.016 and 0.018) (Table 4).

4. Discussion

Instability in the occipitocervical junction from different causes (degenerative disease, trauma, etc.) had been, for a long period, the primary indication for POCF [32–35] and has been successfully used in adults and the elderly suffering from unstable UCI, degenerative upper cervical spine, and inflammatory C1-C2 instability [10, 11, 13, 36, 37].

In this cohort, POCF restored immediately and maintained sufficiently the sagittal cervical and occipitocervical alignment. This correction was associated with low or no neck disability.

Contemporary POCF includes plate-screw-rod constructs that provide immediate postoperative stability [37, 38]. However, POCF in young adults reduces the motion of the C0 upper cervical spine, and subsequently, "occipitium sparing" posterior fusion techniques have been introduced by some authors [14, 33–36]. On the other hand, other authors postulated that the "occipitium sparing" surgery with C1-C2 fixation exposes a patient at a potential of highly increased intraoperative bleeding, while the sacrifice of the degenerated C0 upper cervical spine junction in adult or even elderly people may not make a significant clinical difference in the final functional outcome [33–36]. The aforementioned was also shown in these series where 12 and 8 adult and elderly patients had no or mild disability despite the occipitocervical immobilization.

There is a paucity of data regarding the sagittal occipitocervical parameters that determine good and pertinent clinical outcomes in old and elderly patients undergoing POCF for fresh unstable UCI.

The cervical spine is remarkably mobile and adapts its sagittal alignment to that of the thoracolumbar spine in order to maintain horizontal gaze [38–44]. Because of these adaptation movements, the physiological cervical spine in asymptomatic populations may not be necessarily lordotic but rather flat (45.8%) or kyphotic (21.7–33%) [19, 20, 41–44]. In this study, C2-C7lordosis averaged to −22 ± 15° in the controls, and that is significantly more lordotic than the −9.9 ± 20° that was measured in our patients (P = 0.019).

C0-C2 angle expresses the functional and balanced position of the head on the cervical spine in which an individual feels most comfortable [45]. In this study, patients showed postoperatively a lordotic C0-C2 angle close to that of the age-matched controls, indicating a sufficient restoration of the sagittal balance in upper cervical spine. The lordotic C0-C2 angle was achieved by the position of the patient's head during surgery, the appropriate contouring of the rods connecting the scull with the upper cervical spine and the intraoperative control of the desired occipitocervical junction position using an image intensifier [30, 31]. It is recommended that the C0-C2 angle to be set even more lordotic than the preoperative value in order to avoid dysphagia and respiratory disturbance [17, 22]. Because of the trauma mechanism, no preoperative standing lateral roentgenograms of the patients were available in order to make such comparisons.

In this study patients, C2-C7 lordosis was increased as the C0-C2 angle was increasing, indicating that the fixed C0-C2 angle following POCF "forces" the free segments below fusion to adapt their sagittal alignment to restore via the POCF C0-C2 angle.

In the recent literature, the most important parameter for good clinical outcomes following cervical surgery is to get T1-slope <40° [18–20]. In this study's patients, the T1-slope was <40° and it did not differ (P = 0.31) from the controls' T1-slope. Previous studies [18, 19, 44] showed that T1-slope increases as thoracic kyphosis increases, compensatory to maintain horizontal gaze, and this change affects the C2-C7lordosis. In our patients, T1-slope was positively correlated with C2-C7 lordosis (P = 0.006), which possibly indicates an adaptation of C2-C7 lordosis to preexisted thoracic kyphosis.

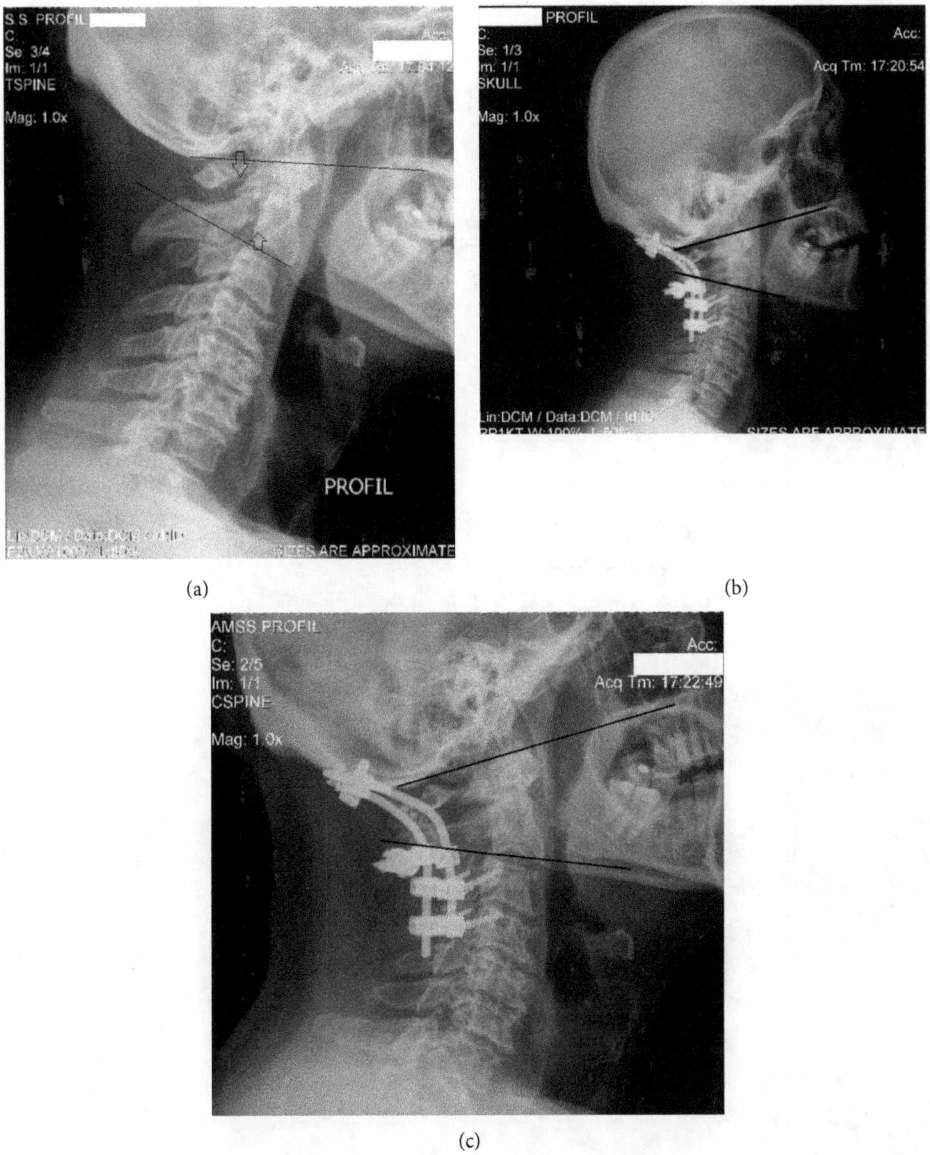

FIGURE 3: (a) Lateral roentgenogram of a 61-year-old man with C2 Levine IIb traumatic spondylolisthesis with >5 mm diastasis (lower arrow) and comminuted Jefferson fracture (upper arrow). The degeneration in the upper most cervical spine is evident. (b) Postoperative lateral roentgenogram following surgery showing reduction of the injury and POCF. There is an improved lordotic C0-C2 angle compared to the preoperative angle in (a). (c) Follow-up observation 36 months postoperatively showing a complete spinal fusion and a lordotic C0-C2 angle.

All cervical spines in both patients and controls were well balanced in the sagittal plane since C2-C7 SVA was <40 mm [46].

Chen et al. [20] showed that both T1-slope (>40 mm) and C2-C7 SVA negatively influence functional outcome scores (ED, 5Q, and HRQOL) in asymptomatic population [46]. Iver et al [47] showed that high C2-C7 SVA and low T1-slope are independent predictors of the high preoperative NDI score. NDI scores were not measured in our asymptomatic controls, but in our patients there was observed a tendency for high NDI scores with increasing T1-slope ($P = 0.097$). In this series, the postoperative NDI did not correlate with C2-C7SVA ($P = 0.5$). We speculate that this finding may explain the low disability (NDI <12) scores in our patients.

The center of gravity of the head is located at the posterior corner of the sella turcica, and therefore, SCA is a good marker to analyze the head positioning [46, 48, 49]. Some authors [19, 46, 50] reported that SCA averages to $83^\circ \pm 9^\circ$ in symptomatic population and is correlated with the cervical lordosis [50] while the combination of C7 or T1-slope < 40° with an SCA ($83 \pm 9^\circ$) was associated with an economical balance [19]. In our patients, the SCA was $75.9 \pm 7^\circ$, close to the economical balance limits, previously reported [19].

Lee et al. [29] described the TIA as the sum of NT + T1-slope in patients with the ankylosing cervical spine, but later,

TABLE 2: Correlation matrix between age, gender, and roentgenographic parameters in 29 asymptomatic individuals.

Parameters	Gender	C2-C7 lordosis	T1-slope	Spinocranial angle	C2-C7 SVA	Neck tilt	Thorax inlet angle	Cervical tilt	Cranial tilt	C0-C2 angle
Age	$r = -0.169$, $P = 0.382$	**r = −0.470, P = 0.01**	**r = 0.452, P = 0.014**	$r = -0.174$, $P = 0.365$	$r = 0.244$, $P = 0.201$	$r = 0.077$, $P = 0.693$	**r = 0.450, P = 0.014**	$r = 0.357$, $P = 0.057$	$r = 0.293$, $P = 0.122$	$r = 0.021$, $P = 0.914$
Gender	1	**r = 0.435, P = 0.018**	$r = 0.094$, $P = 0.628$	**r = −0.441, P = 0.017**	**r = 0.453, P = 0.014**	**r = 0.109, P = 0.575**	$r = 0.158$, $P = 0.412$	**r = −163, P = 0.399**	**r = 0.354, P = 0.059**	**r = 0.258, P = 0.177**
C2-C7 lordosis		1	$r = -0.481$, $P = 0.08$	$r = -0.12$, $P = 0.269$	$r = 0.161$, $P = 0.403$	$r = 0.215$, $P = 0.264$	$r = -0.271$, $P = 0.155$	**r = −667, P ≤ 0.001**	$r = 0.043$, $P = 0.823$	**r = 0.482, P = 0.008**
T1-slope			1	$r = -0.348$, $P = 0.06$	**r = 0.468, P = 0.011**	$r = -0.210$, $P = 0.273$	**r = 0.728, P ≤ 0.001**	**r = 0.790, P ≤ 0.001**	**r = 0.649, P ≤ 0.001**	$r = -0.059$, $P = 0.762$
Spinocranial angle				1	**r = −0.663, P ≤ 0.001**	$r = -0.172$, $P = 0.372$	**r = −0.426, P = 0.021**	$r = 0.102$, $P = 0.6$	**r = −0.693,** $P \leq$ **0.001**	**r = −0.407, P = 0.029**
C2-C7 SVA					1	$r = 0.230$, $P = 0.229$	**r = 0.571, P = 0.001**	$r = -0.114$, $P = 0.557$	**r = 0.902,** $P \leq$ **0.001**	$r = 0.204$, $P = 0.288$
Neck tilt						1	**r = 0.517, P = 0.04**	$r = -0.361$, $P = 0.055$	$r = 0.104$, $P = 0.591$	$r = 0.173$, $P = 0.368$
Thorax inlet angle							1	**r = 0.439, P = 0.017**	**r = 0.642,** $P \leq$ **0.001**	$r = 0.173$, $P = 0.368$
Cervical tilt								1	$r = 0.046$, $P = 0.82$	$r = -0.294$, $P = 0.121$
Cranial tilt									1	$r = 0.269$, $P = 0.269$

The results in bold present statistical significance with $P < 0.05$; r = Pearson correlation coefficient; P = probability value.

TABLE 3: Correlation matrix between age, gender, and final follow-up roentgenographic parameters in 20 operated patients.

Parameters	Age	C2-C7 lordosis	Spinocranial angle	T1-slope	C2-C7 SVA	Neck tilt	Thorax inlet angle	Cervical tilt	Cranial tilt	C0-C2 angle
Gender	*r* = 0.340, *P* = 0.182	*r* = 0.131, *P* = 0.616	*r* = 0.179, *P* = 0.492	*r* = −0.026, *P* = 0.921	*r* = −0.148, *P* = 0.572	*r* = −0.178, *P* = 0.493	*r* = -0.163, *P* = 0.533	**r = 0.124, P = −0.636**	*r* = −0.230, *P* = 0.374	*r* = −0.111, *P* = 0.672
Age	1	*r* = −0.107, *P* = 0.682	*r* = −0.022, *P* = 0.933	*r* = 0.284, *P* = 0.270	*r* = 0.070, *P* = 0.791	*r* = 0.020, *P* = 0.940	*r* = 0.304, *P* = 0.236	*r* = 0.291, *P* = 0.256	*r* = −0.014, *P* = 0.957	*r* = 0.263, *P* = 0.307
C2-C7 lordosis		1	*r* = −0.77, *P* = 0.770	**r = −0.638, P = 0.006**	*r* = 0.468, *P* = 0.058	*r* = 0.213, *P* = 0.412	**r = −0.487, P = 0.047**	**r = −0.663, P = 0.004**	*r* = 0.044, *P* = 0.866	**r = 0.555, P = 0.021**
Spinocranial angle			1	*r* = −0.412, *P* = 0.101	*r* = −0.068, *P* = 0.796	*r* = 0.383, *P* = 0.130	*r* = −0.127, *P* = 0.626	*r* = 0.051, **P = 0.847**	**r = −0.708, P = 0.001**	*r* = −0.231, *P* = 0.372
T1-slope				1	*r* = 0.016, *P* = 0.950	*r* = −0.398, *P* = 0.114	**r = 0.714, P = 0.001**	**r = 0.788, P ≤ 0.001**	*r* = 0.319, *P* = 0.213	*r* = −0.265, *P* = 0.304
C2-C7 SVA					1	*r* = −0.123, *P* = 0.637	*r* = −0.077, *P* = 0.768	*r* = −0.255, *P* = 0.238	*r* = 0.414, *P* = 0.099	*r* = 0.123, *P* = 0.637
Neck tilt						1	*r* = 0.357, *P* = 0.159	*r* = −0.106, *P* = 0.686	*r* = −0.447, *P* = 0.072	*r* = 0.247, *P* = 0.339
Thorax inlet angle							1	**r = 0.766, P ≤ 0.001**	*r* = −0.16, *P* = 0.951	*r* = −0.081, *P* = 0.757
Cervical tilt								1	*r* = −0.333, *P* = 0.192	*r* = −0.336, *P* = 0.187
Cranial tilt									1	*r* = 0.112, *P* = 0.668

The results in bold present statistical significance with $P < 0.05$; r = Pearson correlation coefficient; P = probability value.

TABLE 4: Pearson correlation matrix between roentgenographic parameters and the subfusion angle 3 months postoperatively and in the last follow-up, in 20 operated patients.

Parameters	Subfusion lordosis 3 months postoperatively	Subfusion lordosis in the last follow-up
C2-C7 lordosis	**r = 0.705, *P* = 0.0022**	**r = 0.816, *P* = 0.0001**
SCA	*r* = −0.333, *P* = 0.208	*r* = −0.083, *P* = 0.761
T1-slope	*r* = −0.325, *P* = 0.219	**r = −0.521, *P* = 0.038**
C2-C7 SVA	*r* = 0.369, *P* = 0.160	*r* = 0.174, *P* = 0.519
NT	*r* = −0.341, *P* = 0.197	*r* = −0.070, *P* = 0.797
TIA	*r* = −0.495, *P* = 0.122	*r* = −0.364, *P* = 0.271
CT	**r = −0.698, *P* = 0.016**	**r = −0.693, *P* = 0.018**
CrT	*r* = 0.223, *P* = 0.406	*r* = 0.050, *P* = 0.854
C0-C2 angle	**r = 0.78, *P* = 0.019**	**r = 0.559, *P* = 0.024**

The results in bold present statistical significance with $P < 0.05$; SCA: spinocranial angle; NT: neck tilt; TIA: thorax inlet angle; CT: cervical tilt; CrT: cranial tilt; r = Pearson correlation coefficient; P = probability value.

Janusz et al [39] postulated that TIA is not accurate in patients with symptomatic cervical degenerative disease. This was also justified in our patients, where TIA was postoperatively only 50% of the sum of NT + T1-slope. Our study showed that the functional outcome measure (NDI) in our patients was better in individuals with low TIA angle ($P = 0.023$).

The subfusion angle (SA), which was defined and used first in this study, seems to adapt to the C2-C7lordosis and C0-C2 angle, and it remained unchanged till the final observation indicating no subadjacent segment degeneration.

Only few studies reported on the complications following POCF for pure unstable traumatic cervical injuries [17, 21, 22, 34]. The reported complication rate averages to 52% in patients who received POCF for several causes [23, 30, 51]. A serious complication following UCI and POCF is the airway compromise (4.9%) that is thought to occur secondary to retropharyngeal swelling [51, 52]. No patient in our series showed airway compromise. Another serious complication, the dysphagia [46, 52] following POCF, has a different mechanism than that in anterior cervical surgery. Some authors supported the hypothesis of mechanical stenosis of the airway because of loss of the lordotic C0-C2 angle and suggested the correction of this angle to the lordotic preoperative neutral position or to a slightly more lordotic angle, since dysphagia occurs following POCF [22, 46, 53, 54]. In our series, there was no patient with dysphagia, probably because the C0-C2 angle in the operated patients was sufficiently restored.

The reported screw failure following POCF in nontraumatic instability cases was 7–12.5% [12, 43]. In this series, we did not include patients with loss of occipital plate fixation and/or revision surgery.

There are few limitations in this study: (1) the retrospective design; (2) the relative small number of patients; (3) the lack of standing preoperative roentgenograms for comparison because of the trauma mechanism; (4) postoperative restriction of the head and uppermost cervical spine; and (5) nearly half of the patient who underwent POCF were younger than 60 years.

Because of the lack of preoperative standing X-rays, we used a control group for a more reliable comparison. Supine roentgenograms in the controls would have led us to scientifically not sound results and conclusions, since all spine balance comparisons are currently routinely made in standing position only.

The advantages of this study are as follows: (1) the one surgeon's consecutive series, (2) the homogenous sample of trauma cases, and (3) the age-matched controls for comparison.

We do not advocate POCF in young active individuals without occipitocervical acute or other pathology where a fusion sparing surgical technique is recommended. Since 2017, in our department, we routinely remove the craniocervical hardware (occipital plate, screws, and cranial end of the rods) after radiological cervical fusion is achieved, in young patients, without upper cervical spine symptomatic degenerative disease.

The most important sagittal cervical balance roentgenographic parameters, e.g., C0-C2 lordosis, T1-slope, C2-C7 SVA, TIA, and SCA that are responsible for the clinical outcome measuring, were postoperatively restored and remained till the last evaluation within the "normal" limits.

In conclusion, POCF resulted in sufficient restoration of the sagittal cervical balance, as compared to age-matched controls, without simultaneous decrease of the neck disability score.

References

[1] R. W. Bucholz, W. Z. Burkhead, W. Graham, and C. Petty, "Occult cervical spine injuries in fatal traffic accidents," *Journal of Trauma*, vol. 19, pp. 768–771, 1979.

[2] R. Lador, P. J. Ben-Galim, B. K. Weiner, and J. A. Hipp, "The association of occipitocervical dissociation and death as a result of blunt trauma," *The Spine Journal*, vol. 10, pp. 1128–1132, 2010.

[3] S. L. Tepper, C. L. Fligner, and D. T. Reay, "Atlanto-occipital disarticulation. Accident characteristics," *The American Journal of Forensic Medicine and Pathology*, vol. 11, pp. 193–197, 1990.

[4] D. H. Alander, D. A. Andreychik, and E. S. Stauffer, "Early outcome in cervical spinal cord injured patients older than 50 years of age," *Spine (Phila Pa 1976)*, vol. 19, pp. 2299–2301, 1994.

[5] C. Bellabarba, S. K. Mirza, G. A. West et al., "Diagnosis and treatment of craniocervical dislocation in a series of 17 consecutive survivors during an 8-year period," *Journal of Neurosurgery*, vol. 4, pp. 429–440, 2006.

[6] P. J. Ben-Galim, T. A. Sibai, J. A. Hipp, M. H. Heggeness, and C. A. Reitman, "Internal decapitation:survival after head to neck dissociation injuries," *Spine (Phila Pa 1976)*, vol. 33, pp. 1744–1749, 2008.

[7] NJ. Blackwood III, "Atlo-occipital dislocation: a case of fracture of the atlas and Axis, and forward dislocation of the occiput on the spinal column, life being maintained for thirtyfour hours and forty minutes by artificial respiration, during which a laminectomy was performed upon the third cervical vertebra," *Annals of Surgery*, vol. 47, pp. 654–658, 1908.

[8] S. K. Mendenhall, A. Sivaganesan, A. Mistry, P. Sivasubramaniam, M. J. McGirt, and C. J. Devin, "Traumatic atlantooccipital dislocation: comprehensive assessment of mortality, neurologic improvement, and patient-reported outcomes at a Level 1 trauma center over 15 years," *The Spine Journal*, vol. 15, pp. 2385–2395, 2015.

[9] A. Reis, R. Bransford, T. Penoyar, J. R. Chapman, and C. Bellabarba, "Diagnosis and treatment of craniocervical dissociation in 48 consecutive survivors," *Evidence-Based Spine-Care Journal*, vol. 1, pp. 69-70, 2010.

[10] S. C. Lee, J. F. Chen, and S. T. Lee, "Clinical experience with rigid occipitocervical fusion in the management of traumatic upper cervical spinal instability," *Journal of Clinical Neuroscience*, vol. 13, no. 2, pp. 193–198, 2006.

[11] K. Abumi, T. Takada, Y. Shono, K. Kaneda, and M. Fujiya, "Posterior occipitocervical reconstruction using cervical pedicle screws and plate-rod systems," *Spine*, vol. 24, pp. 1425–1434, 1999.

[12] S. Kukreja, S. Ambekar, A. H. Sin, and A. Nanda, "Occipitocervical fusion surgery: review of operative techniques and results," *Journal of Neurological Surgery*, vol. 76, pp. 331–339, 2015.

[13] P. Korovessis, P. Katonis, P. Aligizakis et al., "Posterior compact Cotrel-Dubousset instrumentation for occipitocervical, cervical and cervicothoracic fusion," *European Spine Journal*, vol. 10, pp. 385–394, 2001.

[14] D. C. Lu, A. C. Roeser, V. P. Mummaneni et al., "Nuances of occipitocervical fixation," *Neurosurgery*, vol. 66, no. 3, pp. 141–146, 2010.

[15] J. C. Wang, P. V. Mummaneni, and R. W. Haid Jr, "Fixation options in the occipitocervical junction," in *Spinal Deformity: A Guide to Surgical Planning and Management*, P. V. Mummaneni, L. G. Lenke, and R. W. Haid Jr, Eds., pp. 223–240, Quality Medical Publishing, St Louis, MO, USA, 2008.

[16] B. J. Garrido and R. C. Sasso, "Occipitocervical fusion," *Orthopedic Clinics of North America*, vol. 43, pp. 1–9, 2012.

[17] M. Miyata, M. Neo, S. Fujibayashi, H. Ito, M. Takemoto, and T. Nakamura, "O-C_2 angle as a predictor of dyspnea and/or dysphagia after occipitocervical fusion," *Spine (Phila Pa 1976)*, vol. 34, pp. 184–188, 2009.

[18] S. Oe, D. Togawa, K. Nakai et al., "The influence of age and sex on cervical spinal alignment among volunteers aged over 50," *Spine*, vol. 40, no. 19, pp. 1487–1494, 2015.

[19] J. C. Le Huec, H. Demezon, and S. Aunoble, "Sagittal parameters of global cervical balance using EOS imaging: normative values from a prospective cohort of asymptomatic volunteers," *European Spine Journal*, vol. 24, no. 1, pp. 63–71, 2015.

[20] Y. Chen, J. Luo, Z. Pan et al., "The change of cervical spine alignment along with aging in asymptomatic population: a preliminary analysis," *European Spine Journal*, vol. 26, no. 9, pp. 2363–2371, 2017.

[21] M. Izeki, M. Neo, H Ito et al., "Reduction of atlantoaxial subluxation causes airway stenosis," *Spine (Phila Pa 1976)*, vol. 38, pp. E513–E520, 2013.

[22] M. Izeki, M. Neo, M. Takemoto et al., "The O-C2 angle established at occipito-cervical fusion dictates the patient's destiny in terms of postoperative dyspnea and/or dysphagia," *European Spine Journal*, vol. 23, pp. 328–336, 2014.

[23] C. D. Winegar, J. P. Lawrence, B. C. Friel et al., "A systematic review of occipital cervical fusion: techniques and outcomes," *Journal of Neurosurgery*, vol. 13, pp. 5–16, 2010.

[24] J. P. Cheung and K. D. Luk, "Complications of anterior and posterior cervical spine surgery," *Asian Spine Journal*, vol. 10, pp. 385–400, 2016.

[25] R. Lehman, D. Riew, and K. Schnake, "AO Classification of upper cervical injuries," *Global Spine Journal*, vol. 9, no. 1, 2019, https://www2.aofoundation.org/wps/portal/surgery.

[26] N. M. Trouli, T. Howard, T. H. Vernon, N. K. Kakavelakis et al., "Translation of the Neck Disability Index and validation of the Greek version in a sample of neck pain patients," *BMC Musculoskelet Disord*, vol. 9, p. 106, 2008.

[27] T. S. Protopsaltis, R. Lafage, S. Vira et al., "Novel angular measures of cervical deformity account for upper cervical compensation and sagittal alignment," *Clinical Spine Surgery*, vol. 30, no. 7, pp. E959–E967, 2017.

[28] C. Amabile, J. C. Le Huec, and W. Skalli, "Invariance of head pelvis alignment and compensatory mechanisms for asymptomatic adults older than 49 years," *European Spine Journal*, vol. 25, pp. 3630–3637, 2016.

[29] S. H. Lee, K. T. Kim, E. M. Seo et al., "The influence of thoracic inlet alignment on the craniocervical sagittal balance in asymptomatic adults," *Journal of Spinal Disorders & Techniques*, vol. 25, no. 2, pp. E41–E47, 2012.

[30] M. Yoshida, M. Neo, S. Fujibayashi, and T. Nakamura, "Upper-airway obstruction after short posterior occipitocervical fusion in a flexed position," *Spine*, vol. 32, pp. 267–270, 2007.

[31] F. M. Phillips, C. S. Phillips, F. T. Wetzel, and C. Gelinas, "Occipitocervical neutral position," *Spine*, vol. 24, pp. 775–778, 1999.

[32] S. M. Papadopoulos, C. Dickman, V. K. H. Sonntag, H. L. Rekate, and R. F. Spetzler, "Traumatic atlanto-occipital dislocation with survival," *Neurosurgery*, vol. 28, pp. 574–579, 1991.

[33] I. H. Lieberman and J. K. Webb, "Occipito-cervical fusion using posterior titanium plates," *European Spine Journal*, vol. 7, no. 4, pp. 308–312, 1998.

[34] M. A. Finn, F. S. Bishop, and A. T. Dailey, "Surgical treatment of occipitocervical instability," *Neurosurgery*, vol. 63, no. 5, pp. 961–968, 2008.

[35] M. Cappuccio, F. De Iure, L. Amendola, S. Paderni, and G. Bosco, "Occipito-cervical fusion in post-traumatic instability of the upper cervical spine and cranio-cervical junction," *European Spine Journal*, vol. 22, no. Suppl 6, pp. S900–S904, 2013.

[36] M. N. Hadley, C. Browner, and V. K. H. Sonntag, "Miscellaneous fractures of the second cervical vertebra," *BHI Q*, vol. 1, pp. 34–39, 1985.

[37] A. R. Vaccaro, M. R. Lim, and J. Y. Lee, "Indications for surgery and stabilization techniques of the occipito-cervical junction," *Injury*, vol. 36, no. Suppl 2, pp. B44–B53, 2005.

[38] M. P. Steinmetz, T. E. Mroz, and E. C. Benzel, "Craniovertebral junction: biomechanical considerations," *Neurosurgery*, vol. 66, no. Suppl 3, pp. 7–12, 2010.

[39] P. Janusz, M. Tyrakowski, P. Glowka et al., "Influence of cervical spine position on the radiographic parameters of the thoracic inlet alignment," *European Spine Journal*, vol. 24, pp. 2880–2884, 2015.

[40] J. S. Smith, V. Lafage, F. J. Schwab et al., "Prevalence and type of cervical deformity among 470 adults with thoracolumbar

deformity," *Spine (Phila Pa 1976)*, vol. 39, pp. E1001–E1009, 2014.

[41] M. Yu, W. K. Zhao, M. Li et al., "Analysis of cervical and global spine alignment under Roussouly sagittal classification in Chinese cervical spondylotic patients and asymptomatic subjects," *European Spine Journal*, vol. 24, no. 6, pp. 1265–1273, 2015.

[42] P. Roussouly, S. Gollogly, E. Berthonnaud, and J. Dimnet, "Classification of the normal variation in the sagittal alignment of the human lumbar spine and pelvis in the standing position," *Spine*, vol. 30, no. 3, pp. 346–353, 2005.

[43] H. W. Hey, E. T. Lau, C. G. Wong, K. A. Tan, G. K. Liu, and H. K. Wong, "Cervical alignment variations in different postures and predictors of normal cervical kyphosis—a new understanding," *Spine*, vol. 42, no. 21, pp. 1614–1621, 2017.

[44] B. G. Diebo, V. Challier, J. K. Henry et al., "Predicting cervical alignment required to maintain horizontal gaze based on global spinal alignment," *Spine*, vol. 41, no. 23, pp. 1795–1800, 2016.

[45] Q. Guo, B. Ni, J. Yang et al., "Relation between alignments of upper and subaxial cervical spine: a radiological study," *Archives of Orthopaedic and Trauma Surgery*, vol. 131, pp. 857–862, 2011.

[46] F. P. Ling and T. Chevillotte, "Which parameters are relevant in sagittal balance analysis of the cervical spine? A literature review," *European Spine Journal*, vol. 27, no. Suppl 1, pp. 8–15, 2018.

[47] S. Iyer, L. G. Lenke, V. M. Nemani, M. Fu et al., "Variations in occipito-cervical and cervico-thoracic alignment parameters based on age: a prospective study of asymptomatic volunteers using full-body radiographs," *Spine*, vol. 41, pp. 1837–1844, 2016.

[48] P. G. Passias, S. Wang, M. Kozanek, S. Wang, and C. Wang, "Relationship between the alignment of the occipitoaxial and subaxial cervical spine in patients with congenital atlantoxial dislocations," *Journal of Spinal Disorders & Techniques*, vol. 26, pp. 15–21, 2013.

[49] J. A. Tang, J. K. Scheer, J. S. Smith et al., "The impact of standing regional cervical sagittal alignment on outcomes in posterior cervical fusion surgery," *Neurosurgery*, vol. 76, no. Suppl 1, pp. S14–S21, 2015, (discussion).

[50] J. M. Vital and J. Senegas, "Anatomical bases of the study of the constraints to which the cervical spine is subject in the sagittal plane. A study of the center of gravity of the head," *Surgical and Radiologic Anatomy*, vol. 8, no. 3, pp. 169–173, 1986.

[51] S. H. Choi, S. G. Lee, C. W. Park, W. K. Kim, C. J. Yoo, and S. Son, "Surgical outcomes and complications after occipito-cervical fusion using the screw-rod system in craniocervical instability," *Journal of Korean Neurosurgical Society*, vol. 53, pp. 223–227, 2013.

[52] S. AlEissa, J. G. Reed, J. B. Kortbeek, and P. T. Salo, "Airway compromise secondary to upper cervical spine injury," *The Journal of Trauma*, vol. 67, pp. 692–696, 2009.

[53] M. J. Lee, R. Bazaz, C. G. Furey, and J. Yoo, "Risk factors for dysphagia after anterior cervical spine surgery: a two-year prospective cohort study," *The Spine Journal*, vol. 7, no. 2, pp. 141–147, 2007.

[54] L. H. Riley 3rd, R. L. Skolasky, T. J. Albert, A. R. Vaccaro, and J. G. Heller, "Dysphagia after anterior cervical decompression and fusion: prevalence and risk factors from a longitudinal cohort study," *Spine (Phila Pa 1976)*, vol. 30, no. 22, pp. 2564–2569, 2005.

33

Computation of Intersegmental Moments during Standing Posture: Can We Neglect the Horizontal Ground Reaction Force? Results from an Experimental Study

Solène Prost,[1,2] Sébastien Pesenti,[2,3] Bertrand Moal,[4] Vincent Pomero,[5] Stephane Fuentes,[1,2] Patrick Tropiano,[1] Virginie Lafage,[6] Jean-Luc Jouve,[2,3] and Benjamin Blondel[1,2]

[1]*Spine Division, Timone, Aix-Marseille University, 13005 Marseille, France*
[2]*Aix Marseille University, Institute of Movement Sciences, CNRS UMR, 7287 Marseille, France*
[3]*Pediatric Orthopedics, Timone Children Hospital, Aix-Marseille University, 264 Rue Saint Pierre, 13005 Marseille, France*
[4]*Bordeaux University, 146 Rue Léo Saignat, 33000 Bordeaux, France*
[5]*Gait Analysis Laboratory, Timone, Aix-Marseille University, 13005 Marseille, France*
[6]*Spine Service, Hospital for Special Surgery, New York, NY, USA*

Correspondence should be addressed to Benjamin Blondel; benjamin.blondel@ap-hm.fr

Academic Editor: Andreas K. Demetriades

Background. The development of postural analysis thanks to force and pressure platforms, in order to determine the center of pressure, can be valuable in the setting of spinal malalignment. The purpose of this study was to compare "pressure" and "force" platforms for the evaluation of the center of pressure. In other words, can we neglect the horizontal ground reaction force in the evaluation of intersegmental moments during standing posture? *Methods.* Postural data from two healthy adult volunteers were analyzed. Analysis of the posture was done according to a protocol providing sagittal intersegmental moments. A set of 36 markers was used to divide the body in 10 segments. Postacquisition calculations were done in order to obtain the sagittal net intersegmental moments. To evaluate the differences in intersegmental moments between force and pressure platforms, the postacquisition calculations were done with a simulated pressure platform. Mean intersegmental moments between each body segment for each volunteer were compared. *Findings.* There were significant differences between the 2 platforms in intersegmental moments for the lumbo-sacral junction, hips, knees, and ankles ($p < 0.005$). All differences were inferior to intrasubject variability measured with the force platform ($p < 0.001$). Results from intra- and interobserver comparisons showed that differences measured with the pressure platform were all inferior to the standard error obtained with the force platform for every intersegmental moment ($p < 0.001$). *Interpretation.* The use of a simulated pressure platform to determine intersegmental moments has the same clinical efficiency as force platforms. Moreover, the possibility to set the platform into the radiograph room will allow in a second time a correlation between radiographic parameters and biomechanical constraints applied to the spine.

1. Introduction

Importance of spinal global sagittal alignment has been widely described in the literature and correlated with clinical outcomes [1–3]. Analysis of these radiographic parameters has led to a better understanding of normal alignment [4] as well as age-related changes [5, 6]. Furthermore, integration of pelvic parameters in spinal assessment was highly correlated with clinical outcomes [7] and helped to understand which factors were related to spinal deformities and which were acting as compensatory mechanism in order to maintain the head over the pelvis and a horizontal gaze [7–10]. The initial change in adult spinal deformity is a loss of lumbar lordosis, leading to an anterior global malalignment, which can potentially be worsen by an increase of thoracic kyphosis. In order to compensate this "anterior fall" of the trunk, pelvis will progressively rotate backward (retroversion) and finally knees will flex in order to maintain body weight over the feet. At the same time, this global malalignment will be associated with an increased cervical lordosis to maintain horizontal gaze [11].

However, one of the limitations of these studies is related to the fact that they are highly dependent on the quality of the spinal radiographs, and it has been shown that this "radiographic posture" does not always represent real alignment of the patient [12], especially in case of significant anterior malalignment. Recent development of the three-dimensional imaging system has improved our ability to assess spinal alignment [13], and significant differences have been revealed between two-dimensional and three-dimensional analyses using a force platform [14, 15]. Standing posture might therefore not be considered as a static condition but more like a permanent control of equilibrium.

On the contrary, various studies have analyzed posture and balance strategies using center of pressure volunteers, patients with chronic low back pain or postoperatively [16–19]. Recently, a new postural analysis protocol was described calculating moments applied on different body segments using a force platform and skin markers [20]. However, this approach is done in a totally free standing position, and it requires a movement analysis laboratory and can be difficult to generalize to clinical centers. Therefore, it may be interesting to adapt this biomechanical postural approach to a more clinically applicable form, using data from full-spine radiographs and a pressure platform. The aim of this study was therefore to evaluate with this protocol the differences between the uses of a pressure platform vs. a force platform. In other words, if we consider the standing posture as a nonstatic condition, can we neglect the horizontal ground reaction force?

2. Methods

2.1. Study Sample. Postural data from two healthy adult volunteers were analyzed for this experimental study.

2.2. Postural Analysis Protocol and Data Acquisitions. Analysis of the posture of each volunteer was done according to a previously described protocol [20] providing sagittal intersegmental moments and summarized hereafter. A set of 36 markers was used to divide the body in 10 segments (head, thorax, abdomen, pelvis, thighs, legs, and feet), and then a mass was attributed to each segment according to Dumas et al. [21] using anthropometric tables and the height/weight of the subject.

Once equipped, the two volunteers were asked to adopt 4 times a free-standing position without external constraint or support, which each foot positioned over a force plate (AMTI, Watertown, MA, USA) in order to collect the ground reaction force of the subject. During acquisition, the location of the markers over time were recorded using a Vicon® (Vicon, Oxford, UK) optoelectronic system with 6 high-resolution infrared cameras and a 100 Hz sampling frequency. Analysis of the acquired data was conducted on a one-second record sample, with the less body sway, in order to calculate mean intersegmental moments in the sagittal plane at each joint center.

Postacquisition calculations were done in order to obtain the sagittal net intersegmental moments (ankles, knees, hips, lumbo-sacral junction, thoraco-lumbar junction, and cervico-thoracic junction) using an ascending manner (i.e., going upward from the ground reaction forces) between each body segment previously identified except for the cervico-thoracic junction, where the sagittal net articular moment was calculated using a descending manner from the center of mass and mass of the head and neck.

2.3. Comparison between Intersegmental Moments and Statistical Analysis. Experimental error measurement of the protocol was done in a previous work according to Schwartz et al. [22] methodology and allowed to obtain intrasubject, intraobserver, and interobserver variability of the protocol. These results were obtained using a force plate giving three-dimensional ground forces and moments (x = anterior-posterior, y = vertical, and z = lateral).

In order to evaluate the differences in terms of intersegmental moments between measurements done using a force or a pressure platform, the postacquisition calculations were done with a simulated pressure platform. Only the vertical component (y) was kept in order to simulate the pressure platform, and results of these "pressure" intersegmental moments were compared to the "force" moments using a t-test with a level of significance set at 5%. Finally, the mean difference between "force" and "pressure" intersegmental moments were compared to the experimental error measurement obtained with the original protocol.

In this study and according to the high correlations between sagittal alignment and clinical outcomes, only sagittal intersegmental moments were analyzed (moments z).

3. Results

3.1. Study Sample. The first volunteer was a 30-year-old male, (180 cm, 80 kg) and the second volunteer was a 26-year-old female (158 cm, 52 kg).

3.2. Comparison between Force vs. Pressure Platform in terms of Mean Intersegmental Moments. After calculation, mean segmental moments ("pressure" and "force") between each body segment for each volunteer were compared. Results from this comparison (Table 1) showed significant differences between the 2 platform configurations in terms of intersegmental moments for the lumbo-sacral junction, hips, knees, and ankles ($p < 0.005$). Significant difference was found neither for the thoraco-lumbar junction ($p = 0.162$) nor for the cervico-thoracic junction but due to the fact that this moment was calculated in a descending manner without taking into account ground reaction force.

TABLE 1: Mean difference (in absolute values) in terms of intersegmental moments between force and pressure platforms (in N·m).

	T-L	L-S	LHip	RHip	LKnee	RKnee	LAnkle	RAnkle
Mean difference	0.161	0.191	1.562	1.774	0.836	1.096	0.062	0.365
p value	0.162	0.048	<0.001	<0.001	<0.001	<0.001	0.006	<0.001

T-L = thoraco-lumbar junction; L-S = lumbo-sacral junction; L/RHip = left/right hip; L/RKnee = left/right knee; L/RAnkle = left/right ankle.

3.3. Comparison between Force vs. Pressure Platform in terms of Experimental Error Measurement. Differences in terms of intersegmental moments (in absolute values) were used in order to compare experimental error measurements with the simulated pressure platform with the previous experimental error measurements obtained with the force platform. Intrasubject comparison revealed that only the variability of hip moments measured with the pressure platform was superior ($p = 0.213$) to the standard error calculated with the force platform, while variability of lumbosacral, knee, and ankle moments calculated with the simulated platform were all inferior to intrasubject variability measured with the force platform ($p < 0.001$).

Results from intra- and interobserver comparisons showed that differences measured with the pressure platform were all inferior to the standard error obtained with the force platform for every intersegmental moment ($p < 0.001$).

4. Discussion

While postural analysis can be done using various protocols, evaluation of intersegmental moments is, to date, a new way to express posture in terms of clinical efforts needed to maintain a stable balance. In order to develop the use of this protocol in clinical practice, a combined analysis with full-spine radiographs and a pressure platform can be a valuable alternative. The aim of this study was to evaluate the comparability of the pressure platform vs. force platform using the same protocol as we described previously. This protocol has shown its accuracy for the calculation of intersegmental moments [20].

To the best of our knowledge, this is the first study describing the use of a simulated pressure platform to calculate the intersegmental moments. According to the findings of the present work, using a pressure platform instead of a force platform leads to significant differences on various intersegmental moments. However, the mean differences between the values obtained with the pressure and the force platforms were almost all significantly inferior to the mean experimental measurement error. In other words, the differences observed between the 2 different ways of measurement are not clinically significant, and horizontal ground reaction force can be neglected for intersegmental moment measurements during the standing posture. Thus, using pressure platforms for the evaluation of the intersegmental moments will represent a valuable alternative to the use of force platforms in daily practice.

A growing number of studies underline the importance of analyzing the center of pressure in patients with spine disorders. Brumagne et al. have shown that patients with chronic low back pain, in addition with changes in postural adaptation, had a significant modification of the position of their center of pressure, in comparison with healthy subjects [23]. Moreover, this kind of data provides information about the constraints that apply at different levels of the spine. Various authors have described the links that exist between low back pain and postural changes of the spine [17, 18, 24]. Analyzing intersegmental moments in these patients could be of great interest. Recently, Bailey et al. [25] reported the results of a biomechanical study that evaluated peak sagittal vertical axis, forces, and muscular moments at various joints. According to their results, a significant improvement of dynamic sagittal balance metrics was observed after surgical correction in the setting of adult spinal deformity.

The advantage of using a pressure platform instead of a force platform is also related to the fact that this device is portative and can be set up in a radiograph room. By this way, correlations between intersegmental moments and radiographic parameters could be analyzed, and correlation with postural adaptation of the spine could be revealed using a simple method in daily practice. Further steps are still needed in order to use these results in daily practice. Among them, we are currently investigating the differences between intersegmental moments using skin markers and simulated markers placed directly on the X-rays. If validated, this point will then allow us to get rid of skin markers and try to correlate intersegmental moments with radiographic parameters.

5. Conclusions

The understanding of postural adaptation of the spine consecutive to degenerative changes is a great issue for the management of age-related spinal disorders. The use of a pressure platform to determine intersegmental moments might have the same clinical efficiency as force platforms. Moreover, these findings may open new possibilities in standing posture evaluation such as the use of a pressure platform into the radiograph room in order to correlate radiographic parameters and biomechanical constraints applied to the spine.

Acknowledgments

Dr Pesenti received grants from SOFCOT, SOFOP, and ADEREM for the funding of a year-long research fellowship.

References

[1] F. Schwab, V. Lafage, A. Patel, and J.-P. Farcy, "Sagittal plane considerations and the pelvis in the adult patient," *Spine*, vol. 34, no. 17, pp. 1828–1833, 2009.

[2] S. D. Glassman, K. Bridwell, J. R. Dimar, W. Horton, S. Berven, and F. Schwab, "The impact of positive sagittal

balance in adult spinal deformity," *Spine*, vol. 30, no. 18, pp. 2024–2029, 2005.

[3] V. Lafage, F. Schwab, W. Skalli et al., "Standing balance and sagittal plane spinal deformity: analysis of spinopelvic and gravity line parameters," *Spine*, vol. 33, no. 14, pp. 1572–1578, 2008.

[4] R. Vialle, N. Levassor, L. Rillardon, A. Templier, W. Skalli, and P. Guigui, "Radiographic analysis of the sagittal alignment and balance of the spine in asymptomatic subjects," *The Journal of Bone and Joint Surgery-American Volume*, vol. 87, no. 2, pp. 260–267, 2005.

[5] J.-M. Mac-Thiong, É. Berthonnaud, J. R. Dimar 2nd, R. R. Betz, and H. Labelle, "Sagittal alignment of the spine and pelvis during growth," *Spine*, vol. 29, no. 15, pp. 1642–1647, 2004.

[6] J.-M. Mac-Thiong, P. Roussouly, É. Berthonnaud, and P. Guigui, "Age- and sex-related variations in sagittal sacropelvic morphology and balance in asymptomatic adults," *European Spine Journal*, vol. 20, no. S5, pp. 572–577, 2011.

[7] V. Lafage, F. Schwab, A. Patel, N. Hawkinson, and J.-P. Farcy, "Pelvic tilt and truncal inclination: two key radiographic parameters in the setting of adults with spinal deformity," *Spine*, vol. 34, no. 17, pp. E599–E606, 2009.

[8] F. Schwab, A. Patel, B. Ungar, J.-P. Farcy, and V. Lafage, "Adult spinal deformity-postoperative standing imbalance: how much can you tolerate? An overview of key parameters in assessing alignment and planning corrective surgery," *Spine*, vol. 35, no. 25, pp. 2224–2231, 2010.

[9] J. C. Le Huec, R. Saddiki, J. Franke, J. Rigal, and S. Aunoble, "Equilibrium of the human body and the gravity line: the basics," *European Spine Journal*, vol. 20, no. S5, pp. 558–563, 2011.

[10] I. Obeid, O. Hauger, S. Aunoble, A. Bourghli, N. Pellet, and J.-M. Vital, "Global analysis of sagittal spinal alignment in major deformities: correlation between lack of lumbar lordosis and flexion of the knee," *European Spine Journal*, vol. 20, no. S5, pp. 681–685, 2011.

[11] J. S. Smith, V. Lafage, E Klineberg, C. I. Shaffrey, F. J. Schwab, and G. Mundis, "Correction of sagittal malalignment following pedicle subtraction osteotomy improves cervical lordosis," in *Proceedings of the International Meeting on Advanced Spine Techniques*, Copenhagen, Denmark, 2011.

[12] M. C. Marks, C. F. Stanford, A. T. Mahar, and P. O. Newton, "Standing lateral radiographic positioning does not represent customary standing balance," *Spine*, vol. 28, no. 11, pp. 1176–1182, 2003.

[13] J. Dubousset, G. Charpak, W. Skalli, G. Kalifa, and J.-Y. Lazennec, "EOS stereo-radiography system: whole-body simultaneous anteroposterior and lateral radiographs with very low radiation dose," *Review of Orthopedic Surgery and Repair of the Motor Apparatus*, vol. 93, no. 6, pp. 141–143, 2007.

[14] N. Gangnet, R. Dumas, V. Pomero, A. Mitulescu, W. Skalli, and J.-M. Vital, "Three-dimensional spinal and pelvic alignment in an asymptomatic population," *Spine*, vol. 31, no. 15, pp. E507–E512, 2006.

[15] N. Gangnet, V. Pomero, R. Dumas, W. Skalli, and J.-M. Vital, "Variability of the spine and pelvis location with respect to the gravity line: a three-dimensional stereoradiographic study using a force platform," *Surgical and Radiologic Anatomy*, vol. 25, no. 5-6, pp. 424–433, 2003.

[16] K. Terry, V. K. Gade, J. Allen, G. F. Forrest, P. Barrance, and W. Thomas Edwards, "Cross-correlations of center of mass and center of pressure displacements reveal multiple balance strategies in response to sinusoidal platform perturbations," *Journal of Biomechanics*, vol. 44, no. 11, pp. 2066–2076, 2011.

[17] M. Salavati, M. R. Hadian, M. Mazaheri et al., "Test-retest reliabty of center of pressure measures of postural stability during quiet standing in a group with musculoskeletal disorders consisting of low back pain, anterior cruciate ligament injury and functional ankle instability," *Gait & Posture*, vol. 29, no. 3, pp. 460–464, 2009.

[18] A. Ruhe, R. Fejer, and B. Walker, "Center of pressure excursion as a measure of balance performance in patients with non-specific low back pain compared to healthy controls: a systematic review of the literature," *European Spine Journal*, vol. 20, no. 3, pp. 358–368, 2011.

[19] V. Sarwahi, O. Boachie-Adjei, S. I. Backus, and G. Taira, "Characterization of gait function in patients with postsurgical sagittal (flatback) deformity," *Spine*, vol. 27, no. 21, pp. 2328–2337, 2002.

[20] B. Blondel, V. Pomero, B. Moal et al., "Sagittal spine posture assessment: feasibility of a protocol based on intersegmental moments," *Orthopaedics & Traumatology: Surgery & Research*, vol. 98, no. 1, pp. 109–113, 2012.

[21] R. Dumas, L. Chèze, and J.-P. Verriest, "Adjustments to McConville et al. and Young et al. body segment inertial parameters," *Journal of Biomechanics*, vol. 40, no. 3, pp. 543–553, 2007.

[22] M. H. Schwartz, J. P. Trost, and R. A. Wervey, "Measurement and management of errors in quantitative gait data," *Gait & Posture*, vol. 20, no. 2, pp. 196–203, 2004.

[23] S. Brumagne, L. Janssens, E. Janssens, and L. Goddyn, "Altered postural control in anticipation of postural instability in persons with recurrent low back pain," *Gait & Posture*, vol. 28, no. 4, pp. 657–662, 2008.

[24] N. W. Mok, S. G. Brauer, and P. W. Hodges, "Hip strategy for balance control in quiet standing is reduced in people with low back pain," *Spine*, vol. 29, no. 6, pp. E107–E112, 2004.

[25] J. F. Bailey, R. P. Matthew, S. Seko et al., "ISSLS prize in bioengineering science 2019: biomechanical changes in dynamic sagittal balance and lower limb compensatory strategies following realignment surgery in adult spinal deformity patients," *European Spine Journal*, vol. 28, no. 5, pp. 905–913, 2019.

34

Not All SLAPs are Created Equal: A Comparison of Patients with Planned and Incidental SLAP Repair Procedures

Mark C. Dougherty,[1] J. Erik Kulenkamp,[2] Haroutioun Boyajian,[3] Jason L. Koh,[4,5] Michael J. Lee,[6] and Lewis L. Shi[6]

[1]*Resident, University of Iowa Hospitals and Clinics, Department of Neurosurgery, Iowa City, IA, USA*
[2]*Resident, University of Minnesota, Department of Ophthalmology and Visual Neurosciences, Minneapolis, MN, USA*
[3]*Resident, Henry Ford Health System, Department of Surgery, Detroit, MI, USA*
[4]*Clinical Professor and Chairman, NorthShore University Health System, Department of Orthopaedic Surgery, Evanston, IL, USA*
[5]*Director, NorthShore Orthopaedic Institute, Evanston, IL, USA*
[6]*Associate Professor, University of Chicago Medicine, Department of Orthopaedic Surgery and Rehabilitation Medicine, Chicago, IL, USA*

Correspondence should be addressed to Lewis L. Shi; lewisshi@uchicago.edu

Academic Editor: Benjamin Blondel

Background. Epidemiological studies have shown a progressive increase in the rate of superior labrum anterior-posterior (SLAP) repair surgery after the year 2000. However, it is not clear whether this is due to increased recognition of isolated SLAP tears or increased SLAP repair performed secondarily during arthroscopy for other purposes. *Hypothesis/Purpose.* We hypothesized that both isolated SLAP repair and secondary SLAP repair increased with time and that patient age influenced the pathway to SLAP diagnosis and surgery—such that younger patients were more likely to have isolated SLAP repair surgery after being diagnosed in clinic. *Study Design.* Descriptive epidemiology study. *Methods.* Data were obtained from the MarketScan database from 2003 to 2013. CPT and ICD-9 codes were used to identify SLAP surgery patients and concomitant procedures. The timing of SLAP diagnosis relative to surgery was used to determine whether the injury was recognized preoperatively. *Results.* 64,497 SLAP surgery patients were included. Preoperative SLAP diagnosis increased from 17.1% in 2003 to 44.6% in 2013. Patients diagnosed preoperatively were younger and had fewer concomitant procedures. Increasing age and concomitant rotator cuff tear (RCT) repair corresponded to lower odds of preoperative SLAP diagnosis. *Discussion.* Younger patients were more likely to have their SLAP tear diagnosed prior to surgery. Those diagnosed before surgery had fewer simultaneous procedures during their operations, suggesting that SLAP repair was more likely the primary operation. From 2003 to 2013, SLAP tears were increasingly recognized in the preoperative setting.

1. Introduction

Superior labrum anterior-to-posterior (SLAP) tears can lead to shoulder pain and instability in young and old patients [1]. SLAP diagnosis can be difficult in the office setting due to nonspecific clinical presentations and a high incidence of co-occurrence with other shoulder injuries; as a result, confirmation of the diagnosis often requires arthroscopy [2–9]. There is currently no standardized guideline for the surgical treatment of SLAP tears, but it is generally thought that young patients—especially athletes—should undergo SLAP repair, while older patients benefit more from biceps tenodesis [10–15].

Several large-scale epidemiological studies have identified a dramatic, unexplained increase in the number of SLAP repair surgeries after the year 2000 [16–18]. Work by our group corroborates those findings; we have also found that after 2009, the increased frequency of surgery for SLAP tears was mostly due to increasing rates of biceps tenodesis. It is unlikely that the true incidence of injury has changed with time; rather, the increased rate of SLAP repair is probably due to improved recognition of the injury. Studies have also suggested that many SLAP surgeries over this time period were performed on older patients [16, 18]. Given our knowledge of poorer outcomes for SLAP repair in older patients, we were inclined to further investigate the connection between age and SLAP repair. We wondered whether surgeons who identified and repaired SLAP tears during arthroscopy for another indication could account for a significant portion of the SLAP repair increase—especially among older patients. Perhaps SLAPs are easily missed when they are coincident with other shoulder injuries, as the clinical features of other injuries might mask the SLAP tear.

We therefore hypothesized that there would be several significant differences between SLAP surgery patients who were diagnosed with SLAP preoperatively and those who were not. Specifically, we hypothesized that patients with preoperative SLAP diagnoses were on average younger and had fewer concomitant shoulder procedures at the time of their SLAP repair than patients diagnosed with SLAP tears intraoperatively. With these differences, we aimed to shed light on the evolving epidemiology of SLAP surgery. To the best of our knowledge, no prior study has attempted to differentiate between these two groups of patients. We utilized data from a national database in order to ensure that our findings would be as generalizable as possible.

We also secondarily analyzed the subset of patients who underwent simultaneous rotator cuff tear (RCT) and SLAP repair. We specifically chose RCT repair for further evaluation because rotator cuff tears are easily recognized prior to surgery and have a substantial clinical impact; thus, RCT repair may be one of the more common procedures during which a surgeon might intraoperatively identify and repair a SLAP tear. RCT repairs are also frequently done in older patients, so that situation may contribute to the high rate of SLAP repairs seen in older patients [19]. Given the relative ease of identifying a torn rotator cuff and the high annual rate of RCT repair (substantially higher than SLAP repair), it is likely that RCT repair was the primary indication for surgery in most cases when RCT and SLAP repairs occurred simultaneously. Thus, we hypothesized that patients with concomitant SLAP and RCT repair surgeries were older and less often diagnosed with SLAP preoperatively than those without concomitant RCT repair.

2. Methods

Patient data in this study were obtained from the Truven Health MarketScan Commercial Database with Medicare Supplemental (http://marketscan.truvenhealth.com/; Ann Arbor, MI, USA), a fee-for-service private insurance claims database with approximately 55 million unique patients in the United States from 2003 to 2013. The database contains information on diagnoses, procedures, patient demographic data, and payments made for a given procedure. Current Procedure Technology (CPT) and International Classification of Diseases-Ninth Revision, Clinical Modification (ICD-9) codes were used to identify relevant procedures and diagnoses, respectively. We identified patients in the database who had exactly one arthroscopic SLAP repair surgery coded (CPT code 29807) between 2003 and 2013. Among these patients, we identified those who also had an RCT repair procedure (CPT codes 29827, 23410, 23412, and 23420) coded on the same day as their SLAP repair. Patients with less than 6 uninterrupted months of claims data before and after SLAP surgery were excluded to minimize the risk of missing key diagnosis and procedure codes. The timing of a patient's earliest SLAP diagnosis code (ICD-9 code 840.7) was used to determine whether the SLAP lesion was recognized prior to SLAP surgery. CPT codes were also used to characterize other concomitant shoulder surgeries (e.g., 29826 subacromial decompression).

Two-sample *t*-tests were used to compare the mean ages and mean number of concomitant shoulder procedures of the preoperative and intraoperative SLAP diagnosis groups. A two-sample *t*-test was also used to compare the mean ages of the RCT repair and non-RCT repair groups. Multivariate logistic regression analysis was used to evaluate the odds of preoperative diagnosis based on age and concomitant RCT repair. One-way analysis of variance (ANOVA) with post hoc Scheffe pairwise testing was used to determine the significance of differences between specific age groups (e.g., 10–19, 20–29). Given our large sample size, we used $p < 0.001$ as the cutoff for statistical significance for all calculations. All statistical analyses were performed using Stata 14.0 (College Station, TX).

3. Results

A total of 64,497 SLAP surgery patients were included in our study; of those, 24,438 were diagnosed with a SLAP lesion prior to SLAP surgery, and 40,059 were not. Patients who were diagnosed preoperatively were significantly younger than those who were not (37.6 vs. 43.2 years; $p < 0.0001$). Likewise, logistic regression demonstrated that increasing age (OR 0.982 per year, $p < 0.001$) and concomitant RCT repair (OR 0.594, $p < 0.001$) corresponded to lower odds of preoperative SLAP diagnosis. Figure 1 illustrates the relative proportions of SLAP repair patients who were diagnosed prior to surgery based on the patient's age. The total number of SLAP surgeries based on patient age had a biphasic distribution, with one peak at age 17 years and another from ages 46 to 52 years (Figure 1).

Nearly half of the patients under 30 were diagnosed preoperatively, whereas a substantially smaller percent of older patients was diagnosed preoperatively. Increasing age corresponded to a decreasing percentage of patients whose SLAP was diagnosed prior to surgery (Figure 2). 87.5% of the patients had one or more concomitant shoulder procedures performed at the time of SLAP repair, the most common of which were subacromial decompression (CPT 29826; 56.0% of patients) and capsulorrhaphy (CPT 29806; 26.6% of patients). Patients who were diagnosed with SLAP tear preoperatively had significantly fewer concomitant surgical procedures (2.67 ± 1.26) than those who were not (3.04 ± 1.28; $p < 0.0001$). Similarly, younger patients had fewer concomitant procedures on average than older patients; for example, patients 10–19 years old averaged

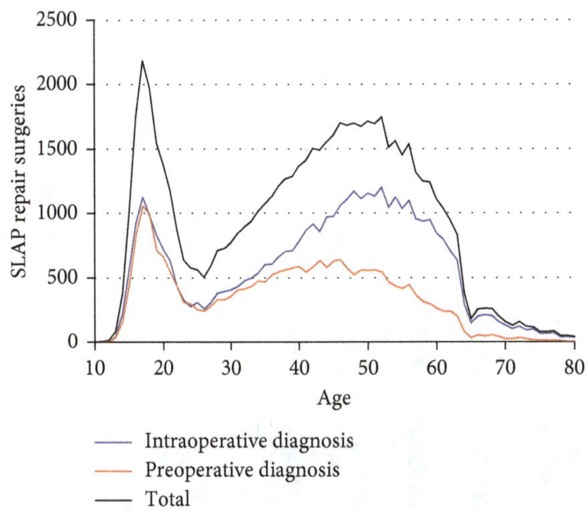

Figure 1: Total number of SLAP repair procedures performed 2003–2013 by patient age, with preoperative diagnosis (red), without preoperative diagnosis (blue), and total (black). The peaks of a biphasic distribution can be seen at ages 17 and 52.

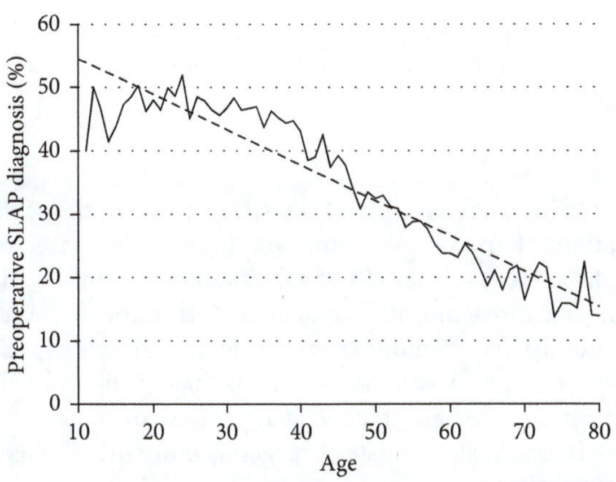

Figure 2: Percentage of patients with SLAP diagnosis prior to surgery. Dashed line represents line of best fit.

2.07 ± 0.90 concomitant shoulder procedures (including SLAP repair), compared to 3.42 ± 1.26 in the 50–59 year age range—a significant difference ($p < 0.001$).

Of the 64,497 SLAP repair patients in our cohort, 17,563 (27.2%) had concomitant RCT repair. However, only 18.2% of the patients with preoperative SLAP diagnosis had concomitant RCT repair compared to 32.7% of the patients without preoperative SLAP diagnosis. Independent of SLAP diagnosis status, patients with concomitant RCT repair were significantly older than non-RCT repair patients (51.6 vs. 37.1 years; $p < 0.0001$) and had more concomitant procedures than non-RCT patients, even without counting the RCT repair (2.00 vs. 1.49, $p < 0.0001$).

As suggested by other studies, we demonstrated that the overall rate of SLAP repair increased over much of the first decade of the new millennium, peaking in 2008 (Figure 3). There was a slight decrease from 2008 to 2013, but rates remained well above 2003 levels. The increase over time was due to increased rates of repair of both diagnosis groups—those with SLAP lesions diagnosed preoperatively and those diagnosed intraoperatively—but the relative contributions of each group changed with time. From 2003 to 2007, the rate of repair in both groups increased substantially. In contrast, from 2008 to 2013, SLAP repairs following intraoperative diagnosis declined, whereas those following preoperative diagnosis remained fairly constant. The percentage of SLAP repair patients that were diagnosed before surgery increased consistently over time, from a low of 17.1% in 2003 to a peak of 45.3% in 2012 (Figure 3).

4. Discussion

While increases in the incidence and repair of SLAP lesions have been noted in the literature, no previously published work has evaluated the impact that age has on how a SLAP tear is diagnosed in those who eventually undergo SLAP repair surgery [16–18, 20]. Our results confirm our suspicion that younger patients were significantly more likely to have their SLAP tear diagnosed prior to surgery. Those who were diagnosed before surgery had significantly fewer concomitant procedures, suggesting that SLAP repair was more likely the primary operation. Ultimately, SLAP repair occurring as a secondary, unplanned procedure may partly explain the high rate of SLAP repair in older patients. Our example of concomitant RCT repair supports this conclusion: RCT repair patients were older, less likely to have a recognized SLAP tear prior to surgery, and had more concomitant procedures than non-RCT repair patients. In other words, these patients were older and had more complicated shoulder pathology than their counterparts. On the one hand, this is a somewhat obvious finding, given that we are comparing patients with one specific procedure (SLAP repair) to others with two specific procedures (SLAP repair and RCT repair). On the other hand, it is easy to imagine why such patients may not have SLAP tears recognized prior to surgery—the more complicated the pathology, the more difficult it is to identify features specific to SLAP tears, which might explain the lower rate of SLAP diagnosis prior to arthroscopy. The corollary is also true: in younger patients, who tend to have less complicated shoulder pathology, SLAP tears are more easily identified without arthroscopy. To confirm these suspicions, further investigation is necessary; this study only evaluated patients who underwent SLAP repair, so we do not have any insight into intraoperative SLAP tear diagnoses that were not subsequently repaired, including those addressed via biceps tenodesis. Furthermore, insurance claims do not contain information on specific symptomatology, so we cannot determine whether SLAP tears identified during surgery were actually symptomatic during preoperative evaluation.

Intraoperative SLAP diagnosis does not fully explain the changing rate of SLAP repair over time because the percentage of SLAP surgeries that had a preoperative SLAP diagnosis actually increased over the period studied. This suggests that, from 2003 to 2013, the orthopaedic community became better at identifying SLAP tears in the preoperative setting. Whether this recognition was due to

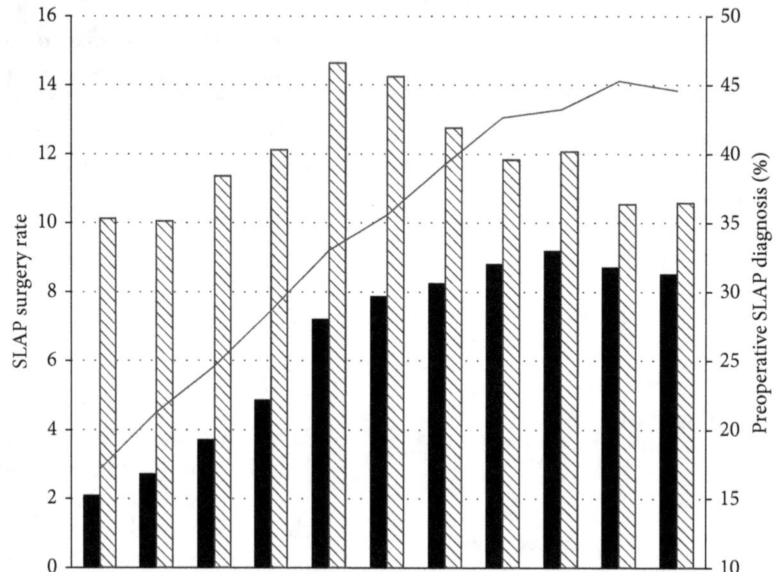

	2003	2004	2005	2006	2007	2008	2009	2010	2011	2012	2013
Preoperative	2.1	2.7	3.7	4.9	7.2	7.9	8.2	8.8	9.2	8.7	8.5
Intraoperative	10.1	10.1	11.4	12.1	14.6	14.2	12.8	11.8	12.1	10.5	10.6
% preoperative	17.1	21.2	24.6	28.6	33.0	35.6	39.3	42.6	43.2	45.3	44.6

FIGURE 3: Left axis: SLAP repairs per 100,000 patients; * with (black) or without (striped) preoperative SLAP diagnosis. Right axis (blue): percent of SLAP repairs with SLAP diagnosis prior to surgery. *2003 and 2013 included only 6 months of data, so numbers from these years were doubled for accurate comparison.

higher clinical suspicion in the office, better physical examination, or improved imaging technology is unclear. Notably, there was a temporary increase in intraoperatively diagnosed SLAP repairs in the middle portion of our study period, peaking in 2007 and 2008, but this increase was essentially gone by 2012 (Figure 3). Although somewhat speculative, our best explanation for this observation is that the orthopaedic community began to identify, and then repair, more and more SLAP lesions before collectively realizing that many SLAP tears should not be repaired. Further investigation showing the rates of SLAP diagnosis independent of SLAP surgery is needed to support this hypothesis.

The MarketScan database allows for a unique analysis of the procedures in question for a variety of reasons. Its national scale reduces the impact of normal variations in physician practices. Its size enables us to identify small differences that smaller datasets cannot. Few studies have utilized a database of this magnitude to evaluate rates of concomitant surgery, and fewer still have stratified specifically by patient age [21–24]. We believe that our findings will therefore help advance our understanding of how patient characteristics affect SLAP repair. In the absence of properly conducted randomized controlled trials, indirectly derived data, such as this, are the best information available for guiding treatment.

5. Limitations

This analysis depends on accurate and consistent billing codification by physicians. We cannot distinguish between true clinical differences and physician-to-physician coding variations. For example, some physicians may enter nonspecific codes such as 719.41 (shoulder pain) until a SLAP lesion is arthroscopically confirmed. Furthermore, surgeons may not list every unique diagnosis while billing—especially in patients with several diagnoses—as they are likely paid the same amount for an office visit regardless of the diagnosis listed; in contrast, we suspect surgeons more often billed for every surgical procedure performed, as doing so probably impacts their payment. Thus, our method of analysis is more likely to miss a suspected diagnosis than a surgical procedure, so we may underestimate the amount of SLAP tears that were suspected prior to surgery. Stated differently, we may overestimate the prevalence of incidental SLAP repairs (SLAPs diagnosed intraoperatively). However, these coding ambiguities are unlikely to vary by age or year, so the differences we found between young and old patients and changes over time are still noteworthy.

Insurance database analyses also lack information on clinical outcome measures, such as pain scores and postoperative functional recovery. Therefore, we cannot directly compare outcome measures between groups, such as old versus young patients, or patients with and without concomitant rotator cuff repair. Finally, although surgeon experience is an obvious and important factor in clinical decision-making, the MarketScan database does not identify individual providers or institutions from which each billing code came. Hence, we cannot comment on whether surgeon experience, institutional volume, private versus academic setting, or various other provider-related factors impact our findings. Although in some ways this is a limitation to our study, it also makes our findings more generalizable since we encompass all practice settings and all ranges of orthopaedic surgeons within the United States.

6. Conclusions

Younger patients were more likely to have their SLAP tear diagnosed prior to surgery. Those who were diagnosed before surgery had fewer operations, suggesting that SLAP repair was more likely the primary operation. From 2003 to 2013, SLAP tears were increasingly recognized in the pre-operative setting.

Disclosure

J. L. K. is a paid consultant for Aesculap/B. Braun, Aperion, and Arthrex, Inc.; a stock holder in Aperion; and a board member or committee member in the American Orthopaedic Society for Sports Medicine, Arthroscopy Association of North America, Illinois Association of Orthopaedic Surgeons, and Patellofemoral Foundation. M. J. L. is a paid consultant for Stryker Spine and DePuy Synthes Spine. L. L. S. is a paid consultant for DePuy; a Shoulder/Elbow Content committee member for the American Association of Orthopaedic Surgery; and a board or committee member for Novation Orthopaedic Council.

References

[1] S. E. Powell, K. D. Nord, and R. K. N. Ryu, "The diagnosis, classification, and treatment of SLAP lesions," *Operative Techniques in Sports Medicine*, vol. 20, no. 1, pp. 46–56, 2012.

[2] N. Aydin, E. Sirin, and A. Arya, "Superior labrum anterior to posterior lesions of the shoulder: diagnosis and arthroscopic management," *World Journal of Orthopedics*, vol. 5, no. 3, pp. 344–350, 2014.

[3] V. P. Chandnani, T. D. Yeager, T. DeBerardino et al., "Glenoid labral tears: prospective evaluation with MRI imaging, MR arthrography, and CT arthrography," *American Journal of Roentgenology*, vol. 161, no. 6, pp. 1229–1235, 1993.

[4] W.-H. Jee, T. R. McCauley, L. D. Katz, J. M. Matheny, P. A. Ruwe, and J. P. Daigneault, "Superior labral anterior posterior (SLAP) lesions of the glenoid labrum: reliability and accuracy of MR arthrography for diagnosis," *Radiology*, vol. 218, no. 1, pp. 127–132, 2001.

[5] W. B. Kibler and A. Sciascia, "Current practice for the diagnosis of a SLAP lesion: systematic review and physician survey," *Arthroscopy: Journal of Arthroscopic & Related Surgery*, vol. 31, no. 12, pp. 2456–2469, 2015.

[6] T. Magee, "Usefulness of unenhanced MRI and MR arthrography of the shoulder in detection of unstable labral tears," *American Journal of Roentgenology*, vol. 205, no. 5, pp. 1056–1060, 2015.

[7] J. W. O'Kane and B. G. Toresdahl, "The evidenced-based shoulder evaluation," *Current Sports Medicine Reports*, vol. 13, no. 5, pp. 307–313, 2014.

[8] D. Popp and V. Schöffl, "Superior labral anterior posterior lesions of the shoulder: current diagnostic and therapeutic standards," *World Journal of Orthopedics*, vol. 6, no. 9, pp. 660–671, 2015.

[9] K. Sheridan, C. Kreulen, S. Kim, W. Mak, K. Lewis, and R. Marder, "Accuracy of magnetic resonance imaging to diagnose superior labrum anterior-posterior tears," *Knee Surgery, Sports Traumatology, Arthroscopy*, vol. 23, no. 9, pp. 2645–2650, 2015.

[10] M. Brockmeyer, M. Tompkins, D. M. Kohn, and O. Lorbach, "SLAP lesions: a treatment algorithm," *Knee Surgery, Sports Traumatology, Arthroscopy*, vol. 24, no. 2, pp. 447–455, 2016.

[11] W. B. Kibler and A. Sciascia, "Current practice for the surgical treatment of SLAP lesions: a systematic review," *Arthroscopy: Journal of Arthroscopic & Related Surgery*, vol. 32, no. 4, pp. 669–683, 2016.

[12] F. McCormick, S. Bhatia, P. Chalmers, A. Gupta, N. Verma, and A. A. Romeo, "The management of type II superior labral anterior to posterior injuries," *Orthopedic Clinics of North America*, vol. 45, no. 1, pp. 121–128, 2014.

[13] B. J. Neuman, C. B. Boisvert, B. Reiter, K. Lawson, M. G. Ciccotti, and S. B. Cohen, "Results of arthroscopic repair of type II superior labral anterior posterior lesions in overhead athletes," *American Journal of Sports Medicine*, vol. 39, no. 9, pp. 1883–1888, 2011.

[14] M. T. Provencher, F. McCormick, C. Dewing, S. McIntire, and D. Solomon, "A prospective analysis of 179 type 2 superior labrum anterior and posterior repairs," *American Journal of Sports Medicine*, vol. 41, no. 4, pp. 880–886, 2013.

[15] J. Erickson, K. Lavery, J. Monica, C. Gatt, and A. Dhawan, "Surgical treatment of symptomatic superior labrum anterior-posterior tears in patients older than 40 years," *American Journal of Sports Medicine*, vol. 43, no. 5, pp. 1274–1282, 2015.

[16] A. L. Zhang, C. Kreulen, S. S. Ngo, S. L. Hame, J. C. Hame, and S. C. Gamradt, "Demographic trends in arthroscopic SLAP repair in the United States," *American Journal of Sports Medicine*, vol. 40, no. 5, pp. 1144–1147, 2012.

[17] I. Onyekwelu, O. Khatib, J. D. Zuckerman, A. S. Rokito, and Y. W. Kwon, "The rising incidence of arthroscopic superior labrum anterior and posterior (SLAP) repairs," *Journal of Shoulder and Elbow Surgery*, vol. 21, no. 6, pp. 728–731, 2012.

[18] R. H. Ablove, A. Allison, and G. Baer, "The incidence and demographics of shoulder repair in Wisconsin, 2002-2010," *WMJ: Official Publication of the State Medical Society of Wisconsin*, vol. 113, no. 6, pp. 223–226, 2014.

[19] N. B. Jain, L. D. Higgins, E. Losina, J. Collins, P. E. Blazar, and J. N. Katz, "Epidemiology of musculoskeletal upper extremity ambulatory surgery in the United States," *BMC Musculoskeletal Disorders*, vol. 15, no. 1, p. 4, 2014.

[20] L. A. Vogel, T. C. Moen, A. A. Macaulay et al., "Superior labrum anterior-to-posterior repair incidence: a longitudinal investigation of community and academic databases," *Journal of Shoulder and Elbow Surgery*, vol. 23, no. 6, pp. e119–e126, 2014.

[21] J. M. Cancienne, S. F. Brockmeier, and B. C. Werner, "Tobacco use is associated with increased rates of infection and revision surgery after primary superior labrum anterior and posterior repair," *Journal of Shoulder and Elbow Surgery*, vol. 25, no. 11, pp. 1764–1768, 2016.

[22] E. Shields, C. Thirukumaran, R. Thorsness, K. Noyes, and I. Voloshin, "An analysis of adult patient risk factors and complications within 30 days after arthroscopic shoulder surgery," *Arthroscopy: Journal of Arthroscopic & Related Surgery*, vol. 31, no. 5, pp. 807–815, 2015.

[23] C. T. Martin, Y. Gao, A. J. Pugely, and B. R. Wolf, "30-day morbidity and mortality after elective shoulder arthroscopy: a

review of 9410 cases," *Journal of Shoulder and Elbow Surgery*, vol. 22, no. 12, pp. 1667.e1–1675.e1, 2013.

[24] M. G. Yeranosian, A. Arshi, R. D. Terrell, J. C. Wang, D. R. McAllister, and F. A. Petrigliano, "Incidence of acute postoperative infections requiring reoperation after arthroscopic shoulder surgery," *American Journal of Sports Medicine*, vol. 42, no. 2, pp. 437–441, 2014.

Possible Improvement of the Sagittal Spinopelvic Alignment and Balance through "Locomotion Training" Exercises in Patients with "Locomotive Syndrome"

Takashi Yurube,[1] Masaaki Ito,[1] Toru Takeoka,[2] Nobuyoshi Watanabe,[3] Hideyo Inaoka,[2] Kenichiro Kakutani,[1] Ryosuke Kuroda,[1] and Kotaro Nishida[1]

[1]*Department of Orthopaedic Surgery, Kobe University Graduate School of Medicine, Kobe 650-0017, Japan*
[2]*Department of Rehabilitation, Kyoto Kujo Hospital, Kyoto 601-8453, Japan*
[3]*Department of Orthopaedic Surgery, Kyoto Kujo Hospital, Kyoto 601-8453, Japan*

Correspondence should be addressed to Takashi Yurube; takayuru-0215@umin.ac.jp

Academic Editor: Benjamin Blondel

On the basis of rapid population aging, in 2007, the Japanese Orthopaedic Association (JOA) proposed a new disease concept "locomotive syndrome" as a degenerative condition of reduced mobility due to the impairment of the musculoskeletal system. Worsened locomotive components, which consist of bones, joints, and intervertebral discs, and muscles and nerves, can lead to symptoms such as pain, limited range of motion, malalignment, impaired balance, and difficulty in walking, ultimately resulting in the requirement of nursing care. "Locomotive syndrome" has gained increased interest in Japan but still not worldwide. Hence, in this brief review, we summarize an updated definition, assessment, and management of "locomotive syndrome". The JOA recommends "locomotion training" exercise intervention to be effective in maintaining motor function that comprises two simple exercises—squatting and single-leg standing. However, the extent to which exercises affect "locomotive syndrome" is unknown. Here, we further report hypothesis-generating patient cases who presented the improved sagittal spinopelvic alignment in standing radiographs and postural stability in piezoelectric force-plate measurements through our 6-month "locomotion training" outpatient rehabilitation program. It is noteworthy that "locomotion training" facilitated these improvements despite the presence of specific disorders including thoracic kyphosis and symptomatic lumbar spinal canal stenosis. This raises the need for further investigations to clarify effects of "locomotion training" exercises on the spinal alignment, global balance, and quality of life in patients with "locomotive syndrome".

1. Introduction

In 2016, the total population of Japan was 127 million, which was the 10th grade ranking country in the world [1]. However, the number of Japanese people in ages of 65 or more (recognized as the old age in Japan) was approximately 35 million, which was 27.3% of the entire population and the highest percentage of the aging rate in the world [2]. Hence, Japan has the most aged society.

In the aged Japanese population, a big issue is the gap between the increased actual life span and the healthy life expectancy. In 2013, this gap was approximately 9 years in Japanese men and 12 years in Japanese women [3]. Furthermore, the primary cause of the requirement of nursing care in elderly Japanese persons was musculoskeletal disorders (24.6% in 2016), which was higher than cerebrovascular disease and dementia [3]. Actually in persons with any subjective symptoms, low back pain, stiff neck and shoulder, and peripheral joint pain occupied the 1st, 2nd, and 5th and 1st, 2nd, and 3rd most frequent complaints in Japanese men and women, respectively [3]. Therefore, the maintenance of healthy musculoskeletal functions is an urgent national concern in Japan.

On the basis of this accelerated population aging, in 2007, the Japanese Orthopaedic Association (JOA) determined a new disease concept "locomotive syndrome" as a condition being restricted in the ability to walk and have a normal life owing to a degenerative dysfunction in one or more of the parts of the musculoskeletal system [4, 5]. The musculoskeletal system which can cause "locomotive syndrome" consists of three major components: (1) bones, (2) joints and intervertebral discs, and (3) muscles and nerves. The age-related impairment of these organs causes (1) osteoporosis and related fragile fractures, (2) osteoarthritis and spondylosis, and (3) sarcopenia and neural disorders. These diseases can lead to symptoms of pain, limited range of joint motion, malalignment, imbalance, and then difficulty in standing-up and walking, finally resulting in reduced activities of daily living (ADL), lower quality of life (QOL), and required nursing care. "Locomotive syndrome" is the basis of musculoskeletal healthcare problems in the present Japanese society.

Degenerative changes in the musculoskeletal system appear before middle ages. The intervertebral disc is one of the earliest organs to develop degeneration in the body [6]. The first unequivocal findings of degeneration in the lumbar discs are seen in the age group 11–16 years [7]. Then, ~40% of people in ages under 30 years and 90% of those in ages over 55 years present lumbar disc degeneration [8]. Furthermore, a Japanese cohort study found that the estimated number of patients with radiographic knee osteoarthritis, lumbar spondylosis, lumbar osteoporosis, and femoral neck osteoporosis were 25, 38, 6.4, and 11 million of 128 million (Japan's 2005 population) [9]. The prevalence of these disorders is quite high, requiring heavy socioeconomic burden. Therefore, health promotion to prevent "locomotive syndrome" is essential.

2. Assessment of "Locomotive Syndrome"

Early diagnosis and recognition are important. To identify people at risk of "locomotive syndrome" and also raise the public interest in the importance of "locomotive syndrome", JOA developed "loco-check" self-completed questionnaire [10]. Although self-assessment by using "loco-check" is not a mandatory step toward the diagnosis with "locomotive syndrome", "loco-check" is a useful self-assessment tool to detect early stages of "locomotive syndrome" and initiate preventive measures. In fact, statistical correlation between the number of positive "loco-check" items and the incidence of falling in the previous year was found [11].

Many functional assessments, such as the hand-grip strength, one-leg standing time, and 6 m walking time, were proposed to evaluate "locomotive syndrome" [12, 13]. These measurements are useful; however, further validations are required. Currently, the stand-up test, two-step test, and 25-question geriatric locomotive function scale (GLFS-25) have been officially introduced for the diagnosis with "locomotive syndrome" [10, 14]. In these assessments, two risk levels of "locomotive syndrome" have been categorized to assess the severity. To determine "locomotive syndrome risk level", all these three tests (stand-up test, two-step test, and GLFS-25) have to be completed. Recent literature has often recognized "locomotive syndrome risk level 2" as patients who have positive "locomotive syndrome" [15].

2.1. Loco-Check. "Loco-check" consists of the following seven statements regarding daily activities: (1) you cannot put your sock on standing on one leg; (2) you often trip up or slip around the house; (3) you need to hold on to the handrail when climbing the stairs; (4) you have difficulty in doing moderately heavy housework; (5) you have difficulty in carrying home 2 kg of shopping; (6) you cannot walk for a quarter of an hour nonstop; and (7) you cannot make it across the road before the light turns red. Persons who meet one or more statements are suspected of having "locomotive syndrome" [10, 11].

2.2. Stand-Up Test. Subjects are asked to stand from stools of varying heights (10, 20, 30, and 40 cm) with a single leg and both legs [16]. First, the trial using the 40 cm stool is performed with both legs. When completed, the 40 cm stool is tried with a single leg, followed by the 30 cm, 20 cm, and then 10 cm stools. When the 40 cm stool with a single leg is not completed in both right and left legs, the 30 cm, 20 cm, and then 10 cm stools are tried with both legs. Consequently, subjects who fail to stand from the 40 cm stool with a single leg in either of bilateral legs are regarded as "locomotive syndrome risk level 1". Then, subjects who fail to stand from the 20 cm stool with both legs are regarded as "locomotive syndrome risk level 2" [10, 14].

2.3. Two-Step Test. Subjects begin the two-step test in an upright posture and move forward for a maximum of two strides without losing his or her balance [16]. The better result after two trials is recorded. The two-slide distance is subsequently standardized according to the subjects' height. Consequently, subjects with the value less than 1.3 and 1.1 are regarded as "locomotive syndrome risk level 1" and "locomotive syndrome risk level 2", respectively [10, 14].

2.4. Twenty-Five-Question Geriatric Locomotive Function Scale. The GLFS-25 is a self-reported tool to assess difficulty and disability in daily activities related to locomotive organs [17]. This questionnaire consists of total 25 questions (4 questions regarding pain, 16 questions regarding ADL, 3 questions regarding social functions, and 2 questions regarding mental health status) that refer to experiences in the preceding month. The answer of each question is rated on a scale of 0–4 points, indicating higher scores as the presence of symptoms and medical conditions resulting from a greater severity of "locomotive syndrome" (total minimum 0–maximum 100). After careful statistical analysis and evaluation [17], patients with 7 or more points of the GLFS-25 score and those with 16 or more points are regarded as "locomotive syndrome risk level 1" and "locomotive syndrome risk level 2", respectively [10, 14].

3. Prevalence of "Locomotive Syndrome"

Nationwide surveys reported the prevalence of "locomotive syndrome (risk level 2 by the GLFS-25 score ≥16)" in Japanese people in ages of 40 years or more as 10.2% (men, 7.9%; women, 12.3%) in 2010 [18] and 11.9% (men, 10.8%; women, 12.9%) in 2014 [19]. The age-specific mean values for GLFS-25 were 5.8, 6.0, 5.9, and 8.8 of 100 points in the 40s, 50s, 60s, and 70s, respectively [18]. The mean value for GLFS-25 was higher in the 70s than in the other age groups and in women than in men [18]. Then, the longitudinal 7-year follow-up survey of the Research on Osteoarthritis/Osteoporosis Against Disability study found the estimated 2013 prevalence in Japan of the indices in "locomotive syndrome risk level 2" including the two-step test score <1.1, difficulty in standing from a 20 cm height using both legs in the stand-up test, and GLFS-25 score ≥16 as 21.1% (men, 20.1%; women, 21.6%), 7.9% (men, 4.9%; women, 9.4% [statistically higher than men]), and 10.6% (men, 9.0%; women, 11.4%), respectively [14]. After the calculation, the estimated Japan's 2013 prevalence of "locomotive syndrome (risk level 2)" was 25.1% (men, 22.7%; women, 26.3%) [20]. This prevalence was significantly higher with aging, although there was no statistical sex difference [20]. Hence, the prevalence of "locomotive syndrome" primarily increases by aging, especially in patients in ages of 70 years or more, which is more likely to develop in women.

4. Intervention in "Locomotive Syndrome"

"Locomotive syndrome risk level 1" indicates that the impairment of locomotive functions has already begun. As muscle strength and posture balance may be deteriorating, JOA recommends to perform daily physical exercises such as "locomotion training" in subjects with "locomotive syndrome risk level 1". In addition, it is recommended to take care to eat a balanced diet with plenty of protein and calcium [10, 21].

"Locomotive syndrome risk level 2" indicates that the impairment of locomotive functions has already progressed. Subjects with "locomotive syndrome risk level 2" are at high risk of having the difficulty in keeping an independent life style. As the subjects may have locomotive organ disorders, JOA recommends to continue exercise training and also medical consultation to orthopaedic clinics [10].

5. "Locomotion Training"

Many studies have reported effectiveness of physical intervention in preventing the loss of mobility, balance, and gait in the geriatric population [22–32], while exercises are generally effective in subjects with mild to moderate disability [24, 33] but not so much in subjects with severe disability [26]. Thus, early detection of "locomotive syndrome" is desirable.

Physical intervention is based on the principles of exercise [34]. First, it is known that the particular body components and skills, which are involved in a given exercise, will demonstrate the improvement (principle of specificity). Second, a high load is required for any functional improvement (principle of overload). Third, it is important to gradually increase the exercise load (principle of progression) with consideration for safety since the majority of people in middle to old ages have chronic degeneration of lumbar spine discs and lower limb cartilages [9].

Therefore, JOA recommends "locomotion training" to improve and sustain standing and gait functions in middle-aged and old-aged subjects [5, 10]. The basic protocol of "locomotion training" just consists of two simple exercises directly related to standing—squatting and single-leg standing [35]. Then, in patients who get used to the basic "locomotion training" exercises, other exercises such as heel raises and front lunges are recommended to be added [10]. Walking is generally recommended [36–38]. However, persons with the GLFS-25 score ≥16 are expected to have trouble in walking and going out [17]. Three "locomotive syndrome risk level" indices—the stand-up test, two-step test, and GLFS-25—all predict immobility significantly and independently, and the accumulation of these indices indicates substantial increases in the risk of immobility [14]. Therefore, overload is unfavourable. The JOA recommends just additional 10-minute mild physical activities which can support the prevention of "locomotive syndrome", e.g., bicycling or walking to work, taking the stairs instead of the elevator or escalator, cleaning, and laundering with zest in addition to stretching when you have a moment, doing "locomotion training" or stretching while watching TV, taking a walk during breaks at the office, walking to a supermarket further away than usual for your shopping, using your local park or sports center, taking part in community sports events, going out to have fun with family or friends on days off, and walking briskly with long strides [5, 10].

5.1. Single-Leg Standing Exercise. The single-leg standing exercise is designed to improve posture balance. This exercise can be done alone [39] or combined with other muscle power training (like chair-rising training) [40]. This test has been demonstrated to be effective in preventing falls [39, 40]. Subjects are instructed to stand on one leg with their eyes open and adjacent to a stable chair or desk for arm support to prevent from falling. Performing one minute for each leg, three times a day (morning, noon, and evening), every day is advised.

5.2. Squatting. The squatting exercise is designed to strengthen leg muscles. Previous studies have demonstrated effectiveness of squatting in reducing bone loss and improving muscle strength and balance in the lower extremities [41, 42]. Subjects slowly move the torso down from the standing position as is done during stand–sit movement. In addition, subjects are instructed to maintain the position of the patella over the toes to prevent overload on the knee. The knee flexion angle should not exceed 90°. Performing slow squats five to six times as one set, three times a day, every day is recommended.

6. Effect of "Locomotion Training"

Only a few English reports describing the improvement of physical function tests (visual analog scale scores of low back pain, single-leg standing time, and 6 m walking time) by "locomotion training" intervention have been published [43]. A prior study demonstrated that "locomotion training" monitored by using serial telephone contacts

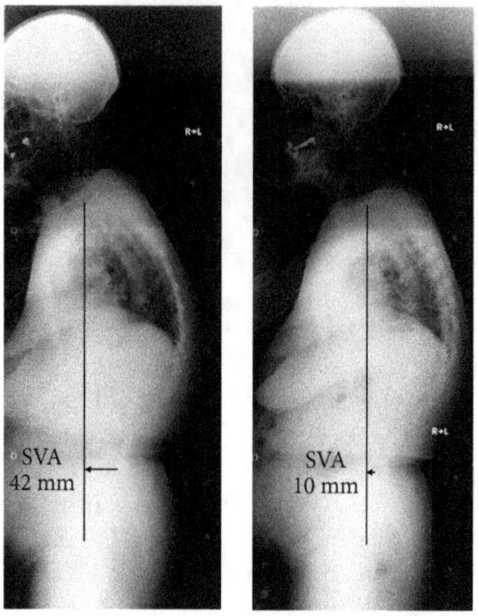

At baseline (a) At 6-month follow-up (b)

Figure 1: A 70-year-old woman with "locomotive syndrome risk level 2" from lumbar spondylosis. Standing whole-spine radiographs showed the sagittal vertical axis (SVA) of 42 mm with thoracic kyphosis (a). After our 6-month "locomotion training" outpatient rehabilitation program, she showed the improvement to "locomotive syndrome risk level 1" with the improved SVA up to 10 mm (<40 mm, normal range) and decreased thoracic kyphosis in radiographs (b).

improved physical function test scores and seven of eight SF-8 subscales [44]. Low back pain decreased in 12.6% of the subjects while it increased only in 2.3%. Knee pain decreased in 17.2% of the participants while it increased only in 1.1%. Hence, evidence is accumulating regarding subjective improvements of physical functions, ADL, and QOL through "locomotion training" exercises. However, multidisciplinary studies regarding objective improvements, e.g., radiography, magnetic resonance imaging, electromyography, and bone densitometry, still need to be conducted. These measurements provide useful information to elucidate effects of "locomotion training" on the spinal and upper and lower extremities' alignment, muscle size and quality, and respective disease severity including osteoarthritis, spinal canal stenosis, sarcopenia, and osteoporosis, as the progress of degenerative disorders is not always symptomatic.

7. Future Directions

In age-related changes in the musculoskeletal system, adult deformity of the spine gains increased attention [45]. Particularly, the loss of lumbar lordosis was associated with increased pain and disability and lower QOL scores [46]. The stronger the back extensors, the smaller the thoracic kyphosis and the larger the lumbar lordosis and sacral inclination [47]. In prior reports studying "Pilates"-based exercises, significant improvement in the sagittal alignment of the head was observed after 6-month exercises; however, this was not the report of radiographic measurements [48].

Based on literature evidence, a prospective cohort study was designed and conducted to assess effects of "locomotion training"-based exercises on the sagittal alignment of the spinopelvic axis in standing radiographs and postural balance in piezoelectric force-plate measurements. All experimental procedures were performed under the approval and guidance of the Institutional Review Board at Kyoto Kujo Hospital (Kyoto, Japan). Written informed consent was obtained from each patient in accordance with the principles of the Declaration of Helsinki and the laws and regulations of Japan. In this paper, we would like to show representative patient cases with varying pathologies who underwent our 6-month "locomotion training" outpatient rehabilitation program.

A 70-year-old woman experienced low back pain lasting over 2 months and then visited our orthopaedic clinic. Her diagnosis was lumbar spondylosis. At baseline, she showed standing-up from a 40 cm height on both legs at her best on the stand-up test (risk level 2), 1.05 on the two-step test (risk level 2), and 14 points on the GLFS-25 score (risk level 1), resulting in the categorization into "locomotive syndrome risk level 2". Then, in standing whole-spine radiographs with the clavicle position, baseline sagittal vertical axis (SVA) was 42 mm, indicating mild sagittal deformity [49]. The lumbar lordosis between L1 and S1 (LL) and pelvic incidence (PI) were 38° and 37°, respectively, causing no mismatch of the PI–LL [49]. The pelvic tilt and sacral slope were 16° and 21°, respectively. Furthermore, C2–C7 angle, T1 slope, and thoracic kyphosis between T5 and T12 (TK) were 16°, 40°, and 51°, respectively, thus suggesting that her sagittal deformity primarily resulted from thoracic kyphosis despite no vertebral fractures (Figure 1(a)). She attended our "locomotion training" outpatient rehabilitation program for 20 minutes, once a week, 6 months to confirm the achievement of exercises and add stretching. At endpoint, she improved "locomotive syndrome" scores to complete standing-up from

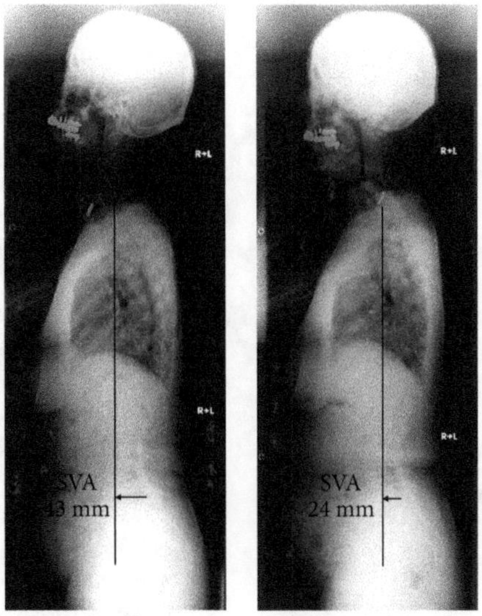

At baseline (a) At 6-month follow-up (b)

FIGURE 2: A 72-year-old woman with "locomotive syndrome risk level 2" from lumbar spinal canal stenosis. Standing whole-spine radiographs showed the sagittal vertical axis (SVA) of 43 mm with decreased thoracic kyphosis (a). After our 6-month "locomotion training" outpatient rehabilitation program, she showed the improvement to "locomotive syndrome risk level 1" with the improved SVA up to 24 mm (<40 mm, normal range) and increased thoracic kyphosis in radiographs (b).

a 20 cm height on both legs on the stand-up test (risk level 1), 1.2 on the two-step test (risk level 1), and 9 points on the GLFS-25 score (risk level 1), corresponding to "risk level 1". The SVA improved up to 10 mm (<40 mm, normal range) [49] with the LL of 42°. Notably, C2–C7 angle, T1 slope, and TK improved to 4°, 29°, and 47°, respectively (Figure 1(b)). The Oswestry Disability Index (ODI) to assess low back pain and related QOL improved from 10 (22.2%, moderate disability) to 7 (15.6%, minimal disability). In piezoelectric force-plate measurements, baseline and endpoint areas of the pressure center, speed, and distance were 7.90 cm^2 and 6.79 cm^2, 3.18 cm/s and 2.00 cm/s, and 190.60 cm and 119.75 cm, respectively, all of which were improved.

A 72-year-old woman experienced low back and bilateral buttock to leg pain worsened only during housework and walking. Her symptoms were relieved after sitting. She visited our orthopaedic clinic, and magnetic resonance imaging analysis found lumbar spinal canal stenosis at L4–L5. Baseline and endpoint "locomotive syndrome" scores were 30 cm on both legs (risk level 2) and 20 cm on both legs (risk level 1) on the stand-up test, 1.1 (risk level 1) and 1.3 (risk level not applicable) on the two-step test, and 8 points (risk level 1) and 5 points (risk level not applicable) on the GLFS-25, respectively (overall risk level 2 $\longrightarrow$ 1). Baseline SVA, LL, and PI–LL were 43 mm, 49°, and +4°, respectively (Figure 2(a)). Then, endpoint SVA, LL, and PI–LL were 24 mm, 48°, and +5°, respectively (Figure 2(b)). Thus, SVA improved to the normal range after "locomotion training" exercises. Also in this case, TK decreased to 26° at baseline but increased up to 38° at endpoint. Baseline and endpoint ODI were 8 (17.8%, minimal disability) and 6 (13.3%, minimal disability), no remarkable deterioration of which was observed. However, she recognized substantial improvement of intermittent claudication. Force-plate examination showed the improvement in part of the area, speed, and distance: 4.47 cm^2 and 2.76 cm^2, 1.53 cm/s and 1.54 cm/s, and 91.69 cm and 92.54 cm at baseline and endpoint, respectively.

The first case's woman had the maintained lumbar lordosis and pelvic parameters but increased thoracic kyphosis. This patient case may be a good candidate of "locomotion training" rehabilitation program. Strengthened leg, hip, and back muscles can facilitate the improvement of the sagittal alignment of the spine. Then, the second case's woman suffered from intermittent claudication. The applied "locomotion training" rehabilitation program improved the sagittal alignment and reduced complaints of intermittent claudication. While the first case decreased the patient's own thoracic kyphosis, the second case increased the thoracic kyphosis. Literature evidence reported a normal range of TK (T5–T12) as 34° ± 11° [50]. Improved power and flexibility of the lower limb, hip, and back muscles might contribute to the normalization of the sagittal alignment of the thoracic spine. It is noteworthy that "locomotion training" facilitated these improvements despite the presence of specific disorders including thoracic kyphosis and symptomatic lumbar spinal canal stenosis.

8. Conclusions

The cases shown raised the need for further prospective cohort studies to clarify multidisciplinary effects of "locomotion training" exercises on the spinal alignment, global balance, and quality of life in patients with "locomotive syndrome". Understanding of "locomotive syndrome" is essential for the future of aging care, which is an important health issue not only in Japan but also in the international society.

References

[1] United Nations Population Division, "World Population Prospects 2017," https://population.un.org/wpp/Download/Standard/Population/.

[2] Government of Japan Cabinet Office, "Annual report on the aging society: 2017," https://www8.cao.go.jp/kourei/english/annualreport/2017/2017pdf_e.html.

[3] Labour and Welfare Ministry of Health, Government of Japan "Annual health, labour and welfare report 2017" https://www.mhlw.go.jp/english/wp/wp-hwl1/index.html.

[4] K. Nakamura, "A "super-aged" society and the "locomotive syndrome"," *Journal of Orthopaedic Science*, vol. 13, no. 1, pp. 1-2, 2008.

[5] K. Nakamura, "The concept and treatment of locomotive syndrome: Its acceptance and spread in Japan," *Journal of Orthopaedic Science*, vol. 16, no. 5, pp. 489–491, 2011.

[6] J. P. Urban and S. Roberts, "Degeneration of the intervertebral disc," *Arthritis Research & Therapy*, vol. 5, no. 3, pp. 120–130, 2003.

[7] N. Boos, S. Weissbach, H. Rohrbach, C. Weiler, K. F. Spratt, and A. G. Nerlich, "Classification of age-related changes in lumbar intervertebral discs: 2002 Volvo Award in basic science," *Spine (Phila Pa 1976)*, vol. 27, no. 23, pp. 2631–2644, 2002.

[8] K. M. C. Cheung, J. Karppinen, D. Chan et al., "Prevalence and pattern of lumbar magnetic resonance imaging changes in a population study of one thousand forty-three individuals," *Spine (Phila Pa 1976)*, vol. 34, no. 9, pp. 934–940, 2009.

[9] N. Yoshimura, S. Muraki, H. Oka et al., "Prevalence of knee osteoarthritis, lumbar spondylosis, and osteoporosis in Japanese men and women: the research on osteoarthritis/osteoporosis against disability study," *Journal of Bone and Mineral Metabolism*, vol. 27, no. 5, pp. 620–628, 2009.

[10] K. Nakamura and T. Ogata, "Locomotive syndrome: definition and management," *Clinical Reviews in Bone and Mineral Metabolism*, vol. 14, pp. 56–67, 2016.

[11] M. Akahane, A. Maeyashiki, S. Yoshihara, Y. Tanaka, and T. Imamura, "Relationship between difficulties in daily activities and falling: loco-check as a self-assessment of fall risk," *Interactive Journal of Medical Research*, vol. 5, no. 2, p. e20, 2016.

[12] N. Yoshimura, H. Oka, S. Muraki et al., "Reference values for hand grip strength, muscle mass, walking time, and one-leg standing time as indices for locomotive syndrome and associated disability: the second survey of the ROAD study," *Journal of Orthopaedic Science*, vol. 16, no. 6, pp. 768–777, 2011.

[13] M. Nakamura, H. Hashizume, H. Oka et al., "Physical performance measures associated with locomotive syndrome in middle-aged and older Japanese women," *Journal of Geriatric Physical Therapy*, vol. 38, no. 4, pp. 202–207, 2015.

[14] N. Yoshimura, S. Muraki, H. Oka et al., "Association between new indices in the locomotive syndrome risk test and decline in mobility: third survey of the ROAD study," *Journal of Orthopaedic Science*, vol. 20, no. 5, pp. 896–905, 2015.

[15] T. Ikemoto and Y.-C. Arai, "Locomotive syndrome: clinical perspectives," *Clinical Interventions in Aging*, vol. 13, pp. 819–827, 2018.

[16] T. Ogata, S. Muranaga, H. Ishibashi et al., "Development of a screening program to assess motor function in the adult population: a cross-sectional observational study," *Journal of Orthopaedic Science*, vol. 20, no. 5, pp. 888–895, 2015.

[17] A. Seichi, Y. Hoshino, T. Doi, M. Akai, Y. Tobimatsu, and T. Iwaya, "Development of a screening tool for risk of locomotive syndrome in the elderly: the 25-question geriatric locomotive function scale," *Journal of Orthopaedic Science*, vol. 17, no. 2, pp. 163–172, 2012.

[18] A. Kimura, A. Seichi, S. Konno, S. Yabuki, and K. Hayashi, "Prevalence of locomotive syndrome in Japan: a nationwide, cross-sectional Internet survey," *Journal of Orthopaedic Science*, vol. 19, no. 5, pp. 792–797, 2014.

[19] A. Seichi, A. Kimura, S. Konno, and S. Yabuki, "Epidemiologic survey of locomotive syndrome in Japan," *Journal of Orthopaedic Science*, vol. 21, no. 2, pp. 222–225, 2016.

[20] N. Yoshimura, S. Muraki, K. Nakamura, and S. Tanaka, "Epidemiology of the locomotive syndrome: The research on osteoarthritis/osteoporosis against disability study 2005–2015," *Modern Rheumatology*, vol. 27, no. 1, pp. 1–7, 2017.

[21] H. A. Bischoff-Ferrari, B. Dawson-Hughes, W. C. Willett et al., "Effect of vitamin D on falls: a meta-analysis," *Journal of the American Medical Association*, vol. 291, no. 16, pp. 1999–2006, 2004.

[22] R. S. Schwartz and W. J. Evans, "Effects of exercise on body composition and functional capacity of the elderly," *The Journals of Gerontology. Series A, Biological Sciences and Medical Sciences*, vol. 50A, no. Special, pp. 147–150, 1995.

[23] R. G. Cumming, "Intervention strategies and risk-factor modification for falls prevention: A review of recent intervention studies," *Clinics in Geriatric Medicine*, vol. 18, no. 2, pp. 175–189, 2002.

[24] E. F. Binder, K. B. Schechtman, A. A. Ehsani et al., "Effects of exercise training on frailty in community-dwelling older adults: results of a randomized, controlled trial," *Journal of the American Geriatrics Society*, vol. 50, no. 12, pp. 1921–1928, 2002.

[25] J. L. Helbostad, O. Sletvold, and R. Moe-Nilssen, "Effects of home exercises and group training on functional abilities in home-dwelling older persons with mobility and balance problems. A radomized study," *Aging Clinical and Experimental Research*, vol. 16, no. 2, pp. 113–121, 2004.

[26] M. J. Faber, R. J. Bosscher, M. J. Chin A Paw, and P. C. van Wieringen, "Effects of exercise programs on falls and mobility in frail and pre-frail older adults: a multicenter randomized controlled trial," *Archives of Physical Medicine and Rehabilitation*, vol. 87, no. 7, pp. 885–896, 2006.

[27] S. Karinkanta, A. Heinonen, H. Sievänen et al., "A multi-component exercise regimen to prevent functional decline and bone fragility in home-dwelling elderly women: randomized, controlled trial," *Osteoporosis International*, vol. 18, no. 4, pp. 453–462, 2007.

[28] T. E. Howe, L. Rochester, F. Neil, D. A. Skelton, and C. Ballinger, "Exercise for improving balance in older people," *Cochrane Database of Systematic Reviews*, no. 11, Article ID CD004963, 2011.

[29] L. D. Gillespie, M. C. Robertson, W. J. Gillespie et al., "Interventions for preventing falls in older people living in the community," *The Cochrane Database of Systematic Reviews*, no. 9, Article ID CD007146, 2012.

[30] C.-H. Chou, C.-L. Hwang, and Y.-T. Wu, "Effect of exercise on physical function, daily living activities, and quality of life in the frail older adults: a meta-analysis," *Archives of Physical Medicine and Rehabilitation*, vol. 93, no. 2, pp. 237–244, 2012.

[31] D. Kendrick, A. Kumar, H. Carpenter et al., "Exercise for reducing fear of falling in older people living in the community," *The Cochrane Database of Systematic Reviews*, no. 11, Article ID CD009848, 2014.

[32] R. Dodds and A. A. Sayer, "Sarcopenia and frailty: new challenges for clinical practice," *Clinical Medicine*, vol. 15, no. Suppl. 6, pp. s88–s91, 2015.

[33] R. Daniels, E. Van Rossum, L. de Witte, G. I. J. M. Kempen, and W. van den Heuvel, "Interventions to prevent disability in frail community-dwelling elderly: a systematic review," *BMC Health Services Research*, vol. 8, article 278, 2008.

[34] B. C. Ammann, R. H. Knols, P. Baschung, R. A. de Bie, and E. D. de Bruin, "Application of principles of exercise training in sub-acute and chronic stroke survivors: a systematic review," *BMC Neurology*, vol. 14, no. 1, p. 167, 2014.

[35] E. Y. Ishigaki, L. G. Ramos, E. S. Carvalho, and A. C. Lunardi, "Effectiveness of muscle strengthening and description of protocols for preventing falls in the elderly: a systematic review," *Brazilian Journal of Physical Therapy*, vol. 18, no. 2, pp. 111–118, 2014.

[36] W. J. Strawbridge, R. D. Cohen, S. J. Shema, and G. A. Kaplan, "Successful aging: Predictors and associated activities," *American Journal of Epidemiology*, vol. 144, no. 2, pp. 135–141, 1996.

[37] M. C. Devries, L. Breen, M. Von Allmen et al., "Low-load resistance training during step-reduction attenuates declines in muscle mass and strength and enhances anabolic sensitivity in older men," *Physiological Reports*, vol. 3, no. 8, p. e12493, 2015.

[38] A. R. Smith, C. Chen, P. Clarke, and N. A. Gallagher, "Trajectories of outdoor mobility in vulnerable community-dwelling elderly: the role of individual and environmental factors," *Journal of Aging and Health*, vol. 28, no. 5, pp. 796–811, 2016.

[39] K. Sakamoto, T. Nakamura, H. Hagino et al., "Effects of unipedal standing balance exercise on the prevention of falls and hip fracture among clinically defined high-risk elderly individuals: a randomized controlled trial," *Journal of Orthopaedic Science*, vol. 11, no. 5, pp. 467–472, 2006.

[40] J. Iwamoto, H. Suzuki, K. Tanaka et al., "Preventative effect of exercise against falls in the elderly: A randomized controlled trial," *Osteoporosis International*, vol. 20, no. 7, pp. 1233–1240, 2009.

[41] C. M. Young, B. K. Weeks, and B. R. Beck, "Simple, novel physical activity maintains proximal femur bone mineral density, and improves muscle strength and balance in sedentary, postmenopausal Caucasian women," *Osteoporosis International*, vol. 18, no. 10, pp. 1379–1387, 2007.

[42] L. B. Seitz, A. Reyes, T. T. Tran, E. S. de Villarreal, and G. G. Haff, "Increases in lower-body strength transfer positively to sprint performance: a systematic review with meta-analysis," *Sports Medicine*, vol. 44, no. 12, pp. 1693–1702, 2014.

[43] H. Hashizume, N. Yoshimura, and K. Nagata, "Development and evaluation of a video exercise program for locomotive syndrome in the elderly," *Modern Rheumatology*, vol. 24, no. 2, pp. 250–257, 2014.

[44] K. Aoki, M. Sakuma, N. Ogisho, K. Nakamura, E. Chosa, and N. Endo, "The effcts of self-directed home exercise with serial telephone contacts on physical functions and quality of life in elderly people at high risk of locomotor dysfunction," *Acta Medica Okayama*, vol. 69, no. 4, pp. 245–253, 2015.

[45] F. Schwab, A. Dubey, L. Gamez et al., "Adult scoliosis: prevalence, SF-36, and nutritional parameters in an elderly volunteer population," *Spine (Phila Pa 1976)*, vol. 30, no. 9, pp. 1082–1085, 2005.

[46] F. Schwab, J.-P. Farcy, K. Bridwell et al., "A clinical impact classification of scoliosis in the adult," *Spine (Phila Pa 1976)*, vol. 31, no. 18, pp. 2109–2114, 2006.

[47] M. Sinaki, E. Itoi, J. W. Rogers, E. J. Bergstralh, and H. W. Wahner, "Correlation of back extensor strength with thoracic kyphosis and lumbar lordosis in estrogen-deficient women," *American Journal of Physical Medicine & Rehabilitation*, vol. 75, no. 5, pp. 370–374, 1996.

[48] A. Cruz-Ferreira, J. Fernandes, Y.-L. Kuo et al., "Does pilates-based exercise improve postural alignment in adult women?" *Journal of Women and Health*, vol. 53, no. 6, pp. 597–611, 2013.

[49] F. Schwab, B. Ungar, B. Blondel et al., "Scoliosis research society-schwab adult spinal deformity classification: a validation study," *Spine (Phila Pa 1976)*, vol. 37, no. 12, pp. 1077–1082, 2012.

[50] D. E. Gelb, L. G. Lenke, K. H. Bridwell, K. Blanke, and K. W. McEnery, "An analysis of sagittal spinal alignment in 100 asymptomatic middle and older aged volunteers," *Spine (Phila Pa 1976)*, vol. 20, no. 12, pp. 1351–1358, 1995.

Permissions

 Every chapter published in this book has been scrutinized by our experts. Their significance has been extensively debated. The topics covered herein carry significant findings which will fuel the growth of the discipline. They may even be implemented as practical applications or may be referred to as a beginning point for another development.

The contributors of this book come from diverse backgrounds, making this book a truly international effort. This book will bring forth new frontiers with its revolutionizing research information and detailed analysis of the nascent developments around the world.

We would like to thank all the contributing authors for lending their expertise to make the book truly unique. They have played a crucial role in the development of this book. Without their invaluable contributions this book wouldn't have been possible. They have made vital efforts to compile up to date information on the varied aspects of this subject to make this book a valuable addition to the collection of many professionals and students.

This book was conceptualized with the vision of imparting up-to-date information and advanced data in this field. To ensure the same, a matchless editorial board was set up. Every individual on the board went through rigorous rounds of assessment to prove their worth. After which they invested a large part of their time researching and compiling the most relevant data for our readers.

The editorial board has been involved in producing this book since its inception. They have spent rigorous hours researching and exploring the diverse topics which have resulted in the successful publishing of this book. They have passed on their knowledge of decades through this book. To expedite this challenging task, the publisher supported the team at every step. A small team of assistant editors was also appointed to further simplify the editing procedure and attain best results for the readers.

Apart from the editorial board, the designing team has also invested a significant amount of their time in understanding the subject and creating the most relevant covers. They scrutinized every image to scout for the most suitable representation of the subject and create an appropriate cover for the book.

The publishing team has been an ardent support to the editorial, designing and production team. Their endless efforts to recruit the best for this project, has resulted in the accomplishment of this book. They are a veteran in the field of academics and their pool of knowledge is as vast as their experience in printing. Their expertise and guidance has proved useful at every step. Their uncompromising quality standards have made this book an exceptional effort. Their encouragement from time to time has been an inspiration for everyone.

The publisher and the editorial board hope that this book will prove to be a valuable piece of knowledge for researchers, students, practitioners and scholars across the globe.

List of Contributors

Mahmoud Ganjifard, Amir Sabertanha and Batool Zeinali
Department of Anesthesia, Faculty of Medicine, Birjand University of Medical Sciences, Birjand, Iran

Samaneh Kouzegaran
Clinical Immunology and Allergy, Faculty of Medicine, Birjand University of Medical Sciences, Birjand, Iran

Reza Abdi
Department of Orthopedics, School of Medicine, Ghaem Hospital, Mashhad University of Medical Sciences, Mashhad, Iran

Mohsen Naseri
Cellular and Molecular Research Center, Birjand University of Medical Sciences, Birjand, Iran

Elahe Allahyari
Social Determinants of Health Research Center, Department of Epidemiology and Biostatistics, Faculty of Health, Birjand University of Medical Sciences, Birjand, Iran

Vahhab Zarei
PhD Student, University of Minnesota, 2450 Riverside Ave. S R200, Minneapolis, MN 55454, USA

Sharon C. Yson
Spine Research Associate, University of Minnesota, 2450 Riverside Ave. S R200, Minneapolis, MN 55454, USA

Joan E. Bechtold
Vice Chair, Research, Gustilo Professor of Orthopaedic Research, Department of Orthopedic Surgery, University of Minnesota, 2450 Riverside Ave. S R200, Minneapolis, MN 55454, USA

Jonathan N. Sembrano
Associate Professor, Department of Orthopaedics, University of Minnesota, 2450 Riverside Ave. S R200, Minneapolis, MN55454, USA

Mir Sadat-Ali, Abdallah S. AlOmran, Sulaiman A. AlMousa, Hasan N. AlSayed and Khalid W. AlTabash
Department of Orthopaedic Surgery, Imam AbdulRahman Bin Faisal University, Dammam, Saudi Arabia
King Fahd Hospital of the University, AlKhobar, Saudi Arabia

Mohammed Q. Azam
Orthopaedic Surgery, All India Institute of Medical Sciences, Rishikesh, India

Tarek M. Hegazi
King Fahd Hospital of the University, AlKhobar, Saudi Arabia
Radiology, Imam AbdulRahman Bin Faisal University, Dammam, Saudi Arabia

Sadananda Acharya
King Fahd Hospital of the University, AlKhobar, Saudi Arabia
College of Public Health, Imam AbdulRahman Bin Faisal University, Dammam, Saudi Arabia

Seyed Ali Hashemi, Mohammad Reza Ranjbar and Mohammad Tahami
Research Center for Bone and Joint Diseases, Department of Orthopedic Surgery, Chamran Hospital, Shiraz University of Medical Sciences, Shiraz, Iran

Reza Shahriarirad and Amirhossein Erfani
Student Research Committee, Shiraz University of Medical Sciences, Shiraz, Iran
Thoracic and Vascular Surgery Research Center, Shiraz University of Medical Sciences, Shiraz, Iran

Naohisa Miyakoshi
Department of Orthopedic Surgery, Akita University Graduate School of Medicine, 1-1-1 Hondo, Akita 010-8543, Japan

Yosuke Iwamoto, Hiroaki Kijima, Shin Yamada, Masashi Fujii and Itsuki Nagahata
Department of Orthopedic Surgery, Akita University Graduate School of Medicine, 1-1-1 Hondo, Akita 010-8543, Japan
Akita Hip Research Group, 1-1-1 Hondo, Akita 010-8543, Japan

Yoichi Shimada
Department of Orthopedic Surgery, Akita University Graduate School of Medicine, 1-1-1 Hondo, Akita 010-8543, Japan
Akita Hip Research Group, 1-1-1 Hondo, Akita 010-8543, Japan
Akita Hand Group, Akita 010-8543, Japan
Department of Orthopedic Surgery, Akita University Graduate School of Medicine, Akita 010-8543, Japan

Hiroshi Tazawa, Natsuo Konishi, Hitoshi Kubota, Takayuki Tani, Keiji Kamo, Norio Suzuki, Yoshihiko Okudera, Ken Sasaki and Tetsuya Kawano
Akita Hip Research Group, 1-1-1 Hondo, Akita 010-8543, Japan

Kivanc Atesok and Efstathios Papavassiliou
Harvard University, Beth Israel Deaconess Medical Center, Department of Neurosurgery, Boston, MA, USA

Shepard Hurwitz
University of North Carolina, Department of Orthopaedic Surgery, Chapel Hill, NC, USA

Donald D. Anderson, Geb W. Thomas and J. Lawrence Marsh
University of Iowa, Department of Orthopaedics and Rehabilitation, Iowa City, IA, USA

Richard Satava
University of Washington, Department of Surgery, Seattle, WA, USA

Ted Tufescu
University of Manitoba, Section of Orthopaedic Surgery, Winnipeg, MB, Canada

Michael J. Heffernan
Children's Hospital of New Orleans, LSU Health Science Center, Department of Orthopaedic Surgery, New Orleans, LA, USA

Steven Theiss
University of Alabama at Birmingham, Department of Orthopaedic Surgery, Birmingham, AL, USA

ChaoFeng Guo and YuXiang Wang
Department of Spine Surgery, Xiangya Hospital of Central South University, Changsha 410008, Hunan Province, China

Daudi R. Manini
Department of Spine Surgery, Xiangya Hospital of Central South University, Changsha 410008, Hunan Province, China
Department of Orthopedic Surgery, Mwananyamala Regional Referral Hospital, Dar-es-Salaam, Tanzania

Frank D. Shega
Department of Spine Surgery, Xiangya Hospital of Central South University, Changsha 410008, Hunan Province, China
Department of Orthopedic Surgery, Mount Meru Regional Referral Hospital, Arusha, Tanzania

Ofir Uri, Yoram Folman, Gil Laufer and Eyal Behrbalk
Department of Orthopedic Surgery, Hillel Yaffe Medical Center, Hadera, Israel

David Ruiz-Picazo, Plácido Jiménez-Ortega, Francisco Doñate-Pérez, Natalia Gaspar-Aparicio, Victor García-Martín, José Ramírez-Villaescusa and Sergio Losa-Palacios
Department of Pediatric Orthopaedics Surgery, Complejo Hospitalario Universitario de Albacete, Spain

S. Pesenti, S. Prost, A. Muñoz McCausland, K. Farah, P. Tropiano, S. Fuentes and B. Blondel
Aix-Marseille Universite, APHM, CNRS, ISM, Hôpital de La Timone, Spine Unit 264 Rue Saint Pierre, Marseille 13005, France

Máté Burkus, Ádám T. Schlégl, Kristóf József, Ian O'Sullivan, István Márkus and Miklós Tunyogi-Csapó
Department of Orthopedics, Medical School, University of Pécs, H-7623 Pécs, Akác St. 1., Hungary

Gregory S. DiFelice
Orthopaedic Trauma Service, Department of Orthopaedic Surgery, Hospital for Special Surgery, NewYork-Presbyterian, Weill Medical College of Cornell University, New York, NY, USA

Jelle P. van der List
Orthopaedic Trauma Service, Department of Orthopaedic Surgery, Hospital for Special Surgery, NewYork-Presbyterian, Weill Medical College of Cornell University, New York, NY, USA
Spaarne Gasthuis Hospital, Department of Orthopaedic Surgery, Hoofddorp, Netherlands
Amsterdam UMC, University of Amsterdam, Department of Orthopaedic Surgery, Amsterdam, Netherlands

Douglas N. Mintz
Department of Radiology, Hospital for Special Surgery, New York-Presbyterian, Weill Medical College of Cornell University, New York, NY, USA

Adrián Borja-Flores, Eloy Reyes-Martínez and Josè Belzazar-Castillo de la Torre
HGZ 5 Con MF, Delegaci´on Estatal Morelos, Zacatepec, Morelos, Mexico

Salvador I. Macías-Hernández
Orthopedic Rehabilitation Division, Instituto Nacional de Rehabilitaci´on Luis Guillermo Ibarra, Mexico City, Mexico

Gabriela Hernández-Molina and Janette Furuzawa-Carballeda
Department of Immunology and Rheumatology, Instituto Nacional de Ciencias Médicas y Nutrición Salvador Zubirán, Mexico City, Mexico

Andric Perez-Ortiz
Escuela de Medicina, Universidad Panamericana, Donatello 59, Insurgentes Mixcoac, Benito Juárez, Mexico City 03920, Mexico

Laura Ávila-Jimènez and María Cristina Vázquez-Bello
Coordinaci´on de Planeaci´on y Enlace Institucional, Jefatura de Servicios de Prestaciones Médicas, Delegación Estatal Morelos, Cuernavaca, Morelos, Mexico

Marco Antonio Leòn-Maòn and Cidronio Albavera-Hernández
Centro de Investigación Educativa y Formación Docente, Coordinación de Planeación y Enlace Institucional, Jefatura de Servicios de Prestaciones Médicas, Delegación Estatal Morelos, Cuernavaca, Morelos, Mexico

Gonzalo Torres-Villalobos and Fernanda Romero-Hernández
Departments of Experimental Surgery and Surgery, Instituto Nacional de Ciencias Médicas y Nutrición Salvador Zubirán, Mexico City, Mexico

Jesùs Pèrez-Correa
Department of Traumatology and Orthopedics, Hospital "Dr. Victorio de la Fuente Narváez ", Mexico City, Mexico

Hilda A. Castro-Rocha
Siracusa No. 51 Col. Lomas Estrella, Mexico City, Mexico

Kunio Ebata and Kentaro Ouchi
Department of Orthopedic Surgery, Yokote Municipal Hospital, Akita 013-8602, Japan

Tatsuru Tomioka
Department of Orthopedic Surgery, Yokote Municipal Hospital, Akita 013-8602, Japan
Akita Hand Group, Akita 010-8543, Japan

Seietsu Senma, Yuichiro Narita, Masakazu Urayama, Satoshi Yumoto, Hiroki Ito, Toshiaki Aizawa, Tsuyoshi Shirahata, Hiroshi Aonuma, Nozomi Kaga, Norimitsu Masutani and Yusuke Yuasa
Akita Hand Group, Akita 010-8543, Japan

Hikaru Saito Naohisa Miyakoshi
Akita Hand Group, Akita 010-8543, Japan
Department of Orthopedic Surgery, Akita University Graduate School of Medicine, Akita 010-8543, Japan

Safa Yousif, Afraa Musa and Ammar Ahmed
Department of Physiology, Faculty of Medicine, University of Khartoum, Khartoum, Sudan

Ahmed Abdelhai
Department of Orthopaedics Surgery and Traumatology, Faculty of Medicine, University of Khartoum, Khartoum, Sudan

Du Hyun Ro, Joonhee Lee, Jangyun Lee, Jae-Young Park, Hyuk-Soo Han and Myung Chul Lee
Department of Orthopaedic Surgery, Seoul National University College of Medicine, Seoul, Republic of Korea

Anna Raciborska, Iwona Malesza, Katarzyna Bilska, Tomasz Koziński and Bartosz Pachuta
Department of Oncology and Surgical Oncology for Children and Youth, Institute of Mother and Child, Warsaw, Poland

Koichiro Ono, Kazuo Ohmori and Takeshi Hori
Center for Spinal Surgery, Nippon Koukan Hospital, Kawasaki 210-0852, Japan

Joseph Maalouly, Fouad Jabbour, Elias Saidy, Georgio Lati, Dany Aouad, Rami Ayoubi and Alexandre Nehme
Department of Orthopedic Surgery and Traumatology, Saint George Hospital University Medical Center, Balamand University, Achra ieh, Beirut 1100 2807, Lebanon

Gerard El-Hajj
Department of Radiology, Saint George Hospital University Medical Center, Balamand University, Achra ieh, Beirut 1100 2807, Lebanon

Zbigniew Żęgota
Zbigniew Żęgota Specjalistyczny O´srodek Leczniczo-Badawczy, Ostróda, Poland

Joanna Goździk
Silmedic Ltd., Katowice, Poland

Joanna Głogowska-Szeląg
Silmedic Ltd., Katowice, Poland
Department of Pathophysiology and Endocrinology, Medical University of Silesia, Zabrze, Poland

Thorsten Jentzsch and Mazda Farshad
Department of Orthopedics, Balgrist University Hospital, University of Zurich, Zurich, Switzerland

Claudio Dora
Swiss Orthopaedics, Bourg-en-Lavaux, Switzerland

Urs Müller
Onaxis Ltd, Bern, Switzerland

HongQi Zhang, MingXing Tang and ShaoHua Liu
Department of Spine Surgery, Xiangya Hospital of Central South University, Changsha City 410008, Hunan Province, China

Shaahin Hajivandi
Department of Orthopedic Surgery, Dezful University of Medical Sciences, Dezful, Iran

Atousa Dachek
Student Research Committee, Dezful University of Medical Sciences, Dezful, Iran

Amirhossein Salimi
Student Research Committee, Shahid Sadoughi University of Medical Sciences, Yazd, Iran

Hesan Jelodari Mamaghani and Seyed Peyman Mirghaderi
Students' Scientific Research Center (SSRC), Tehran University of Medical Sciences, Tehran, Iran

Javad Dehghani
Bone and Joint Diseases Research Center, Department of Orthopedic Surgery, Shiraz University of Medical Sciences, Shiraz, Iran

Roham Borazjani
Trauma Research Center, Shahid Rajaee (Emtiaz) Ttauma Hospital, Shiraz University of Medical Sciences, Shiraz, Iran

Amirmohammad Babaniamansour
Department of Orthotics and Prosthetics, School of Rehabilitation Sciences, Iran University of Medical Sciences, Tehran, Iran

Rojin Sarallah and Salar Javanshir
Islamic Azad University Medical Branch of Tehran, Tehran, Iran

Maryam Salimi
Bone and Joint Diseases Research Center, Department of Orthopedic Surgery, Shiraz University of Medical Sciences, Shiraz, Iran
Student Research Committee, Shiraz University of Medical Sciences, Shiraz, Iran

Achmad Fauzi Kamal and Didi Saputra Ramang
Department of Orthopaedic and Traumatology, Faculty of Medicine Universitas Indonesia, Cipto Mangunkusumo General Hospital, Jakarta, Indonesia

Marcel Prasetyo
Department of Radiology, Faculty of Medicine Universitas Indonesia, Cipto Mangunkusumo General Hospital, Jakarta, Indonesia

Vincenzo De Luna, Fernando De Maio, Alessandro Caterini, Martina Marsiolo, Lidio Petrungaro, Ernesto Ippolito and Pasquale Farsetti
Department of Clinical Sciences and Traslational Medicine, Division of Orthopaedic Surgery, University of "Tor Vergata", Rome, Italy

Mohamad Azwan Aziz and Azmi Mohamed Mohd Nahar
Sports Medicine Department, University Malaya Medical Centre, Kuala Lumpur, Malaysia

Redzal Abu Hanifah
Sports Medicine Unit, Queen Elizabeth Hospital, Kota Kinabalu, Sabah, Malaysia

Alvin Hernandez, Mamer Rosario, Romina Mendoza-Torres, Carl Ryan Marino Taguba, Abigail Garcia and Geoffrey Battad
Department of Orthopaedics, East Avenue Medical Center, East Avenue, Diliman, Quezon City 1101, Metro Manila, Philippines

Kaoru Tada, Seigo Suganuma, Mika Nakada, Masashi Matsuta, Atsuro Murai and Hiroyuki Tsuchiya
Department of Orthopaedic Surgery, Graduate School of Medical Science, Kanazawa University, 13-1 Takaramachi, Kanazawa 920-8641, Japan

Panagiotis Korovessis, Vasileios Syrimpeis, Evangelia Mpountogianni, Ioannis Papaioannou and Vasileios Tsekouras
Orthopaedics Department, General Hospital of Patras, Patras 26335, Greece

Patrick Tropiano
Spine Division, Timone, Aix-Marseille University, 13005 Marseille, France

Solène Prost, Stephane Fuentes and Benjamin Blondel
Spine Division, Timone, Aix-Marseille University, 13005 Marseille, France
Aix Marseille University, Institute of Movement Sciences, CNRS UMR, 7287 Marseille, France

Sèbastien Pesenti and Jean-Luc Jouve
Aix Marseille University, Institute of Movement Sciences, CNRS UMR, 7287 Marseille, France
Pediatric Orthopedics, Timone Children Hospital, Aix-Marseille University, 264 Rue Saint Pierre, 13005 Marseille, France

Bertrand Moal
Bordeaux University, 146 Rue Léo Saignat, 33000 Bordeaux, France

Vincent Pomero
Gait Analysis Laboratory, Timone, Aix-Marseille University, 13005 Marseille, France

Virginie Lafage
Spine Service, Hospital for Special Surgery, New York, NY, USA

Mark C. Dougherty
Resident, University of Iowa Hospitals and Clinics, Department of Neurosurgery, Iowa City, IA, USA

J. Erik Kulenkamp
Resident, University of Minnesota, Department of Ophthalmology and Visual Neurosciences, Minneapolis, MN, USA

Haroutioun Boyajian
Resident, Henry Ford Health System, Department of Surgery, Detroit, MI, USA

Jason L. Koh
Clinical Professor and Chairman, NorthShore University Health System, Department of Orthopaedic Surgery, Evanston, IL, USA
Director, NorthShore Orthopaedic Institute, Evanston, IL, USA

Michael J. Lee and Lewis L. Shi
Associate Professor, University of Chicago Medicine, Department of Orthopaedic Surgery and Rehabilitation Medicine, Chicago, IL, USA

Takashi Yurube, Masaaki Ito, Kenichiro Kakutani, Ryosuke Kuroda and Kotaro Nishida
Department of Orthopaedic Surgery, Kobe University Graduate School of Medicine, Kobe 650-0017, Japan

Toru Takeoka and Hideyo Inaoka
Department of Rehabilitation, Kyoto Kujo Hospital, Kyoto 601 - 8453, Japan

Index